# Innovative Approaches in Knee Arthroscopy

Vikram Arun Mhaskar • J. Maheshwari
Editors

# Innovative Approaches in Knee Arthroscopy

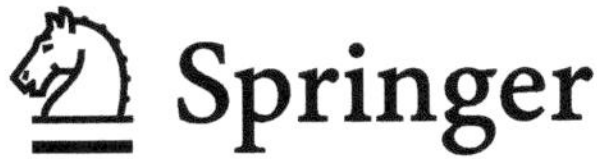

*Editors*
Vikram Arun Mhaskar
F7 East Of Kailash
Knee & Shoulder Clinic
New Delhi, India

JMVM Sports Injury Centre
Sitaram Bhartia Institute of Science & Research
New Delhi, India

J. Maheshwari
F7 East Of Kailash
Knee & Shoulder Clinic
New Delhi, India

JMVM Sports Injury Centre
Sitaram Bhartia Institute of Science & Research
New Delhi, India

ISBN 978-981-99-4380-7 ISBN 978-981-99-4378-4 (eBook)
https://doi.org/10.1007/978-981-99-4378-4



This Springer imprint is published by the registered company Springer Nature Singapore Pte Ltd.
The registered company address is: 152 Beach Road, #21-01/04 Gateway East, Singapore 189721, Singapore

Paper in this product is recyclable.

# Preface

The intention behind my writing of this book was to simplify basic and advanced arthroscopic procedures. It embodies my philosophy of preserving biology wherever possible, improving accuracy and making things more cost-effective. Arthroscopic surgery of the knee has evolved over the years. The instrumentation available these days has managed to not only simplify procedures but also made them more cost-effective. The learning curve is much more arduous in arthroscopic surgery as compared to open surgery as there is immense hand-eye coordination that is required. This book has 27 chapters and close to 1000 illustrations and pictures that take the reader through the step-by-step process of performing relevant arthroscopic surgeries. The illustrations have been created by me personally so as to convey what is being done from a surgeon's perspective. The book also has contributions from authorities in arthroscopic surgery from around the world. I hope you enjoy reading this book and it helps you learn how to do arthroscopic surgeries around the knee more effectively.

This book is dedicated to my mentor and teacher Dr. J Maheshwari, my parents Dr. Rita Mhaskar and Dr. Arun Mhaskar who consistently encouraged my academic pursuits and helped shape what I am today, my wonderful wife Dr. Parul Maheshwari Mhaskar who has always stood by me and last but not least my grandfather late Mr. J. S. Iyer who inspired me to do my best for the society.

New Delhi, India | Vikram Arun Mhaskar

# Contents

# About the Editors

**Vikram Arun Mhaskar, MS, MCh(Orth),** is a fellowship-trained exclusive knee and shoulder surgeon practicing at Sitaram Bhartia Institute of Science and Research where he is the Director of JMVM Sports Injury Center in association with Abhinav Bindra Targeting Performance, New Delhi, India. He has over 20 peer-reviewed publications, 7 book chapters, and 6 original arthroscopic surgical techniques published in several reputed journals. His surgical technique videos are published on many social media channels. He is the co-author of *Essential Orthopedics*, India's leading textbook of orthopedics. He is an honorary visiting professor of clinical orthopedics at DIPSAR, School Of Physiotherapy.

**J. Maheshwari, MS(Orth),** is a knee and shoulder surgeon with over 39 years of experience. He has also served as an additional professor of orthopedics at AIIMS, New Delhi, India. He is an author of *Essential Orthopedics*, sixth edition, published first in 1994. He practices at Sitaram Bhartia Institute of Science and Research where he is the Director of JMVM Sports Injury Center in association with Abhinav Bindra Targeting Performance.

# Part I

# Basic Arthroscopy

# 1 Portals

Vikram Arun Mhaskar

## 1.1 Introduction

Portal placement is essential for a successful surgery. Portals made in the right place provide unobstructed access to various aspects of the knee. Portal making is efficient using a No 11 blade as it has a sharp tip. Portals may be vertical, horizontal, or oblique. Vertical portals have the advantage modularity in a superior to inferior plane but not in the horizontal plane which is just the opposite of a horizontal portal. An 18 G LP needle is an excellent guide that can be used to assess the right direction to the structure that needs to be accessed before the portal is made. The skin is always incised first followed by the deeper layer in the same line. It is best to see the blade tip while making the portal to avoid injury to the surrounding structures. Knowledge of the area to access and surgery to be done as well as a sound knowledge of anatomy is essential for making a proper portal.

## 1.2 Specialised Equipment

1. 7mm Cannula (Arthrex, Naples, FL)
2. Vissinger rod
3. No 11 blade
4. Artery forceps

## 1.3 Types of Portals

1. High anterolateral portal
2. Standard anterolateral portal
3. High anteromedial portal
4. Far medial portal
5. Superolateral portal
6. Superomedial portal
7. Posteromedial portal
8. Posterolateral portal

### 1.3.1 High Anterolateral (AL) Portal

Position: Knee at 70° flexion on an operating table with a side support at the upper thigh and a bolster on the table (Fig. 1.1a).

This is the first portal usually made for viewing the knee and is a blind portal based on landmarks.

#### 1.3.1.1 Important Landmarks

1. Patella inferior pole
2. Lateral aspect of patellar tendon
3. Joint line

This portal is a vertical portal made just above the inferior pole of the patella abutting the lateral margin of the patellar tendon. It is a vertical portal so that it does not violate the patellar tendon.

Step 1: A knife with a No 11 blade is used to incise the skin just lateral to the lateral border of the patellar tendon at the inferior pole of the patella for about 1 cm (Fig. 1.1b).

Step 2: The incision is continued deeper till the joint is entered.

Step 3: A straight artery forceps is then introduced in line with the incision into the notch, directed to the medial compartment along the Medial femoral condyle, the jaws are opened inside and removed slowly in a rotating fashion. This is repeated again (Fig. 1.1c–e).

Step 4: The arthroscope is then introduced in the same direction into the medial compartment of the knee.

V. A. Mhaskar (✉)
F7 East of Kailash, Knee & Shoulder Clinic, New Delhi, India

JMVM Sports Injury Center, Sitaram Bhartia Institute of Science & Research, B16 Qutub Institutional Area, New Delhi, India


V. A. Mhaskar, J. Maheshwari (eds.), *Innovative Approaches in Knee Arthroscopy*,
https://doi.org/10.1007/978-981-99-4378-4_1

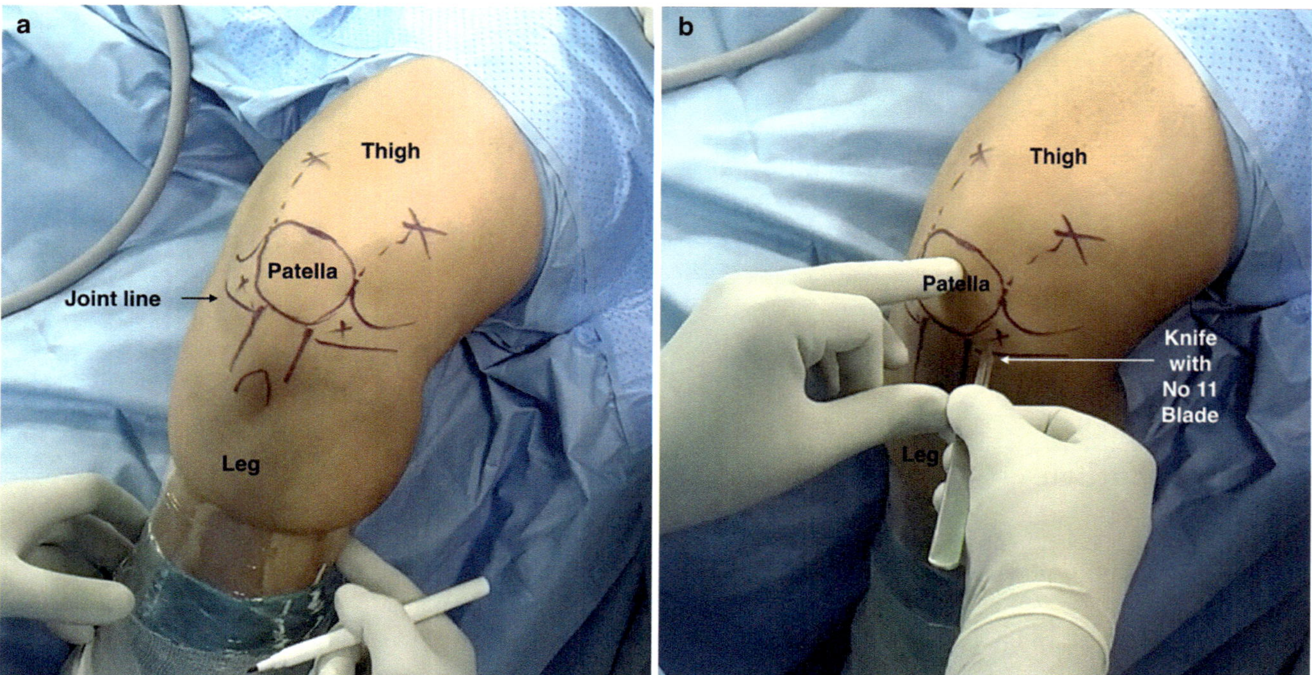


**Fig. 1.1** (**a**) Image of knee with surface markings at 70° flexion on an operating table. (**b**) Image of the No 11 blade used to make the AL portal at the level of the inferior pole of the patella and just lateral to the patellar tendon. (**c**) Image of the knee showing a straight artery forceps being introduced into the portal with its jaws closed towards the notch. (**d**) Image of the knee showing the straight artery introduced into the medial compartment along the medial femoral condyle from the notch. (**e**) Image of the knee showing the straight artery forceps opened in the joint and taken out of the knee in a rotating fashion

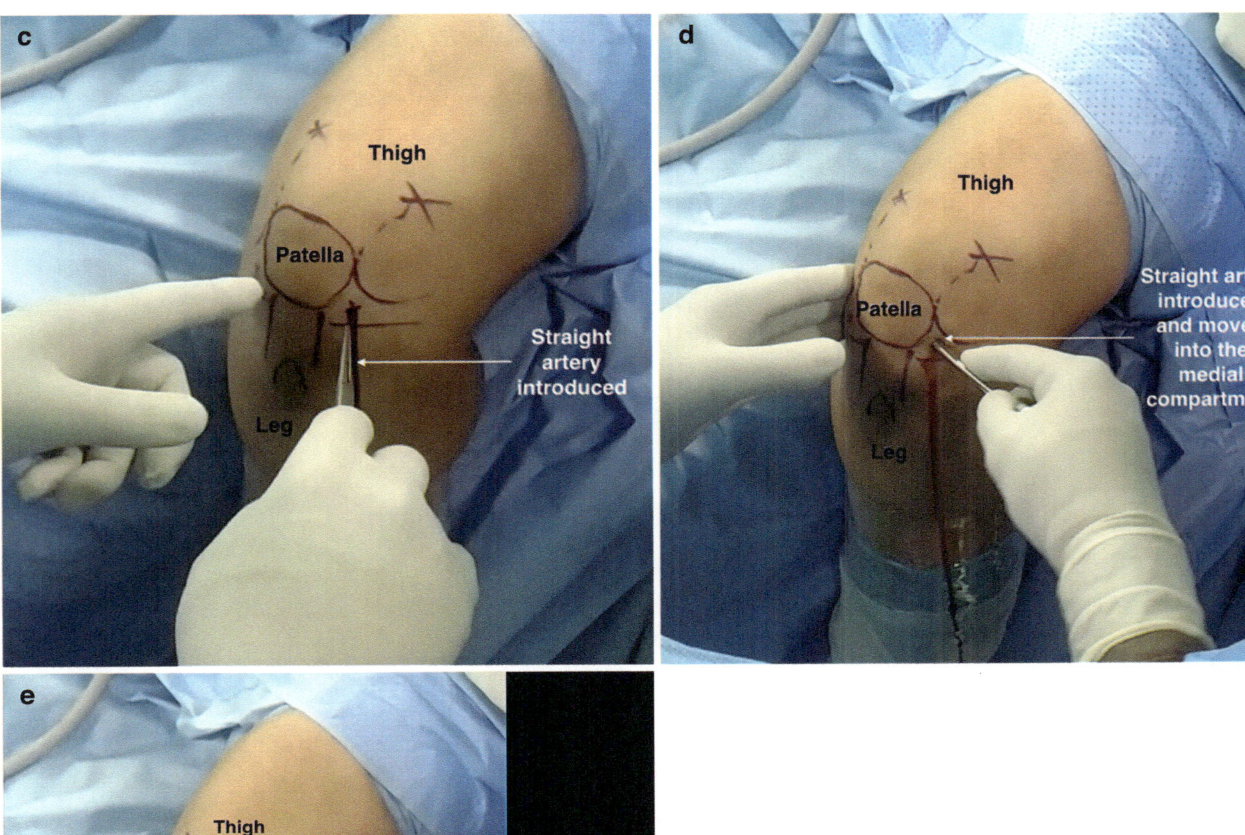


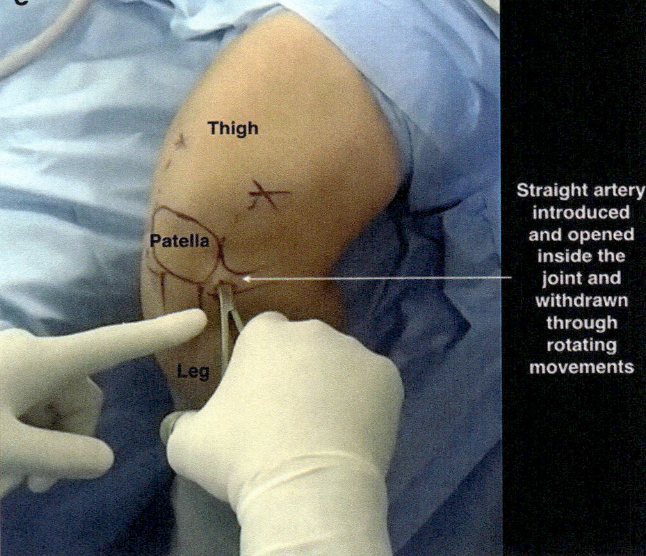


**Fig. 1.1** (continued)

#### 1.3.1.2 Uses

1. Viewing portal for ACL reconstructions as the base of the ACL can also be seen as the portal is high.
2. Working portal for meniscus surgery in the body of the medial meniscus

### 1.3.2 Far Medial Portal

#### 1.3.2.1 Important landmarks

1. Joint line
2. Medial meniscus body
3. Medial Femoral Condyle
4. Medial Tibia Plateau
5. Patellar tendon

**Position** Same as AL portal

This portal is made under vision using an 18G LP needle as a guide.

Step 1: While viewing the medial aspect of the knee, the cable is then rotated 90° to see the medial meniscus and the capsular region. This portal is made just above the medial meniscus and closer to the medial femoral condyle (Fig. 1.2a).

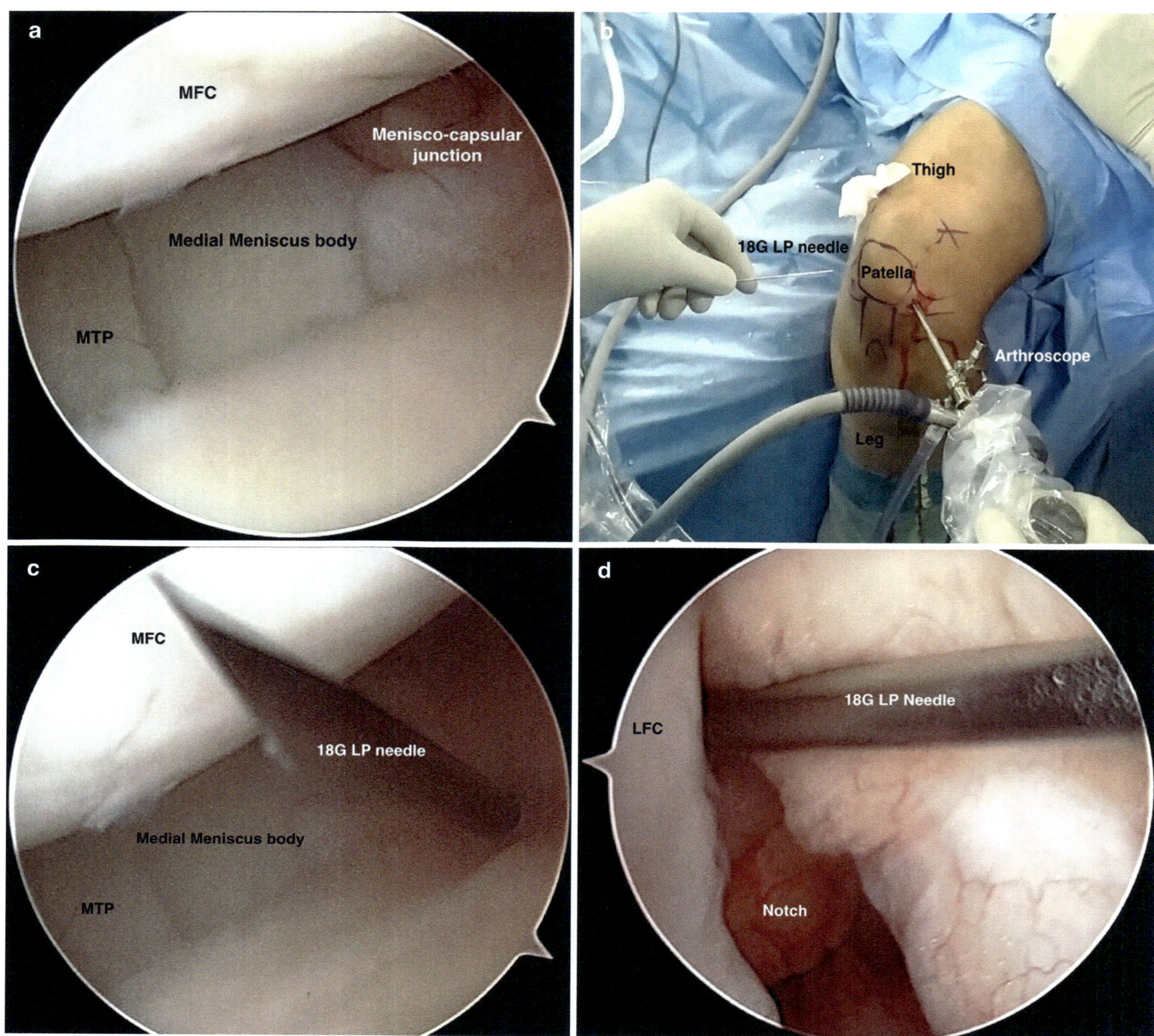


**Fig. 1.2** (**a**) Arthroscopic image showing the medial compartment after rotating the cable 90° while viewing through the AL portal. (**b**) Image showing an 18G LP needle to guide the portal placement on the medial aspect of the knee. (**c**) Arthroscopic image showing the 18 G LP needle entering the knee just above the medial meniscus and near the medial femoral condyle while viewing through the AL portal. (**d**) Arthroscopic image showing the 18G LP needle reaching the notch and away from the medial femoral condyle while viewing through the AL portal. (**e**) Image showing a No 11 blade used to make the far medial portal incising the skin at the level of the 18G LP needle while viewing through the AL portal. (**f**) Arthroscopic image showing the No 11 blade incising the capsule just above the medial meniscus while viewing through the AL portal. (**g**) Image showing a straight artery forceps introduced through the far medial portal and dilating it while viewing from the AL portal. (**h**) Arthroscopic image showing the artery forceps introduced through the medial portal while viewing from the AL portal

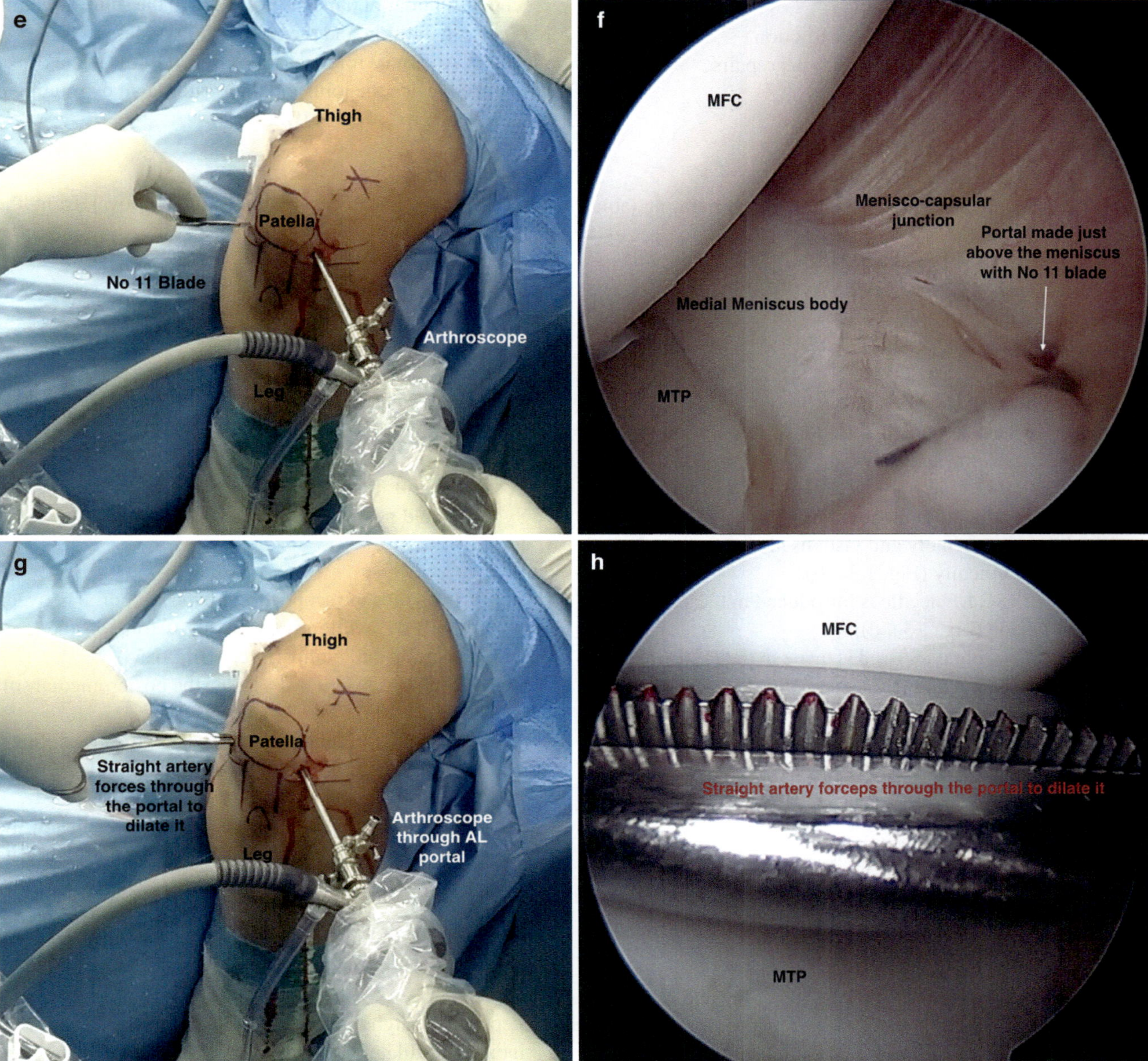


**Fig. 1.2** (continued)

Step 2: Transilluminence can help guide with its approximate location.

Step 3: Then the index finger of the surgeon is used to push the skin externally inwards and while viewing the area arthroscopically in the knee joint the pressure can be seen as the tissue moving inwards arthroscopically.

Step 4: The 18 G LP needle is then introduced holding it near the nozzle in the same direction from outside to inside making sure it is just above the medial meniscus yet away from the medial femoral condyle (Fig. 1.2b, c).

Step 5: The light cable is turned 90° to see if it reaches the ACL footprint on the femur unobstructed or any location you need to access (Fig. 1.2d). It is the removed and the cable is rotated back 90°.

Step 6: The No 11 blade is then used to cut the skin horizontally for about 1cm at the same level seeing the puncture wound that is more accentuated due to transilluminence (Fig. 1.2e, f). The incision is progressed inwards in the same line to cut the capsular tissue horizontally.

Step 7: An artery forceps is introduced in the same direction opened inside the joint and withdrawn in a rotating fashion to dilate the portal while viewing through the AL portal (Fig. 1.2g, h).

#### 1.3.2.2 Uses

1. Working portal for ACL reconstruction
2. Working portal for medial meniscus repairs

### 1.3.3 Superolateral Portal

**Position** Knee in complete extension on an operating table

#### 1.3.3.1 Important Landmarks

1. Superolateral border of patella
2. Lateral femoral condyle
3. Quadriceps tendon

This portal is made under vision.

Step 1: The arthroscope is introduced into the suprapatellar pouch, the lateral aspect of the pouch is visualised by rotating the light cable appropriately and transilluminence seen. Through transilluminence the finger is gently pushed against the skin externally and visualised in the superolateral region arthroscopically (Fig. 1.3a, b).

Step 2: An 18G LP needle is introduced in the same direction from outside (Fig. 1.3c, d).

Step 5: A horizontal incision is made in the same direction first incising the skin and the deeper (Fig. 1.3e, f).

Step 6: An artery forceps is introduced in the same direction opened inside the joint and then withdrawn by rotating it to dilate the portal (Fig. 1.3g, h).

#### 1.3.3.2 Uses

1. Loose body/space occupying lesion removal from gutters or suprapatellar region
2. Synovectomy

### 1.3.4 Superomedial Portal

**Position** Knee in complete extension on an operating table

#### 1.3.4.1 Important Landmarks

1. Superolateral border of patella
2. Medial femoral condyle
3. Quadriceps tendon

This portal is made under vision.

Step 1: The arthroscope is introduced into the suprapatellar pouch. The medial aspect of the pouch is visualised by rotating the light cable appropriately. At the centre of the transilluminence the finger is gently pushed against the skin externally and visualised in the superomedial region arthroscopically (Fig. 1.4a, b).

Step 2: An 18G LP needle is introduced in the same direction from outside (Fig. 1.4c, d).

Step 5: A horizontal incision is made in the same direction first incising the skin and the deeper (Fig. 1.4e, f).

Step 6: An artery forceps is introduced in the same direction opened inside the joint and then withdrawn by rotating it to dilate the portal (Fig. 1.4f).

#### 1.3.4.2 Uses

1. Loose body/space occupying lesion removal from the gutters or suprapatellar region
2. Synovectomy

### 1.3.5 Posteromedial Portal

**Position** Same as anterolateral portal

#### 1.3.5.1 Important Landmarks

1. Posteromedial femoral condyle
2. Synovial fold posteromedially
3. Joint line

Step 1: Introduce the scope through the AL portal between the MFC and PCL while giving a valgus force at the knee into the posteromedial compartment (Fig. 1.5a).

Step 2: Rotate the cable so as to see the posteromedial soft tissue fold (Fig. 1.5b).

Step 3: Apply external pressure where the transilluminence can be seen posteromedially externally and the bulge can be seen arthroscopically.

Step 4: Introduce the 18G LP needle at the centre of the transilluminence and see it exiting internally, can modify its location till it exits just above the fold or below the fold depending on what procedure is intended (Fig. 1.5c, d).

Step 5: A No 11 blade is used to make a vertical portal in the direction of the LP needle and about 1 cm in length (Fig. 1.5e, f).

Step 6: A straight artery is introduced in the direction of the incision to dilate the portal (Fig. 1.5f).

**Alternative** A vissinger rod may be passed and a 7 mm Cannula applied over it.

If used for a RAMP repair by the single portal technique it is made below the synovial fluid and just above the posterior horn of the medial meniscus.

For PCL reconstruction/refixation, synovectomy, etc. it is made above the PM synovial fold.

#### 1.3.5.2 Uses

Arthroscopic PCL reconstruction

Arthroscopic PCL refixation

Arthroscopic RAMP repair

Arthroscopic posterior synovectomy

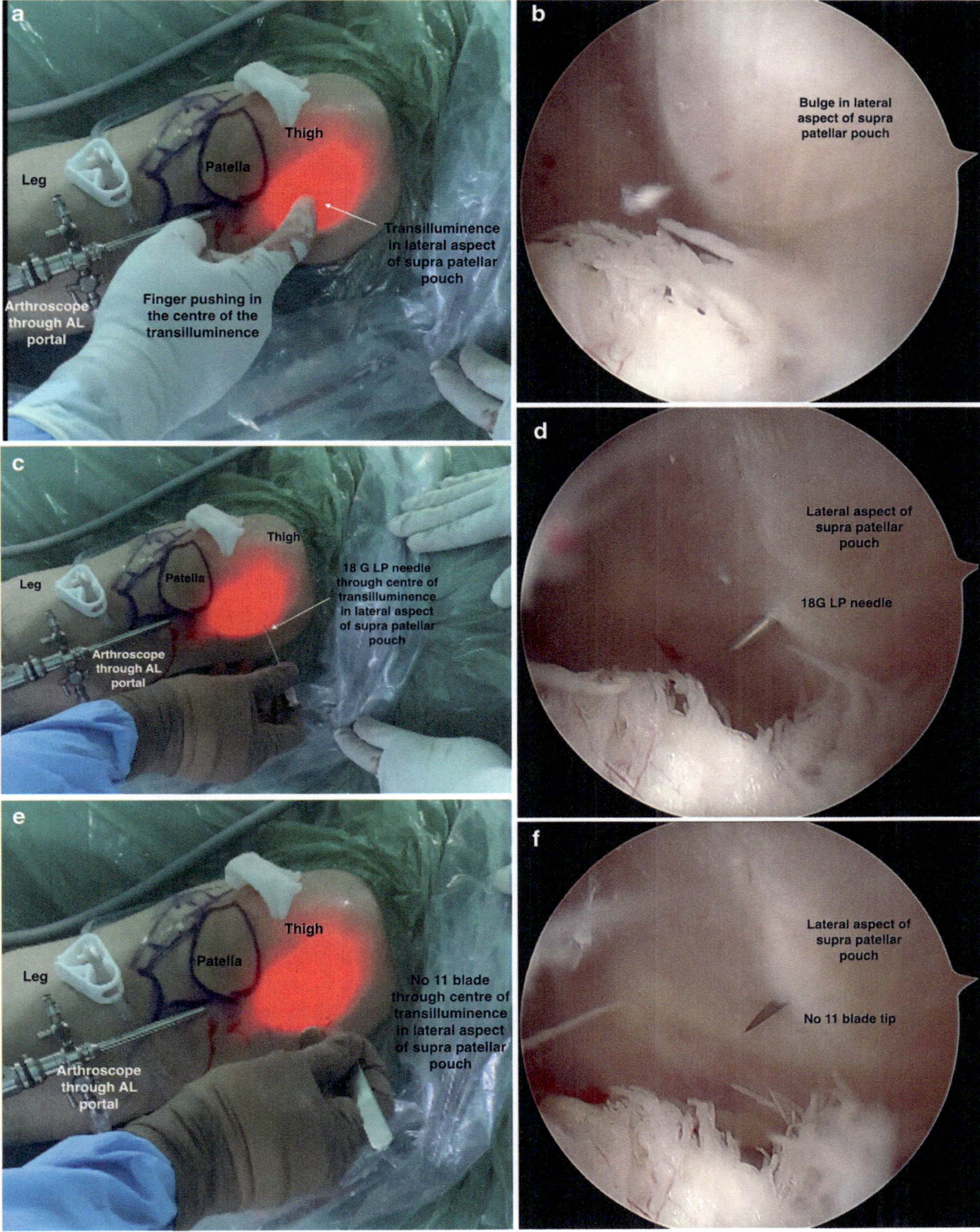


**Fig. 1.3** (**a**) Image of the knee in extension with the scope in the AL portal visualising the lateral aspect of the suprapatellar pouch and transilluminence seen with the finger pressing against the centre of the light shadow. (**b**) Arthroscopic image of the lateral aspect of the suprapatellar pouch and a bulge seen in the capsule as the skin is pressed at the centre of the light shadow while viewing through the AL portal and scope in the lateral aspect of the suprapatellar pouch. (**c**) Image showing the superolateral aspect of the knee and an 18 G LP needle being introduced into the centre of the light shadow while viewing through the AL portal in the suprapatellar pouch. (**d**) Arthroscopic image of the knee showing the 18G LP needle introduced through the centre of the light shadow in the lateral aspect of the suprapatellar pouch while viewing through the AL portal. (**e**) Image of the knee showing the No 11 blade making the portal in the superolateral aspect of the knee while viewing through the AL portal while visualising the lateral aspect of the suprapatellar pouch through the AL portal. (**f**) Arthroscopic image showing the lateral aspect of the suprapatellar pouch where a No 11 blade is entering the capsule through the centre of the light shadow in the direction of the 18G LP needle. (**g**) Image of the knee showing a straight artery forceps entering the lateral aspect of the suprapatellar pouch in the direction of the incision. (**h**) Arthroscopic image showing a straight artery forceps entering through the incision in the lateral aspect of the suprapatellar pouch

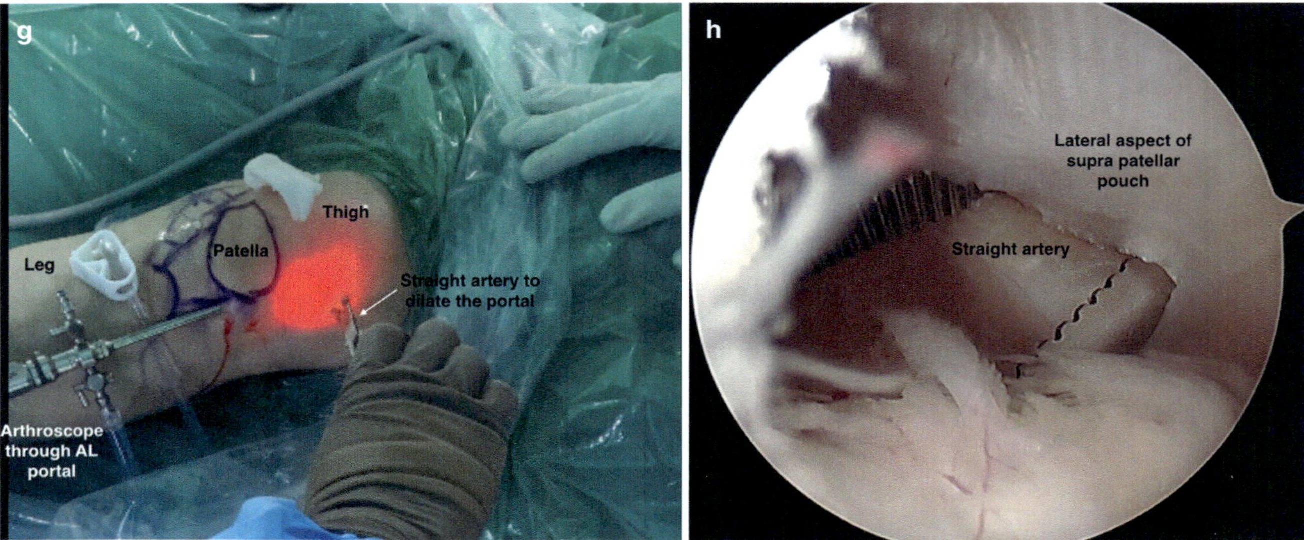


**Fig. 1.3** (continued)

Arthroscopic loose body removal from posterior compartment

Arthroscopic posterior release in a stiff knee

### 1.3.6 Posterolateral Portal

**Position** Knee in 70° flexion like AL portal but while passing the vissinger rod across to the PL compartment knee to be in 90° of flexion

This portal is made inside out through the PM portal while viewing from the AL portal.

#### 1.3.6.1 Important Landmarks

1. Lateral femoral condyle
2. Posterior septum
3. Lateral aspect of the notch

Step 1: The scope in the AL portal is used to visualise the space between the ACL and PCL and a shaver through the AM portal and the space between the ACL and PCL is cleared as well as the septum posteriorly (Fig. 1.6a).

#### 1.3.6.2 Making a Transseptal Portal

Step 1: The arthroscope is in the posterior aspect of the knee in between the ACL and PCL using the AL portal.

Step 2: A vissinger rod is introduced through the PM portal. The rod is visualised and the knee is placed in 100 deg flexion, then under vision it is advanced to the posterolateral compartment of the knee, just along and touching the lateral femoral condyle. This is further advanced till the tip of the rod is seen projecting from the skin above the biceps femoris tendon on the posterolateral aspect of the knee (Fig. 1.6a, b).

Step 2: A 1cm incision is made over it (Fig. 1.6d).

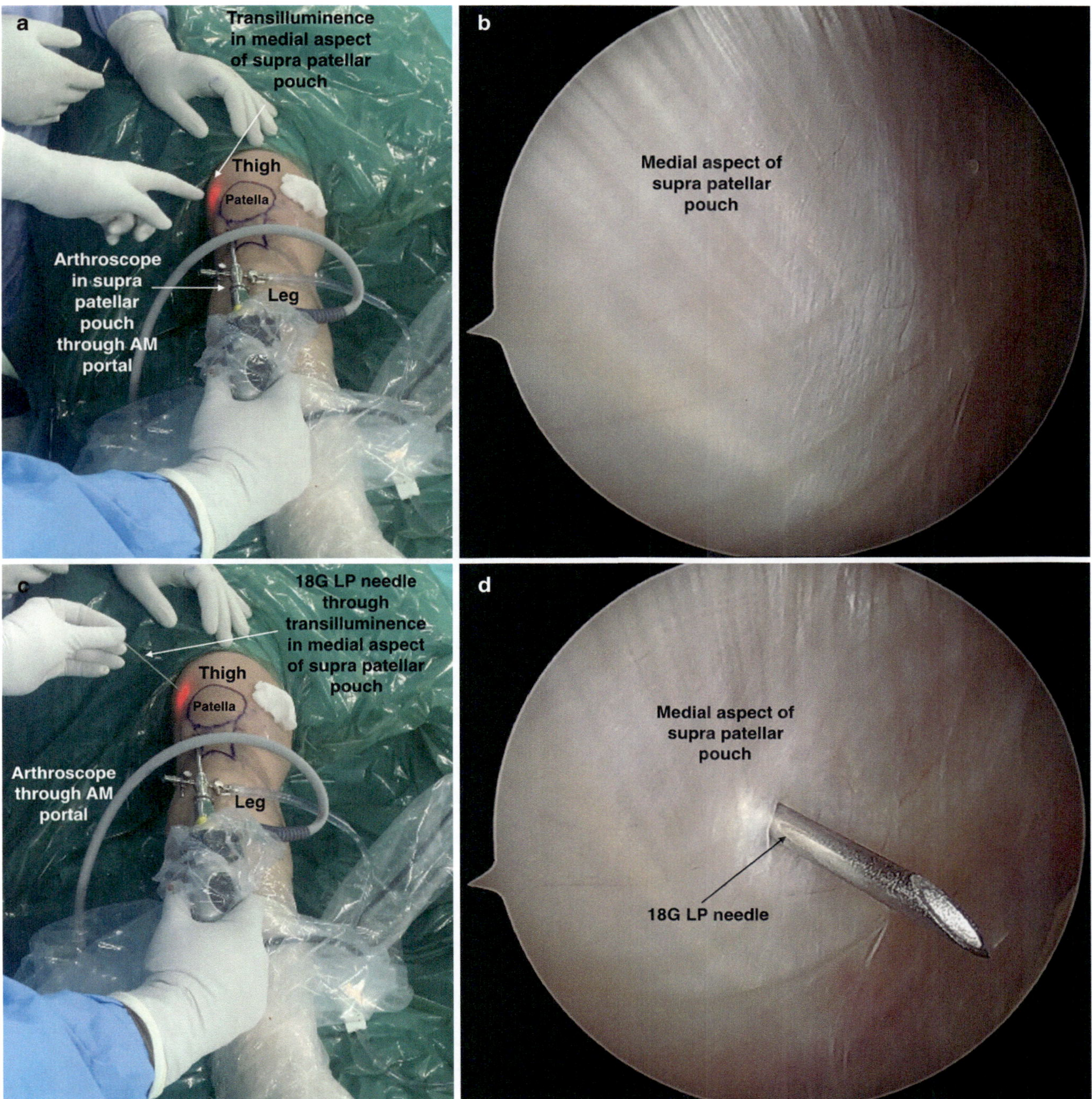


**Fig. 1.4** (**a**) Image of the knee showing the scope from the AM portal visualising the superomedial aspect of the suprapatellar pouch with the knee in extension and finger pressing the centre of the light shadow. (**b**) Arthroscopic image of the medial aspect of the suprapatellar pouch showing the bulge of the index finger in the capsule when pressed at the centre of the light shadow. (**c**) Image of the knee showing the arthroscope in the AM portal visualising the medial aspect of the suprapatellar pouch and an 18G LP needle introduced through the centre of the light shadow. (**d**) Arthroscopic image of the superomedial aspect of the suprapatellar pouch while viewing through the AM portal showing an 18G LP needle coming into the joint through the capsule at the centre of the light shadow. (**e**) Image of the knee showing a No 11 blade incising the skin and making the superomedial portal while viewing the superomedial aspect of the suprapatellar pouch through the AM portal. (**f**) Arthroscopic image of the knee showing a No 11 blade incising the capsule in the direction of the 18 G LP needle in the superomedial aspect of the suprapatellar pouch while viewing from the AM portal. (**g**) Arthroscopic image of the knee showing the straight artery entering the capsule in the superomedial aspect of the suprapatellar pouch while viewing through the AM portal

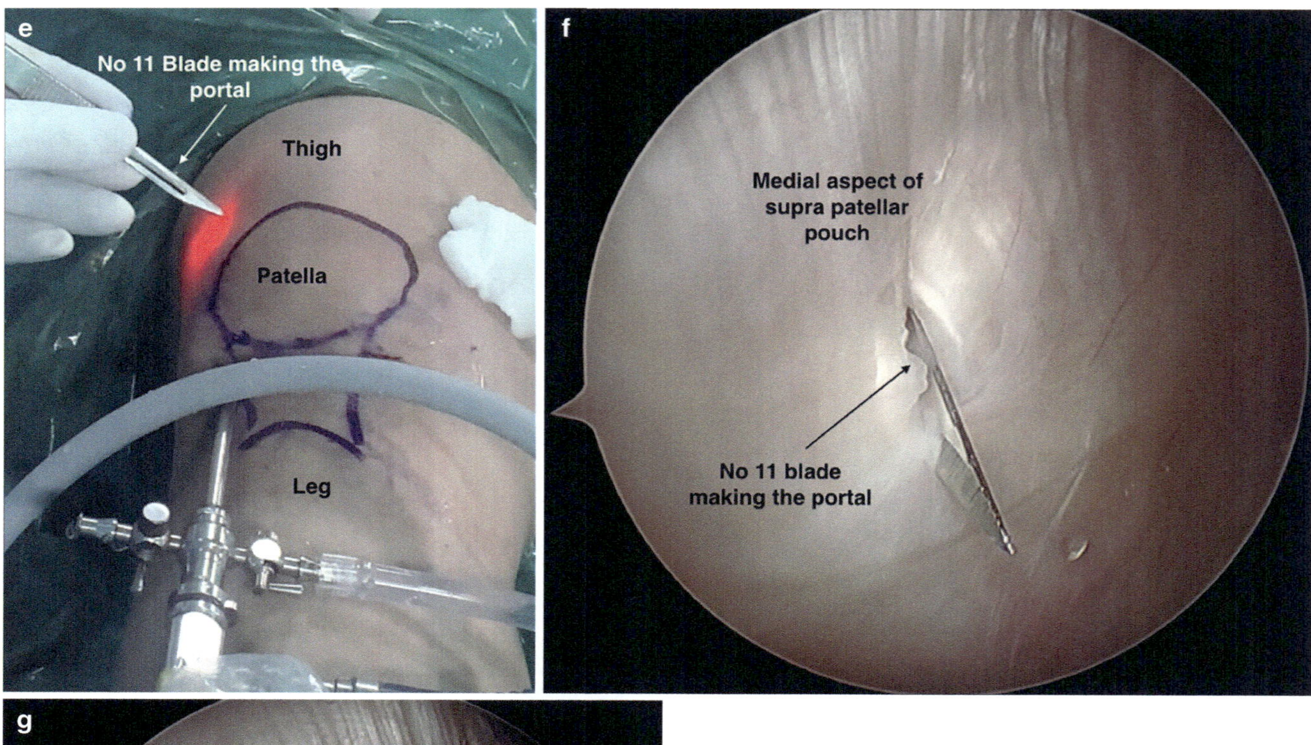


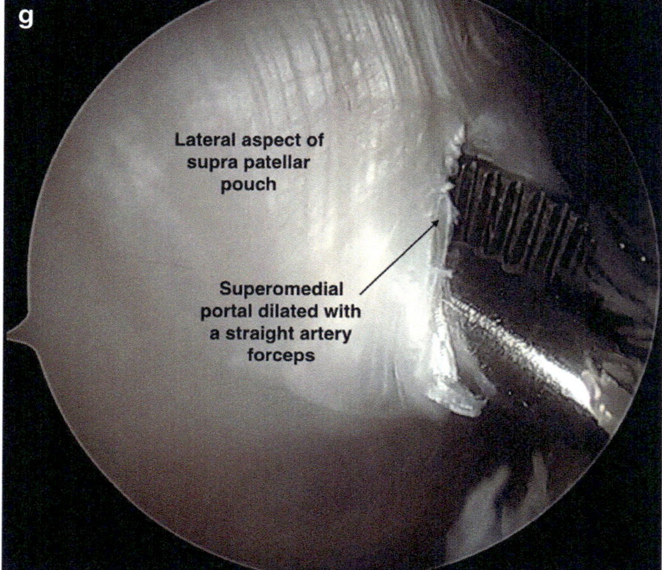


**Fig. 1.4** (continued)

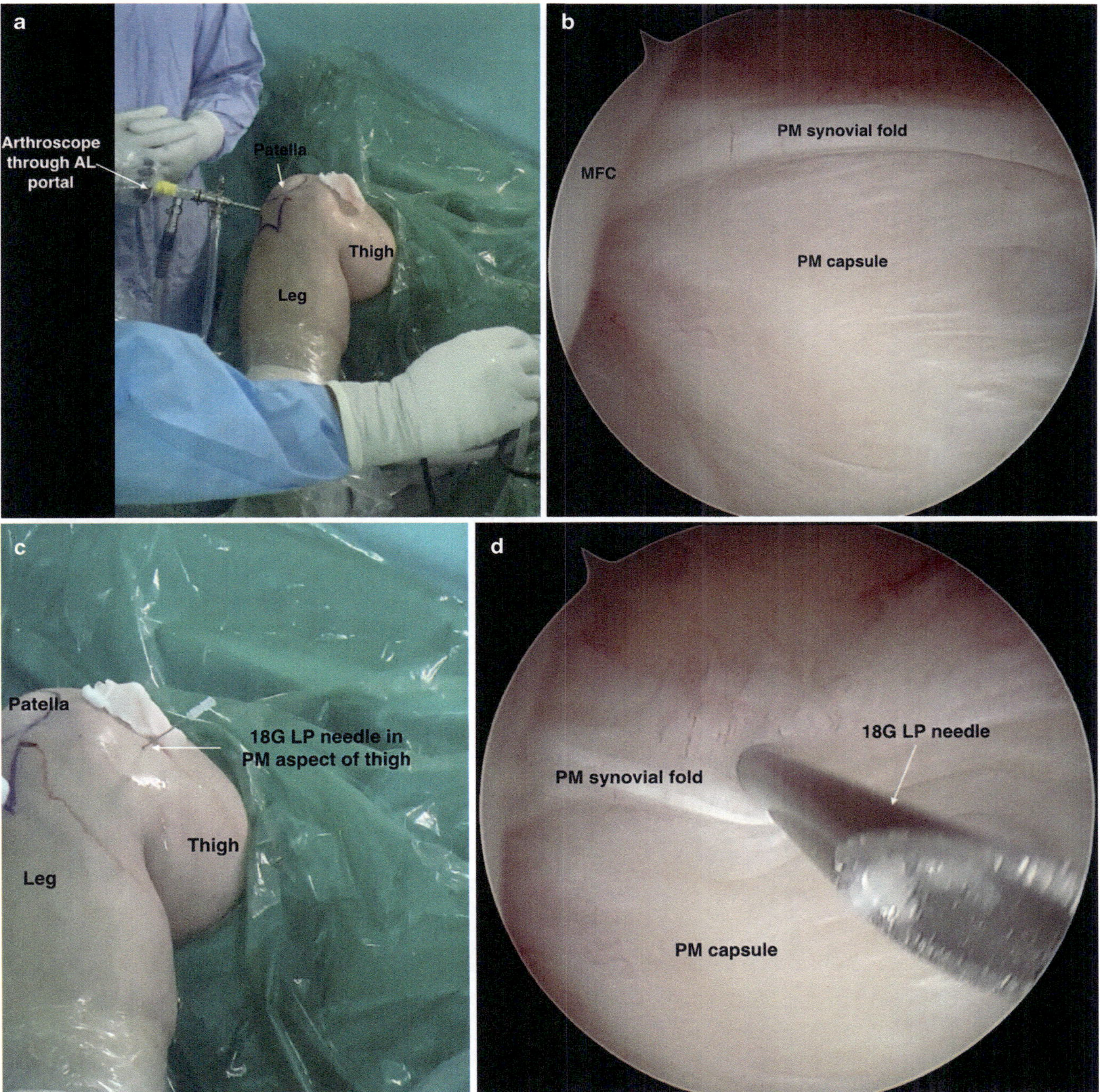


**Fig. 1.5** (**a**) Image of the knee showing the arthroscope in the AL portal entering the posteromedial aspect of the knee between the PCL and medial femoral condyle (MFC). (**b**) Arthroscopic image showing the posteromedial synovial fold while viewing from the AL portal between the PCL and MFC. (**c**) Image of the knee showing the 18G LP needle entering the knee through the PM aspect at the centre of the light shadow. (**d**) Arthroscopic image of the posteromedial aspect of the knee showing an 18 G LP needle entering the knee just above the synovial fold while viewing through the AL portal in between the PCL and MFC. (**e**) Image of the knee showing a No 11 blade making an incision in the centre of the light shadow in the direction of the 18 G LP needle while viewing through the AL portal. (**f**) Arthroscopic image of the knee showing a No 11 blade incising the capsule in the PM aspect just above the synovial fold while viewing through the AL portal. (**g**) Image of the knee showing a straight artery dilating the posteromedial portal while viewing from the AL portal. (**h**) Arthroscopic image showing a straight artery dilating the PM portal while viewing from the AL portal

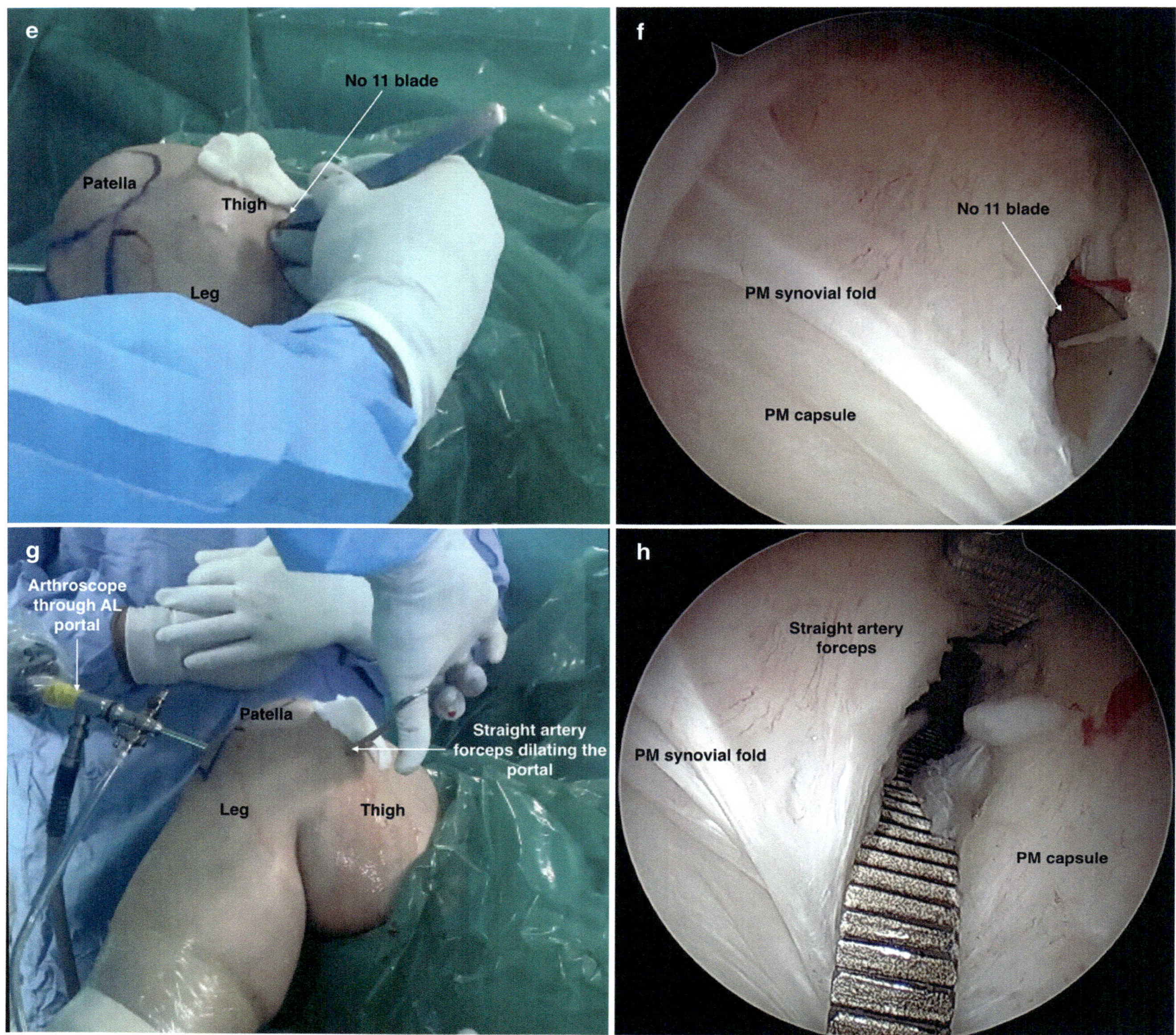


**Fig. 1.5** (continued)

Step 3: The Vissinger rod is advanced from the PM to PL portal with the knee in 100° flexion and scope in AL portal (Fig. 1.6e).

Step 4: Keeping the knee in 100° flexion, the arthroscope sheath is cannulated over the Vissinger rod into the PL compartment (Fig. 1.6f, g).

**Variation** A 7mm cannula can be cannulated over the Vissinger rod too rather than applying the scope directly (Fig. 1.6h–j).

### 1.3.6.3 Uses

1. Arthroscopic PCL reconstruction
2. Arthroscopic PCL avulsion fixation
3. Arthroscopic posterior synovectomy
4. Arthroscopic posterior release

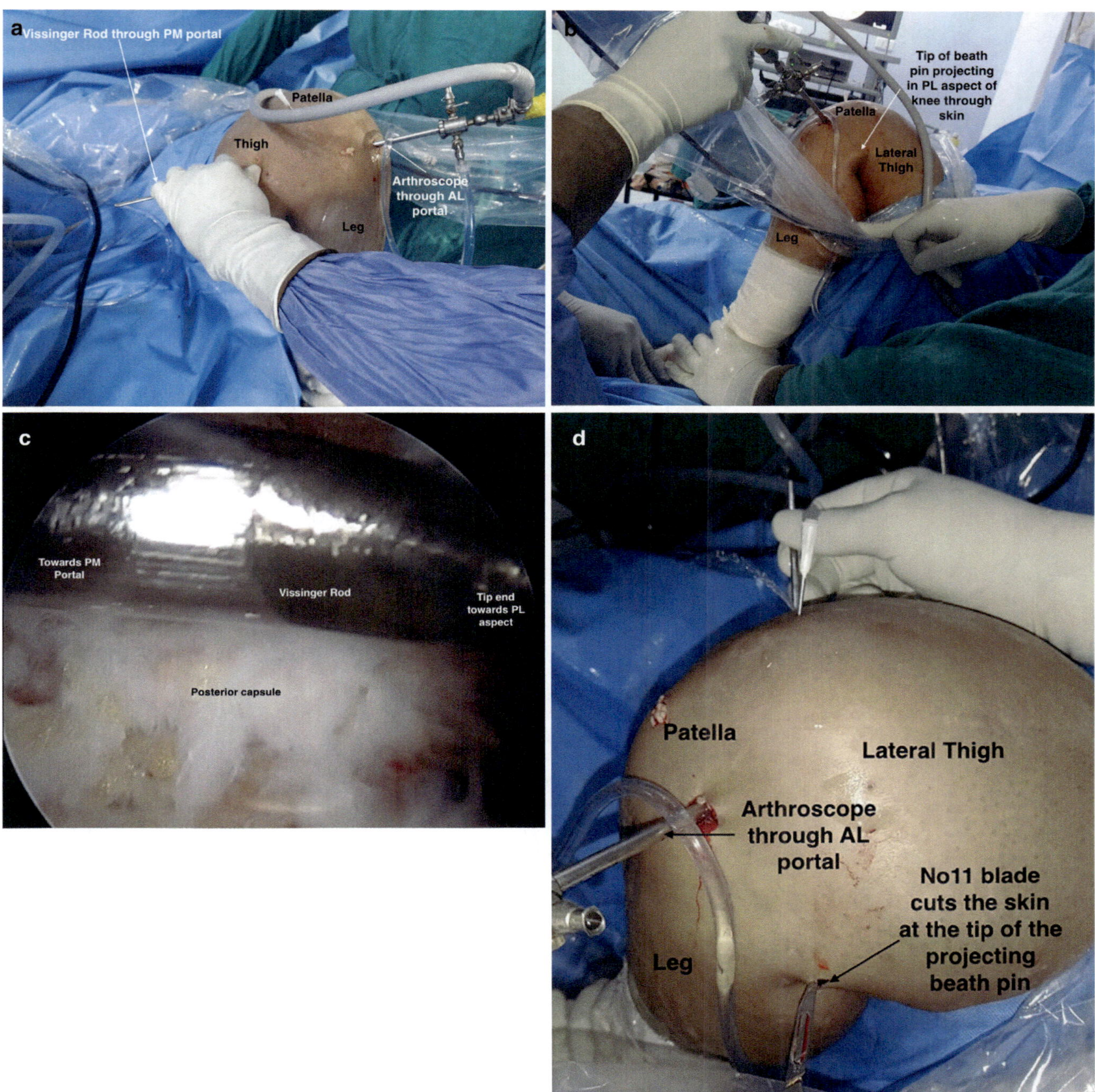


**Fig. 1.6** (**a**) Image of the knee showing a Vissinger rod advanced from the PM portal to the posterolateral aspect of the knee along the femoral condyle. (**b**) Image of the knee showing the Vissinger rod projecting out of the skin in the PL aspect of the knee with the arthroscope in the AL portal and knee in 100° flexion on the operating table. (**c**) Arthroscopic image showing the Vissinger rod going from the PM to PL aspect of the knee while viewing through the AL portal. (**d**) Image of the knee showing an incision made over the tip of the Vissinger rod with a No 11 blade with the scope in the AL portal. (**e**) Image of the knee showing the vissinger rod coming out from the skin in the PL aspect of the knee, arthroscope in AL portal. (**f**) Image of the knee showing the arthroscopic sheath being cannulated over the Vissinger rod to enter the PL aspect of the knee, scope in AL portal. (**g**) Image of the knee showing arthroscope being put into its sheath to visualise the PL compartment after the Vissinger rod has been removed. Scope in AL portal. (**h**) Illustration of the posterior aspect of the knee with the scope between the ACL and PCL and a Vissinger rod introduced through the PM portal along the MFC towards the PL aspect. (**i**) Illustration of the posterior aspect of the knee with the scope through the AL portal between the ACL and PCL showing the Vissinger rod coming out through the PL aspect of the knee and a 6.5 mm cannula applied over it and the knee in 110° flexion. (**j**) View of the posterior aspect of the knee with the scope through the AL portal and between the ACL and PCL showing the PM and PL 6.5 mm cannulas

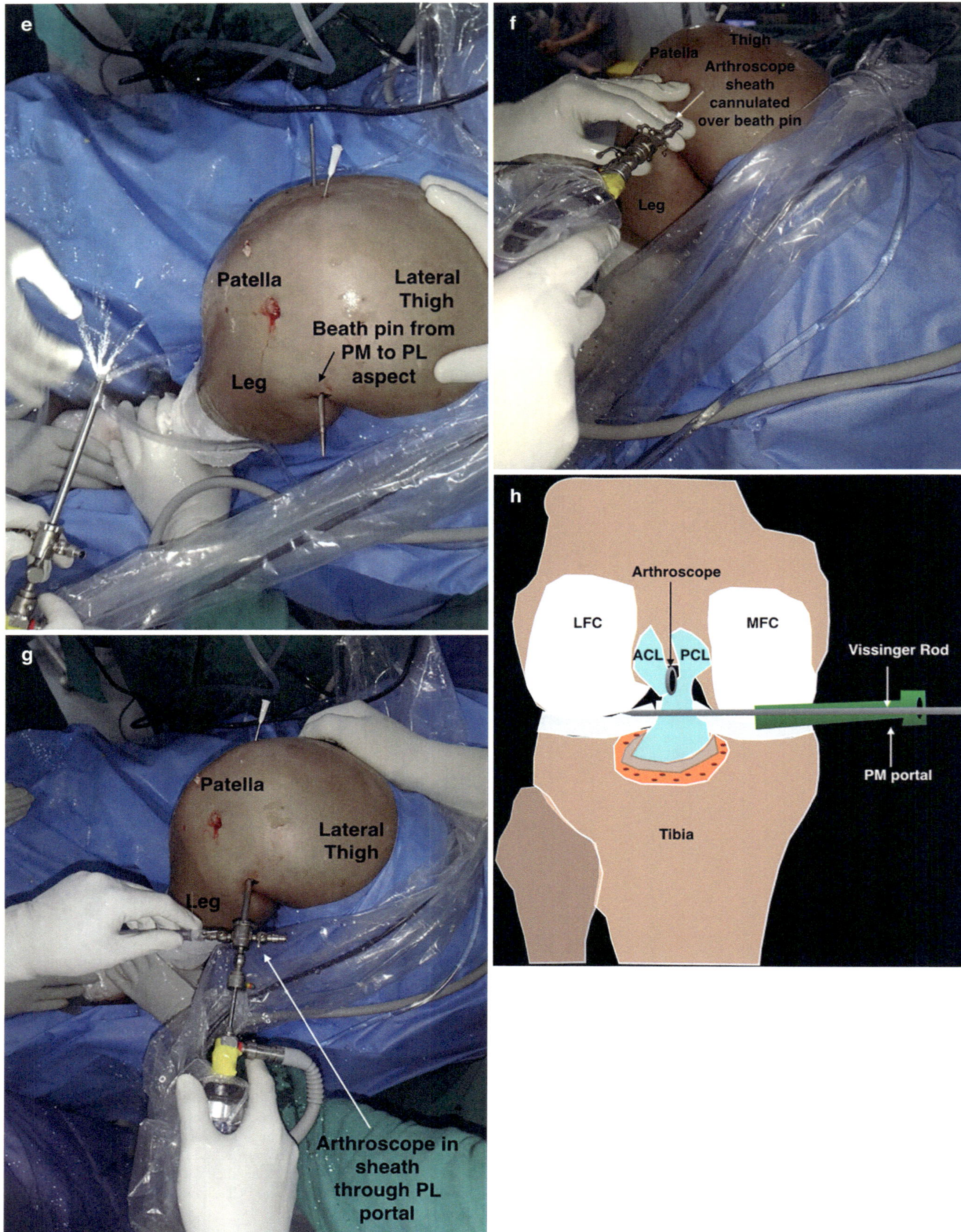


**Fig. 1.6** (continued)

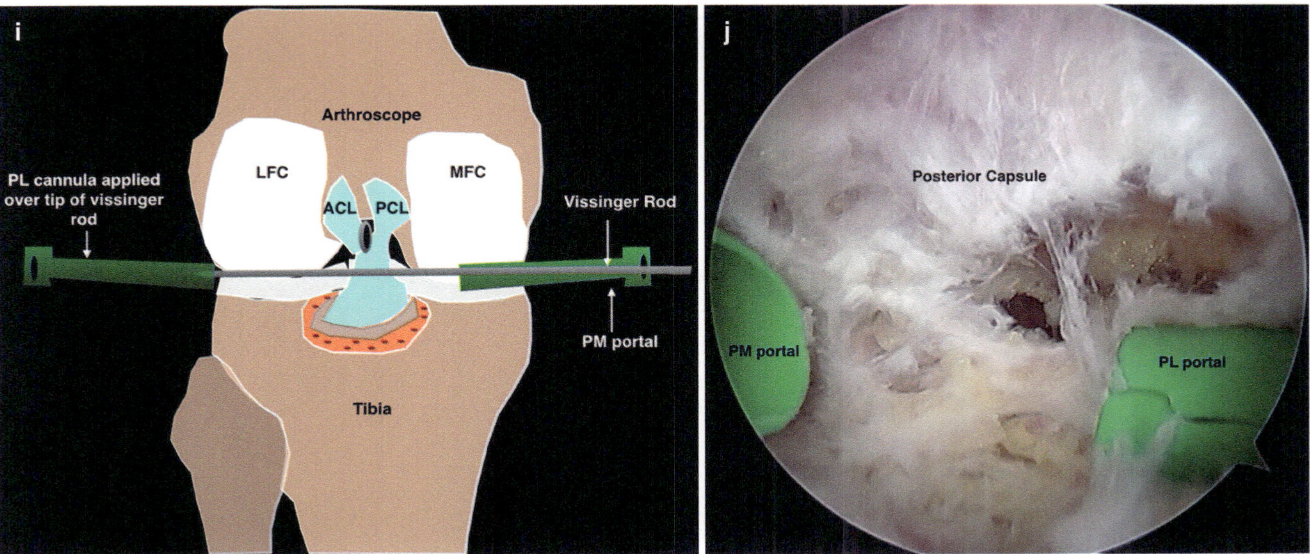


**Fig. 1.6** (continued)

# Arthroscopic Loose Body Removal Using Conventional Open Surgery Instrumentation

2

Vikram Arun Mhaskar

## 2.1 Introduction

Loose bodies can be small pieces of cartilage or osteochondral fragments in the knee. They can be variable in their size. Osteochondral or cartilage lesions are smooth, hence holding them while they are being removed can be tricky and the fragment can slip. Also, because the sizes are variable standard arthroscopic instruments like the grasper may not be able to hold the fragment as a whole. Hence using a normal small artery forceps to remove them can be useful.

## 2.2 Specialised Equipment

1. Small artery forceps

## 2.3 Positioning

Knee bent to 70° flexion on an operating table with side support and bolster at the end of the table.

## 2.4 Portals (Fig. 2.1)

Anterolateral (AL) viewing portal made at the soft spot 5 mm lateral to the patellar tendon (Fig. 2.1).

Anteromedial portal (AM) made in the soft spot 5 mm medial to the patellar tendon and above the medial meniscus.

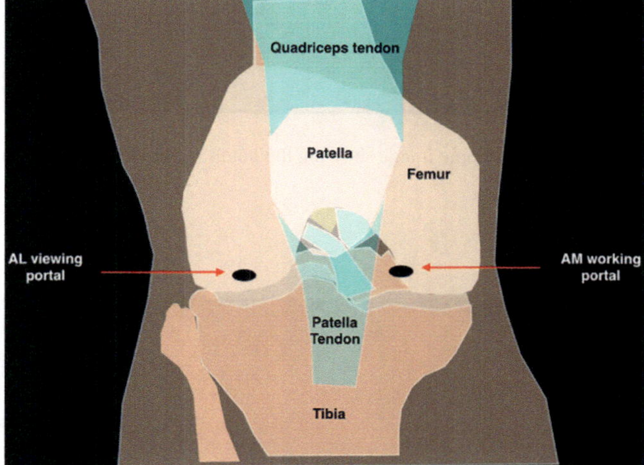


**Fig. 2.1** Illustration showing the AL viewing and AM working portal

## 2.5 Surgical Steps

Step 1: The arthroscope is introduced through the AL and the notch is inspected (Fig. 2.2).

Step 2: Then the arthroscope is moved into the suprapatellar pouch and inspected with the knee in hyperextension and a pillow under the heel (Fig. 2.3).

Step 3: The lateral and medial pouches are inspected in the same position (Fig. 2.4a, b).

Step 4: The fragment is located (Fig. 2.5a, b).

Step 5: If the fragment is in the notch area, a standard AM portal can be made to retrieve the fragment (Fig. 2.1).

Step 6: The size of the fragment is determined and a horizontal AM portal is made with its length approximately the shortest length of the fragment (Fig. 2.6).

Step 7: Making the AM working portal:

1. The skin incision is made such that the length of the incision is approximately size of the fragment.
2. The capsule is then incised in the same direction.

V. A. Mhaskar (✉)
F7 East of Kailash, Knee & Shoulder Clinic, New Delhi, India

JMVM Sports Injury Center, Sitaram Bhartia Institute of Science & Research, New Delhi, India


V. A. Mhaskar, J. Maheshwari (eds.), *Innovative Approaches in Knee Arthroscopy*,
https://doi.org/10.1007/978-981-99-4378-4_2

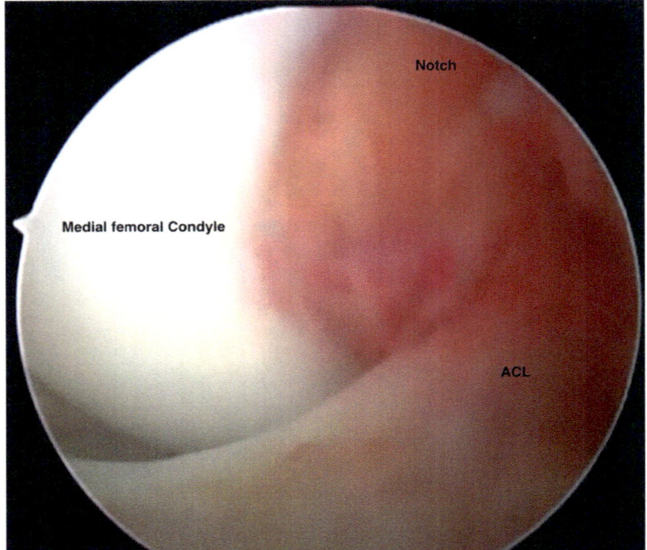


**Fig. 2.2** Arthroscopic image showing the notch while viewing through the AL portal

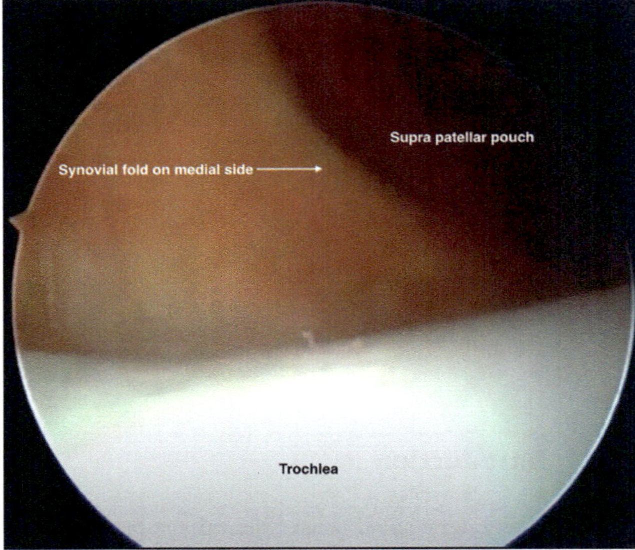


**Fig. 2.3** Arthroscopic image of the suprapatellar pouch while viewing through the AL portal in the suprapatellar pouch

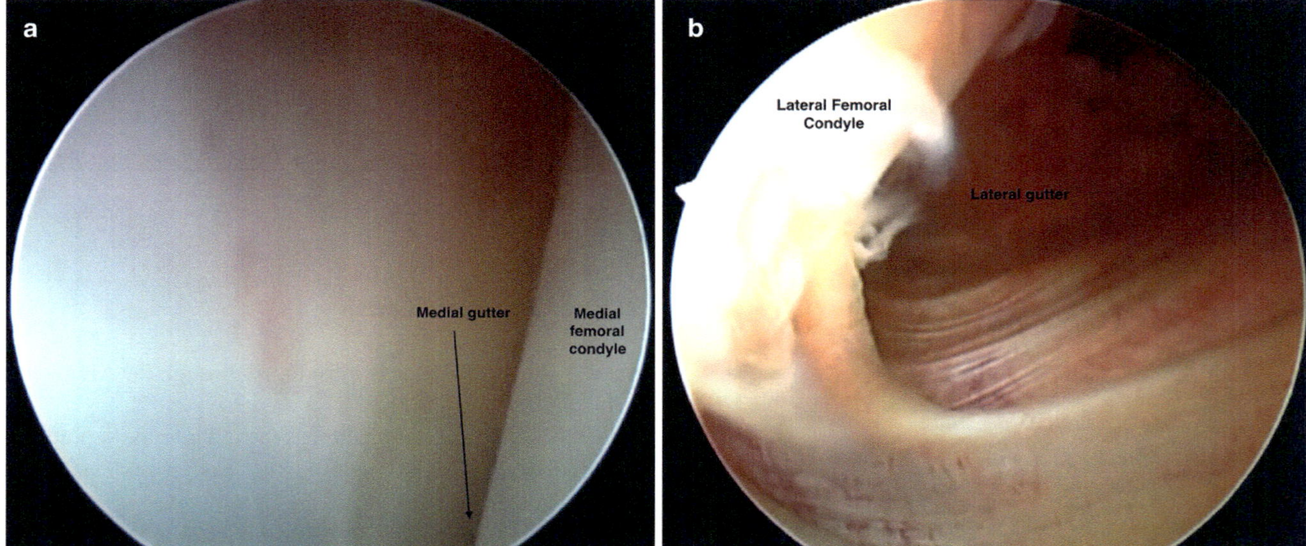


**Fig. 2.4** (**a**) Arthroscopic image of the medial gutter while viewing through the AL portal. (**b**) Arthroscopic image showing the lateral gutter while viewing through the AL portal

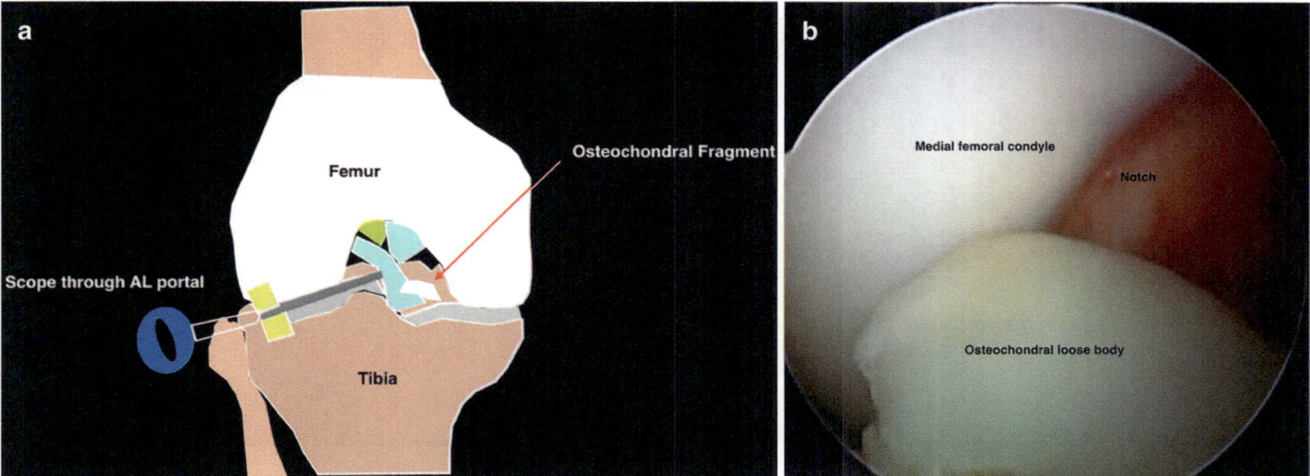


**Fig. 2.5** (**a**) Illustration showing the osteochondral fragment in the notch while viewing through the AL portal. (**b**) Arthroscopic image of the knee showing the osteochondral fragment in the notch while viewing through the AL portal

3. A straight artery forceps in then introduced through the incision with its jaws closed which are opened intra-articularly.
4. With twisting movements the artery forceps is withdrawn outside.

Step 8: The artery forceps is introduced with its jaws closed into the knee (Fig. 2.6a, b).

Step 9: The jaws of the artery forceps are opened when the forceps is near the fragment (Fig. 2.7).

Step 9: The fragment is grasped along its length, such that the breadth corresponds to the length of the portal made (Fig. 2.8a, b).

Step 10. The ratchet on the artery is locked and the fragment removed gradually (Fig. 2.9a, b).

Step 11: If there is any resistance to remove the fragment from the portal, smooth rotating movements can be done while delivering it.

Step 12: If it still does not come out, lengthen the portal incision a little more.

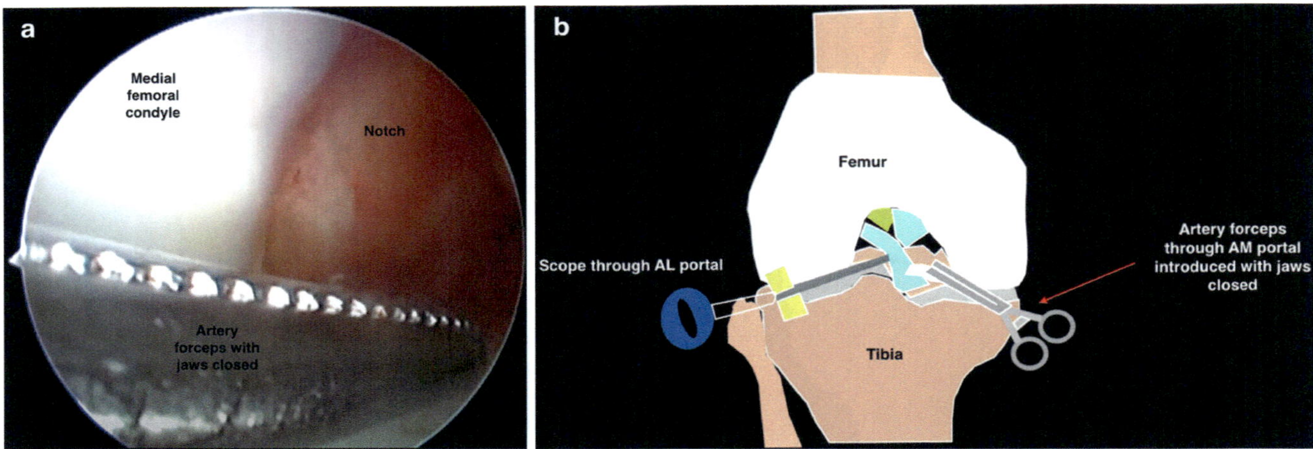


**Fig. 2.6** (**a**) Arthroscopic image of the knee showing the artery forceps through the AM portal in the notch while viewing through the AL portal. (**b**) Illustration of the knee showing the artery forceps introduced through the AM portal while viewing through the AL portal

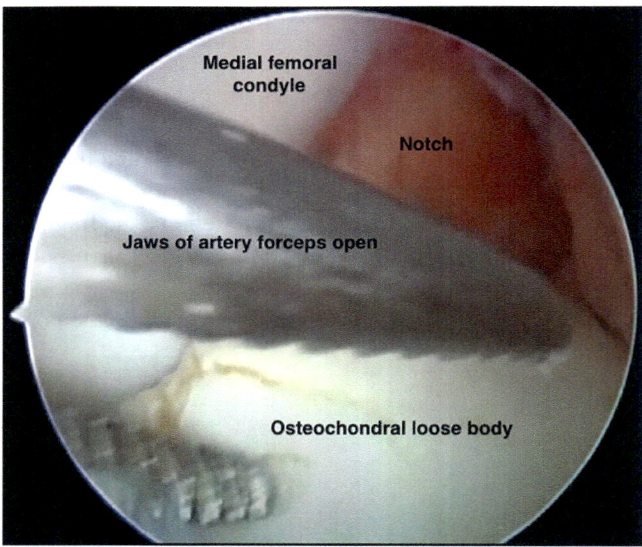


**Fig. 2.7** Arthroscopic image showing the jaws of the artery forceps opened intra-articularly next to the fragment while viewing through the AL portal

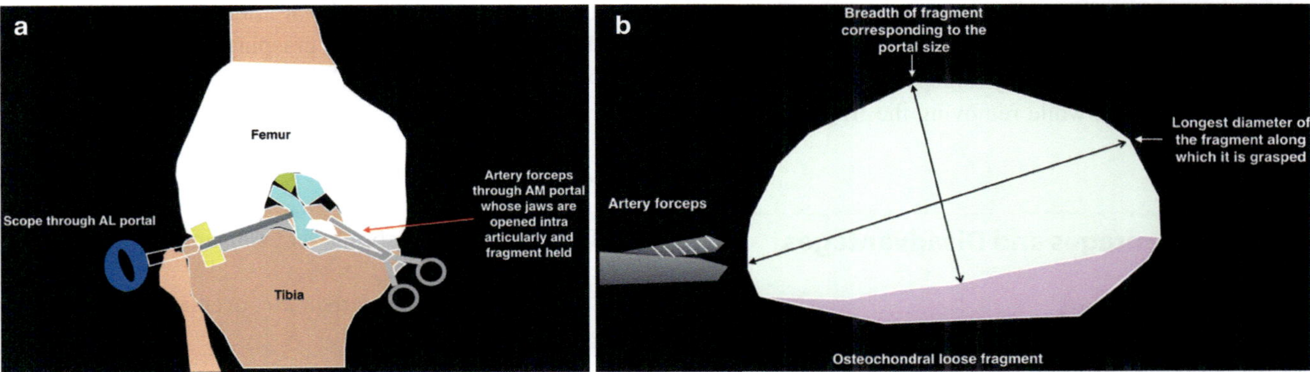


**Fig. 2.8** (**a**) Illustration showing the artery forceps through the AM portal grasping the fragment along its length while viewing through the AL portal. (**b**) Illustration showing the dimensions of the fragment and the way the jaws of the artery forceps should grasp the fragment

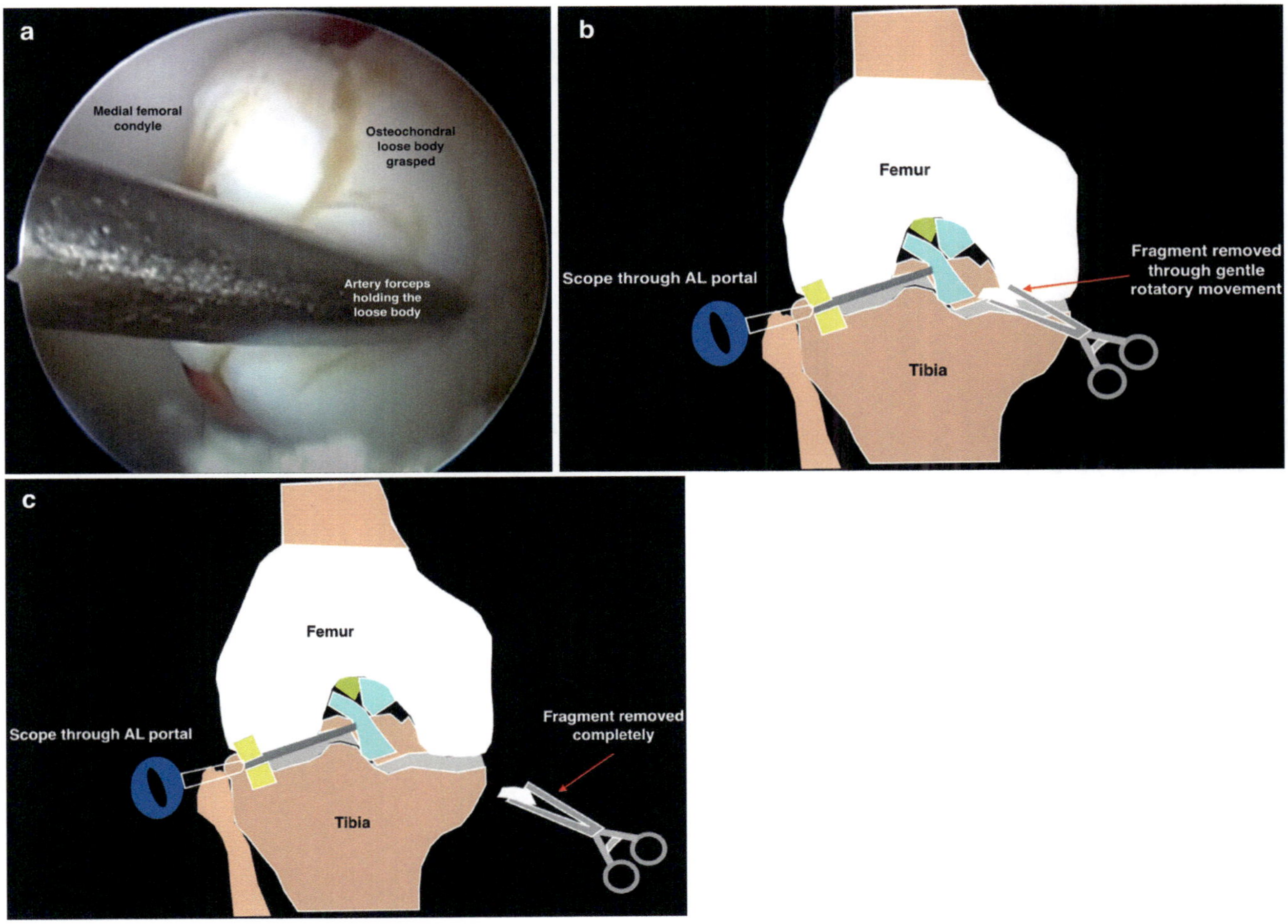

**Fig. 2.9** (**a**) Arthroscopic image of the knee showing the fragment grasped with the artery forceps through the AM portal while viewing through the AL portal. (**b**) Illustration of the knee showing the artery forceps through the AM portal taking out the fragment with gentle rotatory movements while viewing through the AL portal. (**c**) Illustration of the knee showing the fragment being removed from the knee with an artery forceps through the AM portal while viewing through the AL portal

## 2.6 Tips and Tricks

1. Open the jaws of the artery forceps only when in the joint.
2. Lock the ratchet while removing the fragment so that it does not slip.

## 2.7 Advantages and Disadvantages

### 2.7.1 Advantages

1. A conventional straight artery forceps is present in most surgical sets.
2. The jaws of the conventional artery forceps open wider than a grasper and hence grasping larger fragments are possible.

### 2.7.2 Disadvantages

1. The instrument may be harder to manipulate in an arthroscopy setting as
lever arm is shorter than a conventional arthroscopic grasper.

# 3 Arthroscopic MCL Pie Crusting: Single Prick Technique

Vikram Arun Mhaskar

## 3.1 Introduction

Adequate visualisation of the medial joint space in the knee is the key to successful meniscus surgery. In the medial side, releasing the MCL helps in opening the medial compartment. This has not been shown to have any additional risk to causing instability in the future [1]. The technique described uses the principle of pie crusting the medial collateral ligament (MCL) in its mid-substance using an 18G LP needle through a single puncture and multiple internal trephinations so as to stretch the MCL.

## 3.2 Specialised Equipment

1. 18G Lumbar Puncture Needle (Becton, Dickinson and Company, Franklin Lakes, NJ, USA)

## 3.3 Positioning

Patient lying supine on the operating table, with a side support on the upper 1/3 of the thigh with the limb on the bed in extension (Fig. 3.1).

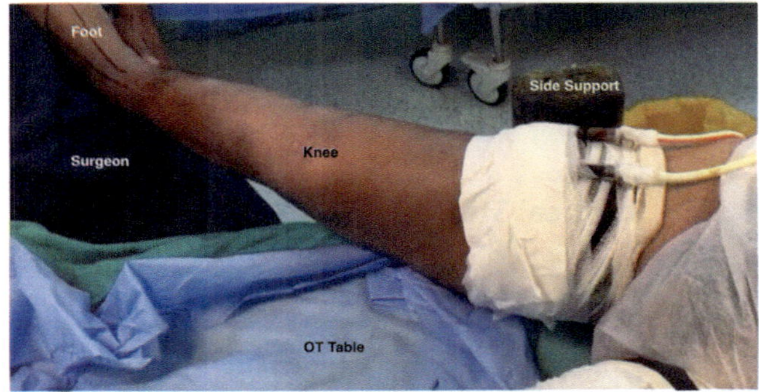


**Fig. 3.1** Position of the right lower limb with a side support, knee in extension with the surgeon standing between the operating table and the patients limb so that he can exert a valgus force on the knee

## 3.4 Portals

Anterolateral (AL) viewing depending on whether ACL is being done can be positioned high or in the soft spot (Fig. 3.2).

V. A. Mhaskar (✉)
F7 East of Kailash, Knee & Shoulder Clinic, New Delhi, India

JMVM Sports Injury Center, Sitaram Bhartia Institute of Science & Research, New Delhi, India


V. A. Mhaskar, J. Maheshwari (eds.), *Innovative Approaches in Knee Arthroscopy*, https://doi.org/10.1007/978-981-99-4378-4_3

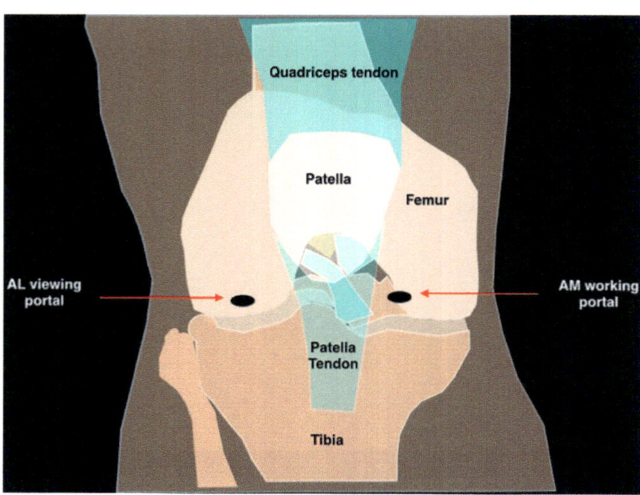


**Fig. 3.2** Standard AM and AL portal positions

## 3.5 Surgical Steps

Step 1: Surface marking of the MCL and joint line is done (Fig. 3.3).

Step 2: The arthroscope is introduced through the AL portal and the medial compartment is visualised (Fig. 3.4).

Step 3: The surgeon stands between the bed and the patient's leg such that the foot is at the level of his hip.

Step 4: The medial portal is made at the required level and a probe introduced into the medial compartment to measure the opening while a valgus force is being exerted.

Step 5: He then exerts an outward thrust with his pelvis to apply a valgus force to the knee with the knee in about 10° of flexion (Fig. 3.5).

Step 6: The foot is externally rotated by the assistant in this position (Fig. 3.6).

Step 7: Keeping the limb in this position the index finger is used to palpate the joint line just below the medial epicondyle corresponding to the deep MCL (Fig. 3.7).

Step 8: An LP needle is introduced just above the joint line at the level of the body of the meniscus and the deep MCL (Fig. 3.8).

Step 9: Through a single entry into the skin with the LP needle, multiple trephinations are made in a at the point of entry, superior and inferior to it while applying the valgus force on the limb (Fig. 3.9).

Step 10: As soon as the MCL stretches there is a sudden pop and gush of blood intra-articularly (Fig. 3.10).

Step 11: The probe is introduced into the medial compartment to measure the opening that is revealed to be more than before the pie crusting (Fig. 3.11).

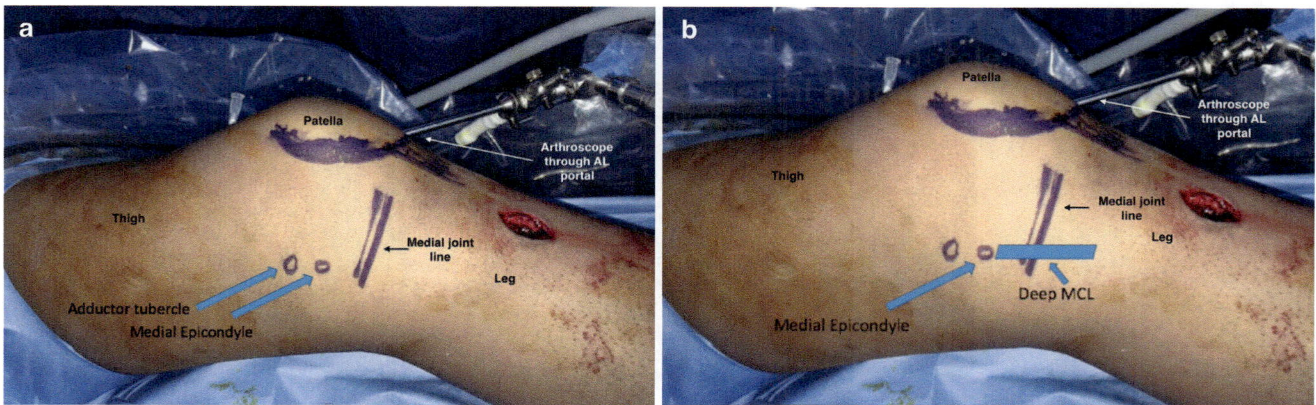


**Fig. 3.3** (**a**) Surface marking of the left knee showing the medial joint line, adductor tubercle, and medial epicondyle. (**b**) Image showing the deep MCL surface marking where the pie crusting is done

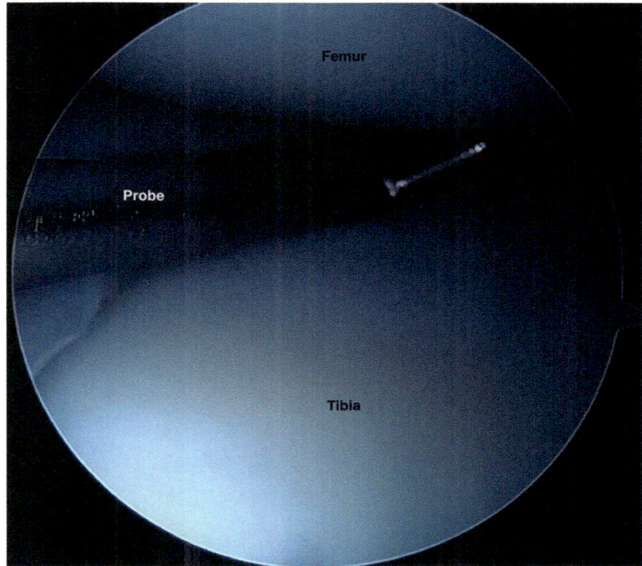


**Fig. 3.4** Arthroscopic image showing the tight medial compartment of the knee with a probe tip to quantify the medial opening

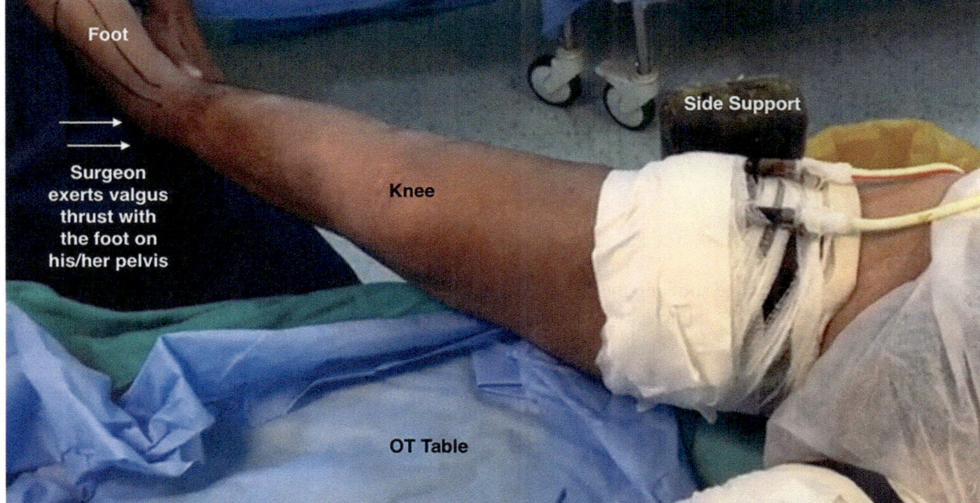


**Fig. 3.5** Image showing the surgeon between the operating table and the limb exerting a valgus force with his pelvis

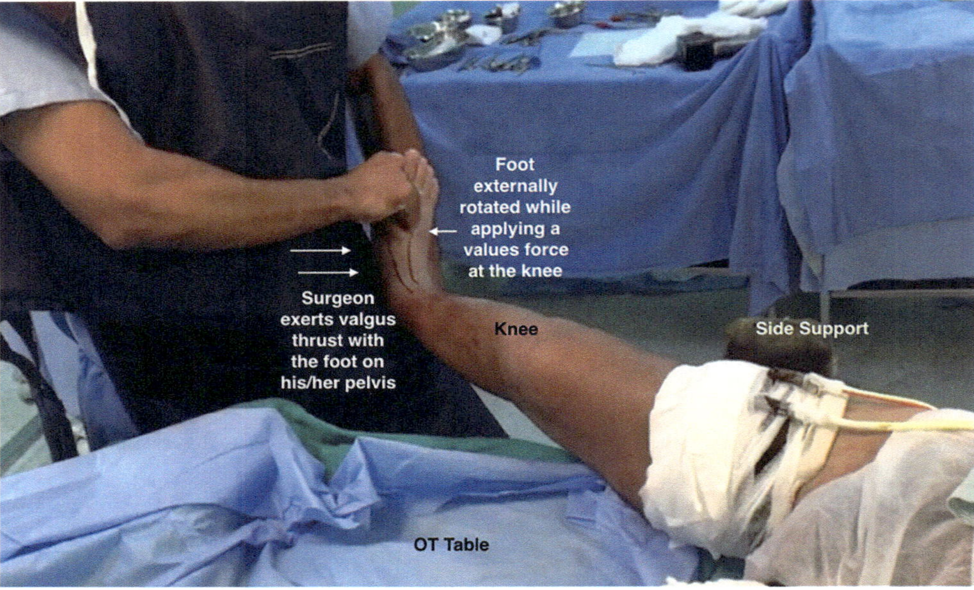


**Fig. 3.6** Image showing valgus force given to the knee and the foot externally rotated for better visualisation of the medial compartment

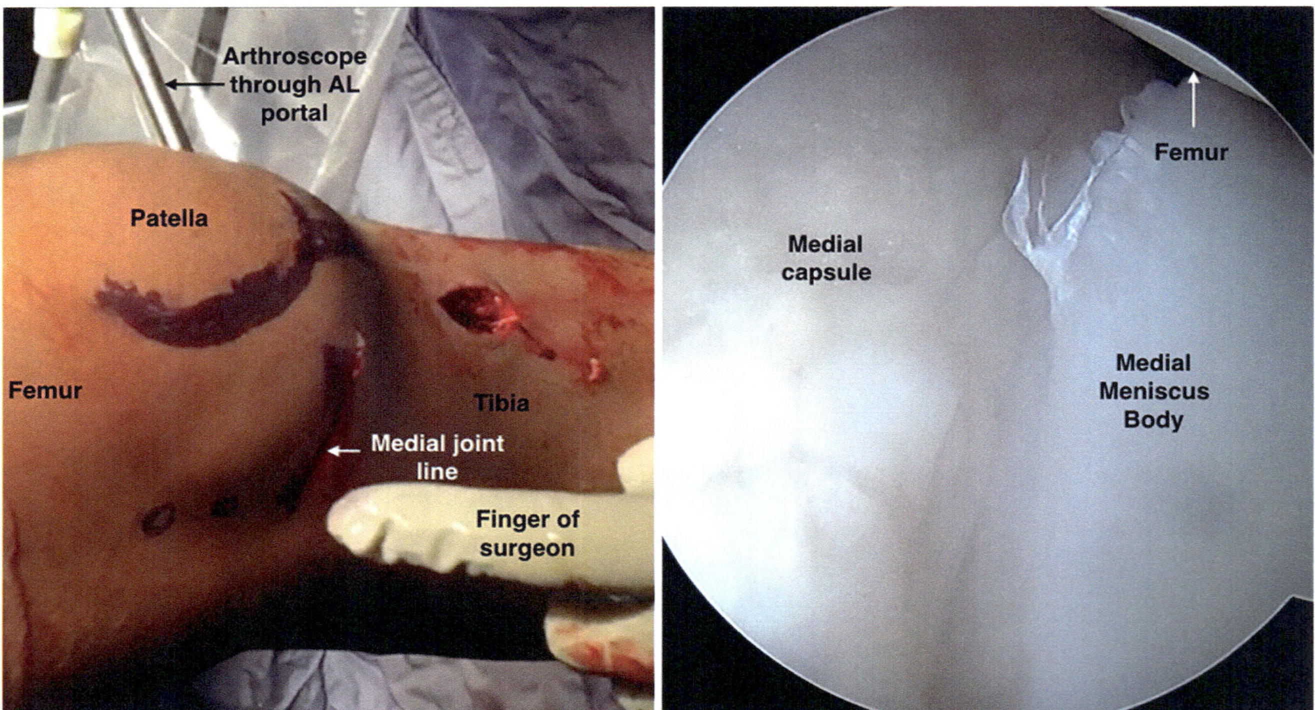


**Fig. 3.7** Left external image showing the index finger of the surgeon palpating the medial joint line and right corresponding area in the knee joint seen arthroscopically and the bulge seen in the capsule internally corresponding to the index finger

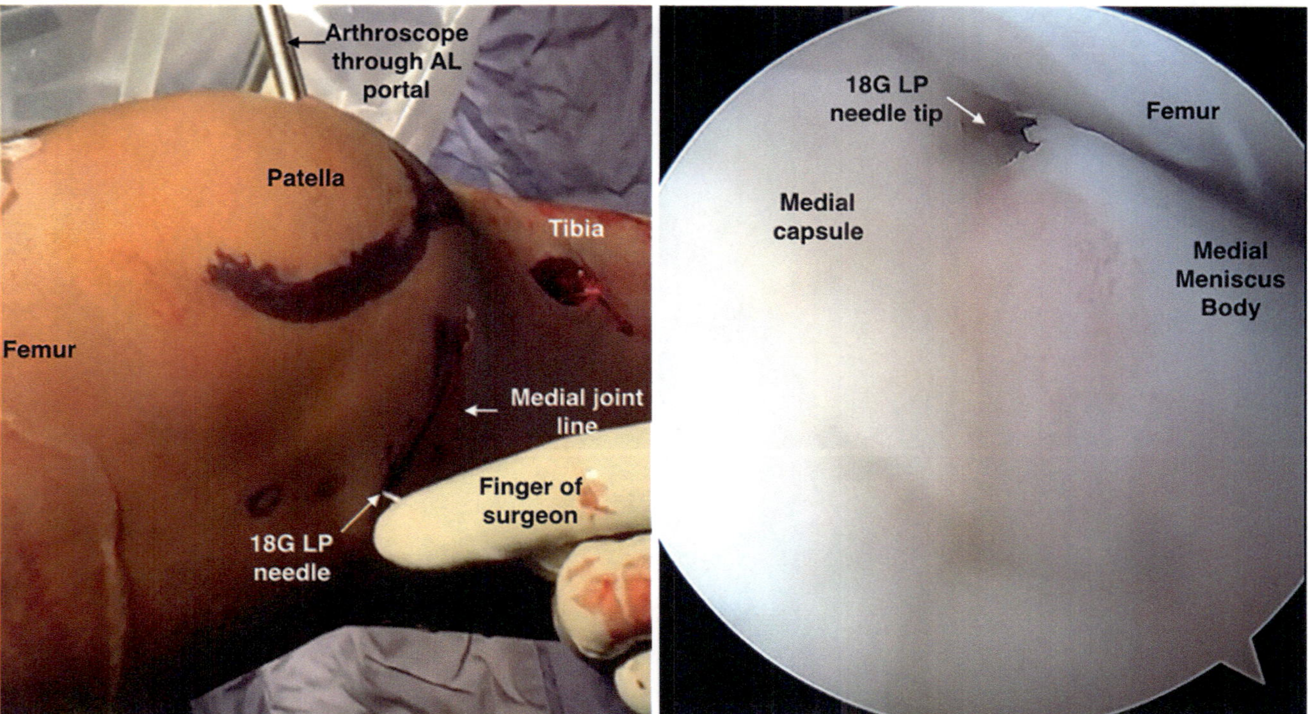


**Fig. 3.8** Left outside image showing the 18G LP needle making trephinations through the deep MCL, right arthroscopic image showing LP needle intra-articularly just above the medial meniscus body corresponding to the deep MCL

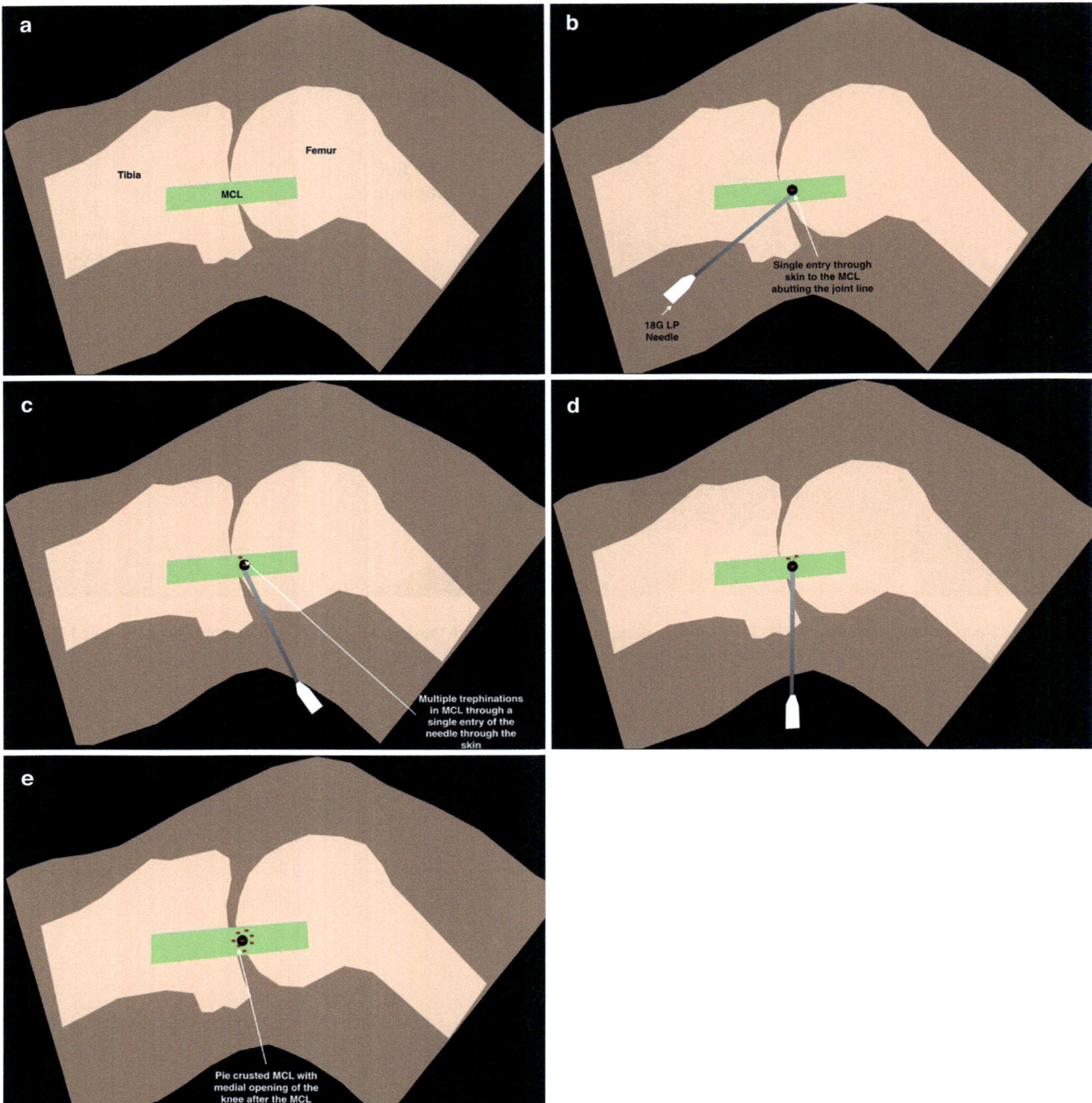


**Fig. 3.9** (**a**) Illustration showing the MCL anatomy. (**b**) Illustration of the knee showing an 18 G LP needle entering the skin and deep MCL through a single entry point. (**c**) Illustration showing the 18 G LP needle making multiple trephinations through a single entry in the deep MCL. A sudden pop can be heard and a gush of blood in the joint indicating the MCL has stretched. (**d**) Illustration showing more trephinations through the MCL using the 18 G LP needle through a single entry in the skin. (**e**) Illustration showing the medial compartment opened and deep MCL stretched by the multiple trephinations through it

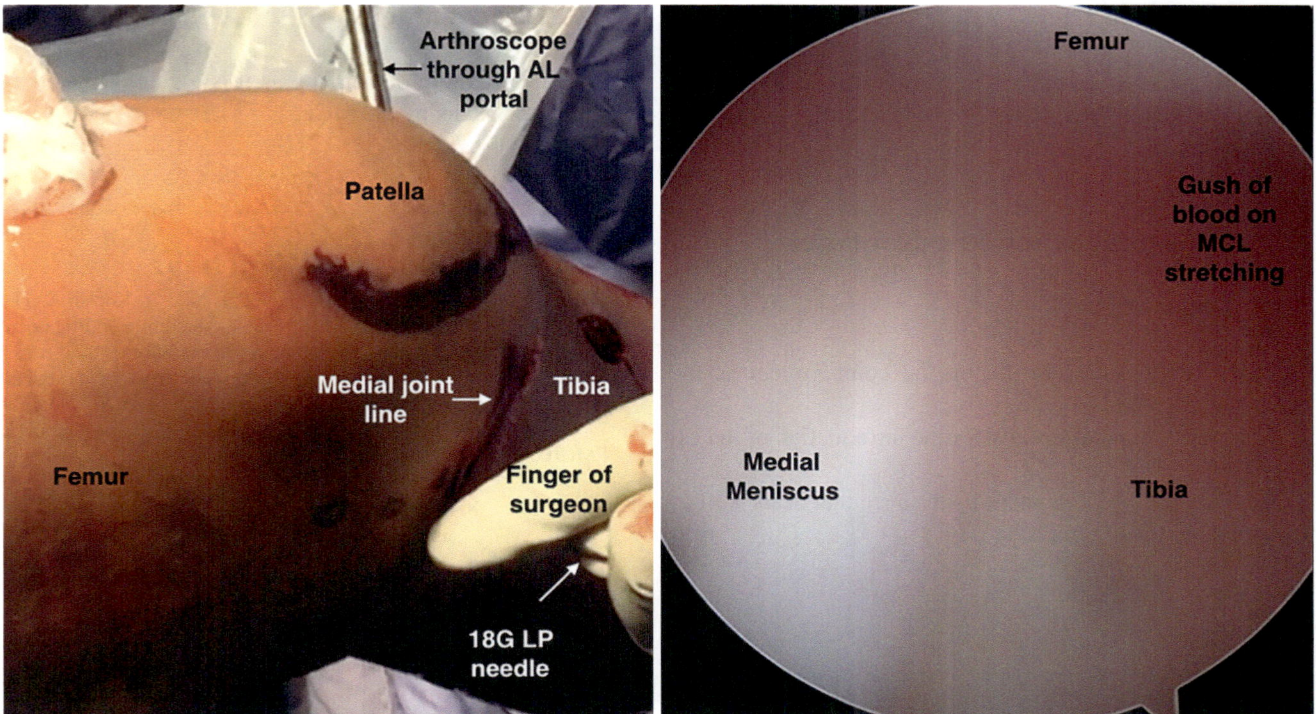


**Fig. 3.10** Left external image showing the 18 G LP needle pie crusting the MCL, right the arthroscopic image of the medial compartment showing the gush of blood and opening of the medial compartment

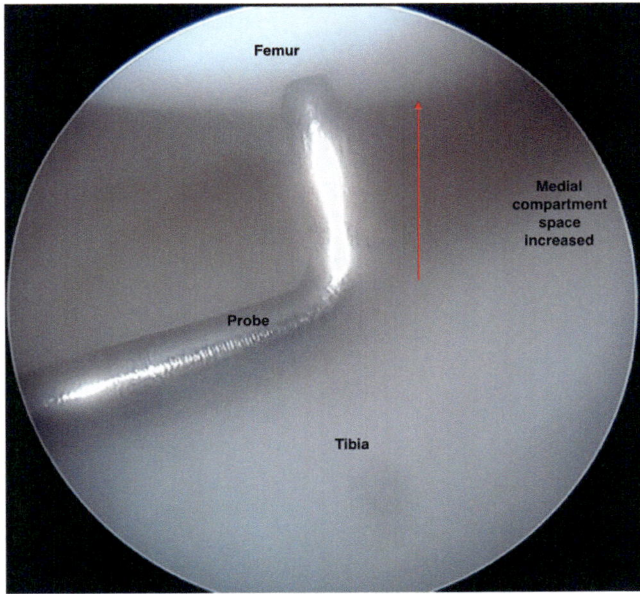


**Fig. 3.11** Arthroscopic image of the medial compartment showing its increased space after pie crusting, quantified by the tip of the probe

## 3.6 Tips and Tricks

1. While pie crusting the MCL, ask the assistant to externally rotate the foot too while giving a valgus force at the knee.

## 3.7 Advantages and Disadvantages

### 3.7.1 Advantages

1. Gives better access to the medial compartment as the space increases.
2. Only one wound externally for the introduction of the LP needle.
3. Releases the MCL in its mid-substance that heals well as compared to the tibial side.

### 3.7.2 Disadvantages

1. Technically more demanding as it is a closed procedure without visualising the MCL.

## Reference

1. Erdem M, Bayam L, Erdem AC, Gulabi D, Akar A, Kochai A. The role of the pie-crusting technique of the medial collateral ligament in the arthroscopic inside-out technique for medial meniscal repair with or without anterior cruciate ligament reconstruction: a satisfactory repair technique. Arthrosc Sports Med Rehabil. 2020;3(1):e31–7. https://doi.org/10.1016/j.asmr.2020.08.005. PMID: 33615245; PMCID: PMC7879191.

# Part II

# Osteochondral Lesions

# 4 Osteochondral Fragment Fixation: Multiple Biopins Technique

Vikram Arun Mhaskar

## 4.1 Introduction

Osteochondral fragments may separate from the femoral condyle as a consequence of injury or osteochondritis dissecans. The intention should be to preserve the fragment and fix it back. This is especially important to prevent degenerative changes from happening. Fixation techniques for these have developed over time and using implants that ultimately absorb while providing adequate stability to the fixation till healing occurs is important.

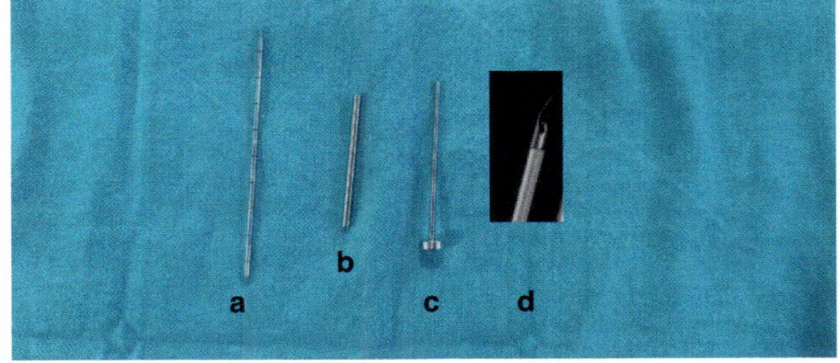


**Fig. 4.1** (**a**) Drill pin, (**b**) Sleeve, (**c**) Tamp, (d) Biopin

## 4.2 Specialised Equipment (Fig. 4.1)

1. Biopins (Arthrex, Naples, FL) (d)
2. Sleeves to introduce the pins (Arthrex, Naples, FL) (b)
3. Mallet
4. Tamp (c)
5. Drill pin (Arthrex, Naples, FL) (a)
6. Drill set (Stryker, Kalamazoo, MI)
7. Standard arthroscopic set (Smith and Nephew, Watford, UK)

## 4.3 Positioning

The patient is positioned supine on the operating table with the knee in 70° flexion with a side support and bolster on the foot end and hyperflexed if the fragment is more distal on the femoral condyle.

## 4.4 Portals (Fig. 4.2)

Portal A: Horizontal anterolateral initial viewing and later working portal at the soft spot just lateral to the patellar tendon.

Portal B: Vertical working portal in the soft spot just medial to the medial aspect of the patellar tendon that is in line with the fragment to be fixed.

Portal C: Additional high anterolateral portal in the soft spot to fix the fragment more superiorly where Portal A cannot reach.

V. A. Mhaskar (✉)
F7 East of Kailash, Knee & Shoulder Clinic, New Delhi, India

JMVM Sports Injury Center, Sitaram Bhartia Institute of Science & Research, New Delhi, India


V. A. Mhaskar, J. Maheshwari (eds.), *Innovative Approaches in Knee Arthroscopy*,
https://doi.org/10.1007/978-981-99-4378-4_4

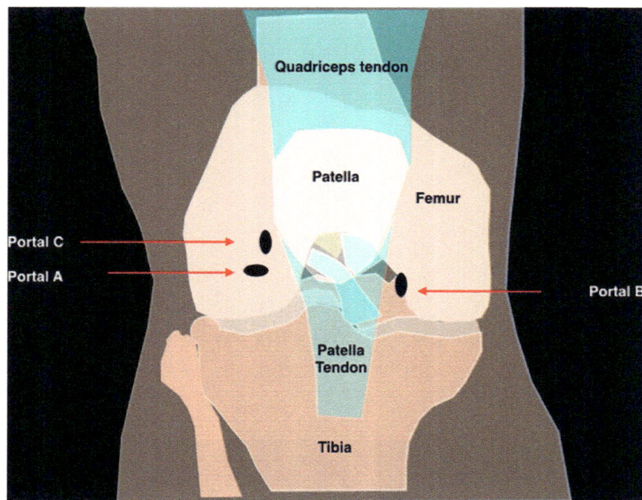


**Fig. 4.2** Portals used: Portal A: medial, Portal B, C: lateral

## 4.5 Surgical Steps

Step 1: While viewing from Portal A, the osteochondral defect is visualised and the fragment identified (Fig. 4.3a–c).

Step 2: A curette is introduced through Portal B and the defect curetted to remove fibrous tissue that has grown over the bed to expose the vascular bed (Fig. 4.4a–c).

Step 3: If the fragment is separated and lying free, manipulate it with a probe to get it to sit on the bed, using a K-wire tip to manipulate it into position in a superior to inferior direction (Fig. 4.5a–d).

Step 4: A guide wire is drilled perpendicular to the fragment next to the K-wire to fix it temporarily on its bed after deciding the position in a superior to inferior direction. Then the fragment can be rotated with a probe to make it sit anatomically in a horizontal plane (Fig. 4.6a, b).

Step 5: A sleeve is applied through Portal B to the temporarily fixed fragment in its middle and a pilot hole drilled with the guidewire to 1cm depth (Fig. 4.7a, b).

Step 6: While keeping the sleeve in position a Biopin (Arthrex, Naples, FL) is then introduced through the sleeve and tapped into the socket (Fig. 4.8a–c).

Step 7: While most of the length of the Biopin has gone in, the tamp is gently withdrawn to see how much more of the pin needs to go in as it is important that it does not go deeper than the fragment thickness. The pin is then tapped back such that it is flush with the remainder cartilage (Fig. 4.9a–d).

Step 8: Multiple pins are then applied at intervals of 0.5cm all around the fragment from the medial side (Fig. 4.10a, b).

Step 9: The arthroscope is then shifted to Portal B and multiple pins are tapped into the fragment in a similar fashion to cover the whole length and breadth of the fragment (Fig. 4.11a–c).

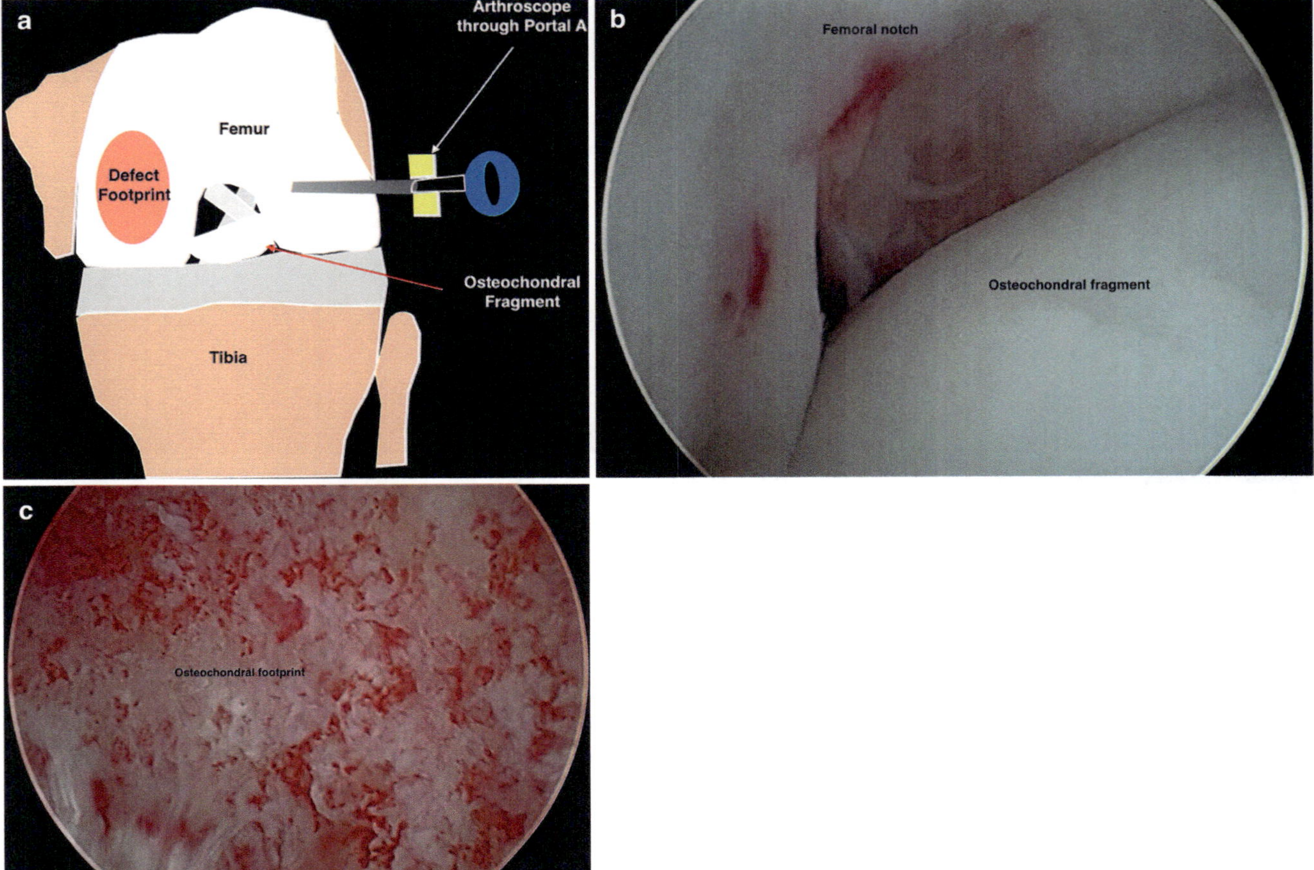


**Fig. 4.3** (**a**) Illustration of the knee showing the osteochondral fragment and the defect on the medial femoral condyle. (**b**) Arthroscopic image showing the osteochondral fragment in the notch. (**c**) Arthroscopic image of the footprint of the osteochondral fragment on the medial femoral condyle

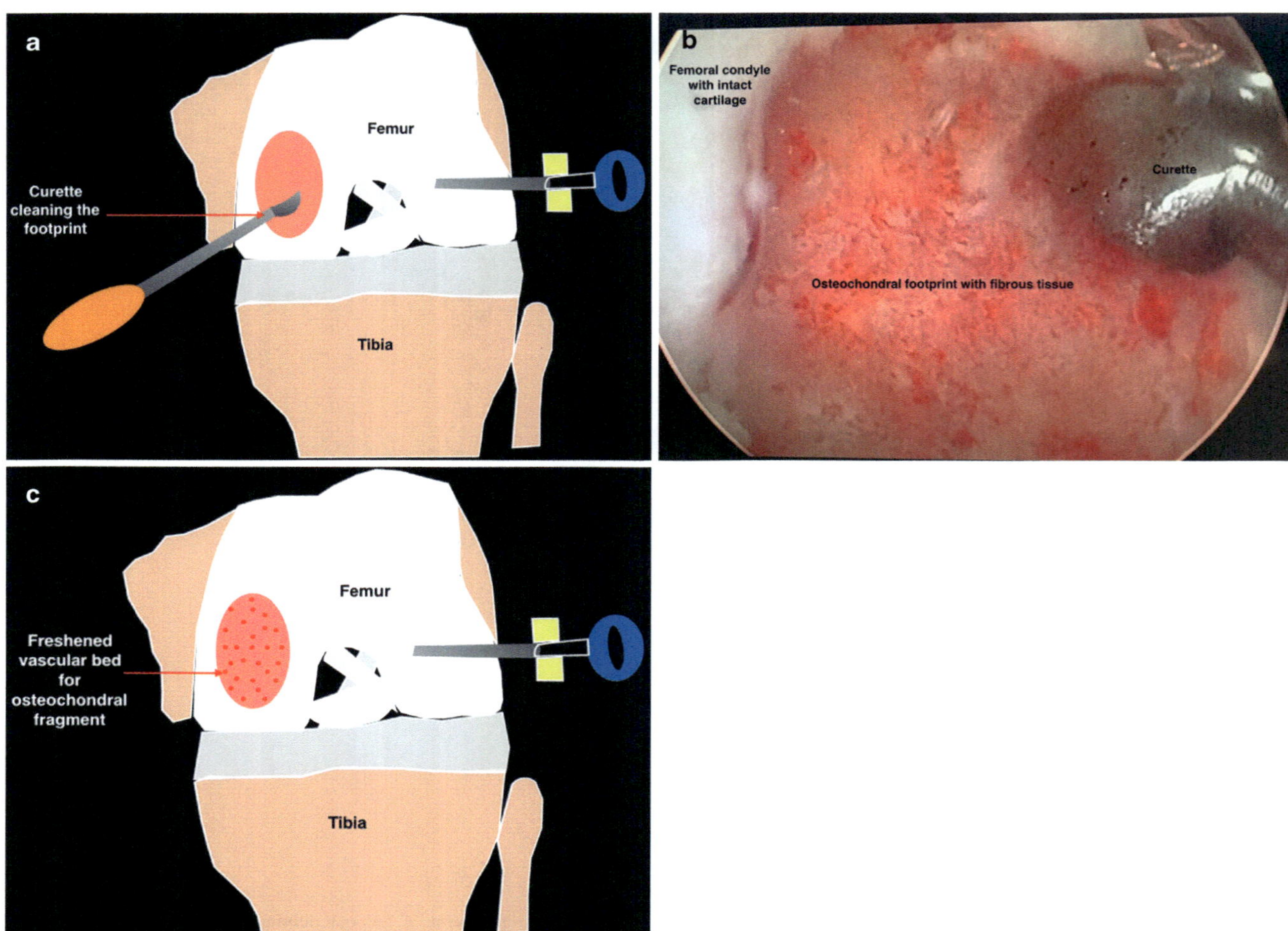


**Fig. 4.4** (**a**) Illustration of the knee showing a curette from Portal B removing fibrous tissue over the osteochondral defect footprint. (**b**) Arthroscopic image showing a curette removing fibrous tissue from the osteochondral defect footprint on the femoral condyle. (**c**) Illustration of the knee showing a freshened vascular bed for the osteochondral fragment

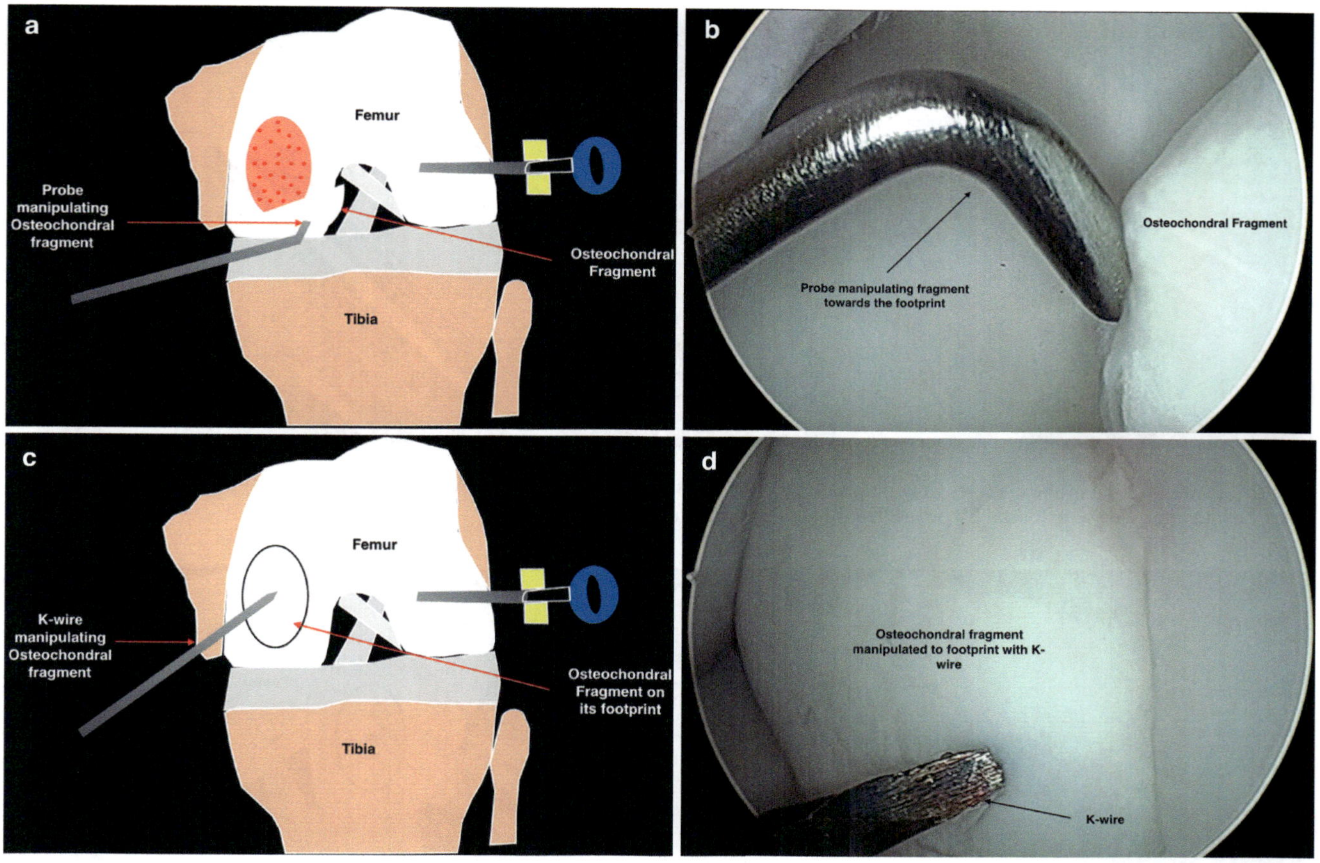

**Fig. 4.5** (**a**) Illustration of the knee showing a probe manipulating the osteochondral fragment to its footprint. (**b**) Arthroscopic image showing the probe manipulating the osteochondral fragment to its footprint. (**c**) Illustration of the knee showing a K-wire manipulating the fragment to its footprint. (**d**) Arthroscopic image of the K-wire manipulating the osteochondral fragment to its footprint

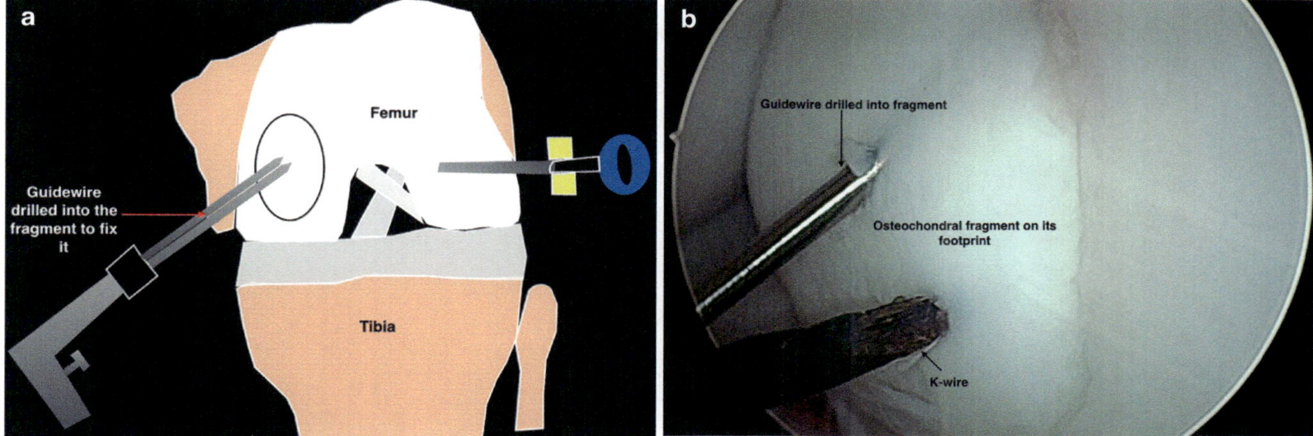


**Fig. 4.6** (**a**) Illustration of the knee showing a guide wire being drilled perpendicular to the fragment. (**b**) Arthroscopic image of the knee showing a guide wire drilled alongside the K-wire into the osteochondral fragment

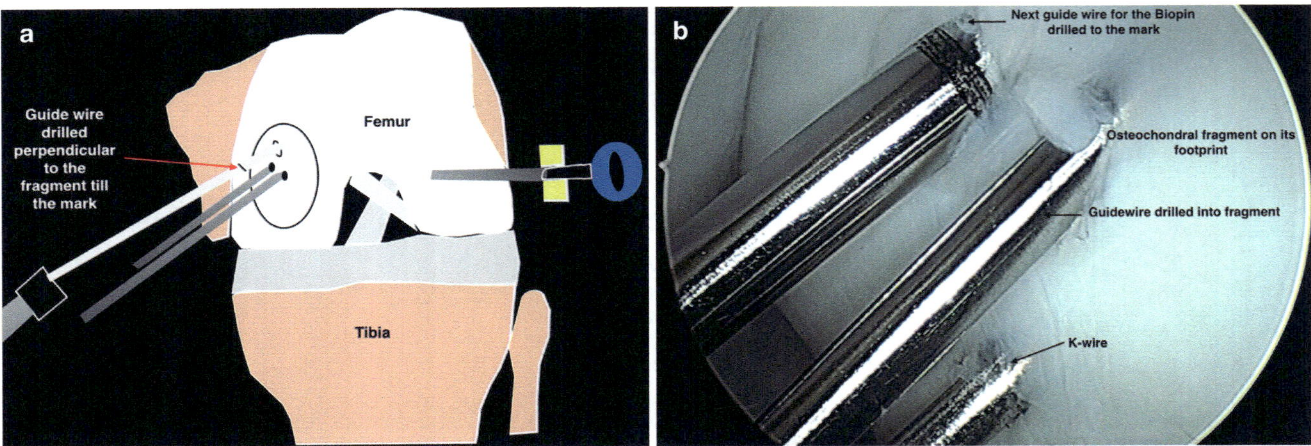


**Fig. 4.7** (**a**) Illustration of the knee showing the guide wire for the Biopin being drilled till the black mark on it. (**b**) Arthroscopic image of the knee showing the guide wire for the Biopin drilled till the black mark on it

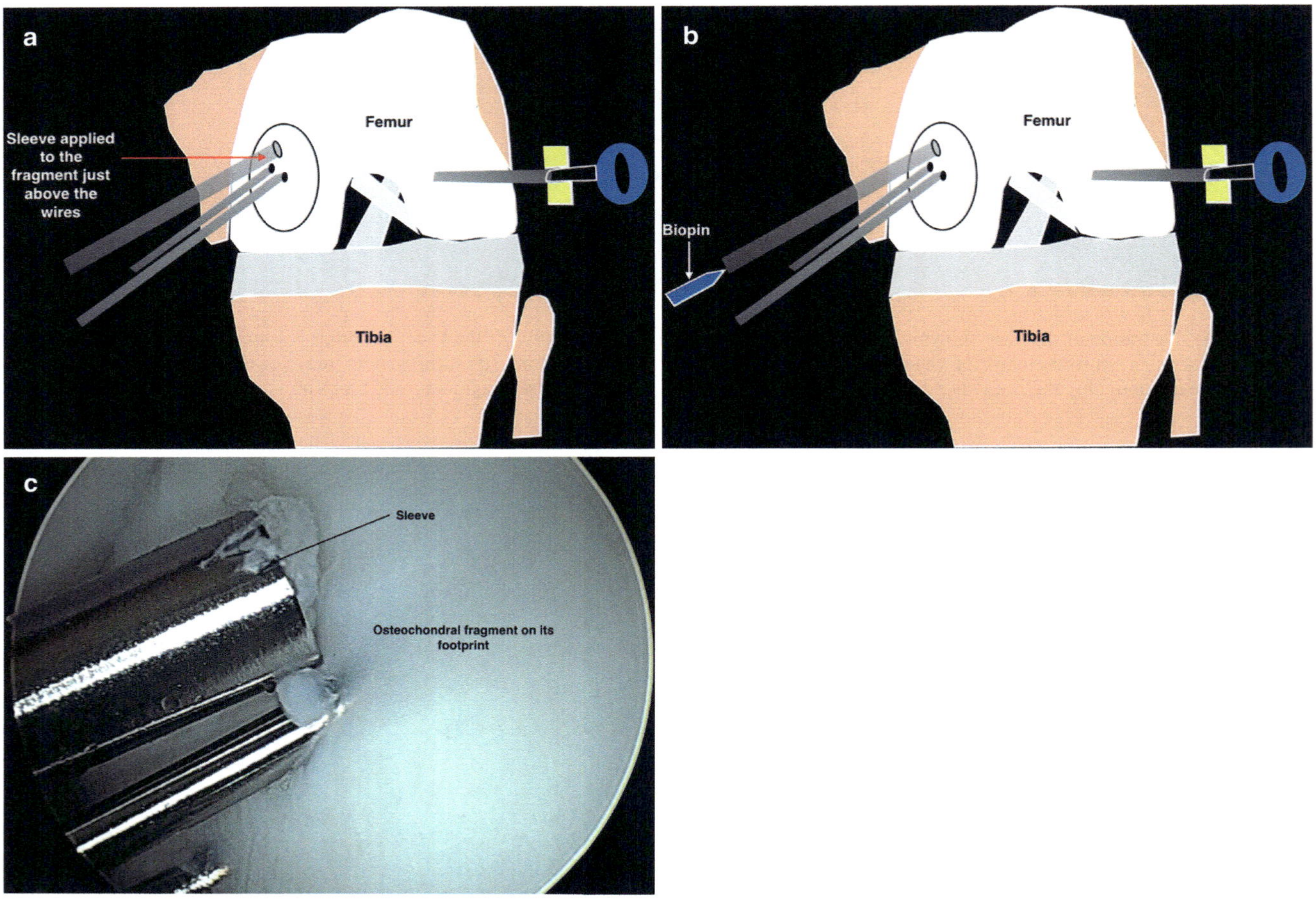

**Fig. 4.8** (**a**) Illustration of the knee showing the sleeve applied to the pilot hole drilled by the guidewire and perpendicular to it. (**b**) Illustration of the knee showing a Biopin being introduced through the sleeve. (**c**) Arthroscopic image of the knee showing the sleeve applied perpendicular to the pilot hole drilled by the guidewire

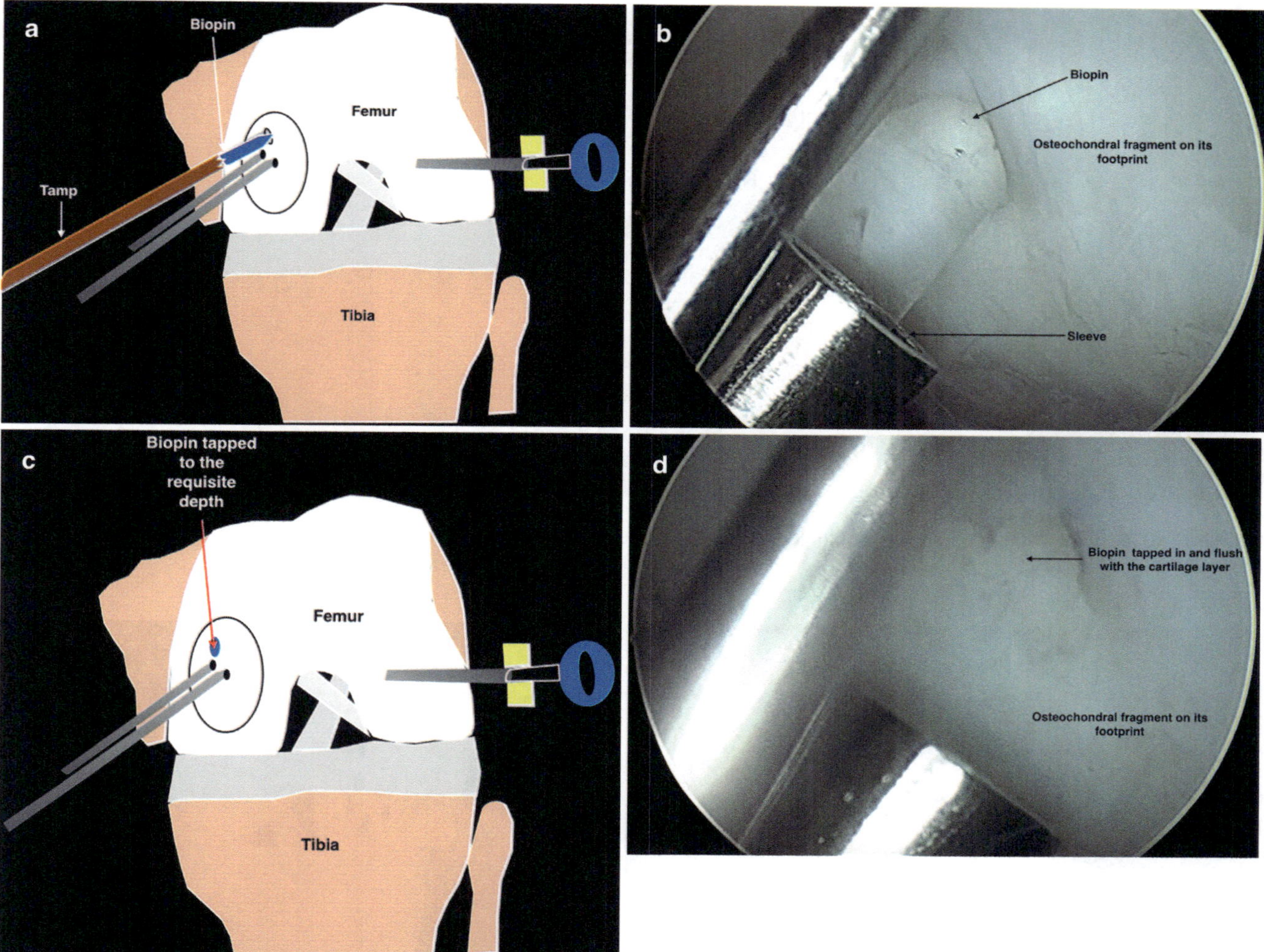


**Fig. 4.9** (**a**) Illustration of the knee showing the Biopin being tapped into the pilot hole through the sleeve using a tamp. (**b**) Arthroscopic image showing the Biopin going through the pilot hole with the sleeve partially withdrawn. (**c**) Illustration of the knee showing the first Biopin in place fixing the osteochondral fragment. (**d**) Arthroscopic image showing the Biopin through the osteochondral fragment and flush with the rest of the cartilage

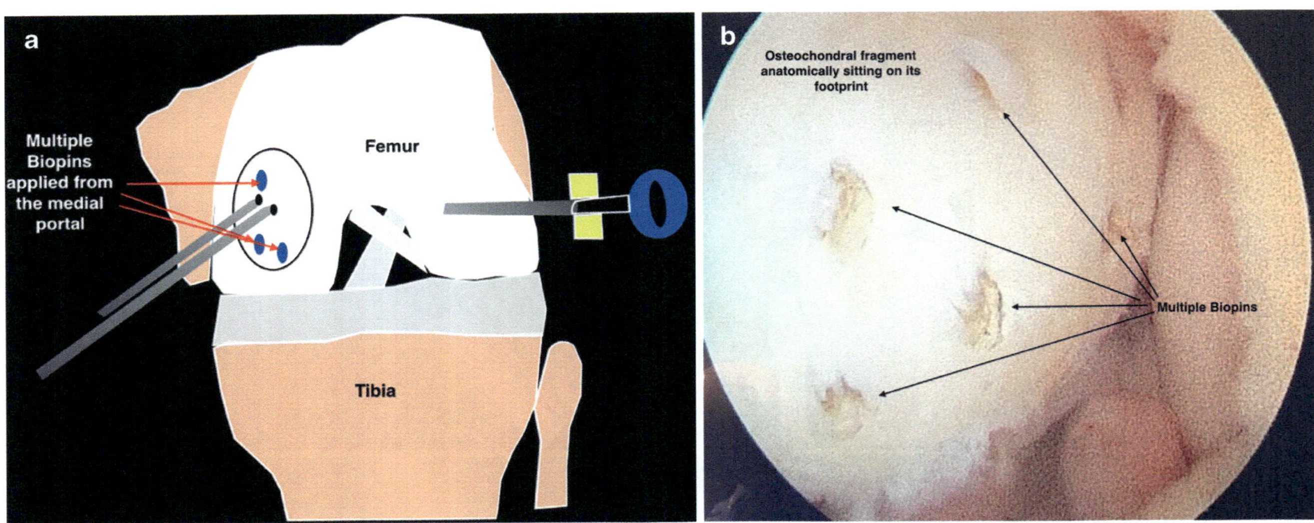


**Fig. 4.10** (**a**) Illustration of the knee showing multiple Biopins fixing the osteochondral fragment while viewing through Portal A. (**b**) Arthroscopic image of the knee showing the osteochondral fragment fixed with multiple Biopins while viewing from Portal A

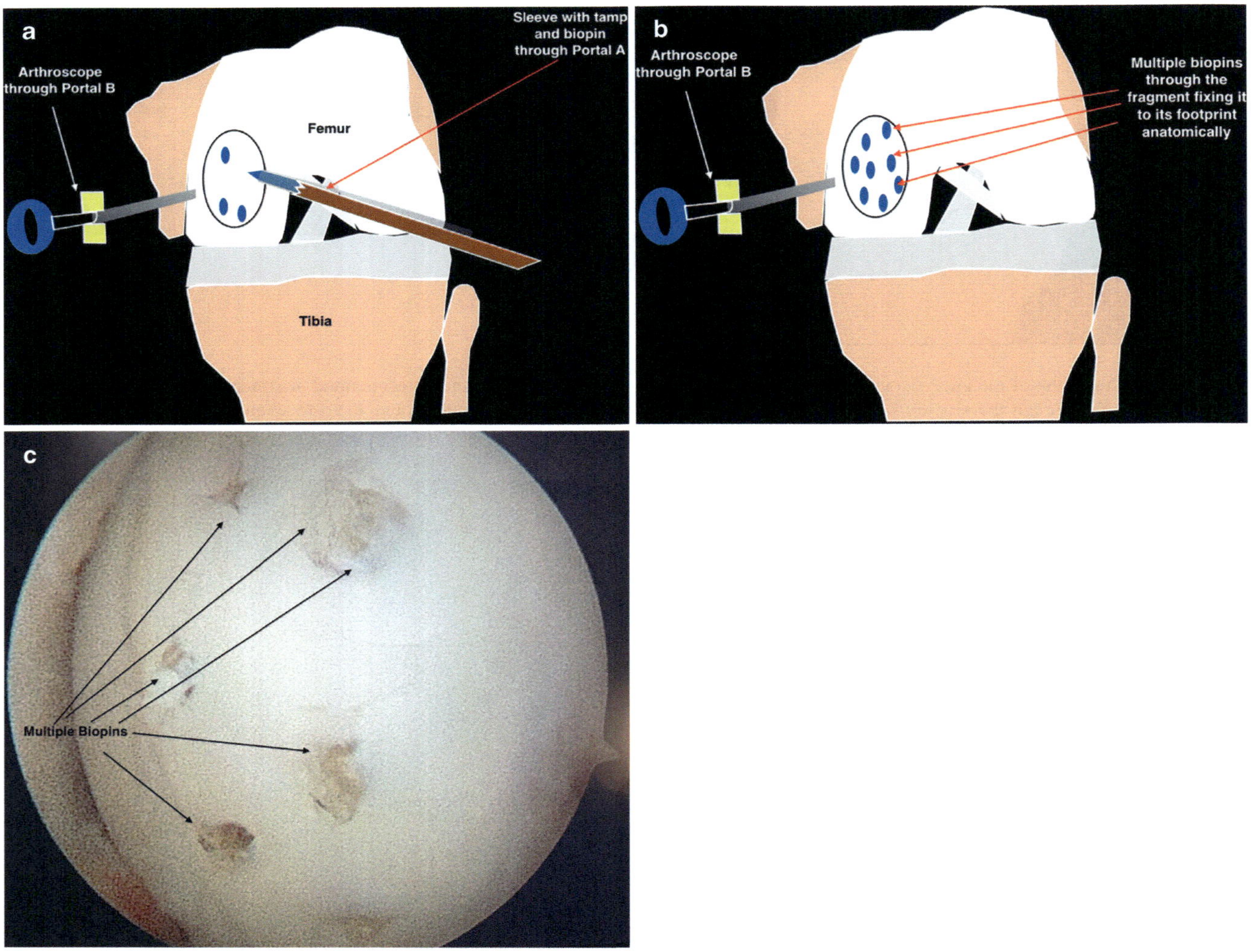

**Fig. 4.11** (**a**) Illustration of the knee showing a Biopin introduced through Portal A while viewing from Portal B. (**b**) Illustration of the knee showing multiple Biopins fixing the osteochondral fragment while viewing through Portal B. (**c**) Arthroscopic image of the knee showing the osteochondral fragment fixed with multiple Biopins while viewing through Portal B

## 4.6 Tips and Tricks

1. A single Biopin can be cut into 3, and each piece sharpened using a No 11 blade like we sharpen the end of a pencil using a blade.
2. Do not hammer the Biopin completely using the sleeve as it may subside more, withdraw the sleeve when there is still some distance for it to go in and tamp it in without the sleeve.
3. Place the pins in various directions perpendicular to the bone for maximum hold.

## 4.7 Advantages and Disadvantages

### 4.7.1 Advantages

1. Completely bioabsorbable implants used.
2. Provides stability throughout the fragment in different directions.

### 4.7.2 Disadvantages

1. Technically demanding
2. Specialised implants and equipment required.
3. Mechanical stability after the pins are absorbed and if the fragment has not united is questionable

# Arthroscopic Suture Bridge Fixation of Osteochondral Fragment

**5**

Vikram Arun Mhaskar and J. Maheshwari

## 5.1 Introduction

Osteochondral fragments can be fixed by a myriad of devices. Using minimal and absorbable implants that provide good stability is the key to a successful result. Using just Vicryl suture in a criss-cross fashion to fix the fragment is an option [1]. The Vicryl suture absorbs over a period of time after the fragment unites and in the end there is no foreign body remaining. This technique can be used in isolation or along with other techniques to stabilise fragments. This technique is described in this chapter.

## 5.2 Specialised Equipment (Fig. 5.1)

1. Beath pin-2 (a, b)
2. Drill (Stryker, Kalamazoo, MI)
3. No 1 Vicryl (Ethicon, Raritan, NJ) (d)
4. Knot Pusher (Arthrex, Naples, FL) (e)
5. Knot Pusher (Arthrex, Naples, FL) (c)

V. A. Mhaskar (✉) · J. Maheshwari
F7 East of Kailash, Knee & Shoulder Clinic, New Delhi, India

JMVM Sports Injury Center, Sitaram Bhartia Institute of Science & Research, New Delhi, India
e-mail: drjmaheshwari@jmvmsportsinjury.com


V. A. Mhaskar, J. Maheshwari (eds.), *Innovative Approaches in Knee Arthroscopy*,
https://doi.org/10.1007/978-981-99-4378-4_5

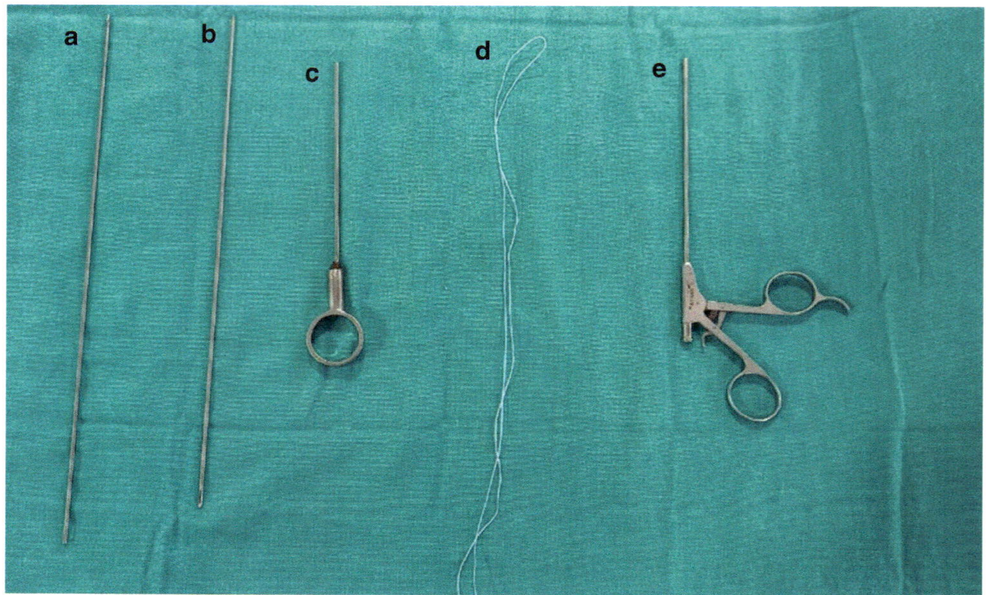


**Fig. 5.1** Instruments used (**a**, **b**) Beath pin, (**c**) Knot Pusher, (**d**) Vicryl, (**e**) Knot Cutter

## 5.3 Positioning

Supine on the operating table with knee at 70° flexion with a bolster at the end of the bed and a side support

## 5.4 Portals (Fig. 5.2)

AL working portal made at the soft spot lateral to the patellar tendon

AM viewing portal made in the soft spot just medial to the patellar tendon

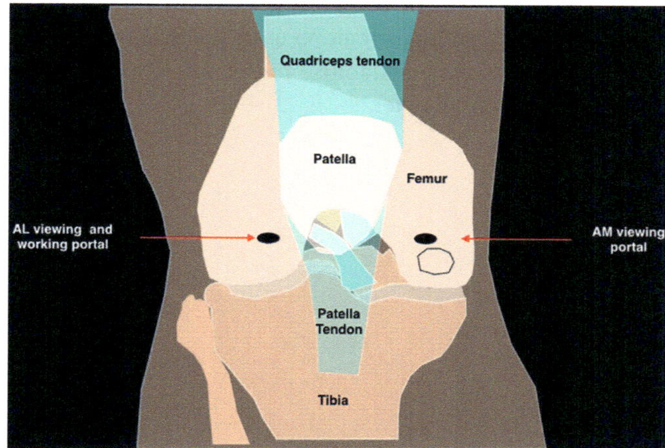


**Fig. 5.2** Illustration of the AM and AL portal position in the soft spot on either side of the patellar tendon

## 5.5 Surgical Steps

Step 1: The osteochondral fragment is visualised by viewing through the AL portal (Fig. 5.3).

Step 2: A probe introduced through the medial portal is used to test its stability (Fig. 5.4).

Step 3: The arthroscope is then shifted to the medial portal and a Beath pin is drilled into the normal cartilage just medial to the equator of the fragment (Fig. 5.5, b).

Step 4: Once drilled across the opposite cortex, it is withdrawn back till the eyelet of the posterior aspect of the Beath pin is just outside the lateral portal.

One end of a No 1 Vicryl suture is then passed through the eyelet and shuttled to the opposite cortex (Fig. 5.6).

Step 5: A Beath pin is drilled in a similar fashion just lateral to the fragment through the normal cartilage and the other end of the No 1 Vicryl suture is shuttled to the opposite cortex (Fig. 5.7a–d).

Step 6: An incision is made on the skin between where the two threads come out on the lateral aspect of the thigh and a straight artery forceps is used to dissect down to the bone and two ends of the Vicryl are delivered through the incision (Fig. 5.8a–e).

Step 7: The two ends of the Vicryl suture are then tied with multiple simple knots using a knot pusher. This stabilises the fragment against its bed (Fig. 5.9a–c).

Step 8: A Beath pin is then drilled through the normal cartilage adjacent to the osteochondral fragment just distal to the line running along its centre in a longitudinal direction (Fig. 5.10).

Step 9: One end of another Vicryl suture is shuttled to the lateral cortex as in Step 4 (Fig. 5.11a, b).

Step 10: The Beath pin is again drilled superior to the osteochondral fragment through the normal cartilage just above the line running through the centre of the fragment in the longitudinal plane (Fig. 5.12).

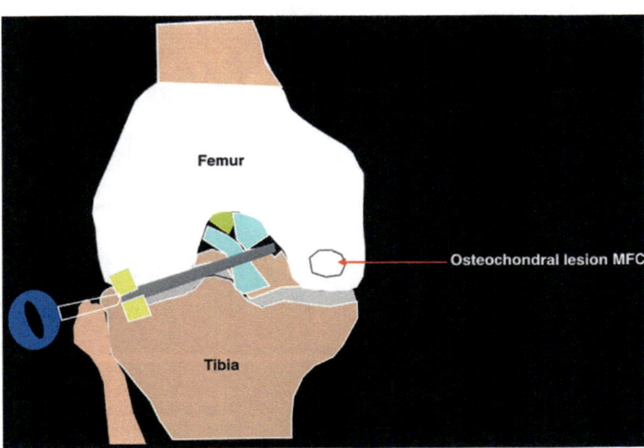


**Fig. 5.3** Illustration of the knee showing the arthroscope through the AL portal visualising the osteochondral lesion on the MFC

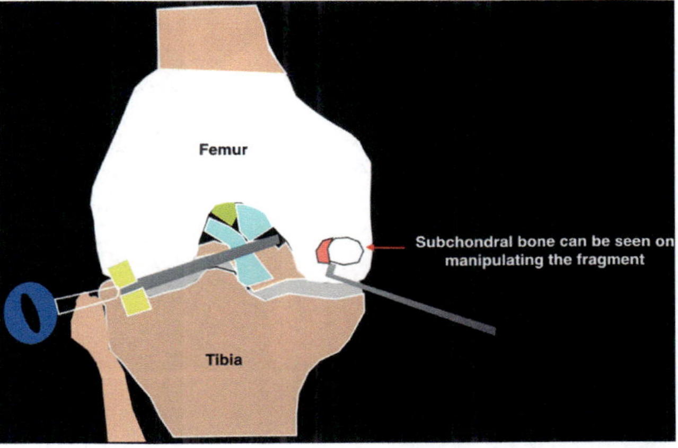


**Fig. 5.4** Illustration of the knees showing the arthroscope through the AL portal and probe through the AM portal manipulating the fragment and exposing its bed

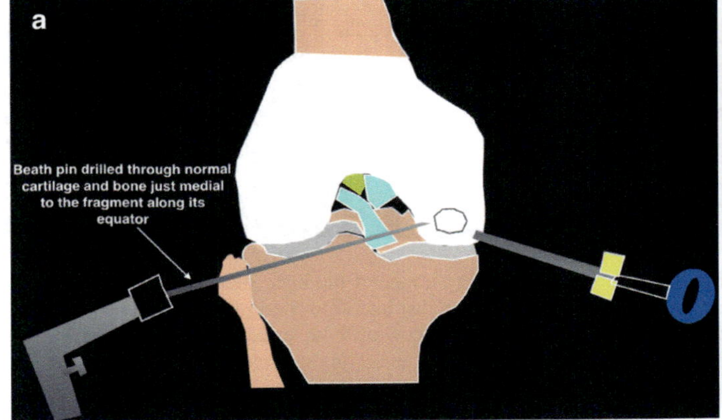


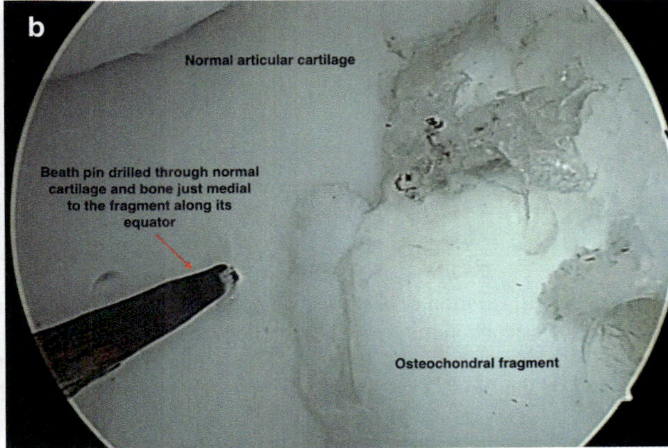


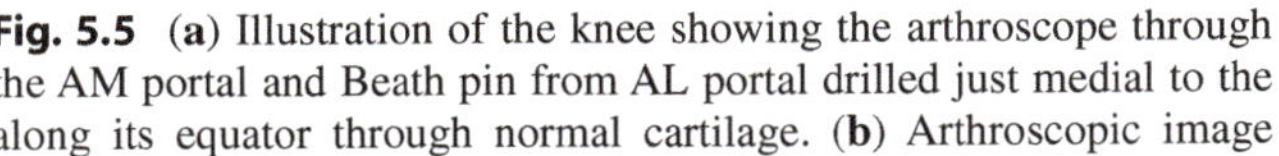

**Fig. 5.5** (**a**) Illustration of the knee showing the arthroscope through the AM portal and Beath pin from AL portal drilled just medial to the along its equator through normal cartilage. (**b**) Arthroscopic image showing the osteochondral fragment while viewing through the AM portal and a Beath pin being drilled just medial to the fragment along its equator through normal cartilage

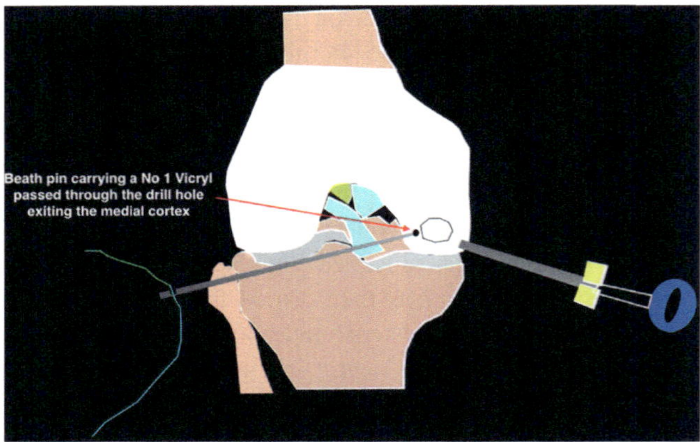


**Fig. 5.6** Illustration of the knee showing the arthroscope through the AM portal and a Beath pin through the AL portal carrying the No 1 Vicryl to be shuttled out of the medial cortex

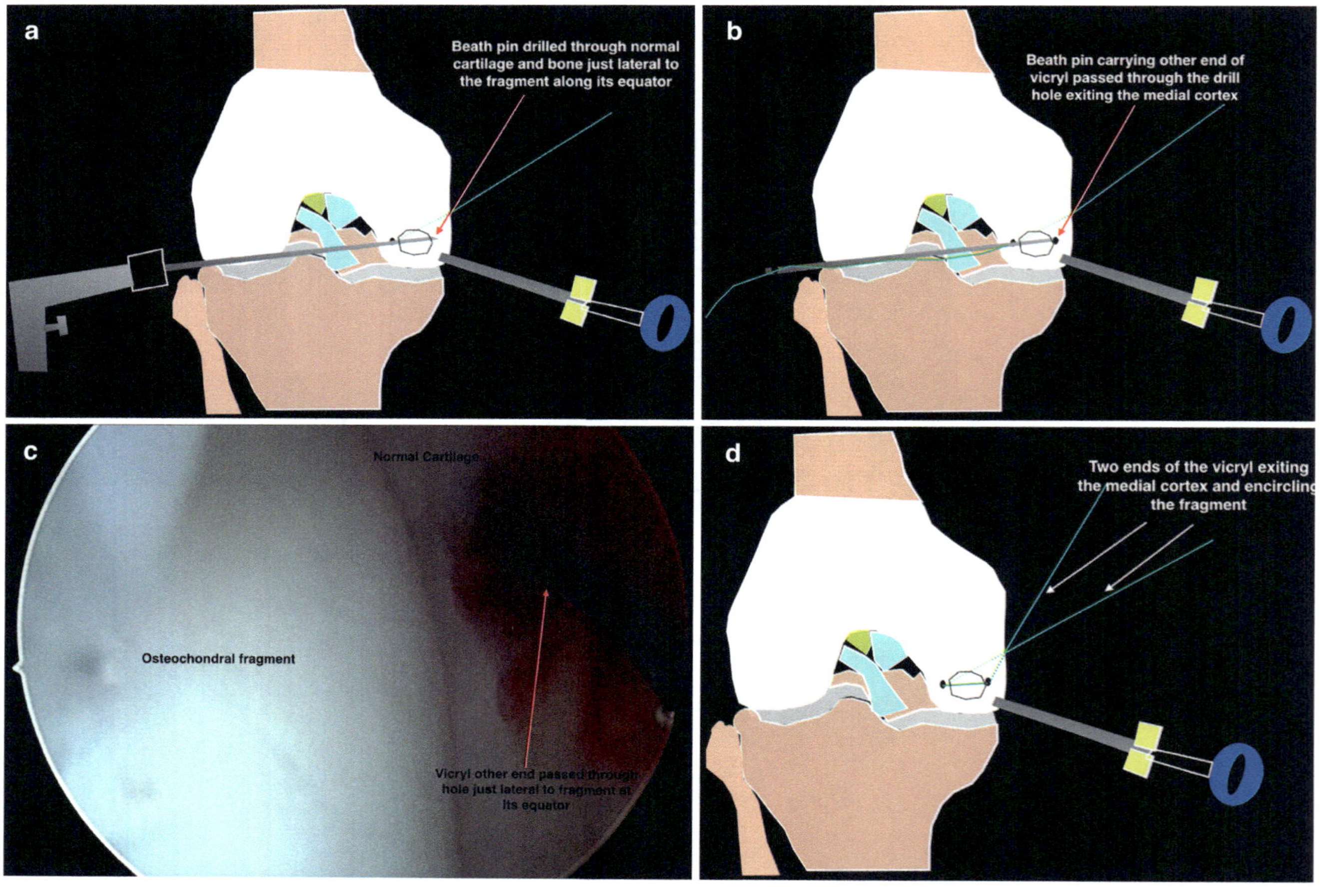

**Fig. 5.7** (**a**) Illustration of the knee showing a Beath pin drilled just lateral to the osteochondral lesion along its equator through normal cartilage. (**b**) Illustration of the knee showing a Beath pin shuttling the other end of the No 1 Vicryl suture across the medial cortex of the femur. (**c**) Arthroscopic image of the knee showing the osteochondral lesion and Vicryl suture just lateral to the lesion along its equator. (**d**) Illustration of the knee showing both ends of the suture exiting the medial cortex of the femur encircling the fragment

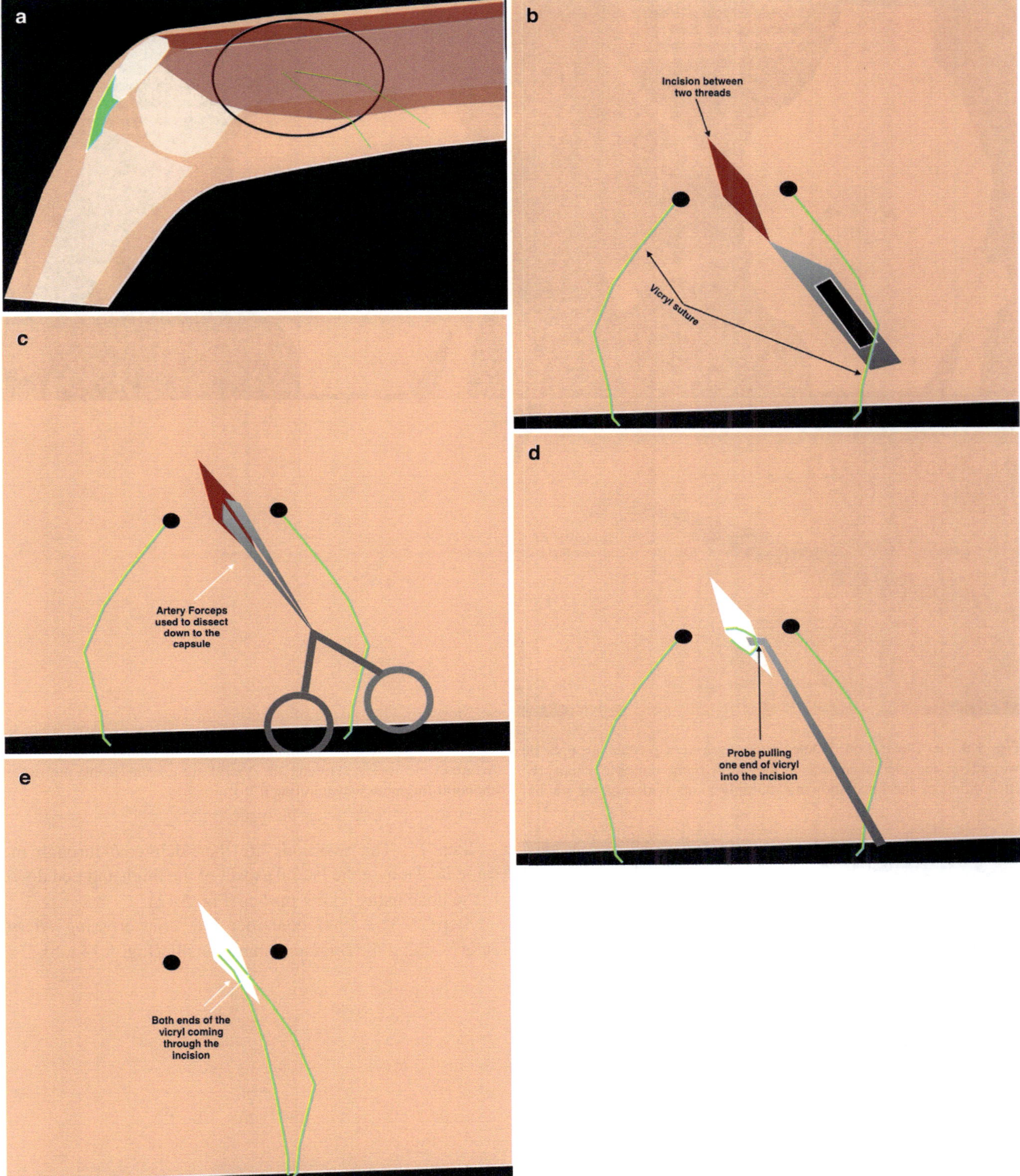


**Fig. 5.8** (**a**) Illustration of the medial side of the knee and thigh showing the two suture ends coming out of the medial cortex of the femur and skin. (**b**) Illustration of the medial aspect of the thigh showing an incision on the skin made between the two ends of the suture. (**c**) Illustration of the medial aspect of the thigh showing an artery forceps dissecting the subcutaneous tissue and muscle till the bone. (**d**) Illustration of the medial aspect of the thigh showing a probe delivering one end of the suture through the wound. (**e**) Illustration of the medial aspect of the thigh showing two ends of the Vicryl suture delivered through the wound

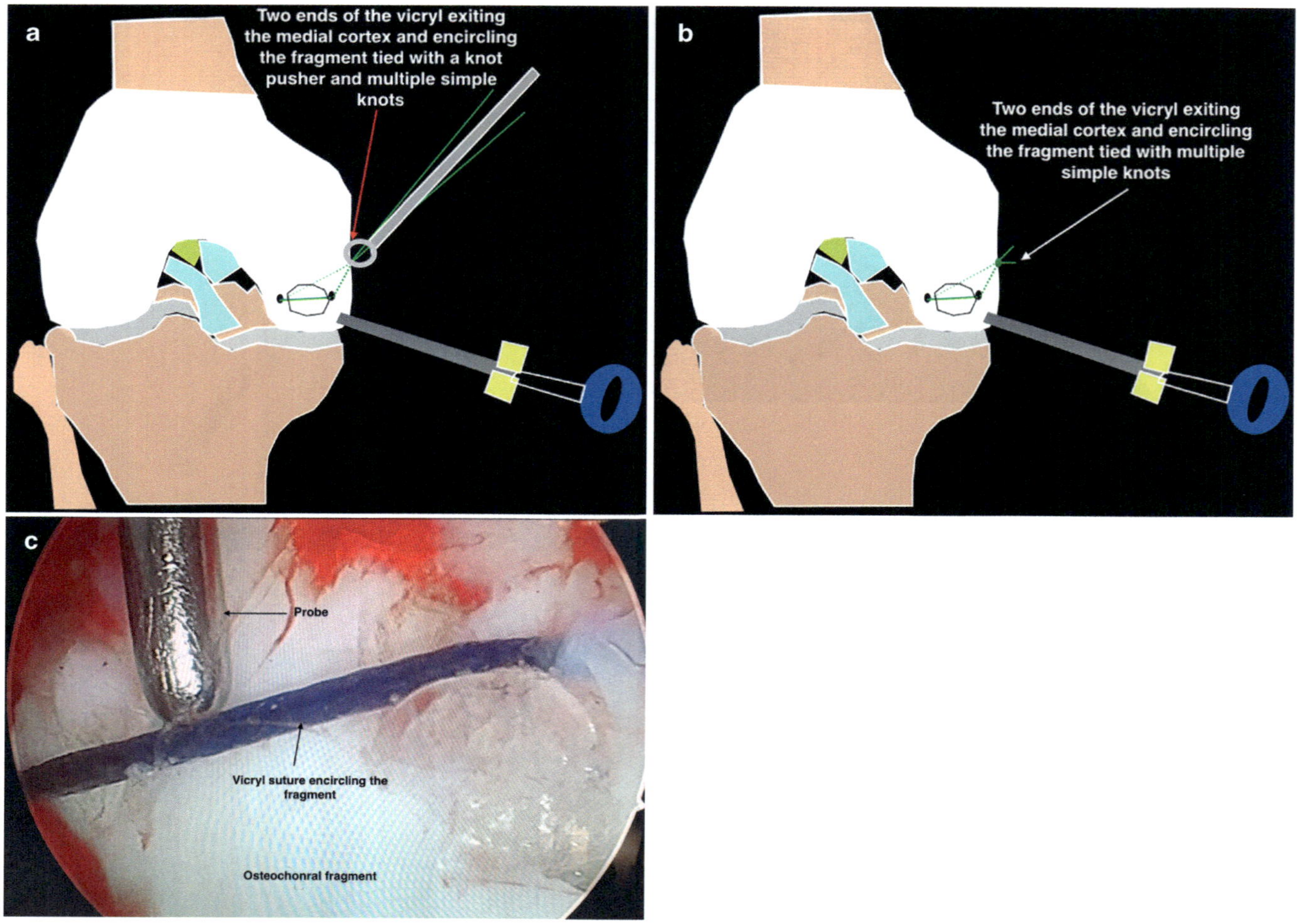

**Fig. 5.9** (**a**) Illustration of knee showing a knot pusher through the wound on the medial aspect of the thigh tying multiple knots. (**b**) Illustration of the knee showing multiple knots tied over the medial aspect of the femur stabilising the osteochondral fragment. (**c**) Arthroscopic image showing the Vicryl suture stabilising the osteochondral fragment by encircling it

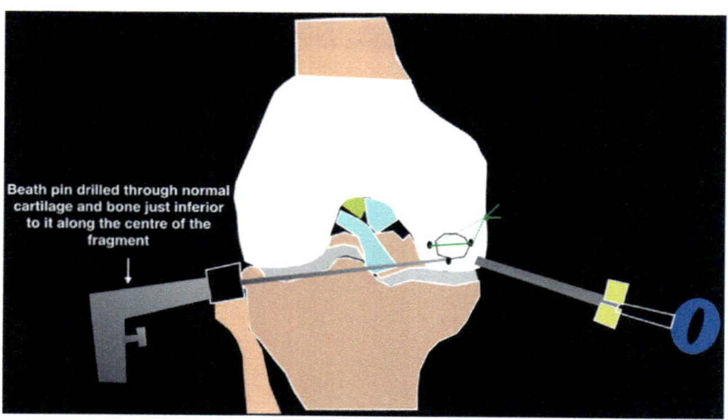


**Fig. 5.10** Illustration of the knee showing a Beath pin drilled through the normal cartilage abutting the osteochondral lesion just distal to it along the line running through the centre of the fragment in the longitudinal plane

Step 11: The two ends are then delivered through the same incision on the lateral aspect of the thigh and tied down to the bone using a knot pusher (Fig. 5.13).

Step12: The final construct has criss-crossing Vicryl sutures fixing the fragment anatomically (Fig. 5.14a, b).

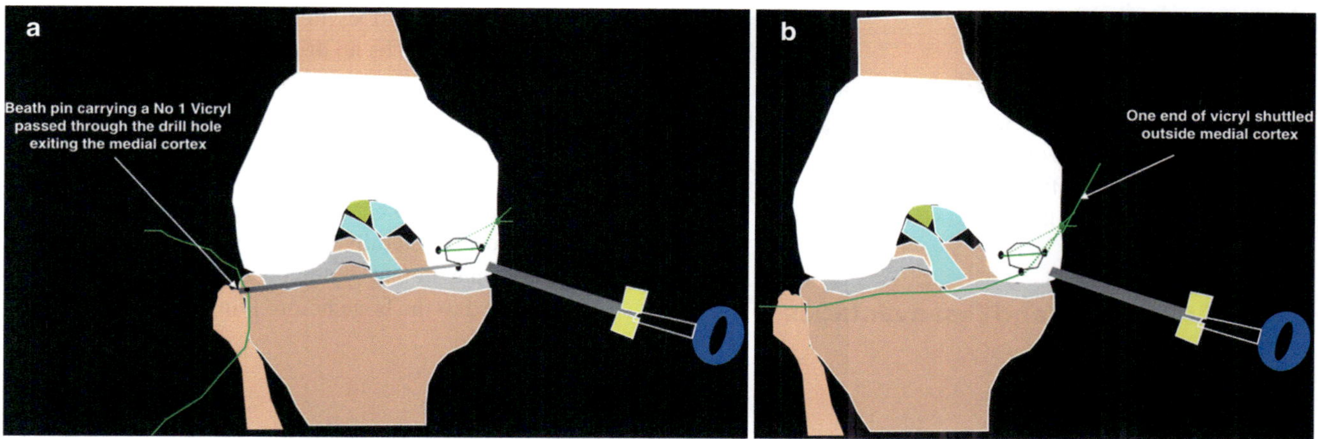


**Fig. 5.11** (**a**) Illustration of the knee showing a Beath pin carrying one end of the Vicryl being shuttled across the medial cortex of the femur. (**b**) Illustration of the knee showing one end of the Vicryl exiting the medial cortex of the femur

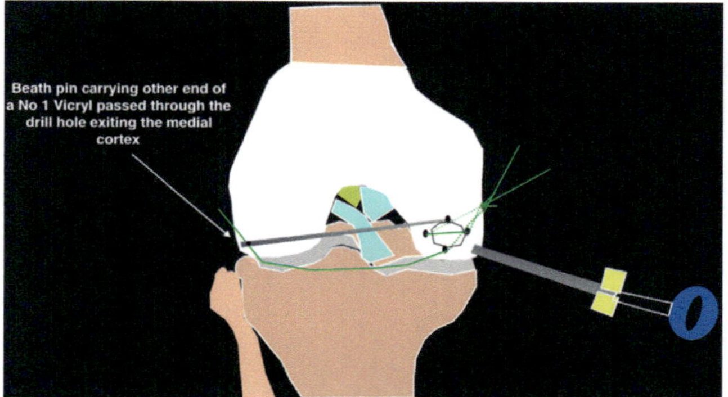


**Fig. 5.12** Illustration of the knee showing the Beath pin carrying the other end of the Vicryl passing through the normal cartilage abutting the fragment along its centre in the longitudinal plane after drilling through across the medial cortex

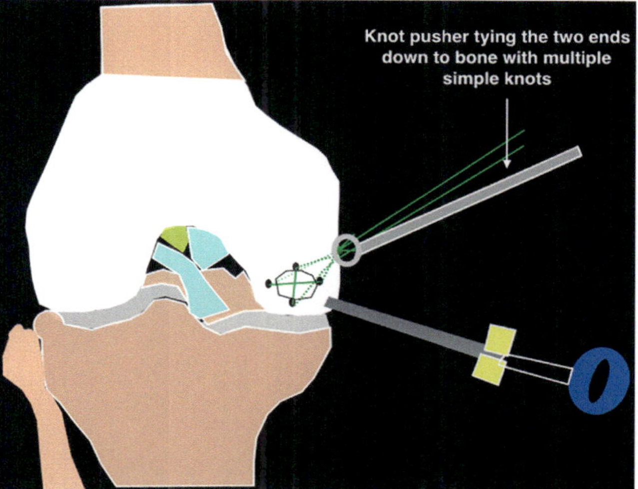


**Fig. 5.13** Illustration of the knee showing a knot pusher tying the two ends of the Vicryl suture with multiple simple knots after delivering both ends of the Vicryl through the same wound

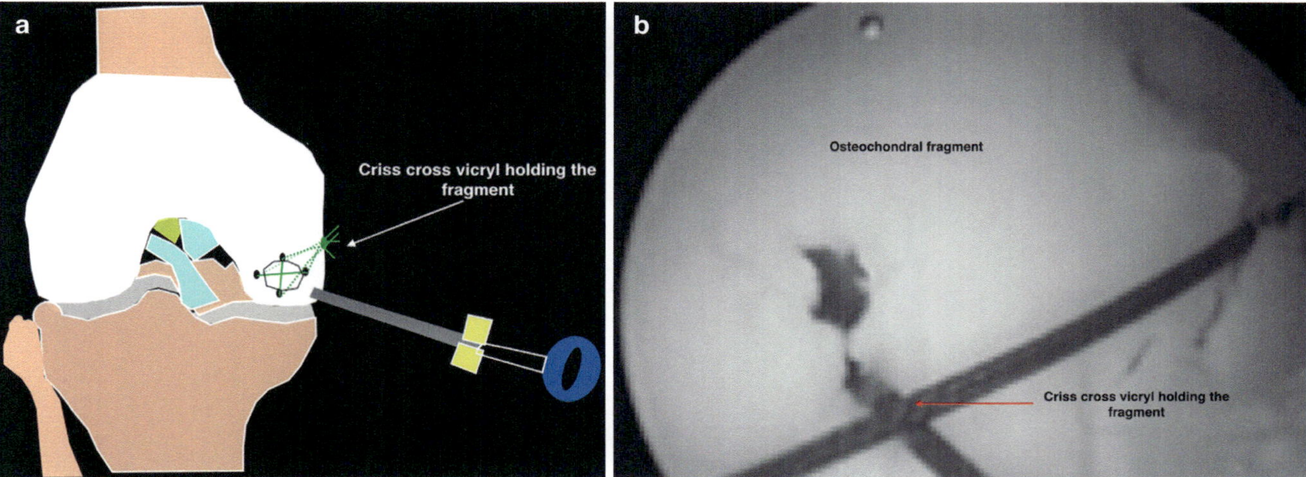


**Fig. 5.14** (**a**) Illustration of the knee showing the final construct with criss-cross Vicryl sutures stabilising the osteochondral fragment. (**b**) Arthroscopic image showing the osteochondral fragment stabilised with criss-cross Vicryl sutures

## 5.6 Tips and Tricks

1. Incise the skin and tissue up to the bone and use an artery forceps to dilate the opening all the way to the bone so that the knots tied sit on the bone directly.
2. Use a probe to keep the fragment opposed to its bed with a probe while tying the sutures so that it does not slip.

## 5.7 Advantages and Disadvantages

### 5.7.1 Advantages

1. No implants other than sutures
2. Sutures are absorbable hence no implant remains after a few months.
3. Stable fixation that does not devitalise the fragment or cause comminution as no drilling happens through it.

### 5.7.2 Disadvantages

1. Sutures may absorb before the fragment unites.
2. Incision needed laterally on the thigh.
3. The knots may not sit on the bone tightly if soft tissue is not dissected to the bone before tying them.

## Reference

1. Maheshwari J, Mhaskar V, Mhaskar PM. Implantless fixation of a large osteocartilaginous fracture of the lateral femoral condyle in a child. Knee Surg Relat Res. 2017;29(1):72.

# Part III

# Meniscus

# 6 Arthroscopic Three Portal Technique to Remove a Bucket Handle Medial Meniscus Tear

Vikram Arun Mhaskar and J. Maheshwari

## 6.1 Introduction

Bucket handle medial meniscus tears are vertical tears where the torn fragment is stuck between the femoral and tibial condyles. Removing them can be challenging as manipulating instruments into a tight medial joint space after reduction of the meniscus can be challenging. We describe a convenient technique of removing a locked bucket handle tear without reducing the meniscus by using three portals [1].

## 6.2 Specialized Equipment

1. Arthroscopic grasper (Smith & Nephew, Watford, UK)
2. Arthroscopic punch (Smith & Nephew, Watford, UK)

## 6.3 Positioning

Knee at 70° flexion on the operating table with a bolster at the end of the bed and a side support.

## 6.4 Portals (Fig. 6.1)

Portal A: Horizontal lateral viewing portal at the soft spot just lateral to the patellar tendon.

Portal B: Vertical high antero-medial working portal for the grasper and arthroscopic punch just medial to the patellar tendon and at the level of the inferior pole of the patella.

Portal C: Horizontal low medial portal just above the medial meniscus and at the end of the anteriorly.

V. A. Mhaskar (✉)
F7 East of Kailash, Knee & Shoulder Clinic, New Delhi, India

JMVM Sports Injury Center, Sitaram Bhartia Institute of Science & Research, New Delhi, India

J. Maheshwari
F7 East of Kailash, Knee & Shoulder Clinic, New Delhi, India
e-mail: dr.maheshwari@jmvmsportsinjury.com

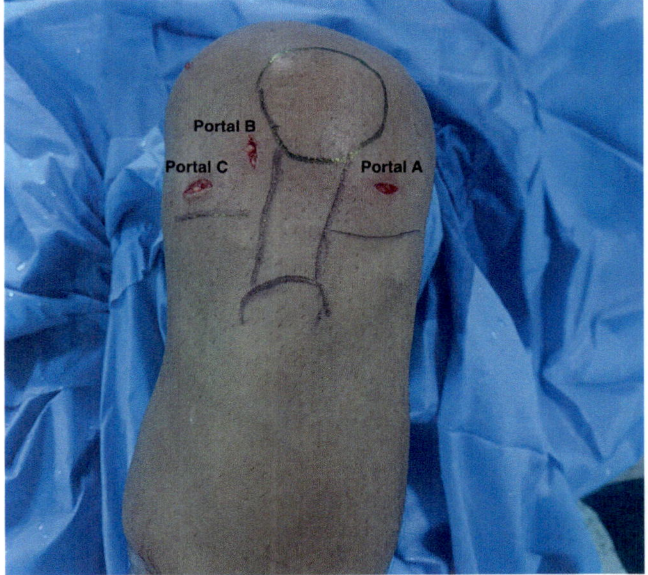


**Fig. 6.1** Portals used for the technique, Portal A: lateral viewing portal in the soft spot, Portal B: high medial working portal, and Portal C: low medial working portal

## 6.5 Surgical Steps

Step 1: The arthroscope is introduced through Portal A and the bucket handle medial meniscus tear is identified (Fig. 6.2a–c).

Step 2: The torn fragment is held at its root close to the notch with an arthroscopic grasper introduced through Portal B and lifted upwards with a little traction to expose its attachment close to the root (Fig. 6.3a, b).

Step 3: A straight arthroscopic punch is introduced through Portal C and the attachment of the torn fragment is


V. A. Mhaskar, J. Maheshwari (eds.), *Innovative Approaches in Knee Arthroscopy*,
https://doi.org/10.1007/978-981-99-4378-4_6

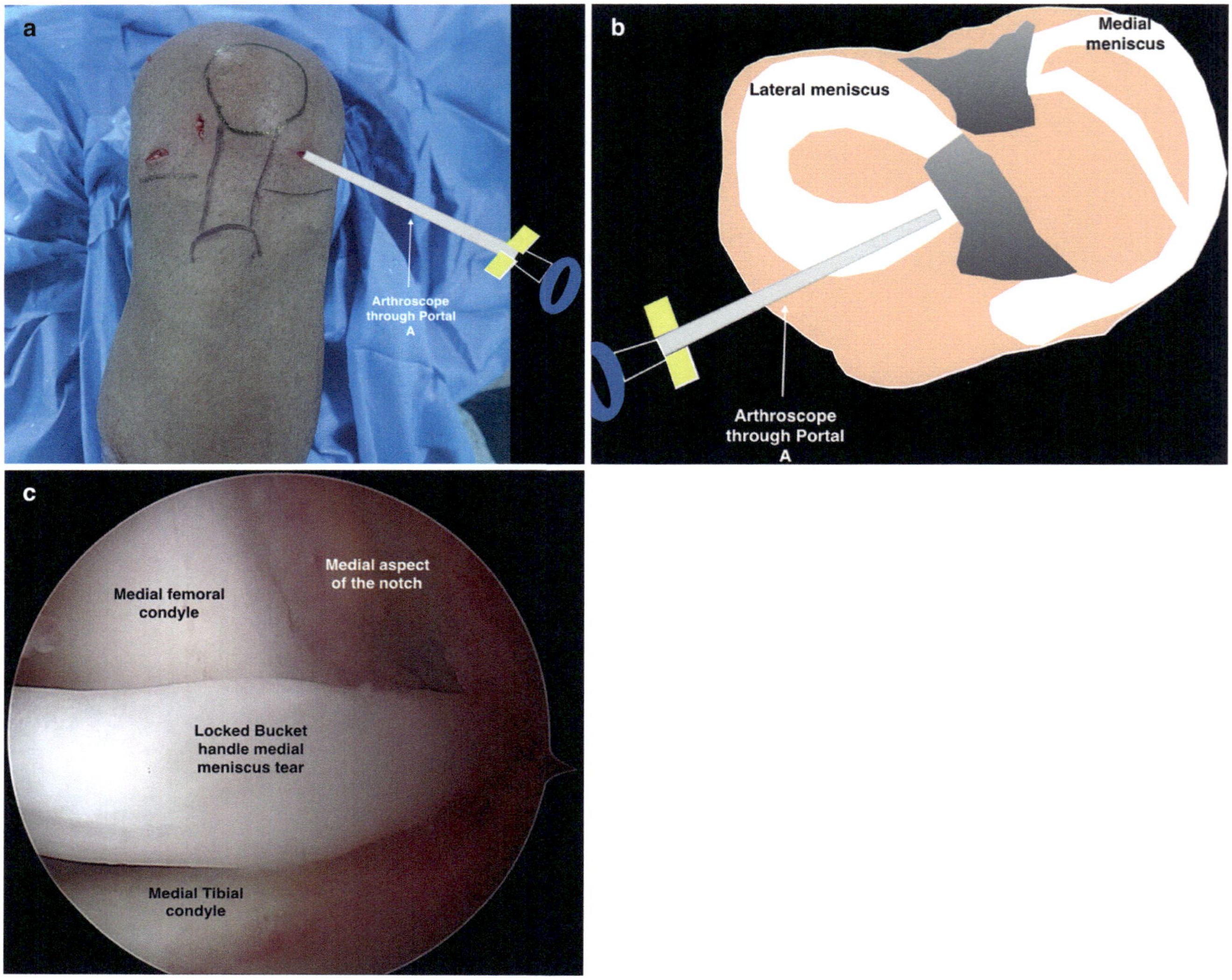

**Fig. 6.2** (**a**) Outside image of left knee showing an arthroscope introduced through Portal A. (**b**) Illustration of knee showing the bucket handle medial meniscus while viewing from Portal A. (**c**) Arthroscopic image of the knee showing a locked bucket handle medial meniscus tear

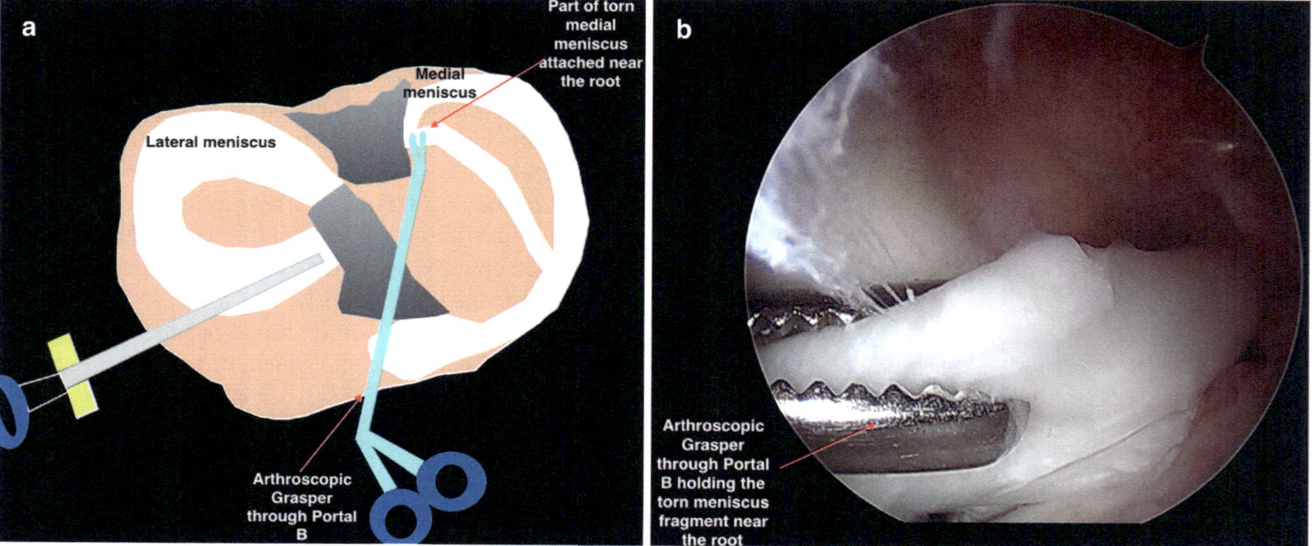


**Fig. 6.3** (**a**) Illustration of the knee showing an arthroscopic grasper through Portal B holding the fragment of torn meniscus near its root attachment. (**b**) Arthroscopic image of the knee showing an arthroscopic grasper through Portal B holding the meniscus fragment at the root

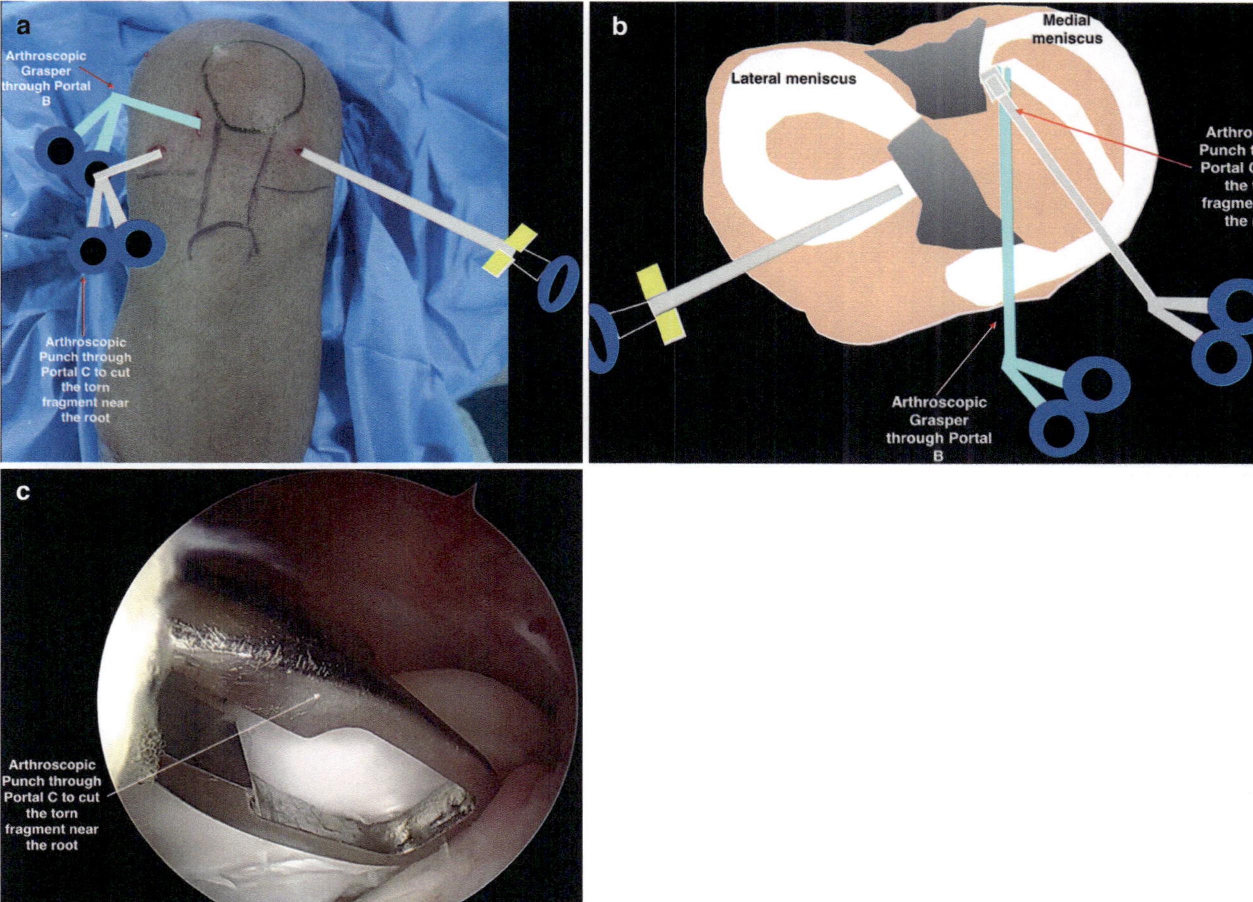


**Fig. 6.4** (**a**) Outside image of the knee showing the arthroscope through Portal A, an arthroscopic grasper through Portal B, and an arthroscopic punch through Portal C. (**b**) Illustration of the knee showing an arthroscopic grasper through Portal B, an arthroscopic punch cutting the meniscus fragment close to the root through Portal C while viewing through Portal A. (**c**) Arthroscopic image showing an arthroscopic punch through Portal C cutting the meniscus fragment close to the root while holding the fragment with an arthroscopic grasper through Portal B and viewing through Portal A

cut as close to the root of the meniscus as possible while grasping it with the maneuver in Step 2 (Fig. 6.4a–c).

Step 4: The part of the fragment left attached at the body, anterior horn junction is then held with an arthroscopic grasper introduced through Portal C.

Step 5: An arthroscopic punch is then introduced through Portal B and the part left attached is cut (Fig. 6.5a–c).

Step 6: The part of the meniscus cut is then pulled out of the medial portal by adjusting the grasper in such a way that the menisectomised fragment is held at one end such that is exits the medial portal longitudinally (Fig. 6.6a–c).

Step 7: The rest of the meniscus left is trimmed with a shaver.

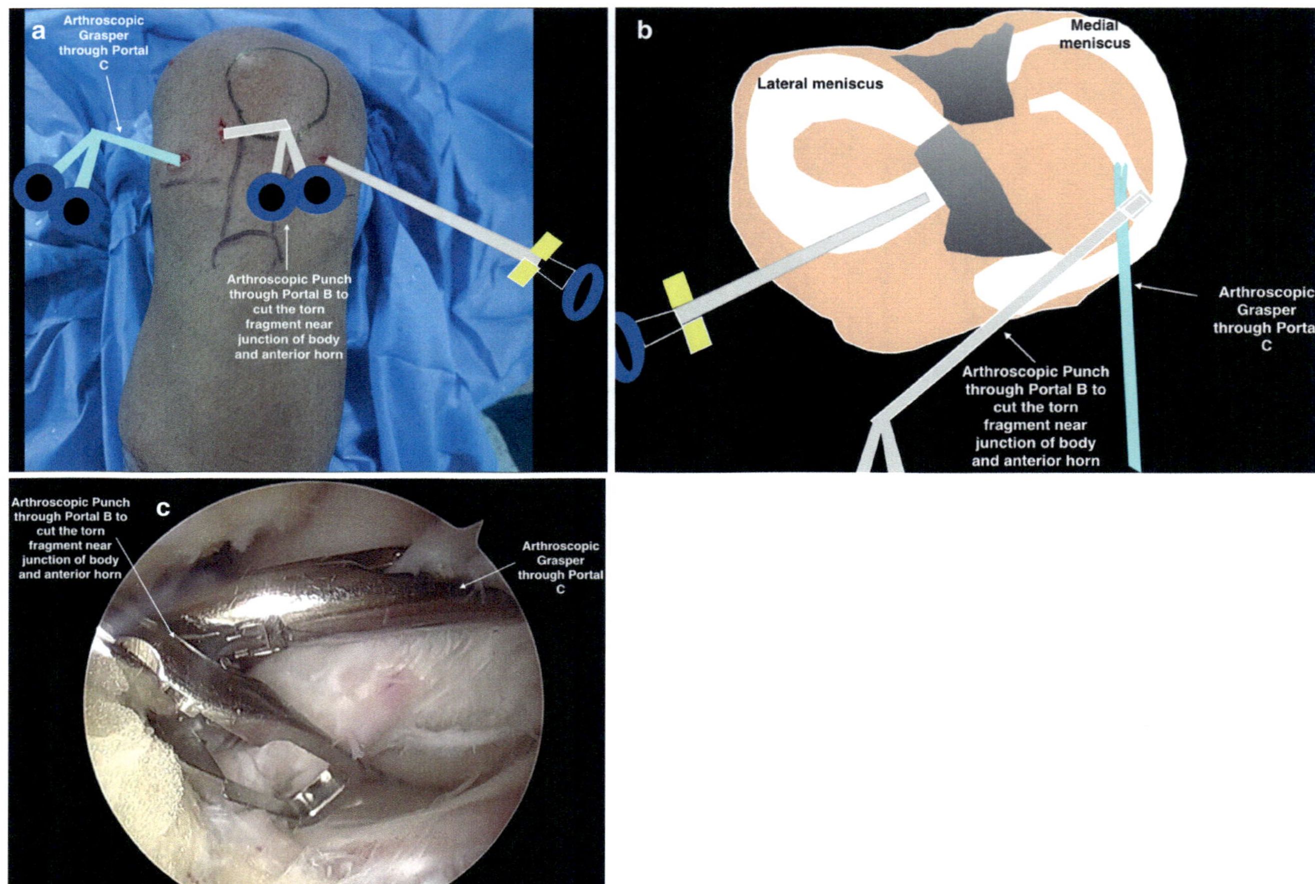


**Fig. 6.5** (**a**) Outside image of the knee showing an arthroscopic grasper through Portal C, arthroscopic punch through Portal B while viewing through Portal A. (**b**) Illustration of the knee showing an arthroscopic grasper through Portal C holding the meniscus fragment near its attachment at the body, anterior horn junction and an arthroscopic punch through Portal B cutting the meniscus at the body, anterior horn junction while viewing through Portal A. (**c**) Arthroscopic image of an arthroscopic grasper through Portal C holding the meniscus fragment near its attachment at the body, anterior horn junction and an arthroscopic punch through Portal B cutting the meniscus at the body, anterior horn junction while viewing through Portal A

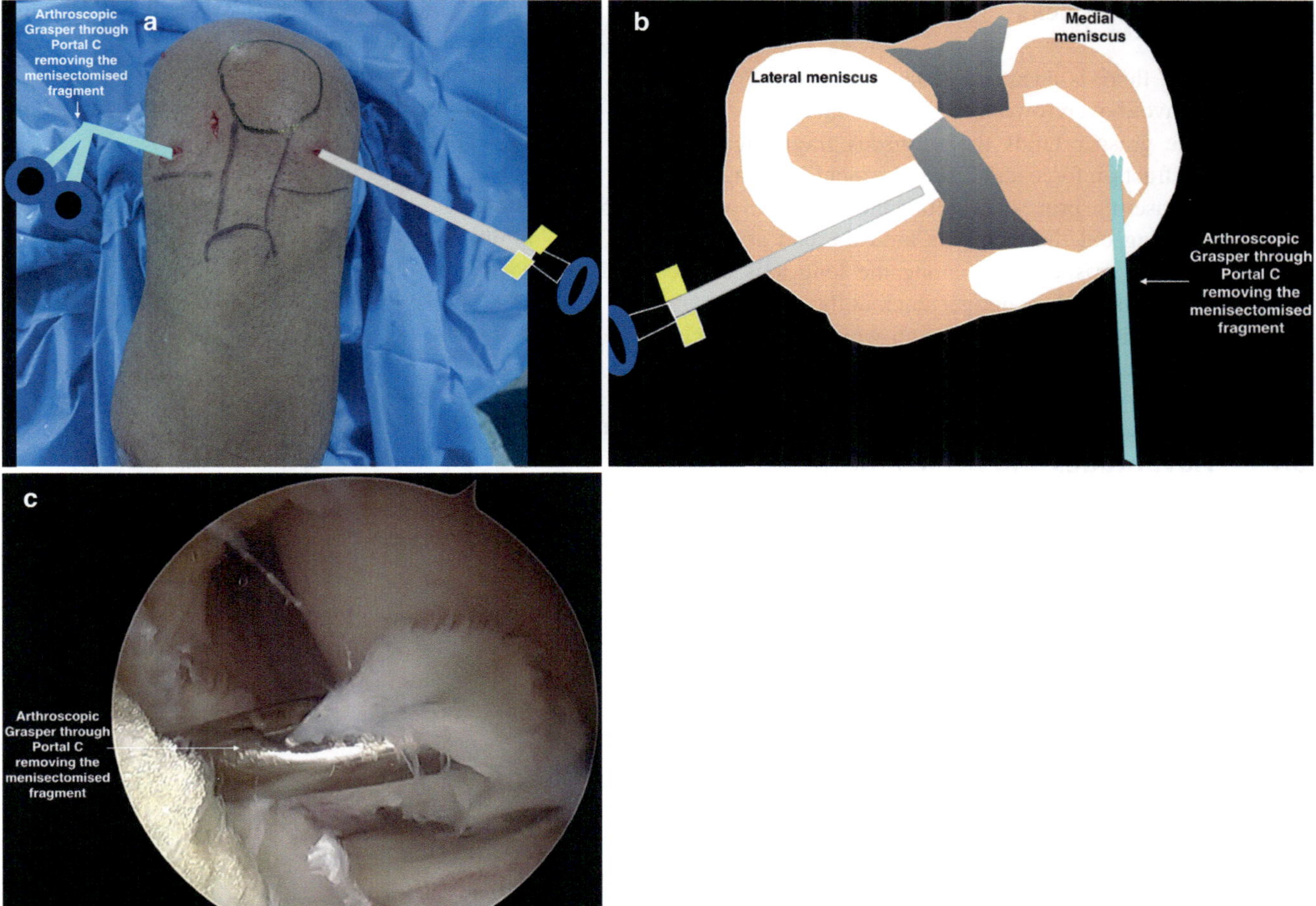


**Fig. 6.6** (**a**) Outside image of the knee showing an arthroscopic grasper through Portal C removing the meniscus fragment while viewing through Portal A. (**b**) Illustration of the knee showing the menisectomised fragment being removed using an arthroscopic grasper through Portal C while viewing through Portal A. (**c**) Arthroscopic image of the knee showing an arthroscopic grasper through Portal C holding the menisectomised fragment at one end and withdrawing it while viewing through Portal A

## 6.6 Tips and Tricks

1. Make sure there is adequate distance between Portal B and C to avoid overcrowding of instruments.
2. When the grasper holds the meniscus fragment to be trimmed, traction force and lifting the meniscus fragment upwards eases the process of cutting the end with a punch.
3. While pulling out the meniscus hold the end at the tip such that the grasper tip is along the long axis of the meniscus so that it does not get stuck in the portal.
4. Adequately dilate Portal B through which the meniscus fragment is delivered with artery forceps.

## 6.7 Advantages and Disadvantages

**Advantages**

1. No need to reduce the meniscus before menisectomising it.
2. Meniscus fragment can be removed as a whole rather than piecemeal.
3. Easier to perform in tight knees on the medial side.
4. Does not require an assistant to give valgus while doing the meniscectomy.

**Disadvantages**

1. Three portals
2. The need for a trained assistant to hold the arthroscope while the arthroscopic grasper and punch are manipulated by the surgeon.

## Reference

1. Mhaskar VA, Maheshwari J. Convenient three portal technique to remove locked bucket handle medial meniscus tear. J Arthrosc Joint Surg. 2019;6(2):128–30.

# 7 All Inside Meniscus Repair Using an Antegrade Suture Passer

Vikram Arun Mhaskar

## 7.1 Introduction

Vertical tears of the meniscus have a good propensity to heal and should be repaired wherever possible. The lateral joint is roomier as compared to the medial side so instrumentation introduction into the joint is easier. The lateral meniscus heals better than the medial side, hence repair should be attempted wherever possible. Conventional all inside devices are convinient but expensive. They also have the added disadvantages of implants on the capsule that can potentially irritate the posterior capsule. Inside out and outside in techniques are useful, cheaper but require another incision to tie the threads on the capsule. The technique presented is a true all inside technique with conventional knot tying and the knot being intra-articular with no devices on the capsule. It has the advantage of being more economical.

## 7.2 Specialised Equipment (Fig. 7.1)

1. Antegrade suture passer (Knee scorpion) for the knee (Arthrex, Naples, FL) (a)
2. 2-0 Fiberwire (Arthrex, Naples, FL) (e)
3. Arthroscopic meniscus rasp
4. Knot pusher (Arthrex, Naples, FL) (e)
5. Arthroscopic Suture Cutter (Arthrex, Naples, FL)
6. Flexible Cannula (Passport Cannula) (Arthrex, Naples, FL) (d)
7. Crochet (Smith & Nephew, Watford,UK) (c)

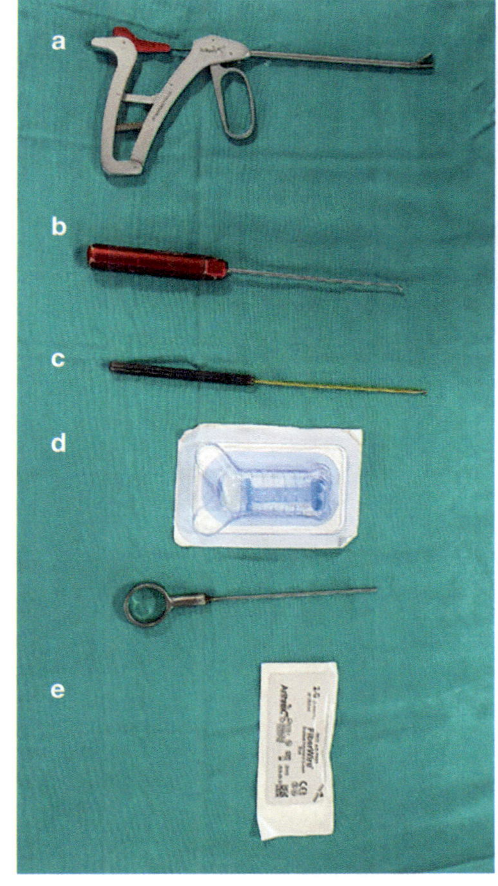


**Fig. 7.1** (**a**) Knee scorpion, (**b**) Arthroscopic meniscus rasp, (**c**) Crochet, (**d**) Passport Cannula, (**e**) Arthroscopic Knot Pusher and 2-0 Fiberwire

## 7.3 Positioning

Patient on the table supine with knee flexed to 90°. While repairing the lateral meniscus the knee is kept in a Figure of four position.

V. A. Mhaskar (✉)
F7 East of Kailash, Knee & Shoulder Clinic, New Delhi, India

JMVM Sports Injury Centre, Sitaram Bhartia Institute of Science & Research, New Delhi, India


V. A. Mhaskar, J. Maheshwari (eds.), *Innovative Approaches in Knee Arthroscopy*,
https://doi.org/10.1007/978-981-99-4378-4_7

## 7.4 Portals (Fig. 7.2)

Portal A: High anterolateral (AL) viewing portal at the level of the inferior pole of the patella just lateral to the patellar tendon.

Portal B: High anteromedial (AM) portal 1 cm medial to the patellar tendon made using an LP needle.

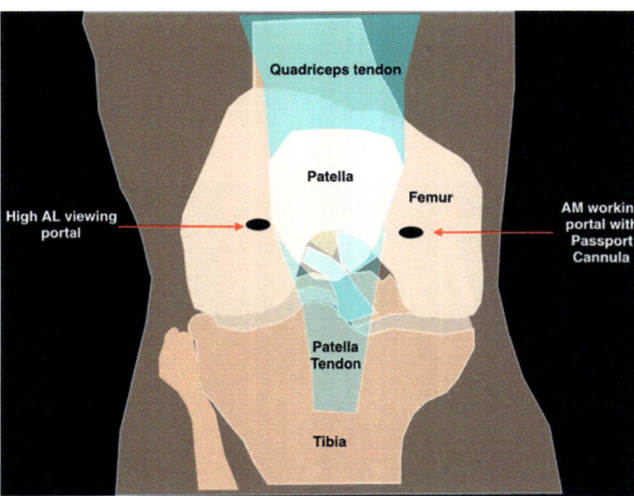


**Fig. 7.2** Illustration showing the AL and high AM working portal positions

## 7.5 Surgical Steps

### 7.5.1 Variation A [1]

Step 1: The arthroscope is introduced through Portal A and the vertical tear of the lateral meniscus is visualised (Fig. 7.3a, b).

Step 2: A flexible cannula is introduced through Portal B.

Step 3: The antegrade suture device (Arthrex, Naples, FL) with a 2-0 Fiberwire (Arthrex, Naples, FL) is introduced through Portal B and advanced to the lateral meniscus posterior horn and the meniscus is grabbed in the jaws of the device such that the far end of the meniscus beyond the tear is captured in the jaws and bite taken to deploy the needle carrying a 2-0 Fiberwire (Fig. 7.4a–e).

Step 4: The lower arm of the 2-0 Fiberwire is then loaded again in the antergrade suture passer and a bite taken through the near end of the meniscus with respect to the tear (Fig. 7.5a, b).

Step 5: The two ends are then tied with a knot pusher using at least four simple knots (Fig. 7.6).

Step 6: The ends of the knot are then cut (Fig. 7.7a, b).

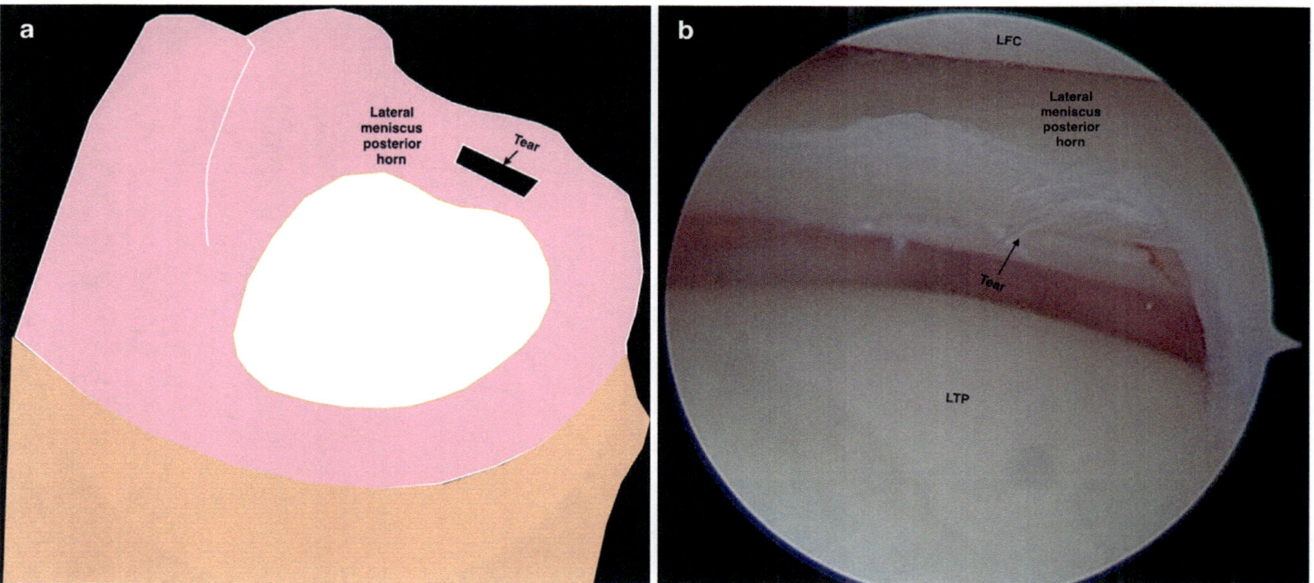


**Fig. 7.3** (**a**) Illustration of the knee showing a vertical tear in the posterior horn of the lateral meniscus. (**b**) Arthroscopic image of the knee showing a vertical tear of the posterior horn of the lateral meniscus

### 7.5.2 Variation B [1]

This is done when the jaws cannot reach the far end of the mensicus (Fig. 7.8).

Step 1: The jaws of the antegrade device through Portal B are introduced through the tear to the far end of the meniscus and bite taken with a 2-0 Fiberwire (Fig. 7.9).

Step 2: A crochet is introduced through Portal B and the lower end of the suture delivered from under the near end of the meniscus through Portal B (Fig. 7.10a, b).

Step 3: A bite is taken through the near end similar to the technique described above (Fig. 7.11a, b).

Step 4: The two ends are then tied with a knot pusher using at least four simple knots (Fig. 7.12a, b).

Step 5: The ends of the knot are then cut.

### 7.5.3 Variation B

Step 1: The antegrade suture device with a 2-0 Fiberwire is introduced through Portal B and advanced to the lateral meniscus posterior horn and the meniscus is grabbed in the jaws of the device such that the far end of the meniscus beyond the tear is captured in the jaws and the needle is

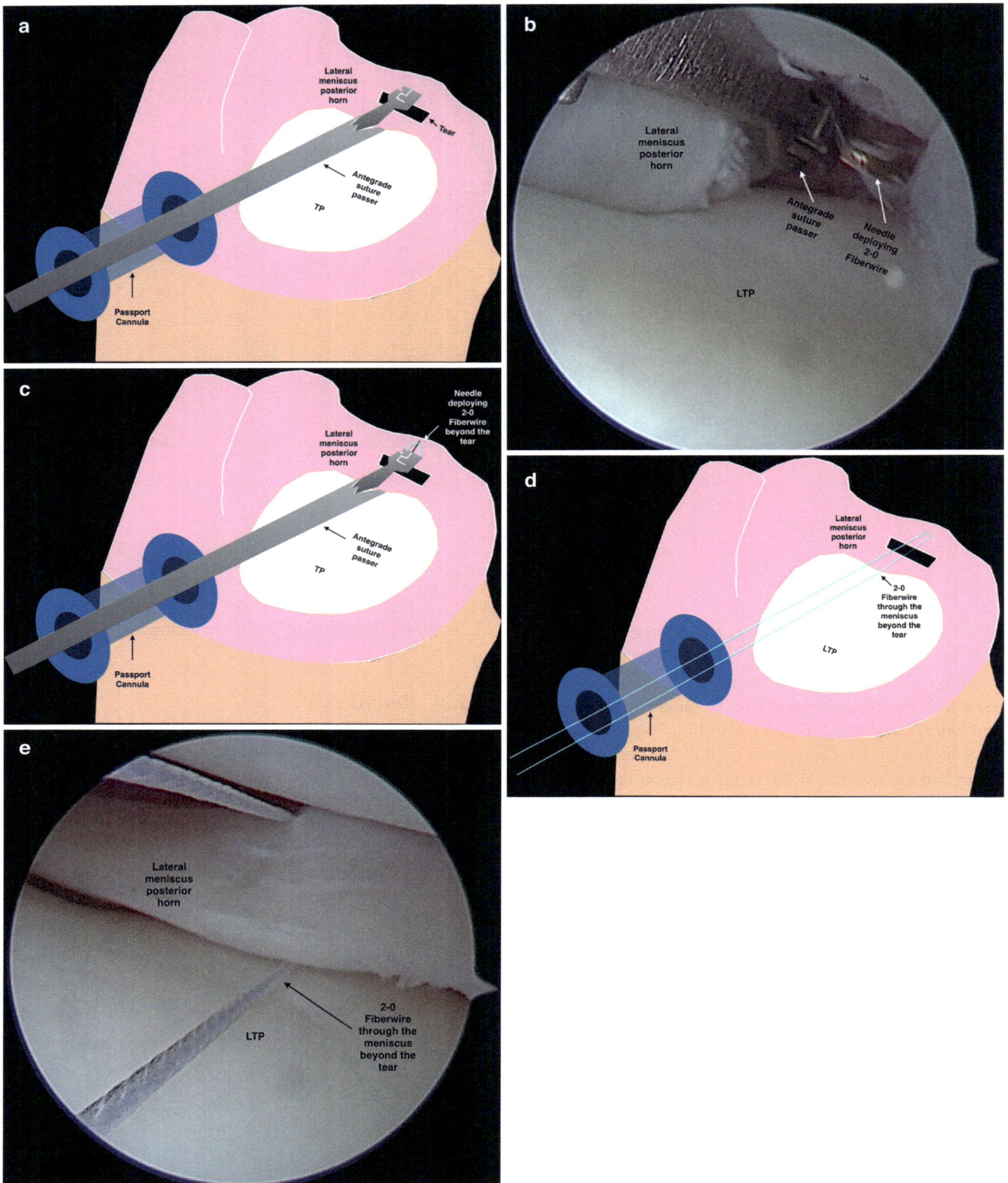


**Fig. 7.4** (**a**) Illustration of the knee showing the antegrade device introduced through Portal B and grasping the meniscus beyond the tear. (**b**) Arthroscopic image of the knee showing the Scorpion device taken a bite through the far end of the posterior horn of the meniscus beyond the tear with a 2-0 Fiberwire. (**c**) Illustration of the knee showing the Scorpion device taken a bite through the far end of the posterior horn of the meniscus beyond the tear with a 2-0 Fiberwire. (**d**) Illustration of the knee showing the 2-0 Fiberwire passing through the far end of the posterior horn of the meniscus beyond the tear. (**e**) Arthroscopic image of the knee showing the 2-0 Fiberwire passing through the far end of the meniscus beyond the tear and coming through Portal B

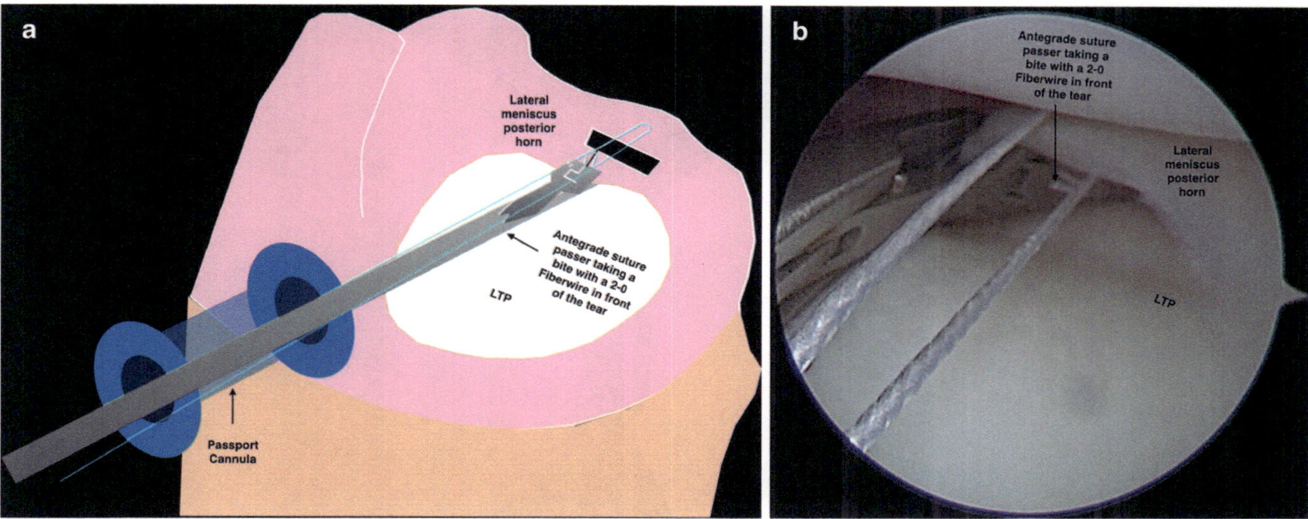


**Fig. 7.5** (**a**) Illustration of the knee showing the lower end of the 2-0 Fiberwire loaded on an antegrade suture passer and bite taken through the near end of the meniscus in front of the tear. (**b**) Arthroscopic image of the knee showing a bite taken with the antegrade suture passer loaded with a 2-0 Fiberwire through the near end of the meniscus in front of the tear

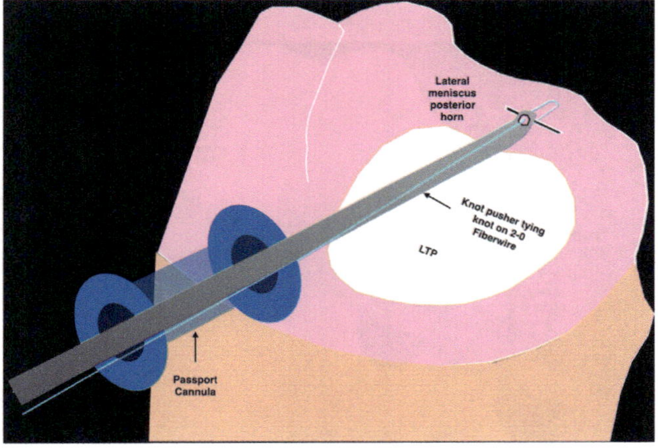


**Fig. 7.6** Illustration of the knee showing simple knots being tied with a knot pusher to approximate the meniscus tear though Portal B

deployed passing on end of the Fiberwire through the far end of the meniscus (Fig. 7.13a–d).

Step 2: The two ends of the suture are tied with a knot pusher and four simple knots (Fig. 7.14a, b).

Step 4: The ends are cut with an arthroscopic suture cutter (Fig. 7.15).

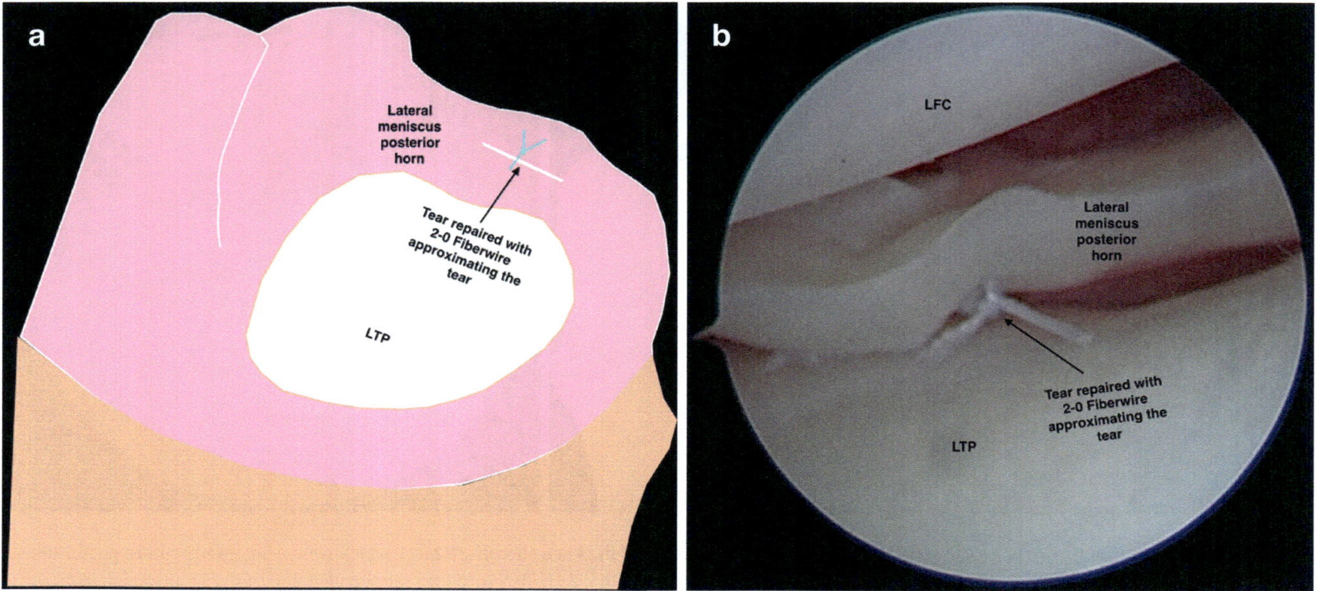


**Fig. 7.7** (**a**) Illustration of the knee showing the repaired tear with the two ends of the 2-0 Fiberwire cut. (**b**) Arthroscopy image of the knee showing the repaired tear with the two ends of the 2-0 Fiberwire cut

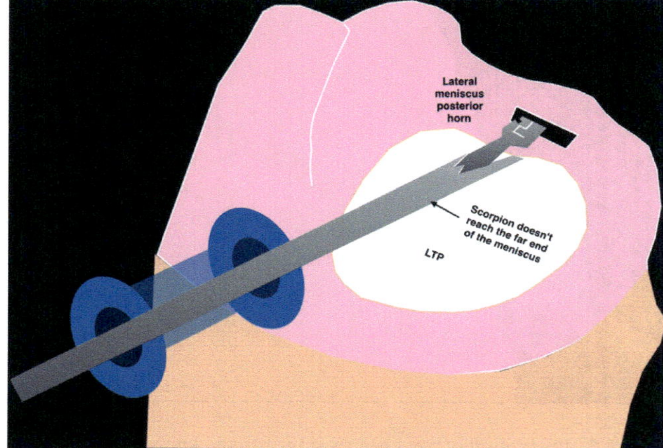


**Fig. 7.8** Illustration showing the jaws of the antegrade suture passer not reaching the far end of the meniscus

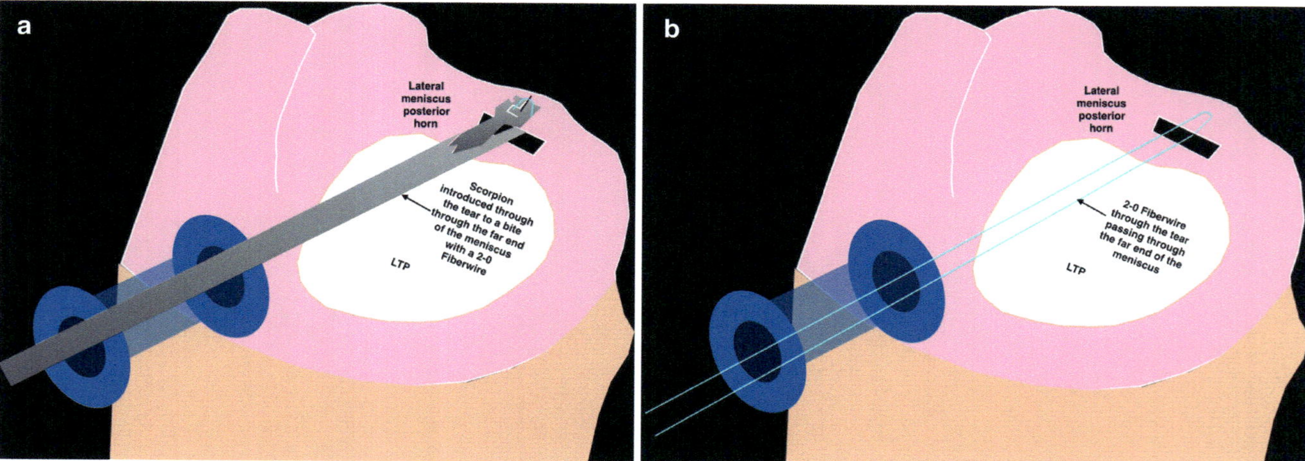


**Fig. 7.9** (**a**) Illustration of the knee showing a bite taken through the far end of the meniscus with the jaws introduced through the tear. (**b**) Illustration of the knee showing a 2-0 Fiberwire passing through the far end of the meniscus with the lower end coming out through the tear

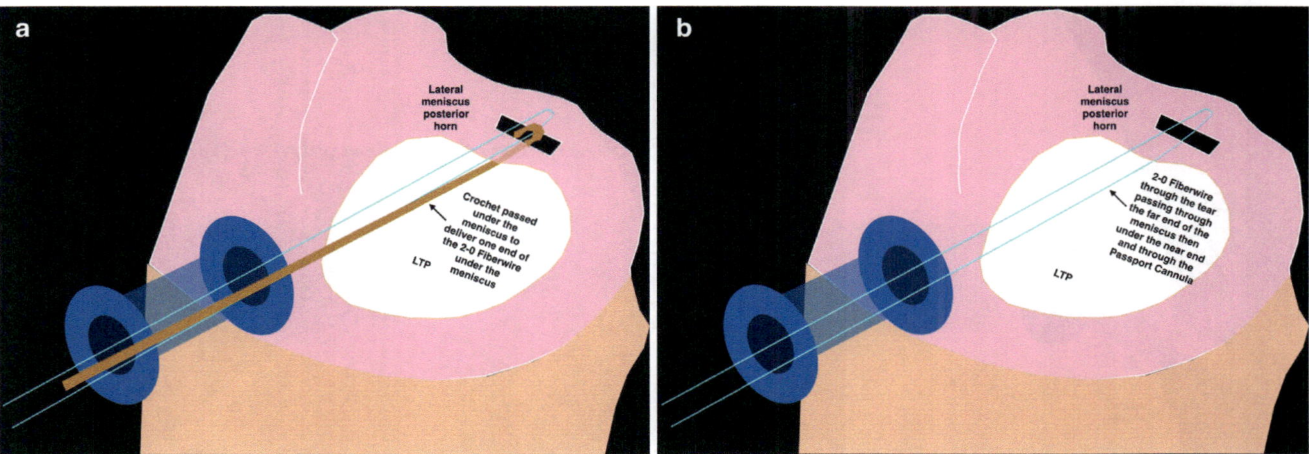


**Fig. 7.10** (**a**) Illustration of the knee showing a crochet introduced under the meniscus and delivering the lower end of the 2-0 Fiberwire from under the meniscus. (**b**) Illustration of the knee showing the 2-0 Fiberwire passing through the far end of the meniscus and lower end coming under the tear and near end of the meniscus

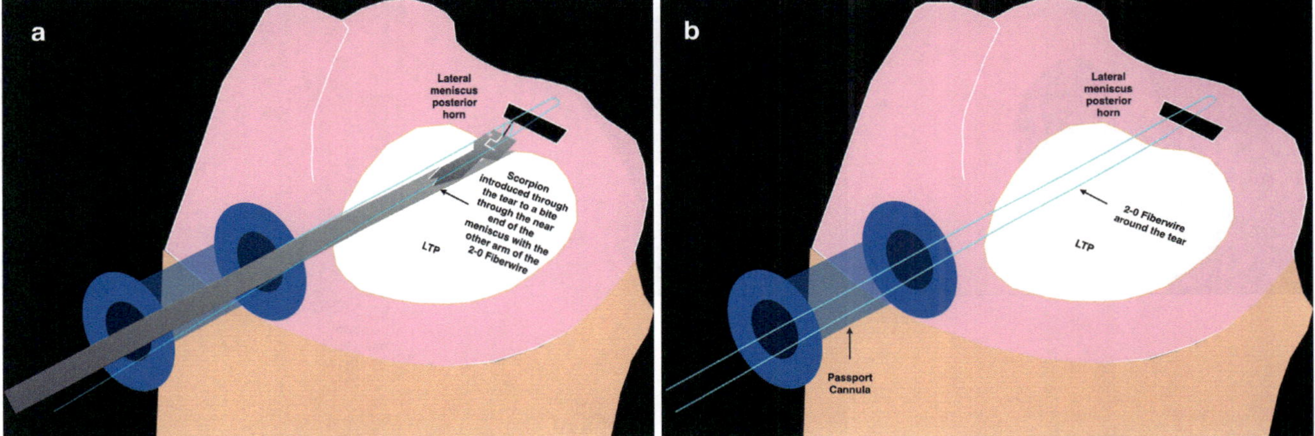


**Fig. 7.11** (**a**) Illustration of the knee showing the antegrade device taking a bite from the near end of the meniscus with the lower end of the 2-0 Fiberwire. (**b**) Illustration of the knee showing the 2-0 Fibewire passing through the far and near end of the meniscus

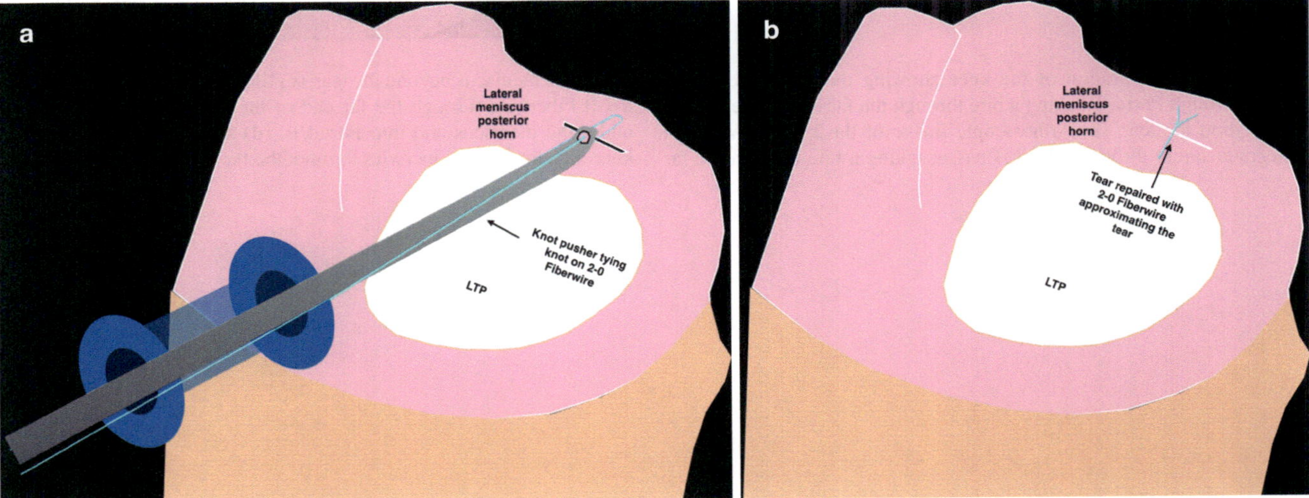


**Fig. 7.12** (**a**) Illustration of the knee showing multiple simple knots tied with a knot pusher through Portal B. (**b**) Illustration of the knee showing the repaired tear with the two ends of the 2-0 Fiberwire cut

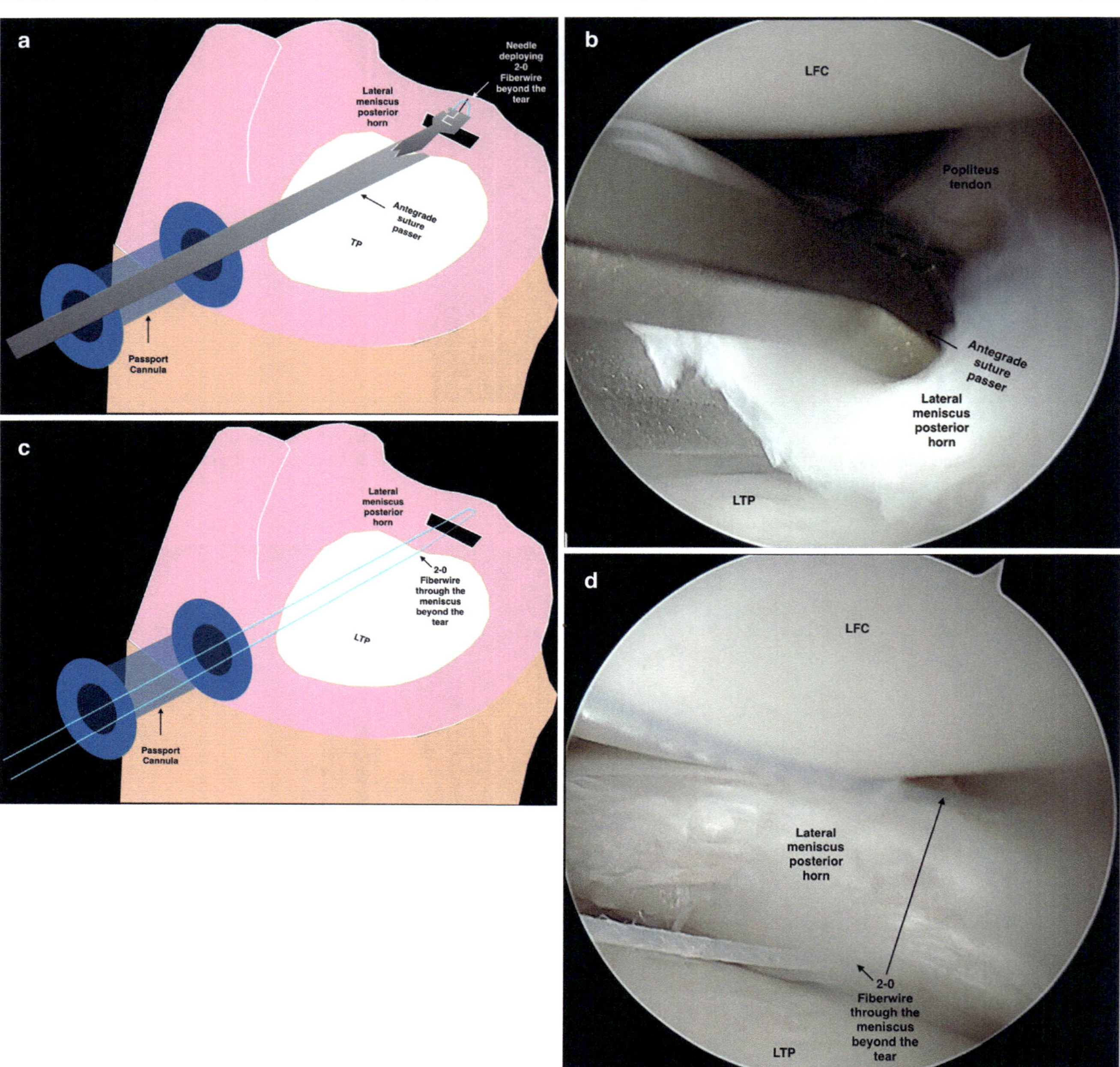


**Fig. 7.13** (**a**) Illustration of the knee showing the antegrade suture device through Portal B taking a bite through the far end of the meniscus beyond the tear. (**b**) Arthroscopic image of the knee showing an antegrade suture through Portal B passer taking a bite through the far end of the meniscus beyond the tear. (**c**) Illustration of the knee showing a 2-0 Fiberwire through the far end of the meniscus and coming out under the meniscus and into Portal B. (**d**) Arthroscopic image of the knee showing a 2-0 Fiberwire through the far end of the meniscus

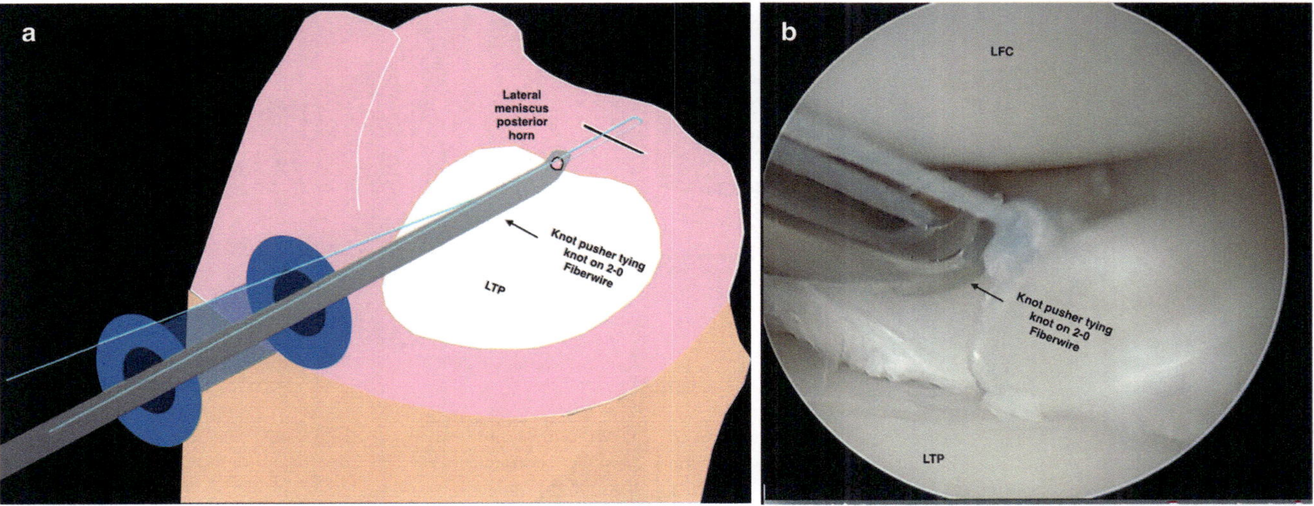


**Fig. 7.14** (**a**) Illustration of the knee showing a knot pusher through Portal B tying multiple simple knots. (**b**) Arthroscopic image of the knee showing a knot pusher through Portal B tying multiple simple knots

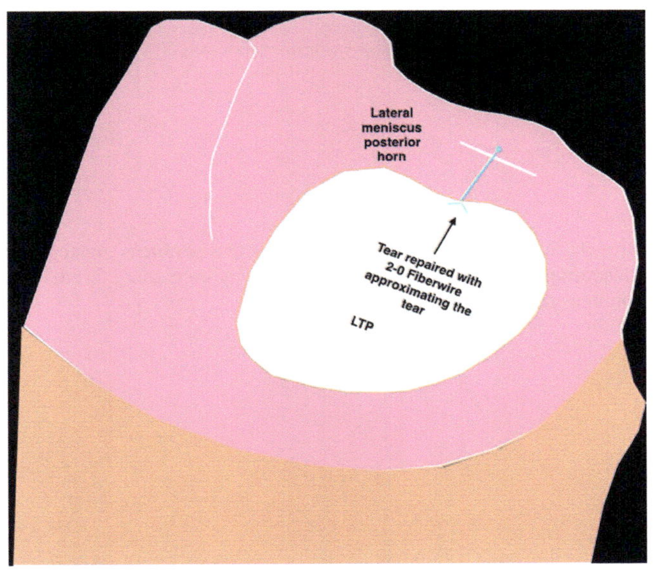


**Fig. 7.15** Illustration of the knee showing the repaired meniscus with a 2-0 Fiberwire

### 7.5.4 Variation C [2]

Step 1: The antegrade suture passer carrying the 2-0 Fiberwire is introduced through Portal B and a bite is taken through the popliteus tendon (Fig. 7.16a–c).

Step 2: One end of the suture is then reloaded and a bite taken through the meniscus tissue anterior to the tear and towards the posterior horn (Fig. 7.17a, b).

Step 3: The other end of the suture is then loaded and a bite taken through the meniscus tissue anterior to the tear and towards the body of the meniscus (Fig. 7.18a, b).

Step 4: Four simple knots are tied using a knot pusher through Portal B (Fig. 7.19).

Step 5: Two ends of the sutures are cut using an arthroscopic suture cutter (Fig. 7.20a, b).

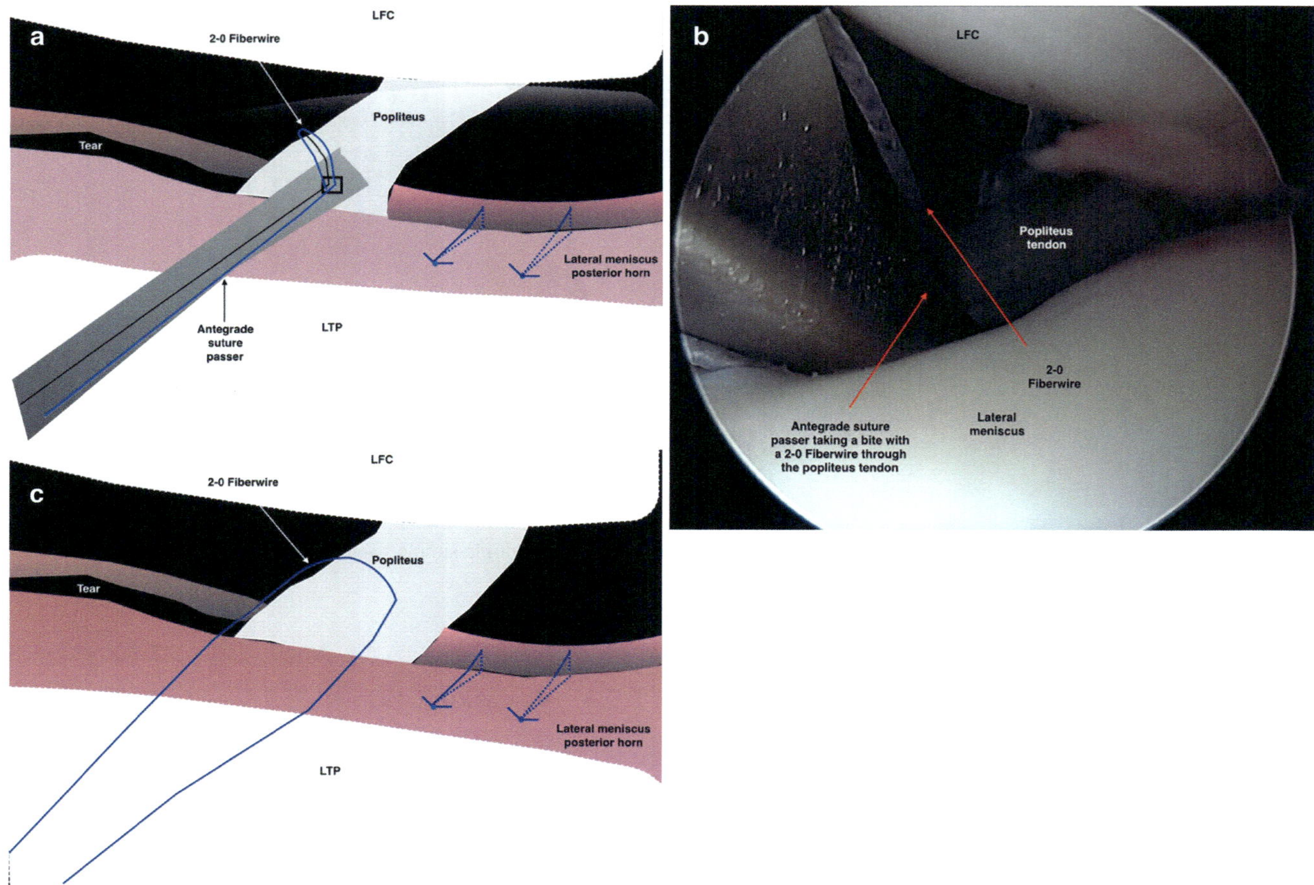


**Fig. 7.16** (**a**) Illustration of the knee showing an antegrade suture passer through Portal B taking a bite with a 2-0 Fiberwire through the popliteus tendon. (**b**) Arthroscopic image of the antegrade suture passer through Portal B taking a bite through the popliteus tendon. (**c**) Illustration of the knee showing the 2-0 Fiberwire passing through the popliteus tendon

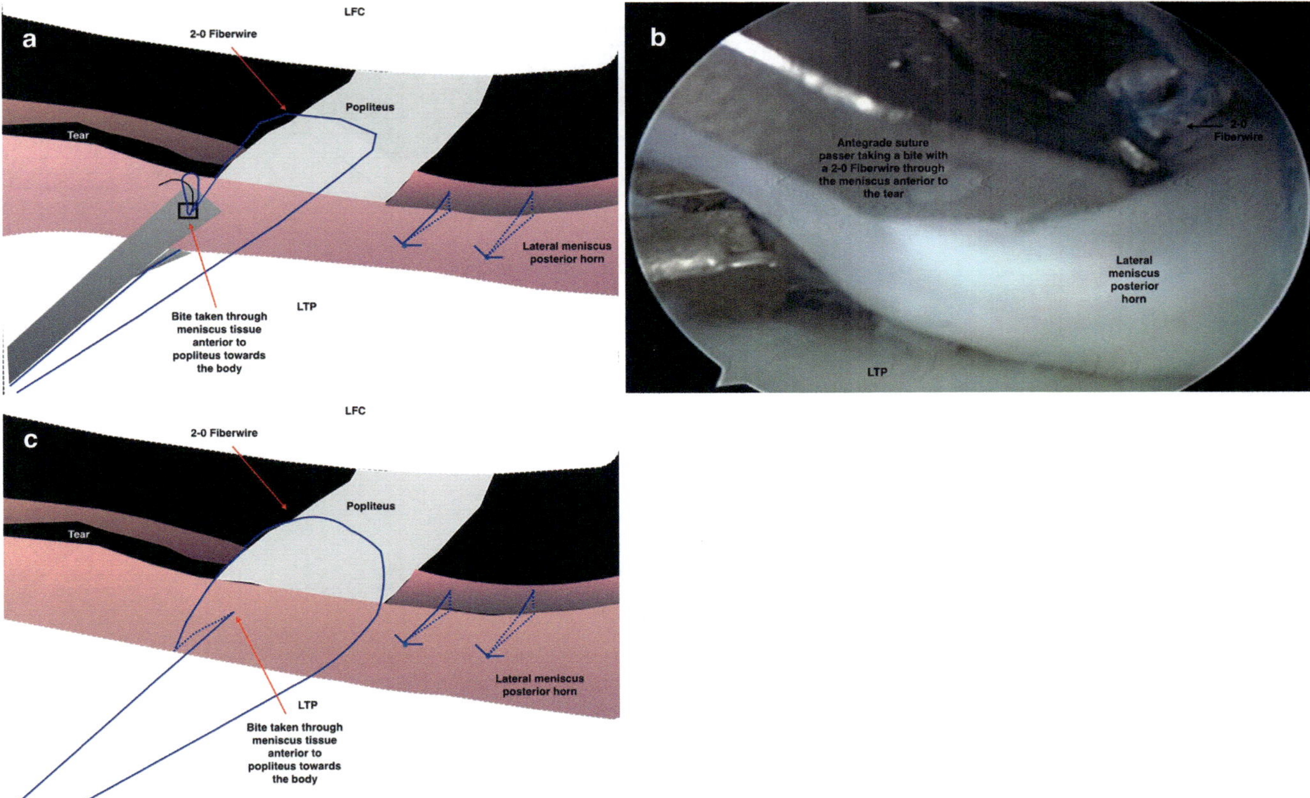


**Fig. 7.17** (**a**) Illustration of the knee showing an antegrade suture passer through Portal B taking a bite through the meniscus anterior to the tear. (**b**) Arthroscopic image of the knee showing a bite taken with an antegrade suture passer through the lateral meniscus anterior to the tear and popliteus tendon. (**c**) Illustration of the knee showing the 2-0 Fiberwire passing through the meniscus anterior to the tear and popliteus tendon

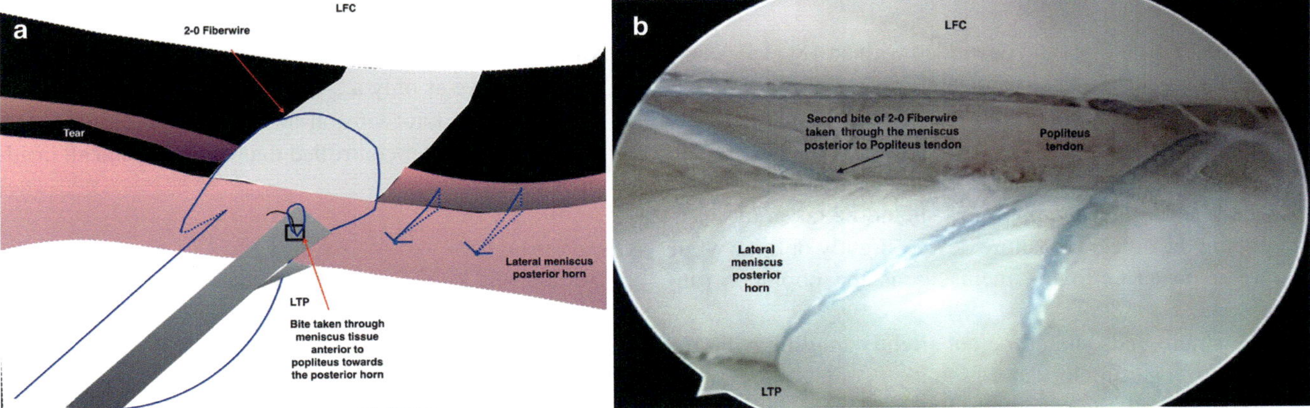


**Fig. 7.18** (**a**) Illustration of the knee showing an antegrade suture passer through Portal B taking a bite through the meniscus posterior to the tear. (**b**) Arthroscopic image of the knee showing the 2-0 Fiberwire passing through the popliteus and two ends through the meniscus anterior and posterior to the tear

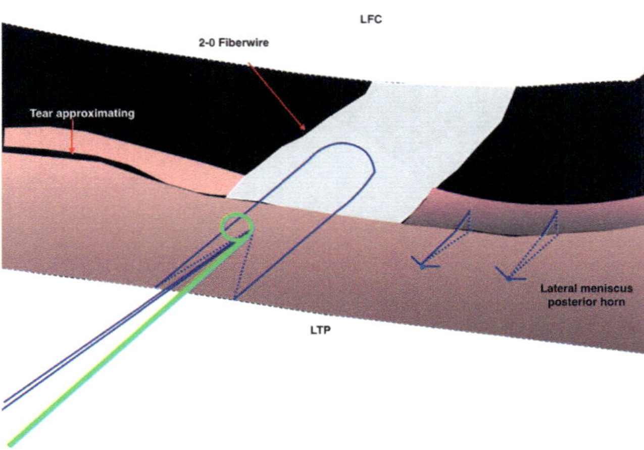


**Fig. 7.19** Illustration of the knee showing a knot pusher through Portal B tying multiple simple knots with the two ends of the 2-0 Fiberwire in front of the popliteus tendon

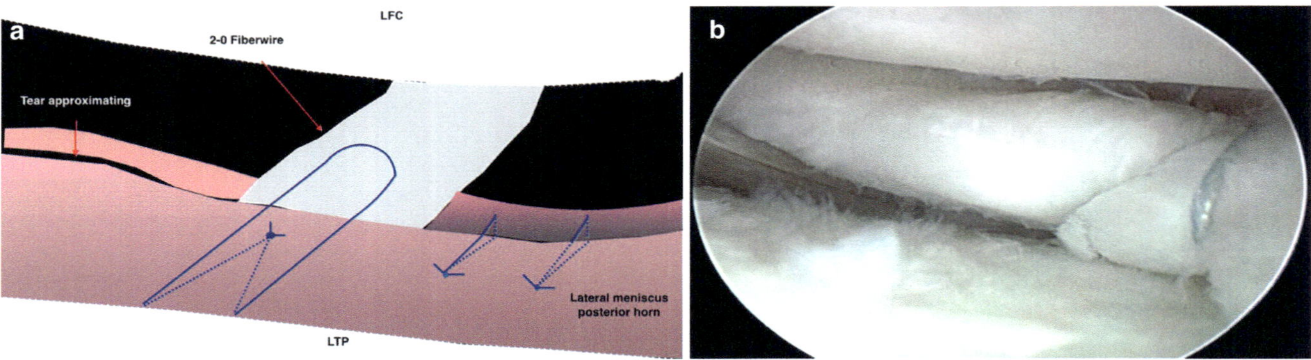


**Fig. 7.20** (**a**) Illustration of the knee showing the final construct after the knot is tied and two ends cut. (**b**) Arthroscopic image showing the final construct after the two ends of the 2-0 Fiberwire are cut

## 7.6 Tips and Tricks

1. Making Portal B should be guided with an 18G LP needle so that it is ideal for instrumentation.
2. While taking a second bite with the other end of the 2-0 Fiberwire keeping the first end slightly pulled and in tension helps in avoiding suture entanglement.
3. The bite through the poplitues should be taken by introducing the antegrade suture device slightly oblique while going posterior to the meniscus as the popliteus runs oblique.
4. The suture ends should be cut slightly long to avoid the knot from getting loose.
5. Sometimes if the antegrade device cannot fit into the space and grasp the meniscus, it can be inverted and a bit can be taken.

## 7.7 Advantages and Disadvantages

**Advantages**

1. Cost effective as only a 2-0 Fiberwire is used.
2. Regulation of knot tension and hence approximation of tear ends are better controlled than conventional all inside devices.

**Disadvantages**

1. Sutures and knots are on the surface of the meniscus and can potentially abrade the cartilage.
2. Technically demanding.

## References

1. Mhaskar VA. Alternative all-inside technique of repairing a vertical meniscus tear. Arthrosc Tech. 2020;9(8):e1181–9.
2. Mhaskar VA, Agrahari H, Maheshwari J. True all inside meniscus repair using the popliteus tendon. Eur J Orthop Surg Traumatol. 2023;33(5):2151–7.

# 8 Inside Out Meniscus Suturing

Vikram Arun Mhaskar

## 8.1 Introduction

Suturing a torn meniscus can be done via inside out, outside in, or all inside techniques. The inside out technique was the original technique to repair meniscus using needles carrying sutures that penetrate the meniscus and are tied over the capsule. These needles are introduced into the joint using specialised cannulas. Inside out suturing is an effective and cheaper technique to repair the meniscus but involves making a safety incision on the medial aspect of the tibia to avoid injury to the saphenous nerve, vessels and also makes sure the sutures are tied over the capsule. The technique can be used to repair any part of the medial meniscus; however, it is largely used to repair only the body and anterior horn of the lateral meniscus.

## 8.2 Specialised Equipment (Fig. 8.1)

1. Single lumen inside out cannulas (a) (Arthrex, Naples, FL)
2. Flat all inside meniscus sleeve (b) (Smith & Nephew, Watford, UK)
3. Inside out suturing needles (c) (Smith & Nephew, Watford, UK)
4. 2-0 Fiberwire (d) (Arthrex, Naples, FL)
5. Knot pusher (e) (Arthrex, Naples, FL)
6. Artery forceps (f)
7. Suture cutter (g) (Arthrex, Naples, FL)

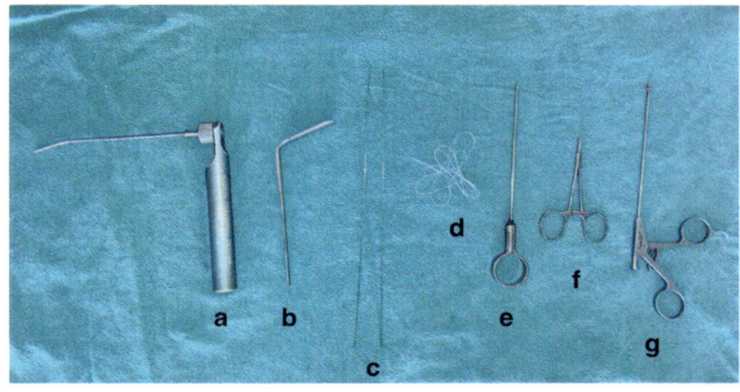


**Fig. 8.1** Image of instruments used in inside out meniscus suturing, (**a**) inside out cannula, (**b**) sleeve, (**c**) meniscus repair inside out needles, (**d**) 2-0 fiberwire, (**e**) knot pusher, (**f**) artery forceps, (**g**) suture cutter

## 8.3 Position (Fig. 8.2a, b)

Supine on an operating table with knee in 70° flexion with a side support and bolster at the end of the table. The limb may be kept on the hip of the surgeon and valgus force given to open the medial compartment while working in the medial compartment or in a figure of four position for the lateral compartment.

V. A. Mhaskar (✉)
F7 East of Kailash, Knee & Shoulder Clinic, New Delhi, India

JMVM Sports Injury Center, Sitaram Bhartia Institute of Science & Research, New Delhi, India


V. A. Mhaskar, J. Maheshwari (eds.), *Innovative Approaches in Knee Arthroscopy*,
https://doi.org/10.1007/978-981-99-4378-4_8

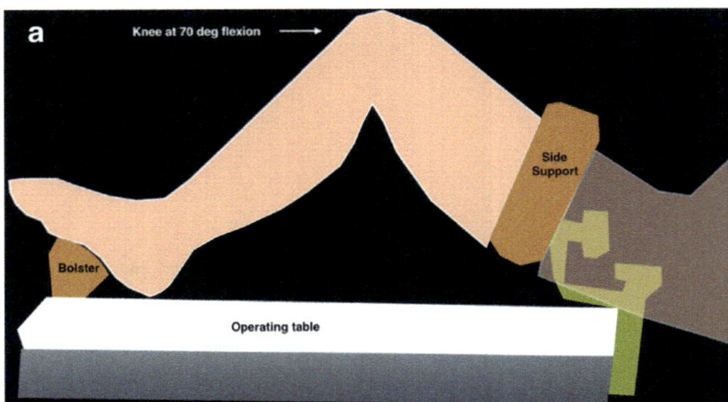


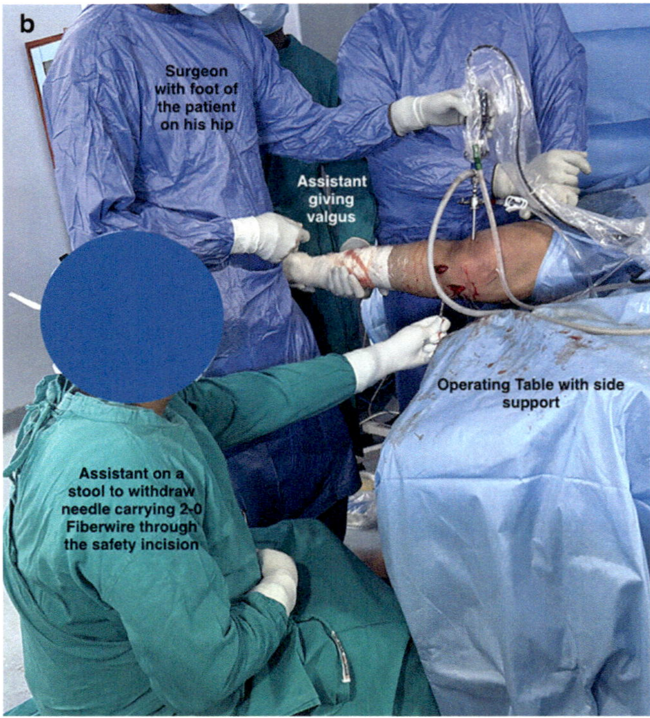


**Fig. 8.2** (**a**) Knee in 70° flexion on an operating table with a side support and bolster at the end of the table. (**b**) Illustration showing the positioning during repair of the medial meniscus with the limb on the operating table with a side support and a valgus force at the knee. One assistant to the side helps in giving valgus and putting the needles carrying the 2-0 Fiberwire, the other sitting down retrieves the needles

## 8.4 Portals (Fig. 8.3)

Anterolateral portal just lateral to the inferior pole of the patella for viewing the posterior horn and as a working portal for the body of the medial meniscus.

Anteromedial portal in the soft spot on the medial side for viewing the body of the medial meniscus and as a working portal for the posterior horn.

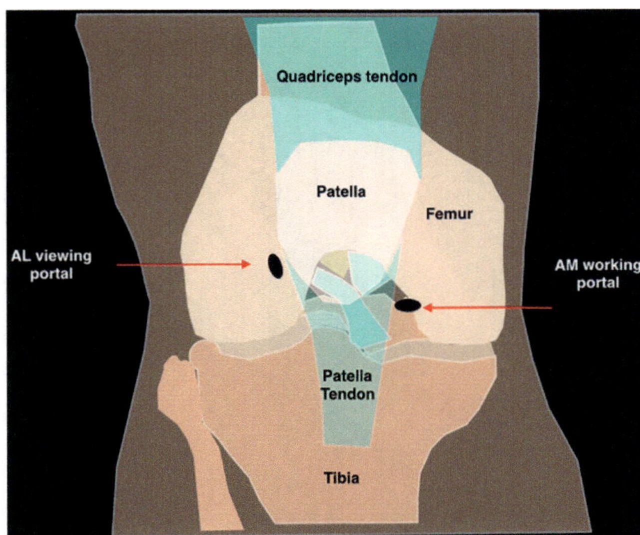


**Fig. 8.3** Illustration showing the two portals used a standard high anterolateral portal and an anteromedial portal

## 8.5 Surgical Steps

Step 1: A safety incision is made on the medial side by placing the knee in flexion. A skin incision is made between the medial border of the tibia and the gastrocnemius. The pes anserinus is retracted to protect the saphenous nerve that lies posteromedial to the tendons (Fig. 8.4a, b).

Step 2: The wound is dissected till the interval between the medial gastrocnemius and the joint capsule. The index finger can be used to dissect between the gastrocnemius and posterior capsule and the joint line felt posteriorly (Fig. 8.5).

Step 3: A sleeve is applied between the medial gastrocnemius and the posterior capsule (Fig. 8.6a, b).

Step 4: The sleeve is applied to the meniscus through the portal of best access that is perpendicular to the meniscus surface that it needs to be applied to (Fig. 8.7a, b).

Step 5: A needle carrying a 2-0 Fiberwire is then passed through this sleeve and into the meniscus through the capsule (Fig. 8.8a, b).

Step 6: The assistant sitting on a stool retrieves this needle (Fig. 8.9a, b).

Step 7: The sleeve is then applied to the capsular portion of the meniscus (Fig. 8.10a, b).

Step 8: The second needle carrying the other end of the suture is then passed through the sleeve and into the meniscus and capsule. While doing this, the suture already passed is kept taut and the needle is passed parallel to it (Fig. 8.11a, b).

Step 9: The assistant sitting on the stool retrieves the needle (Fig. 8.12).

Step 10: The two ends of the meniscus are then tied onto the capsule using multiple half hitches (3–4) (Fig. 8.13a, b).

Step 11: The two ends of the suture are then cut (Fig. 8.14a).

Step 12: The meniscus is visualised arthroscopically to ensure it is repaired satisfactorily (Fig. 8.15a, b).

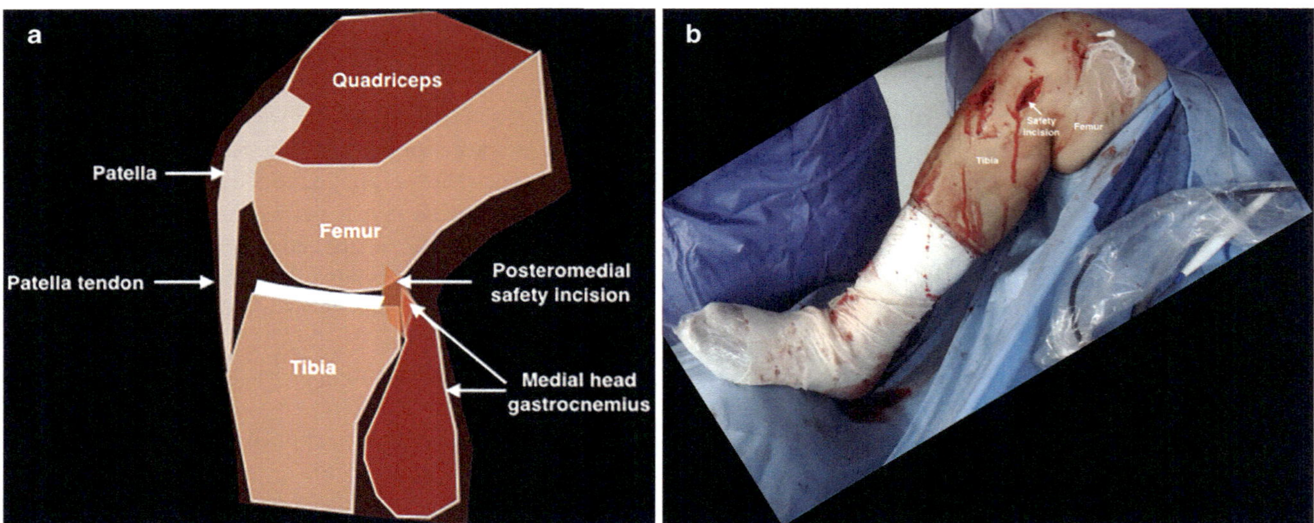


**Fig. 8.4** (**a**) Illustration showing the safety incision landmarks, the medial head of the gastrocnemius, and the posteromedial capsule. (**b**) Image of the knee showing the medial aspect with the safety incision

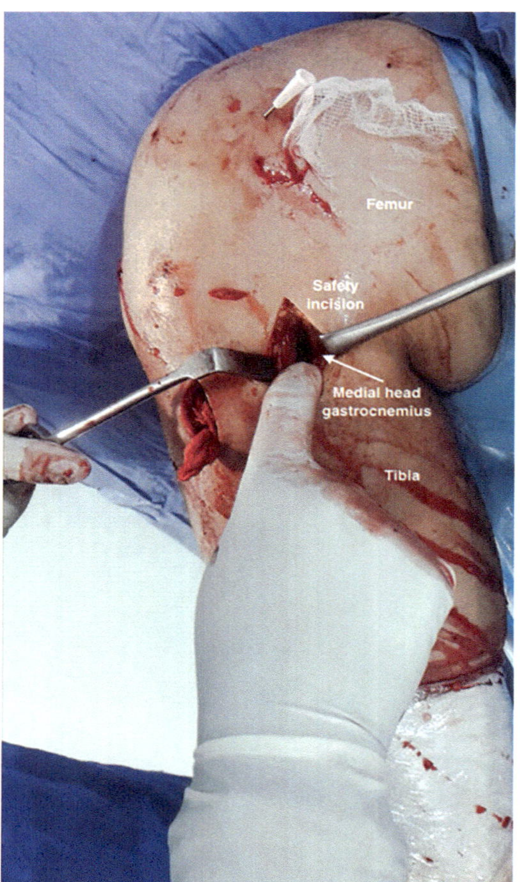


**Fig. 8.5** Image showing index finger applied between the medial gastrocnemius and posterior capsule creating a plane

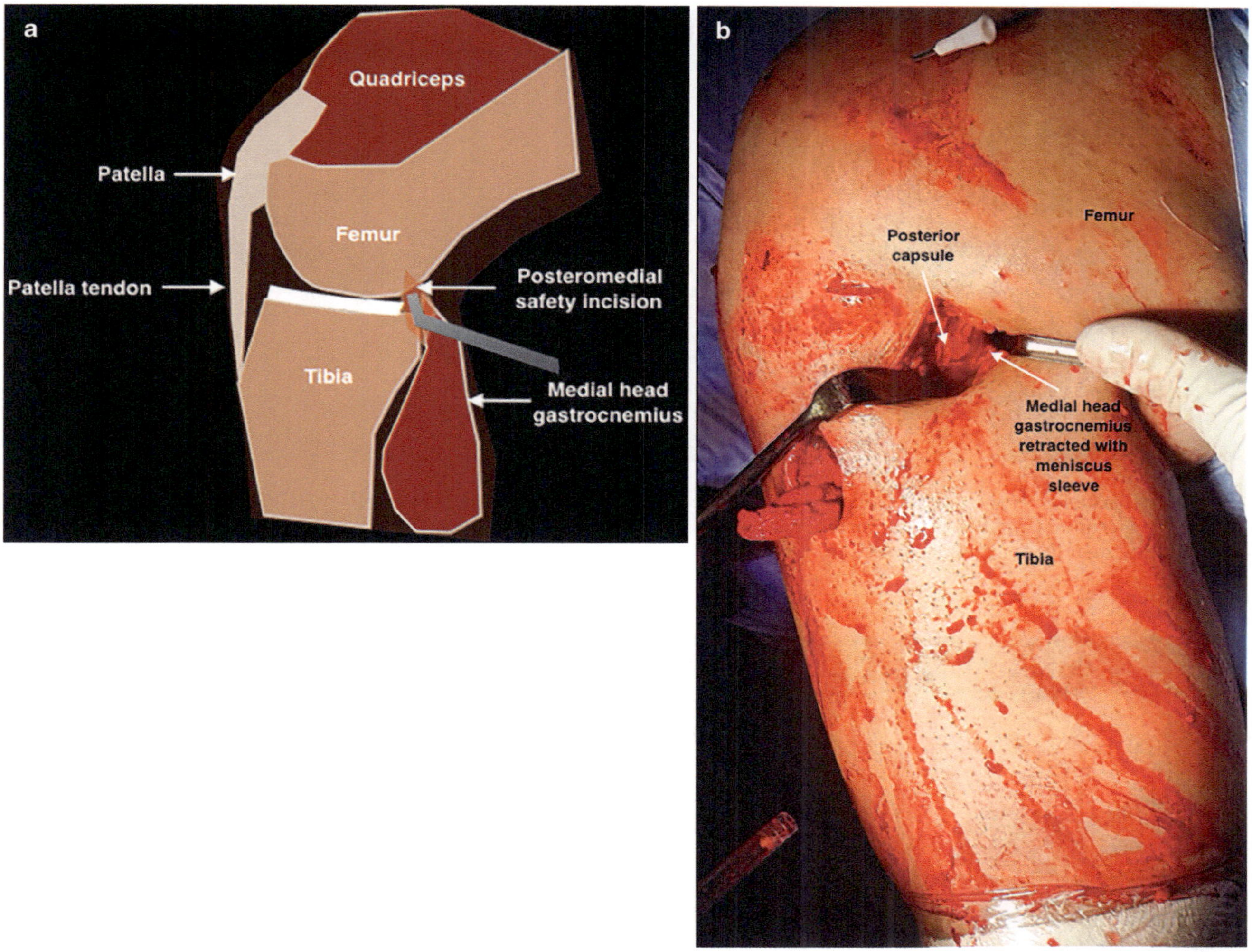

**Fig. 8.6** (**a**) Illustration showing a sleeve applied between the medial gastrocnemius and the posterior capsule in the safety incision. (**b**) Image showing the sleeve applied between the medial gastrocnemius and the posterior capsule in the safety incision

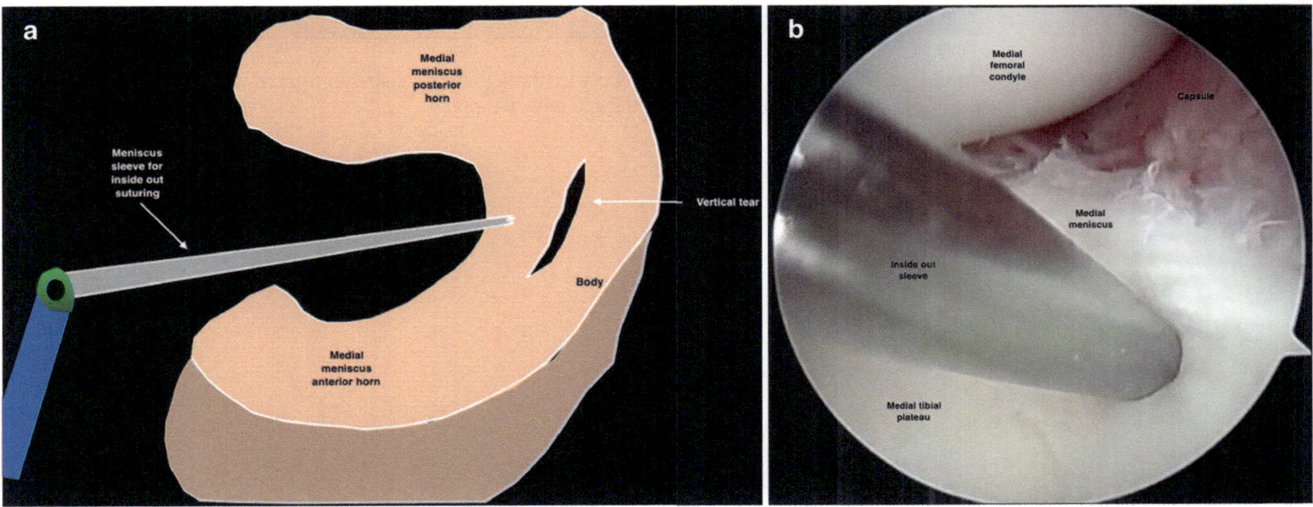


**Fig. 8.7** (**a**) Sleeve applied to the meniscus in front of the tear from the anterolateral portal while viewing from the anteromedial portal. (**b**) Arthroscopic image showing the sleeve from the anteromedial portal applied to the meniscus just in front of the tear while viewing from the anterolateral portal

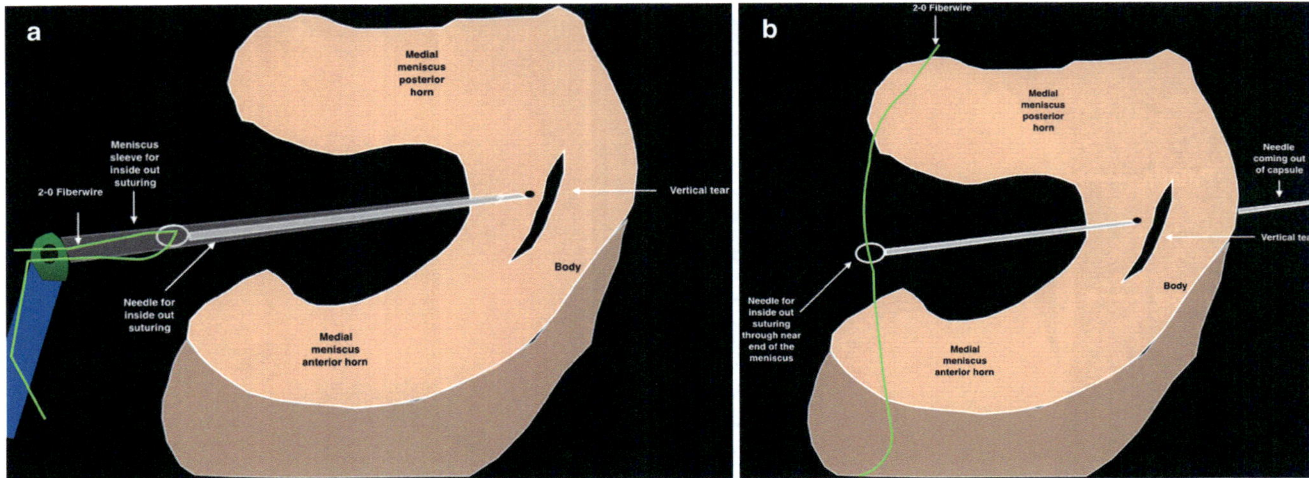


**Fig. 8.8** (**a**) Illustration showing the needle carrying the 2-0 Fiberwire piercing the meniscus in front of the tear from the anterolateral portal while viewing from the anteromedial portal. (**b**) Illustration showing the needle carrying the 2-0 Fiberwire from the anterolateral portal passing through the meniscus anterior to the tear and coming out of the capsule posteriorly through the safety incision

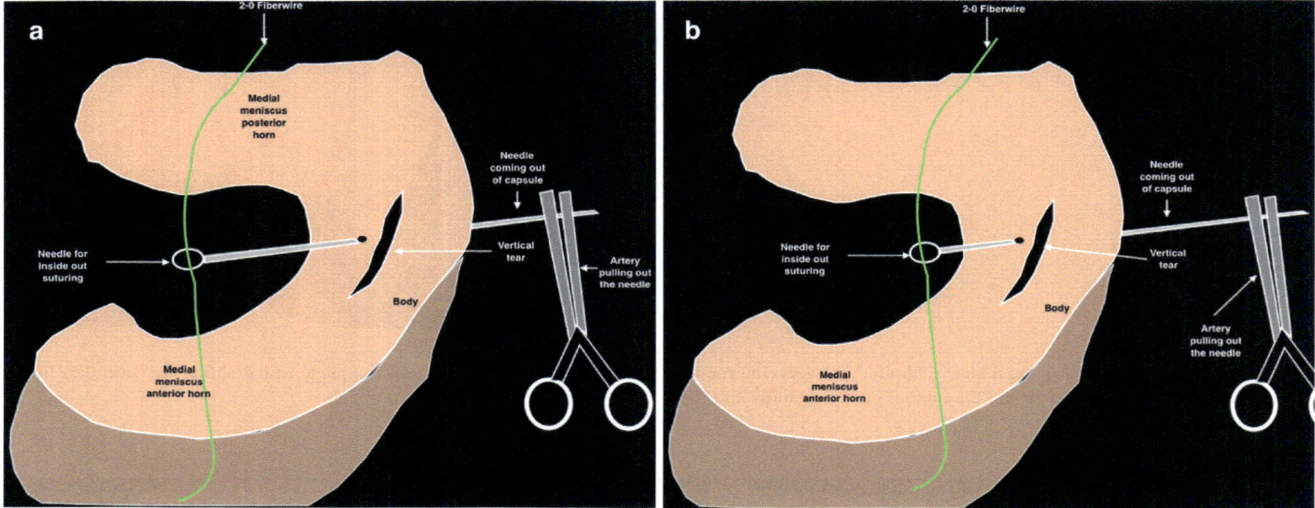


**Fig. 8.9** (**a**) Illustration showing an artery forceps pulling the needle out of the safety incision while viewing from the anteromedial portal. (**b**) Illustration showing the artery pulling the needle carrying the 2-0 Fiberwire through the meniscus in front of the tear while viewing from the anteromedial portal

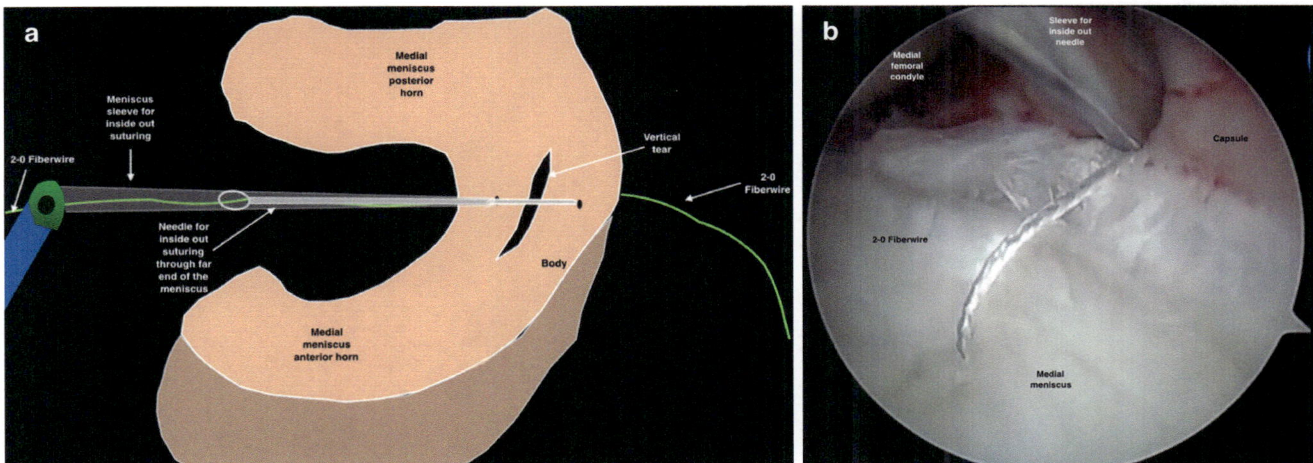


**Fig. 8.10** (**a**) Illustration showing the sleeve applied to the meniscus beyond the tear carrying the needle with a 2-0 Fiberwire from the anterolateral portal while viewing from the anteromedial portal. (**b**) Image showing the sleeve from the anterolateral portal applied to the capsule beyond the meniscus tear while viewing from the anteromedial portal

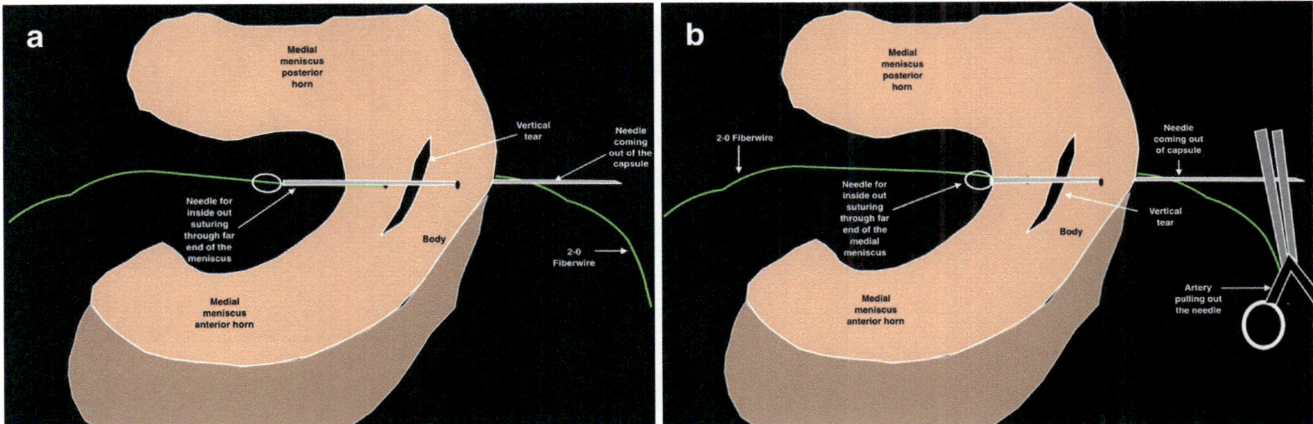


**Fig. 8.11** (**a**) Illustration showing the needle carrying the other end of the 2-0 Fiberwire from the anteromedial portal passing through the meniscus beyond the tear. (**b**) Illustration showing an artery forceps through the safety incision pulling the needle carrying the 2-0 Fiberwire while viewing from the anteromedial portal

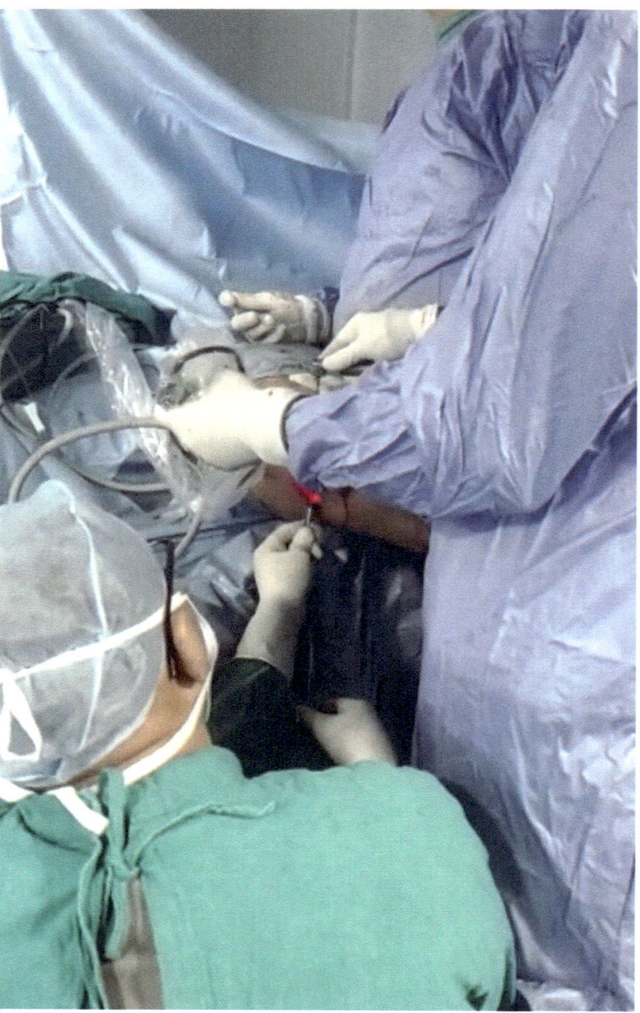

**Fig. 8.12** Image showing the assistant sitting on a stool and retrieving the needle from the safety incision on the medial side

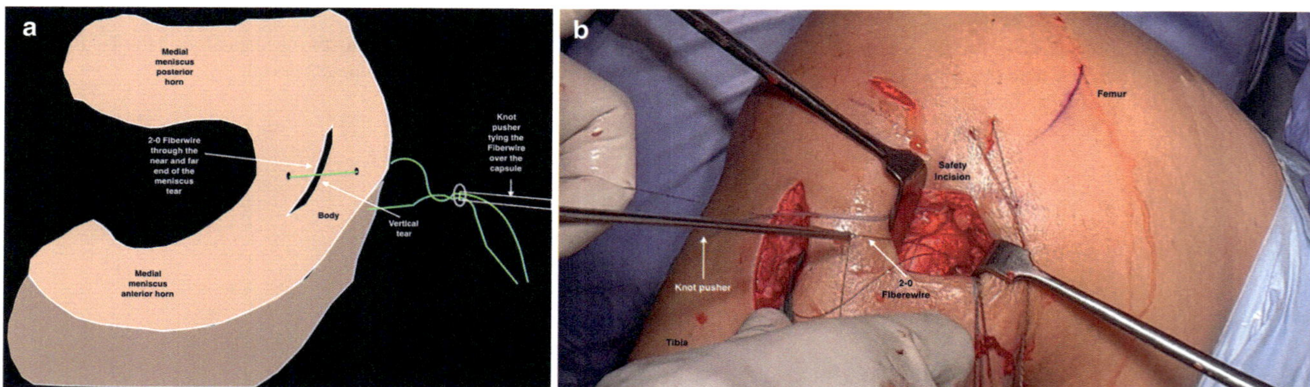


**Fig. 8.13** (**a**) Illustration showing the two ends of the suture being tied onto the capsule using a knot pusher through the safety incision. (**b**) Image showing the two ends of the 2-0 Fiberwire being tied over the capsule through the safety incision using a knot pusher

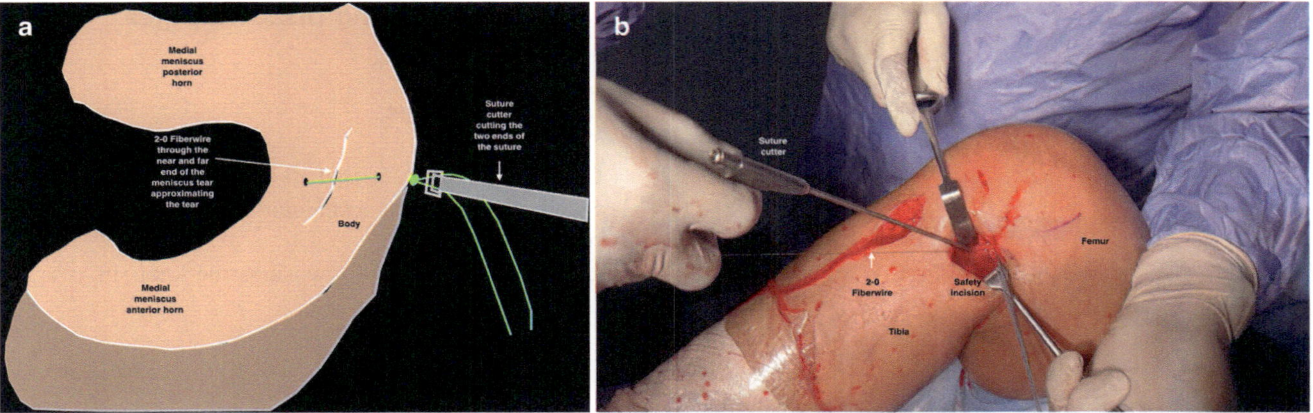


**Fig. 8.14** (**a**) Illustration showing both ends of the suture being cut using a suture cutter through the safety incision. (**b**) External image of the knee showing the ends of the 2-0 Fiberwire being cut in the safety incision after the repair

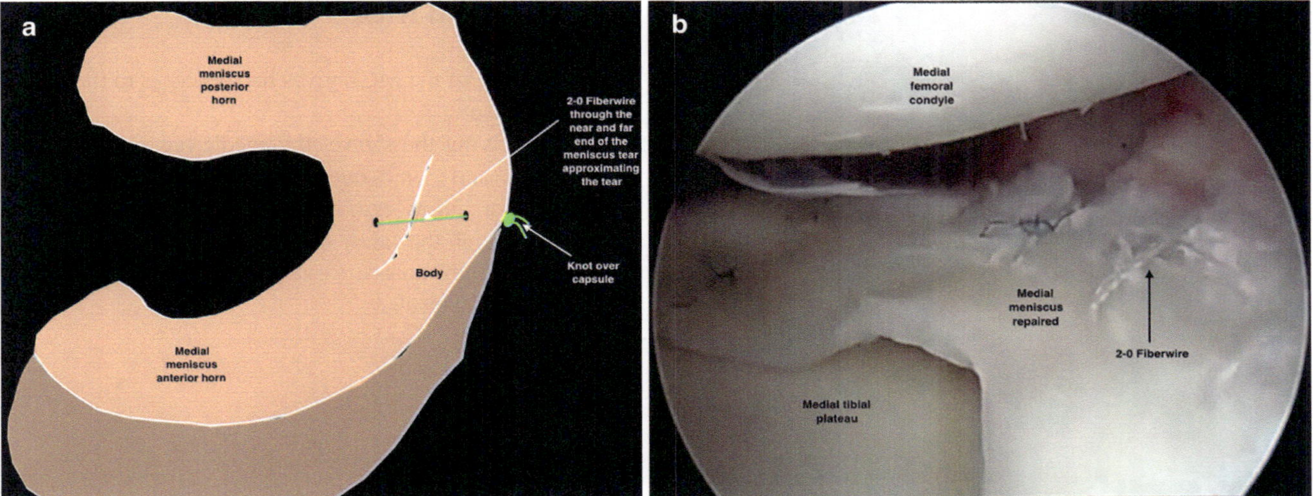


**Fig. 8.15** (**a**) Illustration showing the repaired vertical tear viewing through the anterolateral portal. (**b**) Arthroscopic image of the repaired medial meniscus while viewing through the anterolateral portal

## 8.6 Variation

Same steps are repeated except the sutures are applied to the meniscus tissue side by side in a horizontal mattress configuration (Fig. 8.16).

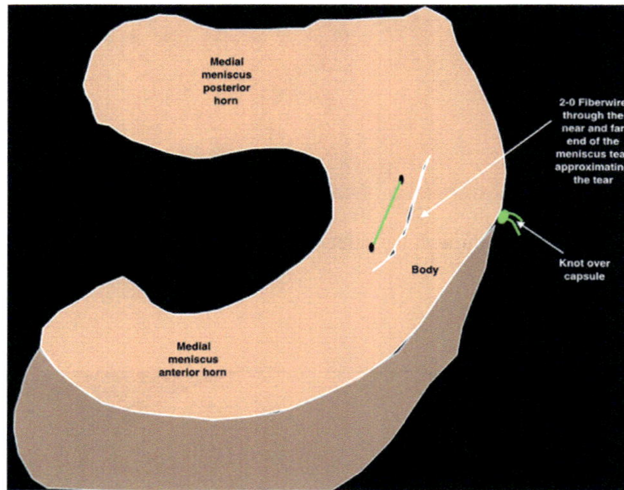


**Fig. 8.16** Illustration showing the repaired medial meniscus with a horizontal mattress inside out repair while viewing through the anterolateral portal

## 8.7 Advantage and Disadvantages

### 8.7.1 Advantages

1. Cheaper than conventional all inside technique.
2. Standard knot tying technique employed that is easily reproducible.
3. Using the safety incision ensures the knot sits over the capsule.

### 8.7.2 Disadvantages

1. Sutures and knots may irritate the knee posteriorly.
2. Saphenous nerve and vein injury can potentially happen.

## 8.8 Tips and Tricks

1. Pie crusting of the MCL gives better access to the medial compartment.
2. After applying the sleeve, the needle has penetrated the meniscus and come out of the capsule, the sleeve is retrieved to allow removal of the needle carrying the suture through the safety incision.
3. Using the light source to view the capsule while tying knots on the capsule.

# 9 Arthroscopic Outside in Meniscus Repair: Suture Shuttle Technique

Vikram Arun Mhaskar

## 9.1 Introduction

Repairing a vertical meniscus tear should be the intention wherever possible. The technique used should be stable and cost-effective. All inside meniscus repair devices are expensive and when the tears are large can be substituted with inside out and outside in repair techniques. Outside in repair is especially useful to repair body and anterior horn tears. The technique described uses standard lumbar puncture (LP) needles and PDS sutures used to shuttle a 2-0 Fiberwire and repair a vertical tear of the meniscus.

## 9.2 Specialised Equipment (Fig. 9.1)

18G LP needle-2 (Becton, Dickinson and Company, Franklin Lakes, NJ) (a)
0 PDS sutures-2 (Ethicon, Raritan, NJ) (b)
2-0 Fiberwire-1 (Arthrex, Naples, FL) (d)
Arthroscopic Grasper (Smith & Nephew, Watford, UK) (c)
Knot pusher-1 (Arthrex, Naples, FL) (e)

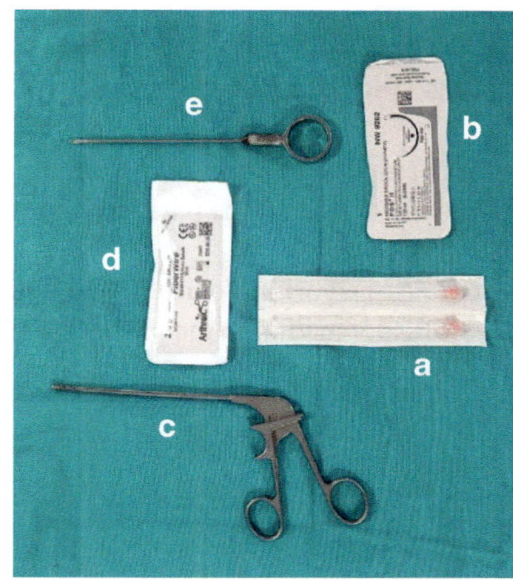


**Fig. 9.1** (**a**) 2, 18G Lumbar puncture needles, (**b**) PDS suture, (**c**) Grasper, (**d**) 2-0 Fiberwire, (**e**) Knot Pusher

## 9.3 Positioning

Patient supine on an operating table with side supports and a bolster on the foot end of the table.

When repairing the medial meniscus, the knee in 30° flexion with the foot on the surgeons hip with a valgus force being given with the surgeon standing between the patients limb and bed (Fig. 9.2).

While tying the knots, the limb is on the table at 70° knee flexion.

V. A. Mhaskar (✉)
F7 East of Kailash, Knee & Shoulder Clinic, New Delhi, India

JMVM Sports Injury Center, Sitaram Bhartia Institute of Science & Research, New Delhi, India


V. A. Mhaskar, J. Maheshwari (eds.), *Innovative Approaches in Knee Arthroscopy*,
https://doi.org/10.1007/978-981-99-4378-4_9

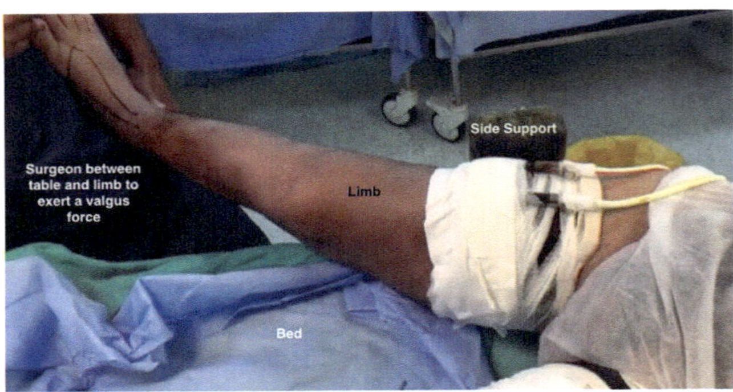


Fig. 9.2 Position of the limb on the operating table with the knee in 30° flexion and a side support to help in exerting a valgus force with the surgeon standing between the limb and the operating table

## 9.4 Portals (Fig. 9.3)

Anterolateral (AL) viewing portal: 1 cm vertical portal made at the level of the lower pole of the patellar tendon just lateral to the patellar tendon.

Anteromedial (AM) working portal, 1 cm horizontal portal made at the soft spot medial to the patellar tendon and just above the medial meniscus.

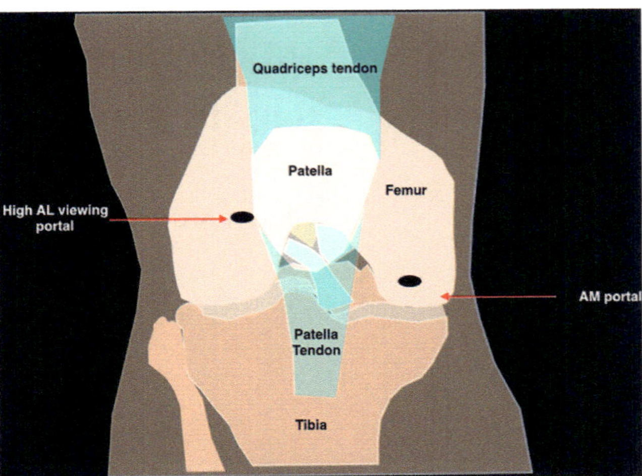


Fig. 9.3 Illustration showing a high AL viewing portal and an AM working portal

## 9.5 Surgical Steps

Step 1: With the arthroscope through the AL portal, the tear is identified (Fig. 9.4a, b).

Step 2: An 18G LP needle is introduced at the level of the meniscus corresponding to the tear from outside to inside the joint, the tip of the needle is used to pierce the meniscus tissue in its peripheral one-third from the inferior to the

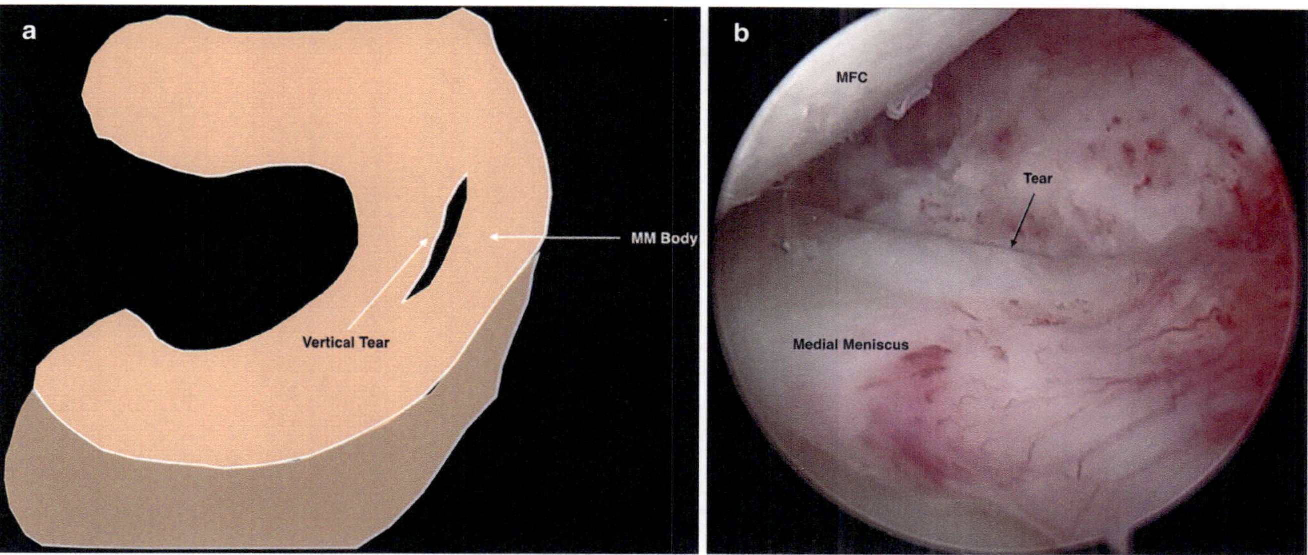


**Fig. 9.4** (**a**) Illustration of the medial meniscus showing a vertical tear in the body viewing through the AL portal. (**b**) Arthroscopic image showing a vertical tear in the body of the medial meniscus while viewing through an AL portal

superior surface till the tip can be seen coming out of the meniscus tissue in the peripheral 1/3 (Fig. 9.5).

Step 3: A second 18G LP needle is introduced at the level of the meniscus corresponding to the tear from outside to inside the joint, the tip of the needle is used to pierce the meniscus tissue in its peripheral one-third from the inferior to the superior surface till the tip can be seen coming out of the meniscus tissue in the peripheral 1/3 (Fig. 9.6a, b).

Step 4: A PDS suture is put through the upper and lower needle from outside in till a long length of suture is intra articular (Fig. 9.7a, b).

Step 5: A grasper is introduced through the AM portal and both PDS suture ends are held simultaneously (Fig. 9.8a, b).

Step 6: The two needles are then withdrawn externally while firmly holding the two PDS ends (Fig. 9.9a, b).

Step 7: The two PDS suture ends are simultaneously retrieved through the AM portal to act as a virtual cannula (Fig. 9.10).

Step 8: Each end of the PDS suture through the AM portal is tied over one end of a 2-0 Fiberwire (Arthrex, Naples, FL) with a simple knot tied firmly (Fig. 9.11).

Step 9: The other two ends of PDS suture coming out of the skin are then pulled through to shuttle the 2-0 Fiberwire through the meniscus and peripheral capsular tissue (Fig. 9.12a, b).

Step 10: A stab incision is made between the points from where the 2-0 Fiberwire is coming out of the skin (Fig. 9.13).

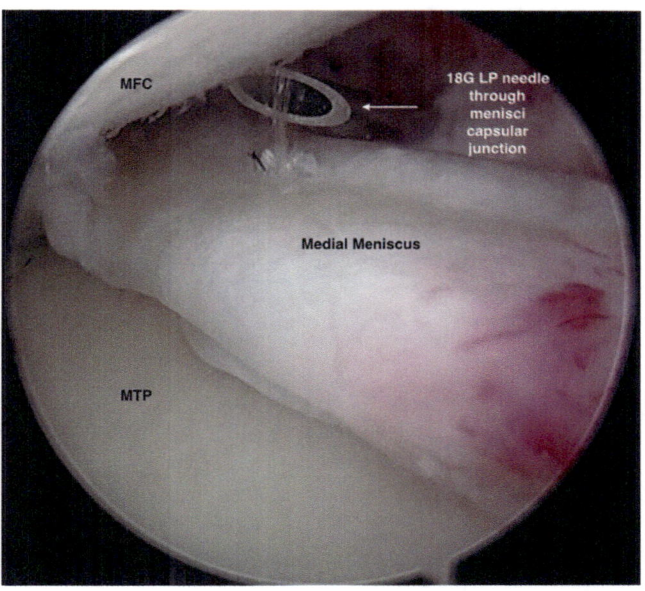


**Fig. 9.5** Arthroscopic image showing the 18G LP needle introduced from externally to the peripheral aspect of the medial meniscus body while viewing through the AL portal

Step 11: A straight artery is introduced through the incision and tissues dissected till the capsule (Fig. 9.14).

Step 12: An arthroscopic probe is used subcutaneously to deliver the two ends of the 2-0 Fiberwire through the same incision (Fig. 9.15a, b).

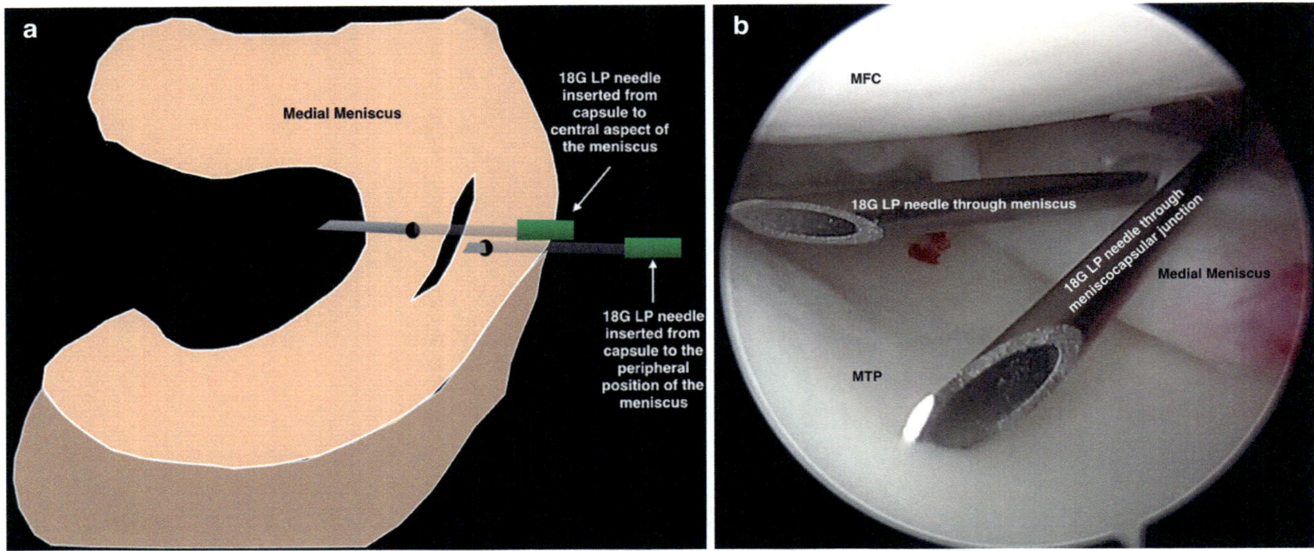


**Fig. 9.6** (**a**) Illustration showing two 18G LP needles on through the peripheral meniscus and the other through the meniscus tissue central to the tear while viewing through the AL portal. (**b**) Arthroscopic image showing the two 18G LP needles one from the peripheral meniscus and the other from the meniscus tissue central to the tear, viewing through the AL portal

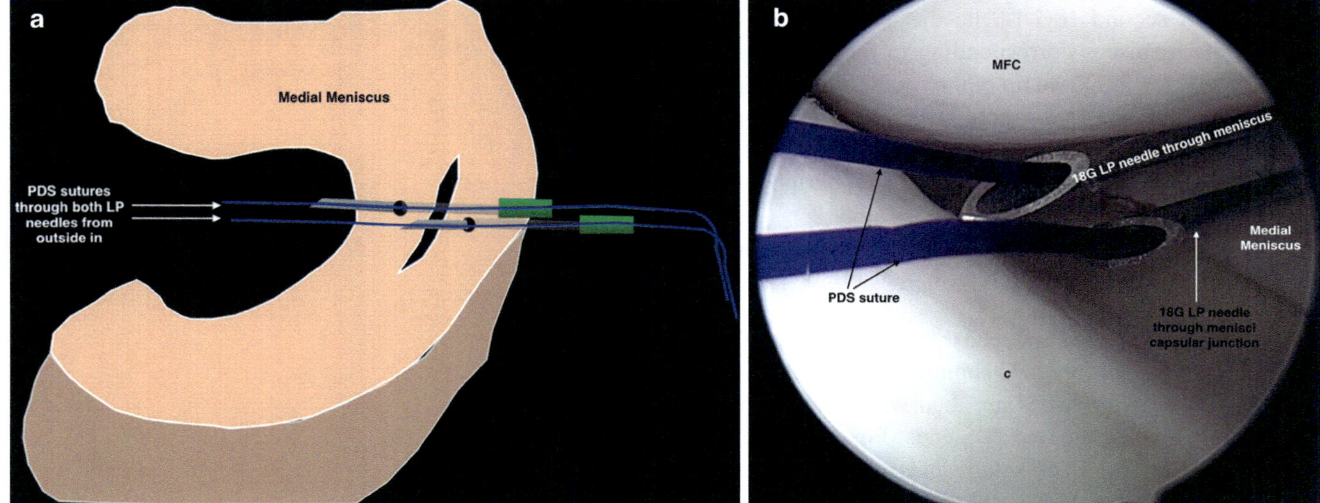


**Fig. 9.7** (**a**) Illustration showing PDS sutures passed through the LP needles from externally to into the joint while viewing through the AL portal. (**b**) Arthroscopic image showing two PDS sutures coming out of the two needles while viewing through the AL portal

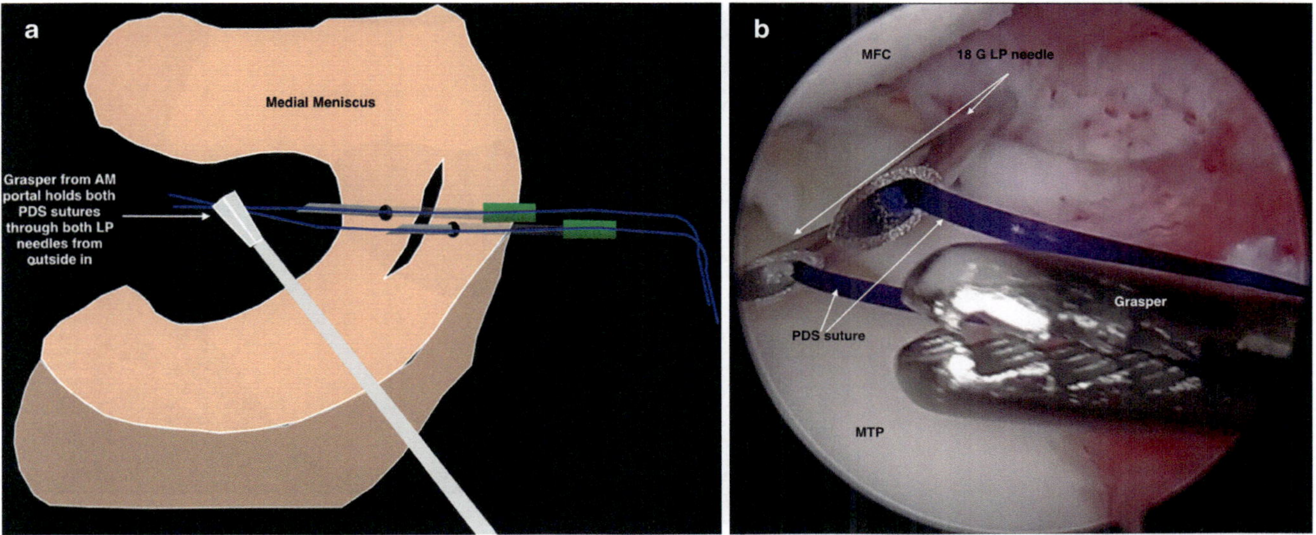


**Fig. 9.8** (**a**) Illustration showing a grasper from the AM portal grasping the two PDS sutures while viewing through the AL portal. (**b**) Grasper holding both PDS sutures while viewing through the AL portal

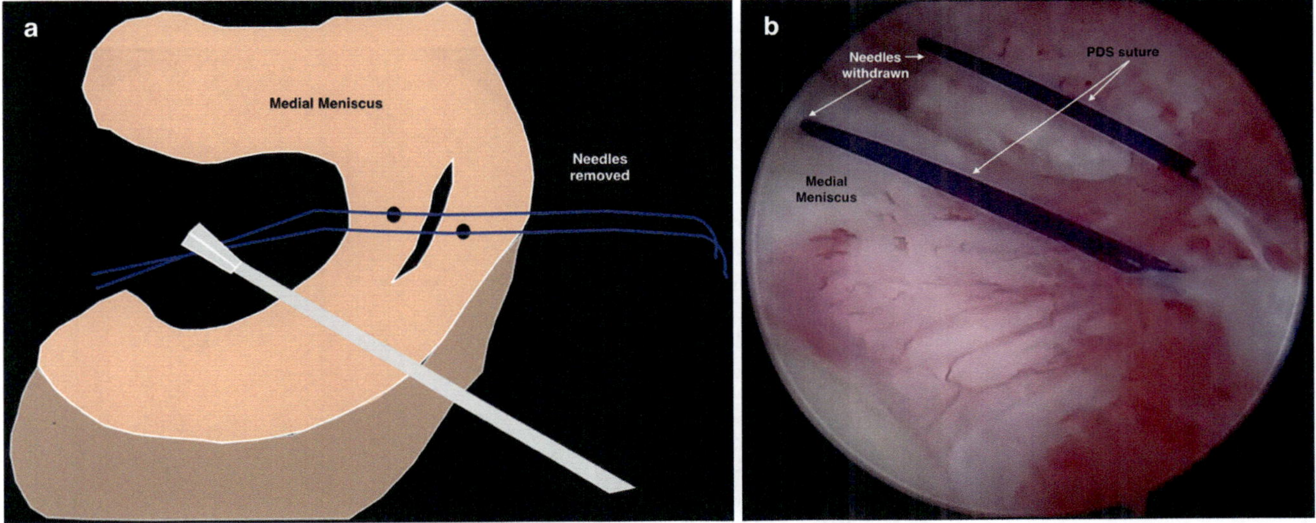


**Fig. 9.9** (**a**) Illustration showing the two needles withdrawn externally as the grasper continues to hold the two PDS sutures while viewing through the AL portal. (**b**) Arthroscopic image of the two needles being withdrawn and showing the two PDS sutures viewing from the AL portal

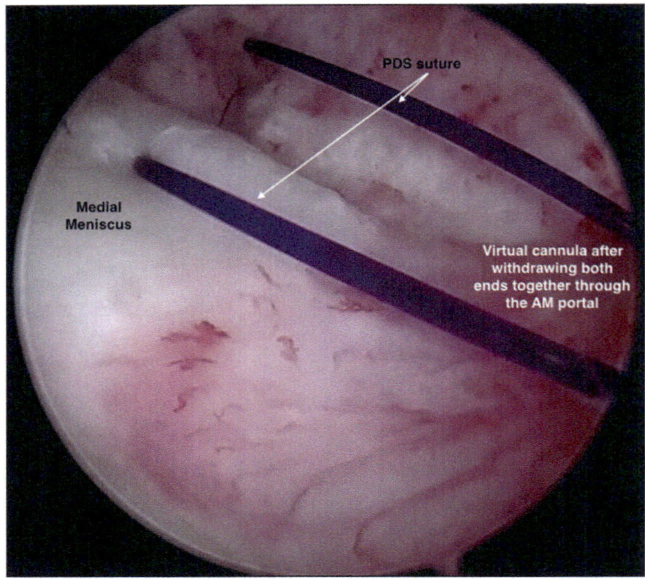


**Fig. 9.10** Arthroscopic view of the two PDS sutures withdrawn simultaneously through the AM portal while viewing through the AL portal

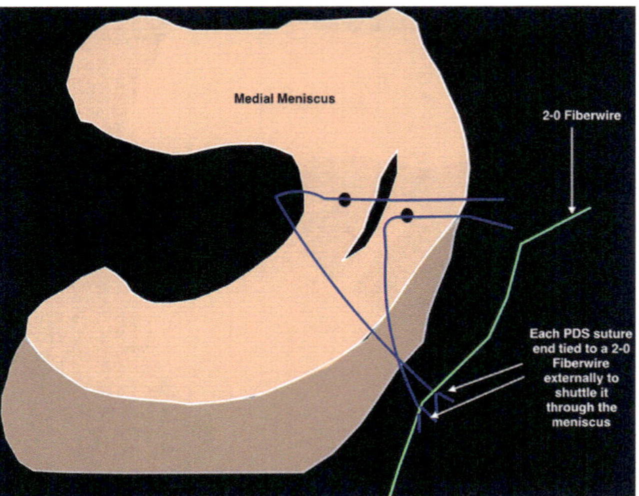


**Fig. 9.11** Illustration showing the two ends of the PDS tied to two ends of a 2-0 Fiberwire to shuttle it in place of the PDS through the medial meniscus

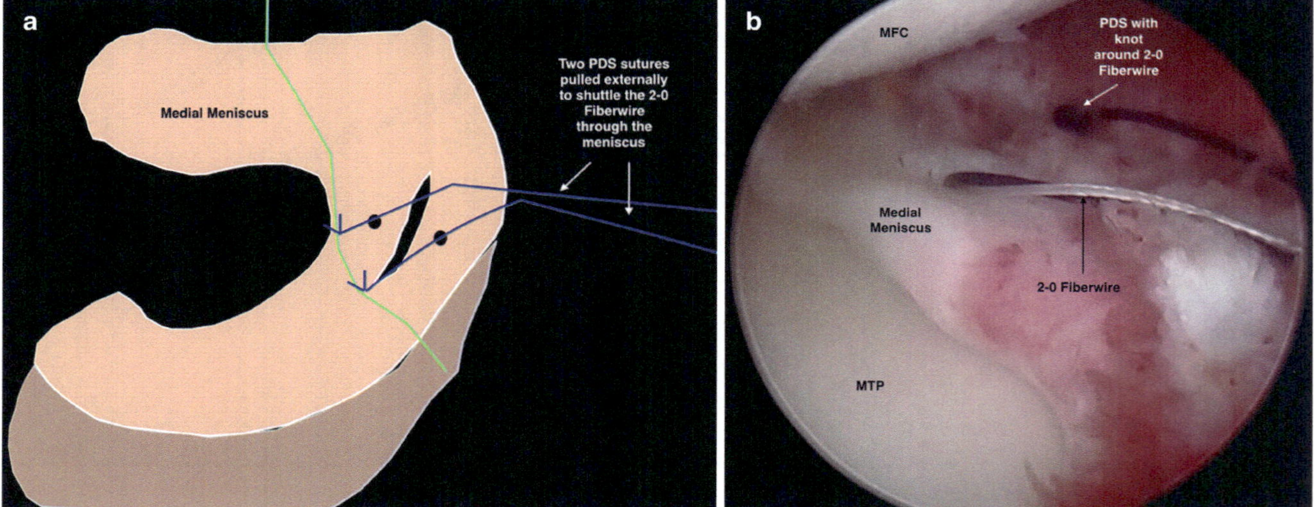


**Fig. 9.12** (**a**) Illustration showing the 2-0 Fiberwire being shuttled through the medial meniscus viewing through the AL portal. (**b**) Arthroscopic image of the knee showing the 2-0 Fiberwire being shuttled through the medial meniscus using the two PDS sutures viewing from the AL portal

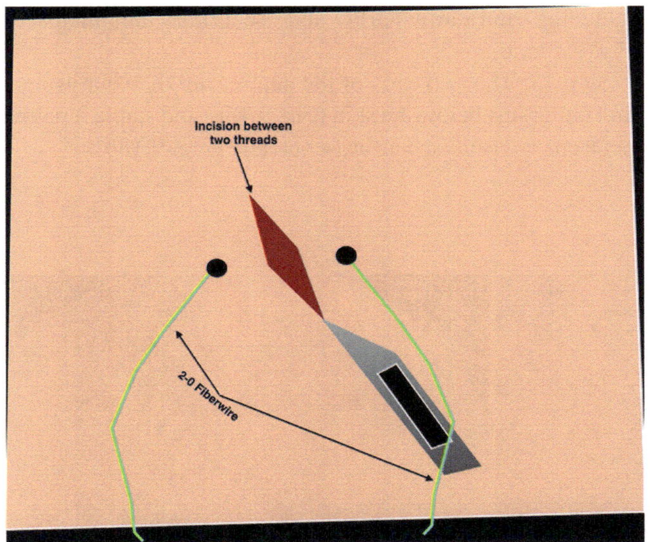


**Fig. 9.13** Illustration showing an incision being made between the points where the two ends of the 2-0 Fiberwire come out of the skin

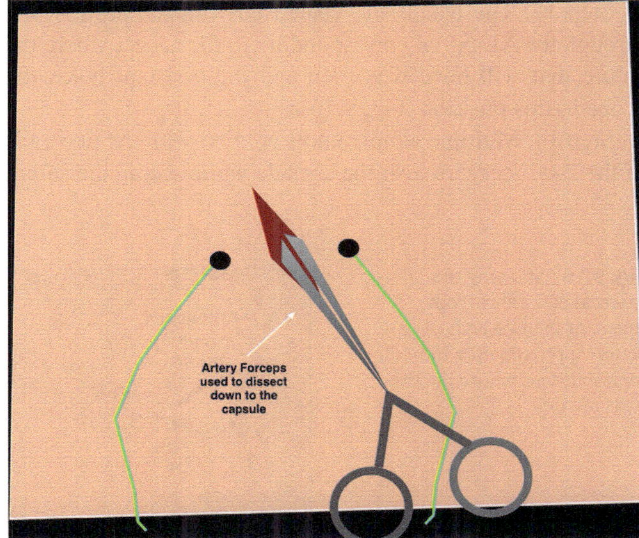


**Fig. 9.14** Illustration showing an artery forceps dissecting the tissue till the capsule corresponding to the repaired area of the meniscus

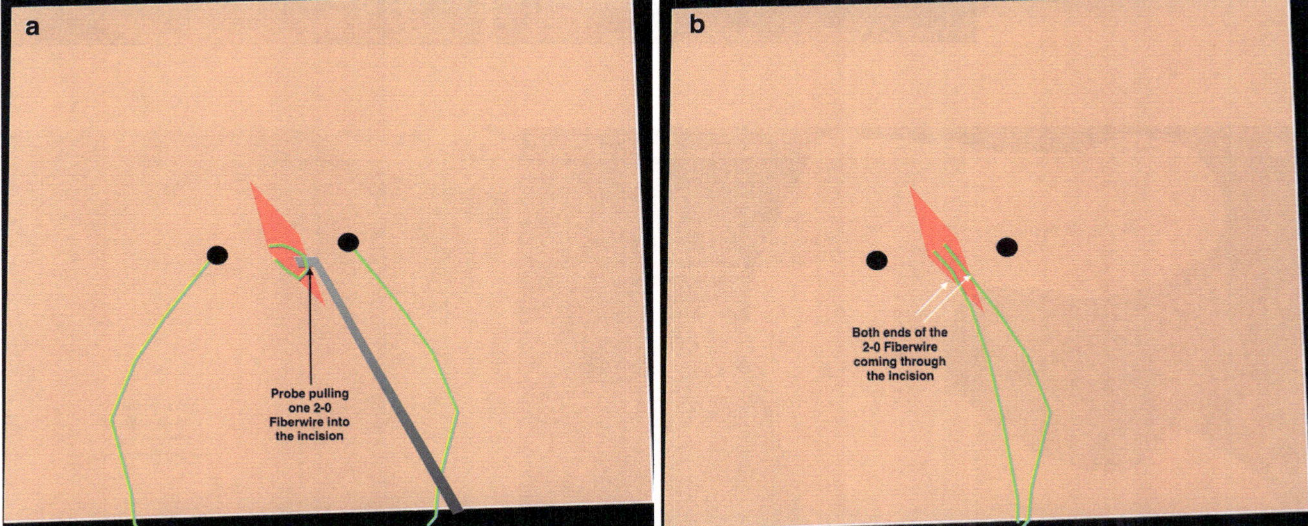


**Fig. 9.15** (**a**) Illustration showing an arthroscopic probe delivering one end of the suture through the incision. (**b**) Illustration showing an arthroscopic probe delivering the other end of the 2-0 Fiberwire through the wound

Step 13: The tear is the visualised with the arthroscope through the AL portal corresponding to the aspect where the suture that will be tied is seen and the assistant holds the scope in this position (Fig. 9.16).

Step 14: Multiple simple knots are tied with the two ends of the 2-0 Fiberwire over the capsule while seeing the suture tightening intra-articularly and securing the meniscus (Fig. 9.17a, b).

Step 15: The two ends of the sutures are then cut using a knot cutter just below the skin (Fig. 9.18a) and stable repaired meniscus is visualised arthroscopically (Fig. 9.18b).

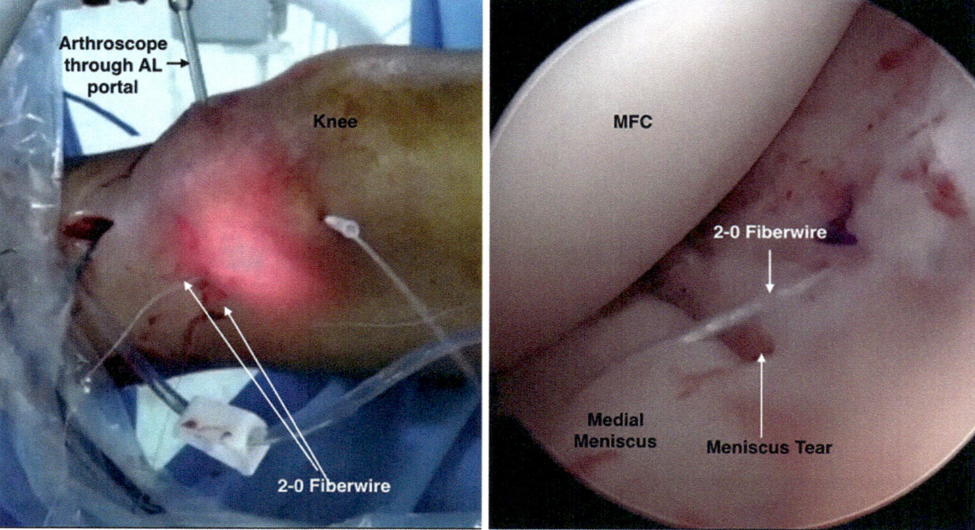


**Fig. 9.16** Showing the external and arthroscopic image of the two ends of suture approximating the meniscus tear before the two ends are tied

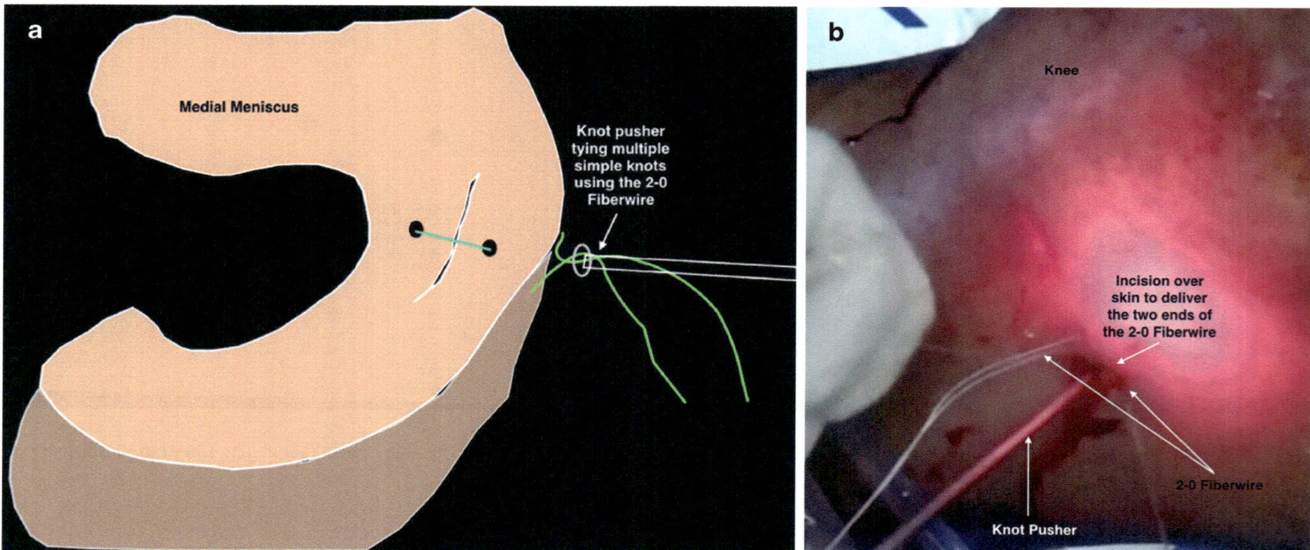


**Fig. 9.17** (**a**) Illustration of the two ends of the 2-0 Fiberwire being tied with a knot pusher while visualising the sutures in the knee through the AL portal. (**b**) External image showing the two ends of the 2-0 Fiberwire being tied with multiple simple knots using a knot pusher while visualising the sutures in the knee through the AL portal. The arthroscope is held by the assistant

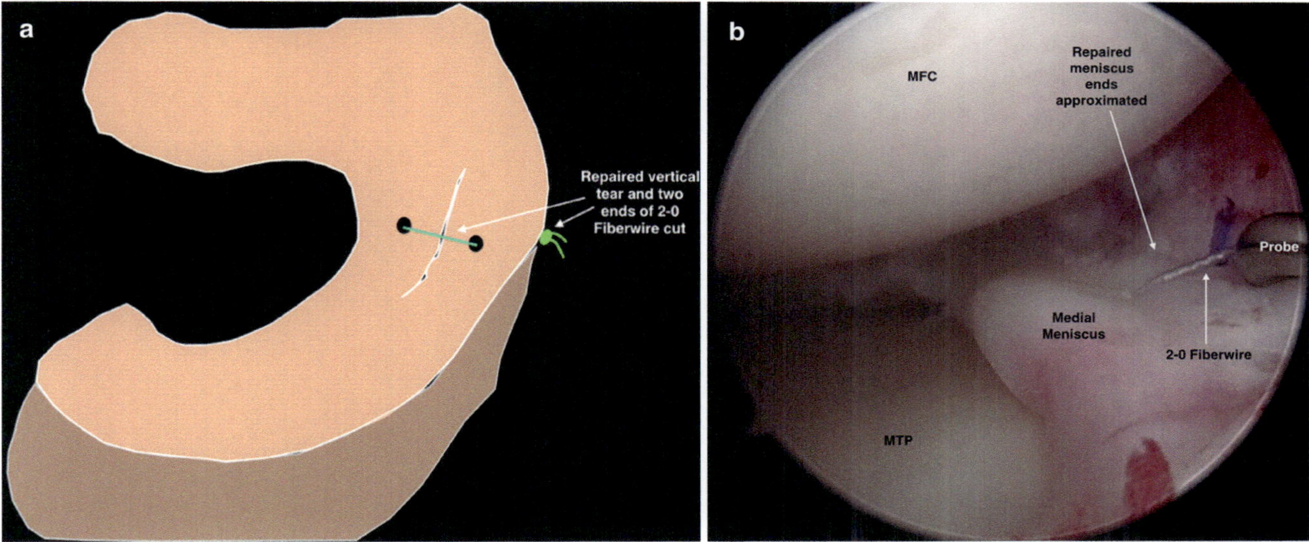


**Fig. 9.18** (**a**) Illustration of the two ends of the 2-0 Fiberwire after being cut by a suture cutter. (**b**) Arthroscopic image of the meniscus tear repaired after tying the knots

## 9.6 Tips and Tricks

1. Transilluminance helps in identifying where to pass the 18G LP needle.
2. Even if the entry is slightly off position, the needle tip can be manipulated in the subcutaneous plane without withdrawing the needle.
3. After holding the two ends of the PDS with a grasper intra-articularly, withdrawing the needle helps in easy passage of the Fiberwire 2-0.

## 9.7 Advantages and Disadvantages

**Advantages**

1. Needles utilised (18G spinal needles) are normal needles available in the OT used for spinal anaesthesia.
2. Technique eliminates trapping a suture with a loop/chia wire intra-articularly that can be technically demanding.
3. Arthroscopic visualisation of the sutures while tying them makes sure that the repair is stable and the tear is approximated securely.

**Disadvantages**

1. Potentially more time consuming than the standard technique
2. The PDS suture knots to shuttle the 2-0 Fiberwire may make the holes in the meniscus larger or may not pass easily through the meniscus.

# Arthroscopic Single Portal RAMP Repair Technique

# 10

Vikram Arun Mhaskar

## 10.1 Introduction

RAMP repairs occur in association with ACL tears and can be a cause of a high grade pivot shift test [1]. They occur in the posteromedial corner of the knee and refer to a type of menisco-tibial separation. They can be repaired either using all inside or inside out devices introduced from the anterior compartment of the knee or using an all inside technique using suture lasso or an antegrade suture passer introduced from the posteromedial compartment. We describe one such technique that uses a single posteromedial portal and a suture lasso to repair the RAMP lesion.

## 10.2 Specialised Equipment (Fig. 10.1)

1. 7 mm transparent cannula (Arthrex, Naples, FL) (a)
2. Suture lasso 45° curved right and left facing (Arthrex, Naples, FL) (b,c)
3. PDS suture (Ethicon, Raritan, NJ) (d)
4. Arthroscopic grasper (Smith & Nephew, Raritan, NJ)

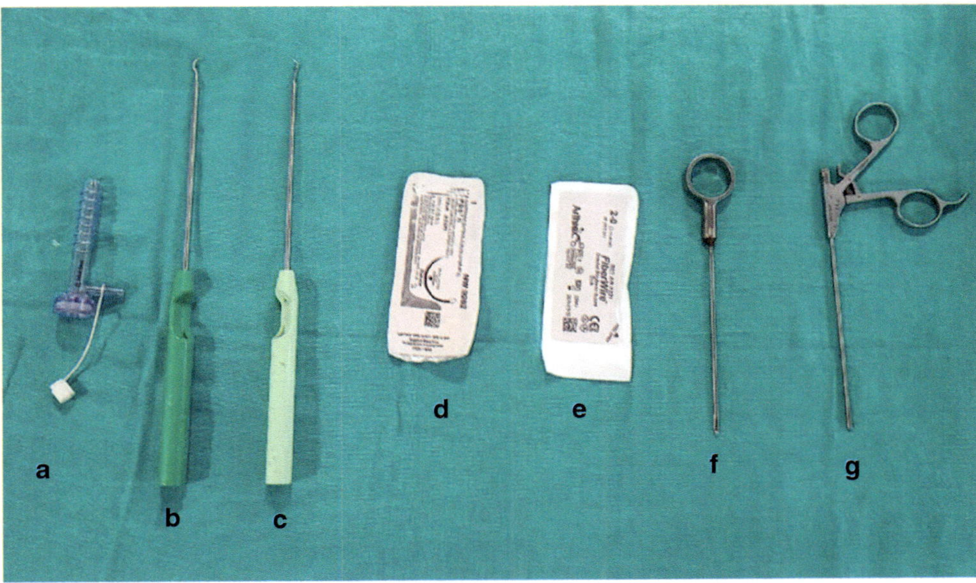


**Fig. 10.1** (**a**) 7 mm cannula, (**b, c**) suture passers, (**d**) PDS suture, (**e**) 2-0 Fiberwire, (**f**) Knot Pusher, (**g**) Suture Cutter

V. A. Mhaskar (✉)
F7 East of Kailash, Knee & Shoulder Clinic, New Delhi, India

JMVM Sports Injury Center, Sitaram Bhartia Institute of Science & Research, New Delhi, India


V. A. Mhaskar, J. Maheshwari (eds.), *Innovative Approaches in Knee Arthroscopy*,
https://doi.org/10.1007/978-981-99-4378-4_10

## 10.3 Positioning (Fig. 10.2)

Patient is kept supine on the operating table with a side support at the level of the upper thigh and a bolster on the OT table such that the knee is in 70° flexion.

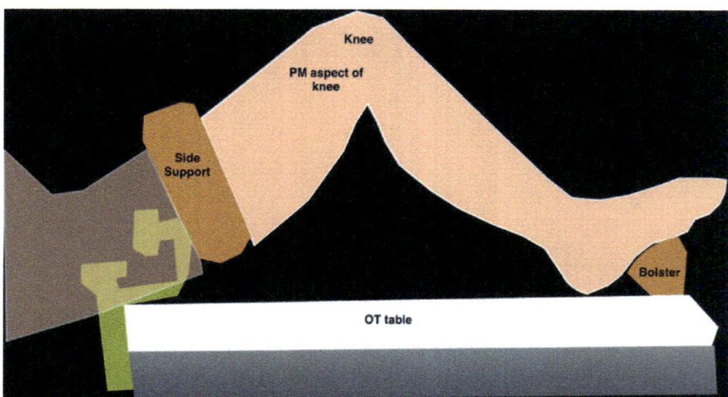


**Fig. 10.2** Illustration of the knee position in 70° flexion with adequate access to the posteromedial and posterolateral aspects of the knee while doing a Ramp repair

## 10.4 Portals (Fig. 10.3a, b)

1. High anterolateral (AL) vertical viewing portal at the level of the lower pole of the patella just adjacent to the patellar tendon.
2. Posteromedial portal just above the synovial fold, first localised by introducing an 18 G LP needle then making the portal. A 7 mm clear cannula is introduced through it.

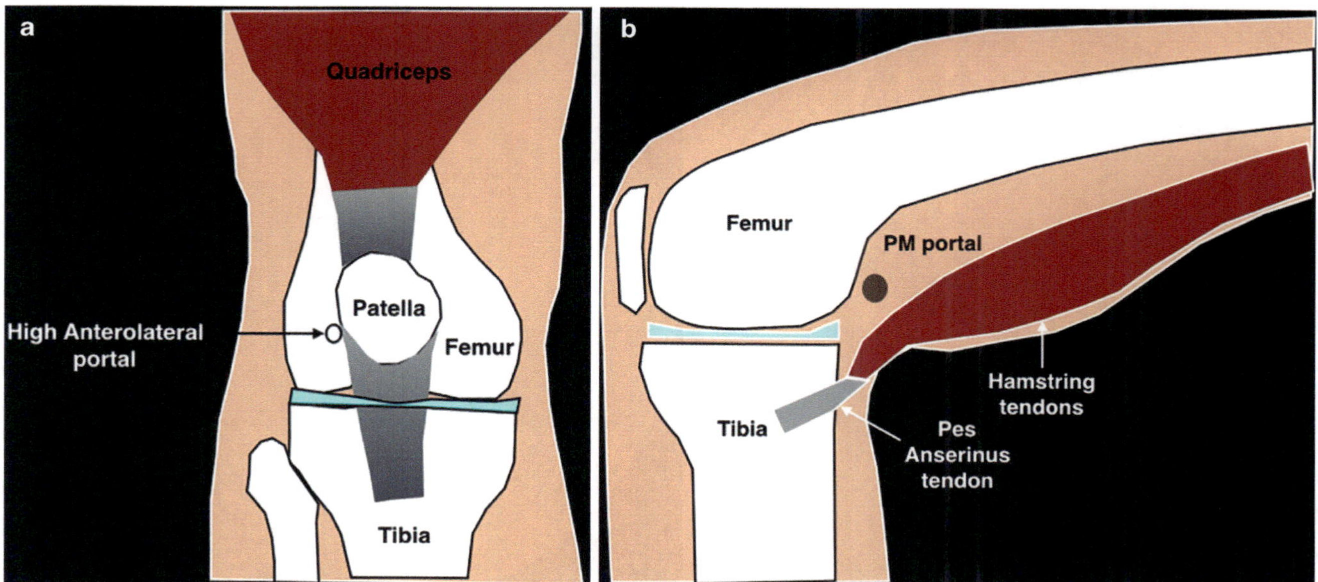


**Fig. 10.3** (**a**) Illustration of the front of the knee showing a high anterolateral viewing portal. (**b**) Illustration of the medial aspect of the knee showing a posteromedial working portal

## 10.5 Surgical Steps

Step 1: The arthroscope is introduced through the anterolateral portal and the scope is manipulated in between the PCL and medial femoral condyle with a slight valgus applied to the knee in 70° flexion (Fig. 10.4).

Step 2: The RAMP tear is visualised (Fig. 10.5a, b).

Step 3: The posteromedial region corresponding to the PM compartment in the knee visualised arthroscopically is identified via transillumination. Using the finger to exert pressure from outside on the skin and visualising it at the level of the synovial fold internally indicating the correct level to make the portal (Fig. 10.6).

Step 4: An 18G LP needle is then introduced at that level such that the tip exits inside the knee just above the synovial fold. An No 11 blade is used to make a vertical incision in the skin and capsule to make the PM portal. A Vissinger rod is then introduced from outside in.

Step 5: A 7 mm clear cannula is then cannulated over this Vissinger rod so that at least two turns of the cannula are intra-articular (Fig. 10.7a, b).

Step 6: A diamond rasp followed by a shaver is introduced through the PM portal while viewing from the AL portal between the tear and it is freshened (Fig. 10.8a–c).

Step 7: A 45° curved lasso loaded with a PDS is then introduced through this cannula (Fig. 10.9a, b).

Step 8: A bite is taken through the capsule and then the posterior horn of the meniscus using this lasso (Fig. 10.10a, b).

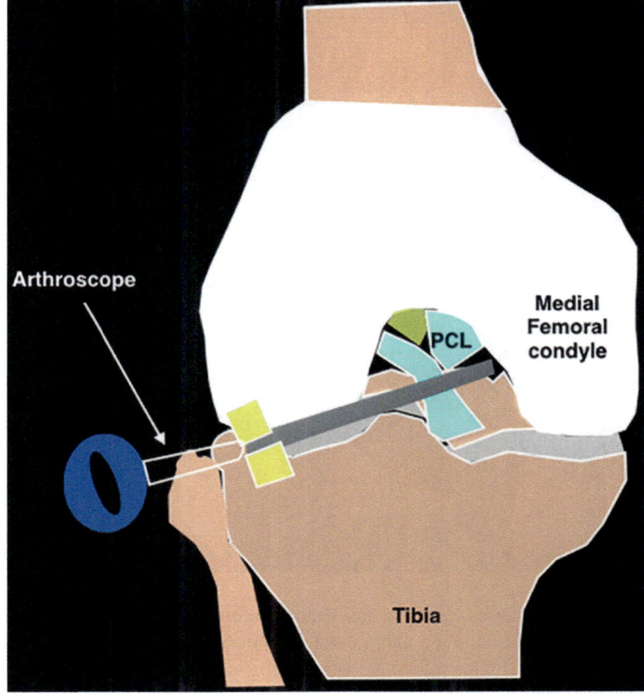


**Fig. 10.4** Illustration of the front of the knee showing the arthroscope being manipulated between the PCL and medial femoral condyle to the posteromedial aspect of the knee

Step 9: Once the tip exits the meniscus tissue, the PDS suture is pushed through till most of its length is intra-articular in the posteromedial compartment (Fig. 10.11a, b).

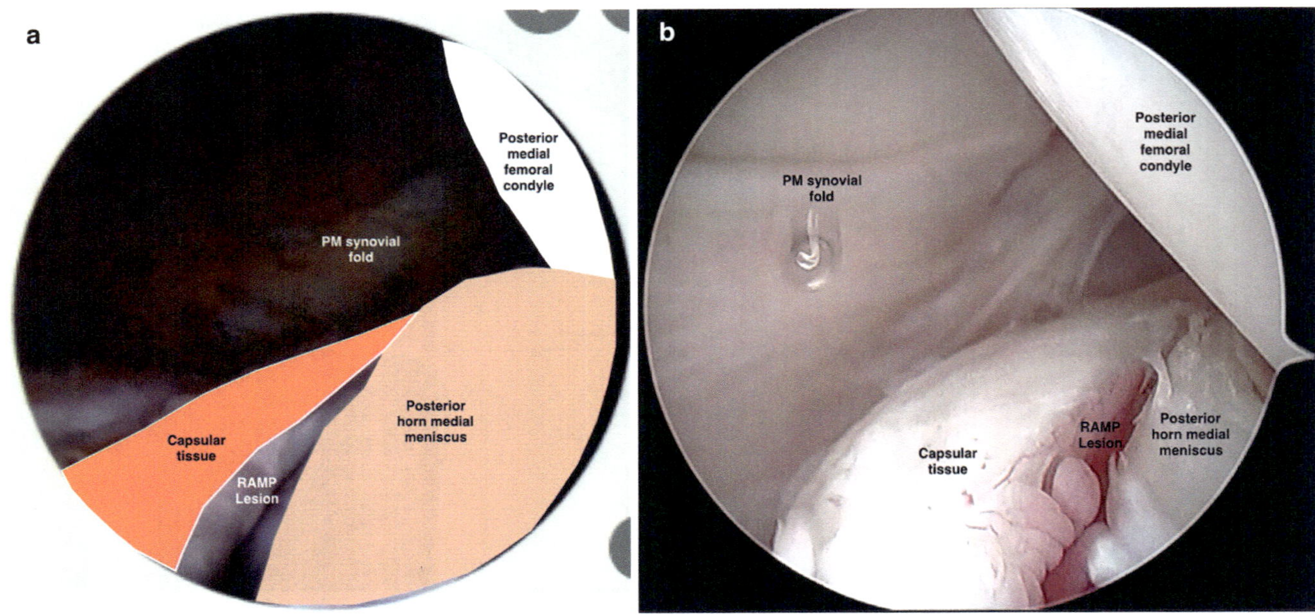


**Fig. 10.5** (**a**) Illustration of the posteromedial aspect of the knee showing a RAMP lesion. (**b**) Arthroscopic image of the posteromedial aspect of the knee showing a RAMP lesion

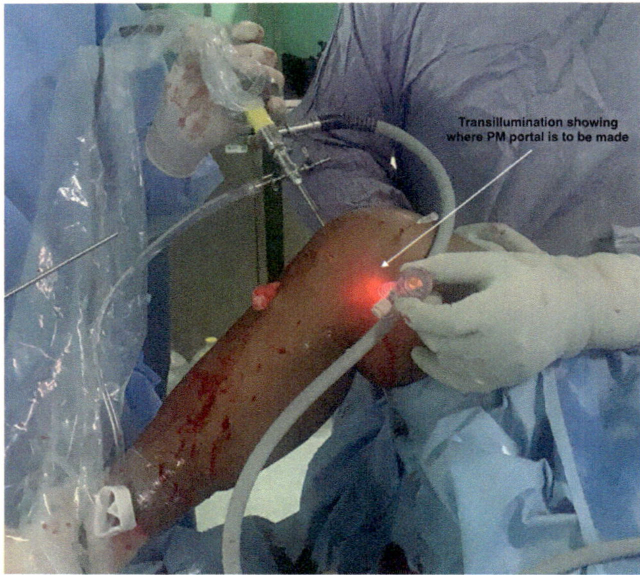


**Fig. 10.6** External image of transillumination of the region where the PM portal is to be made and a cannula applied externally to show the location

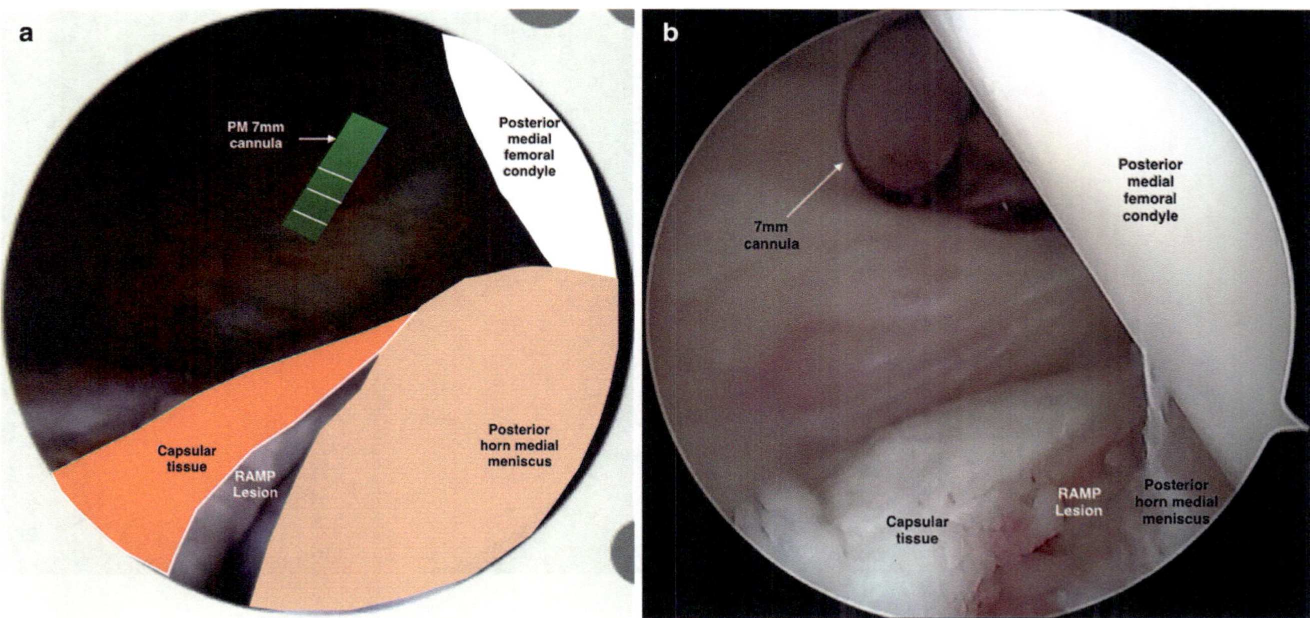


**Fig. 10.7** (**a**) Illustration of posteromedial aspect of the knee showing a 7 mm cannula applied to the PM portal. (**b**) Arthroscopic image of the posteromedial aspect of the knee showing a 7 mm cannula in the PM portal

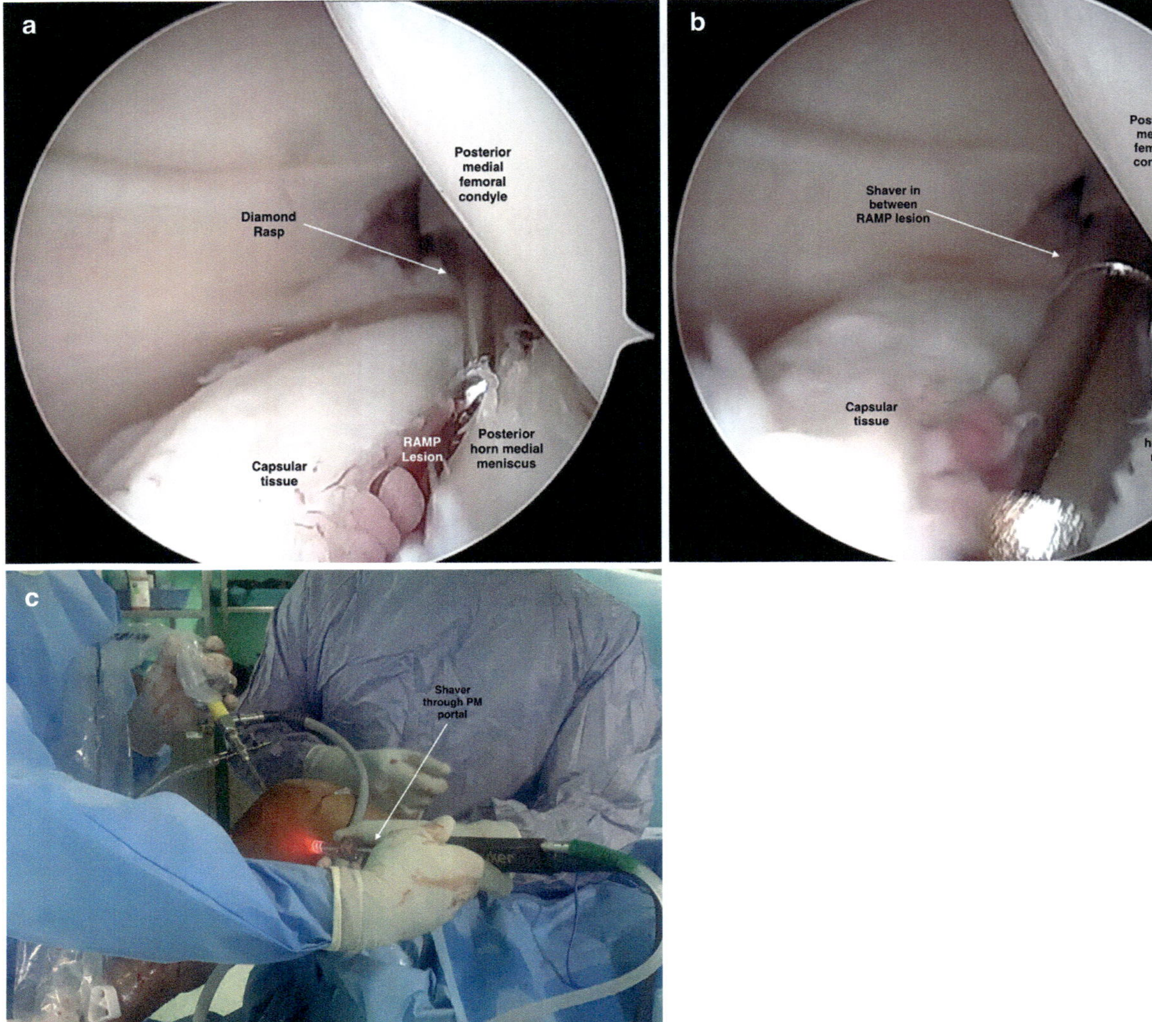


**Fig. 10.8** (**a**) Arthroscopic image of the posteromedial aspect of the knee showing a diamond rasp in the RAMP lesion to freshen it. (**b**) Arthroscopic image of the PM aspect of the knee showing a shaver in the RAMP lesion to freshen it. (**c**) External image of shaver being introduced through the PM portal while viewing through the AL portal

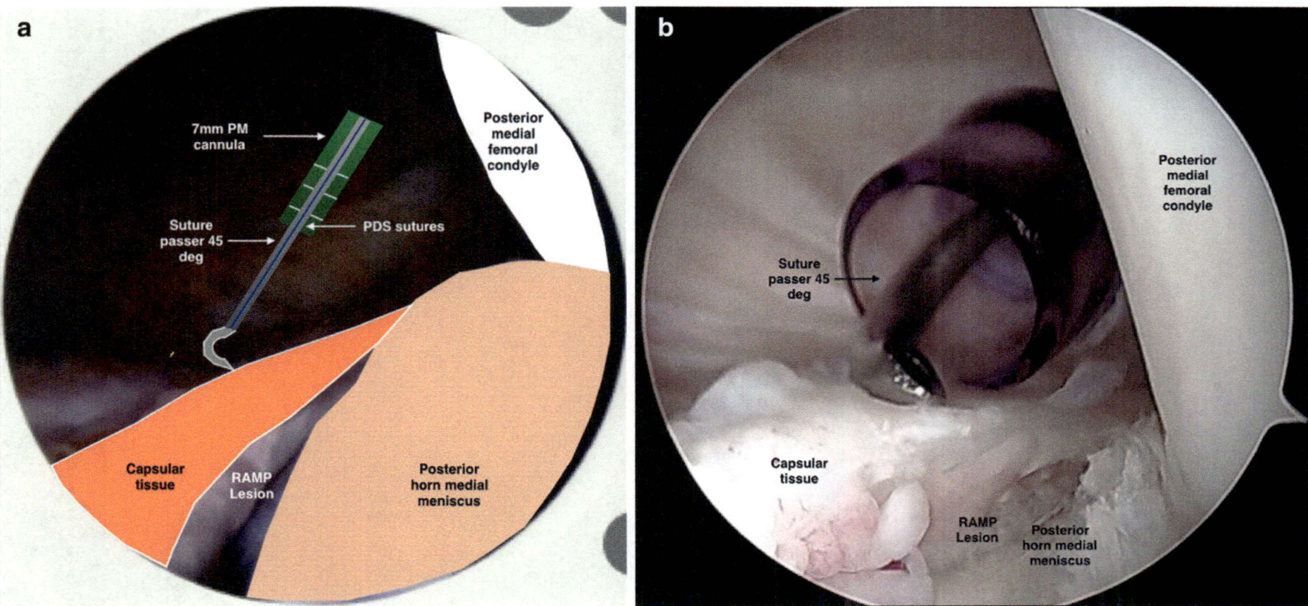


**Fig. 10.9** (**a**) Illustration of the PM aspect of the knee showing a 45° suture lasso introduced through the PM portal. (**b**) Arthroscopic image of the PM aspect of the knee showing a 45° curved suture lasso through the PM portal

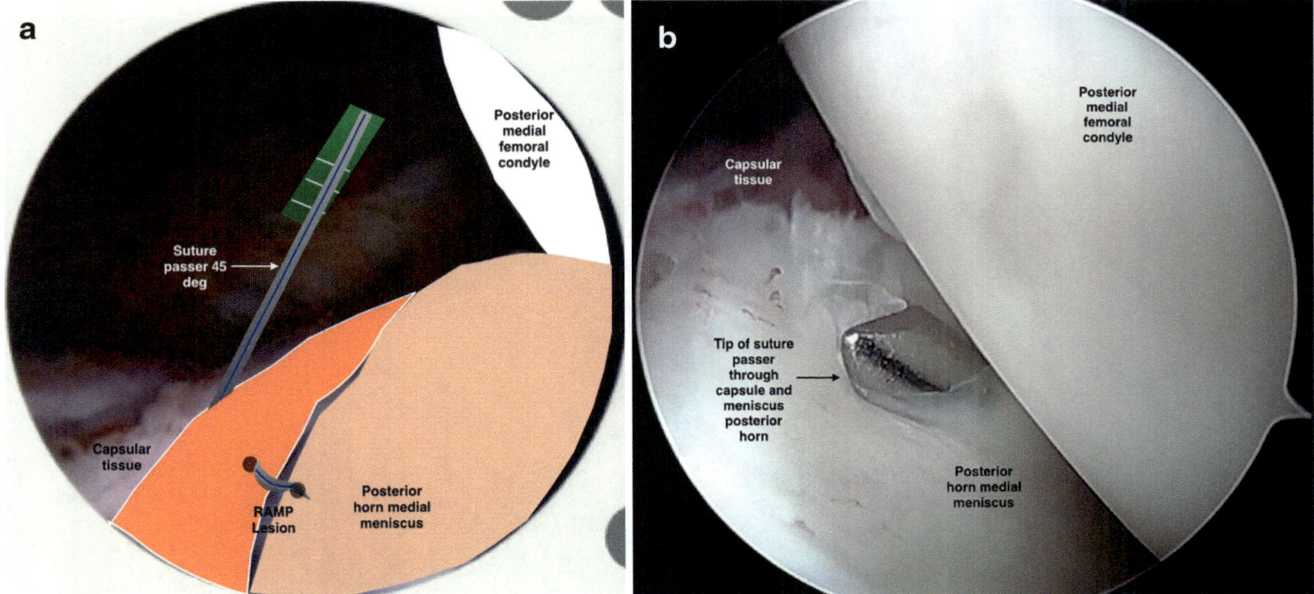


**Fig. 10.10** (**a**) Illustration of the PM aspect of the knee showing the suture lasso taking a bite through the capsular and meniscus tissue adjoining the RAMP lesion. (**b**) Arthroscopic image of the PM aspect of the knee showing the suture lasso tip coming out through the meniscus tissue after passing through the capsular tissue adjoining the RAMP lesion

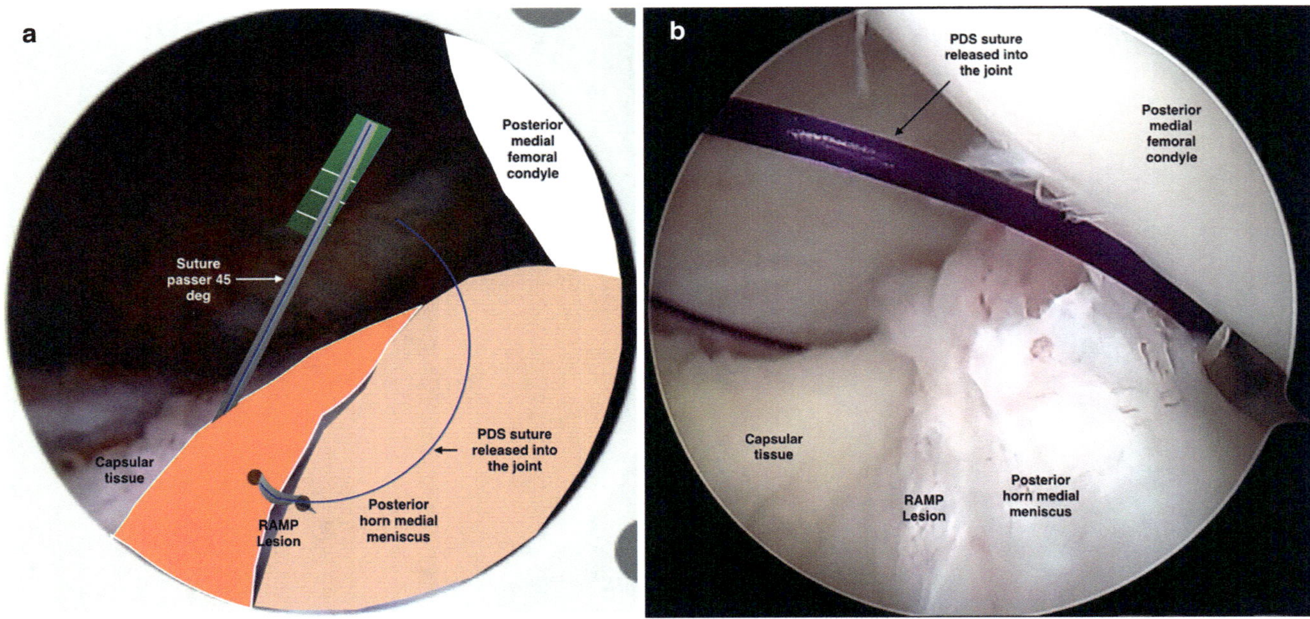


**Fig. 10.11** (**a**) Illustration of the PM aspect of the knee showing the PDS suture being released after taking a bite. (**b**) Arthroscopic image of the PDS suture released into the PM aspect of the knee after taking a bite to

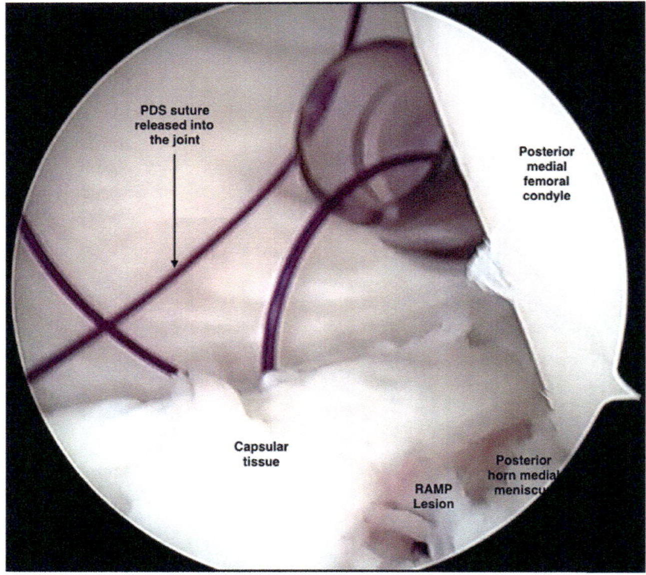


**Fig. 10.12** Arthroscopic image of the PM aspect of the knee showing the PDS suture coming out of the capsule and meniscus and through the PM portal

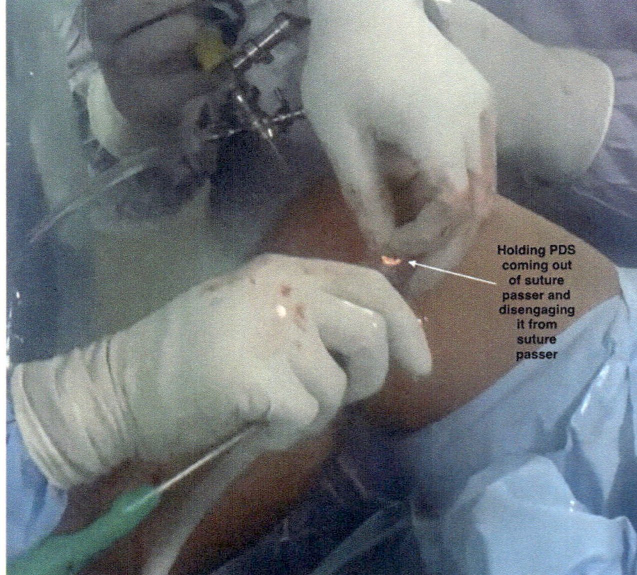


**Fig. 10.13** External image showing the PDS suture coming from the suture passer being disengaged from it close to the cannula mouth so as not to disengage the suture coming from the meniscus after taking a bite

Step 10: The suture passer is then gently removed from the meniscus and capsular tissue by gently twisting it out along the curvature of the end of the suture passer (Fig. 10.12).

Step 11: It is then withdrawn from the cannula till the tip just exits the entry of the cannula, when the PDS just distal to the tip is held firmly and PDS disengaged from the suture passer (Fig. 10.13).

Step 12: One end of the PDS is through the cannula, a grasper is introduced into the cannula to grasp the other end

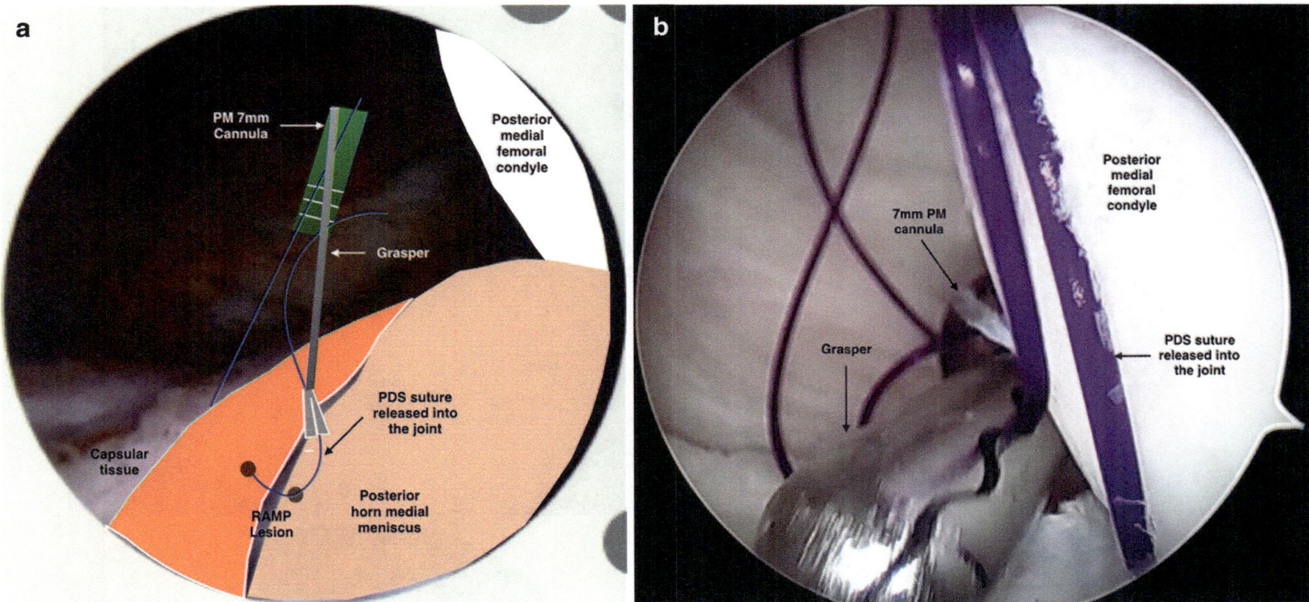


**Fig. 10.14** (**a**) Illustration of the PM aspect of the knee showing a grasper holding the PDS suture coming from the meniscus delivered through the PM portal. (**b**) Arthroscopic image of the PM aspect of the knee showing a grasper in the PM portal holding the PDS coming out from the meniscus tissue

of the PDS and withdraw it through the PM cannula (Fig. 10.14a, b).

Step 13: Multiple simple knots (At least five) are tied using a knot pusher through the PM cannula (Fig. 10.15a–e).

Step 14: An arthroscopic knot cutter is then used to cut the two ends of the suture such that they are at least 0.5 cm long (Fig. 10.16a, b).

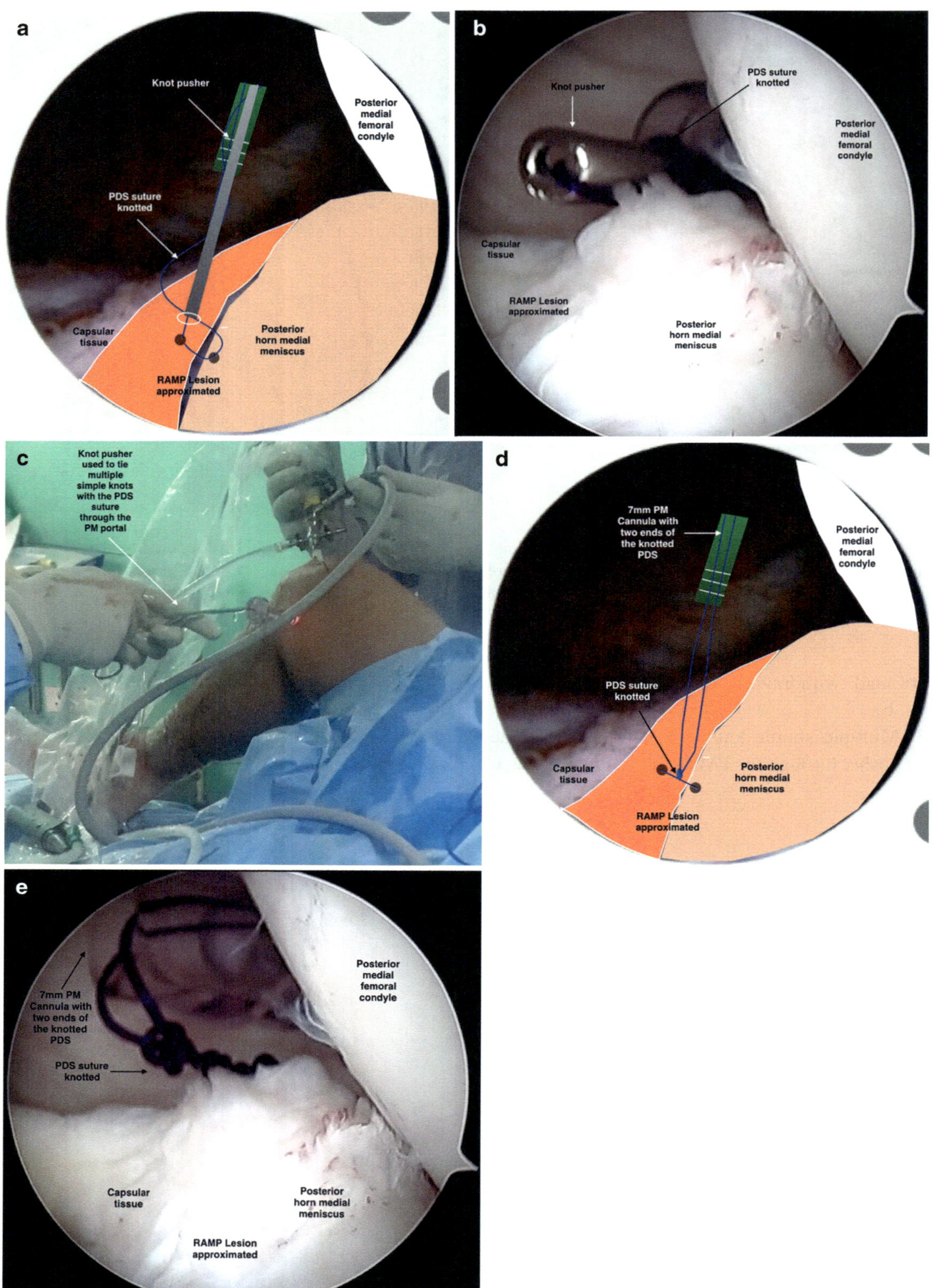


**Fig. 10.15** (**a**) Illustration of the PM aspect of the knee showing a knot pusher tying a simple knot on the two ends of the PDS suture. (**b**) Arthroscopic image of the PM aspect of the knee showing a knot pusher tying simple knots to approximate the RAMP lesion. (**c**) External image of tying multiple simple knots using a knot pusher with the PDS suture through the PM portal while viewing from the AM portal. (**d**) Illustration of the PM aspect of the knee showing multiple simple knots tied to approximate the RAMP tear. (**e**) Arthroscopic image of the PM aspect of the knee showing multiple knots tied to the PDS suture to approximate the RAMP lesion

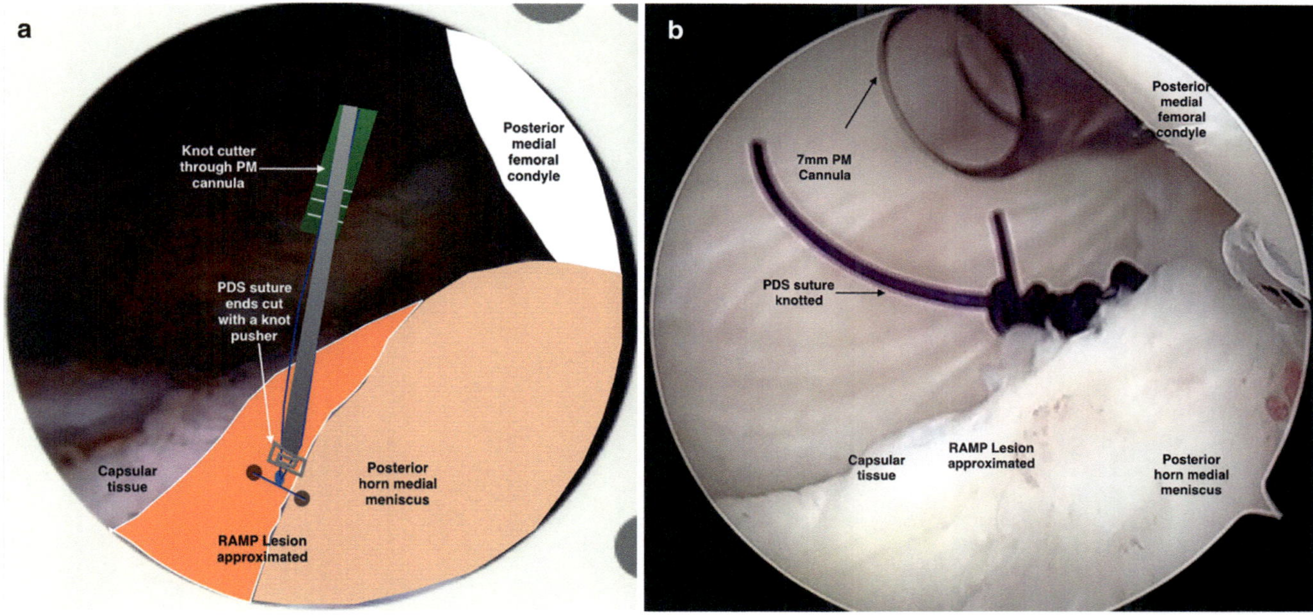


**Fig. 10.16** (**a**) Illustration of the PM aspect of the knee showing a knot cutter through the PM portal cutting the two ends of the PDS suture. (**b**) Arthroscopic image of the PM aspect of the knee showing a repaired RAMP lesion using PDS sutures and multiple simple knots

## 10.6 Tips and Tricks

1. Release a long loop of PDS in the joint so that it does not get disengaged when the lasso is removed.
2. While the lasso is taken out of the cannula, hold the suture at its tip while disengaging the lasso from the suture to avoid the suture from coming out of the tissue.
3. Tie multiple knots with a knot pusher as knot security of the PDS is low and do not over tighten as it may break.

## 10.7 Advantages and Disadvantages

**Advantages**

1. Uses only a single posteromedial portal.
2. Tying simple knots gives more control on the tension of the knots.
3. Uses absorbable sutures.

**Disadvantages**

1. Technically more demanding than all inside devices as one has to make a PM portal.
2. More chances of one end of the PDS suture coming out of the meniscus or capsular tissue when the suture passer is withdrawn.
3. Knot security in a PDS suture is less than Fiberwire so more knots are required.

## Reference

1. Taneja AK, Miranda FC, Rosemberg LA, Santos DCB. Meniscal ramp lesions: an illustrated review. Insights Imaging. 2021;12(1):134. https://doi.org/10.1186/s13244-021-01080-9. PMID: 34564751; PMCID: PMC8464645.

# 11 Arthroscopic Meniscus Root Repair with Centralisation

Vikram Arun Mhaskar

## 11.1 Introduction

Meniscus root tears are comparable to a total meniscectomy. Compromised hoop stresses lead to decreased tibio-femoral contact area and thus increased pressures [1]. Root repairs are the mainstay of treatment in nonarthritic knees. Root repairs have been shown to improve outcomes, decrease extrusion, and in turn decrease the progression of osteoarthritis of the knee. Suture anchor and transtibial pull out sutures are the two main techniques with the latter being more popular [2, 3]. In recent times suture tapes are being used in place of normal sutures, as they do not have a less cheese grating effect on the meniscus, reducing the chances of pull out. Centralisation is a concept that is now popular as it has been shown that extrusion may not be reduced after a root repair. It involves reducing the extrusion by placing a suture anchor to the tibial articular surface just posterior to the MCL, taking bites through the meniscus and tying it down to the anchor [4]. This technique has produced favourable results in reducing extrusion.

## 11.2 Specialised Equipment (Fig. 11.1)

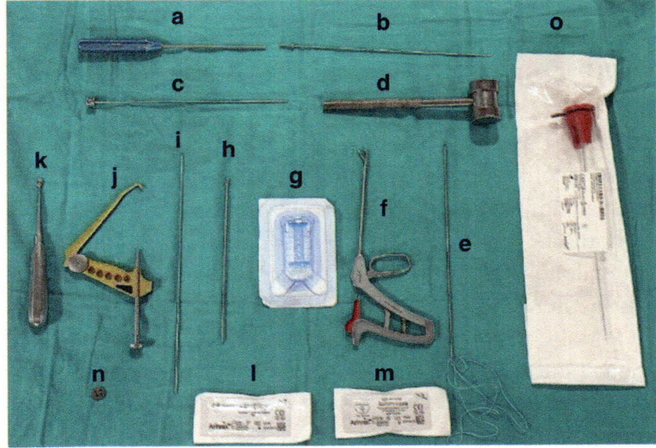


**Fig. 11.1** (**a**) Anchor sleeve, (**b**) drill bit for anchor, (**c**) Tamp, (**d**) Mallet, (**e**) Beath pin with No 5 Ethibond, (**f**) Knee Scorpion, (**g**) Passport Cannula, (**h**) 4.5 mm drill bit, (**i**) Beath pin, (**j**) ACL tibial guide, (**k**) Curette, (**l**) 2-0 Fiberwire, (**m**) Suture Tape, (**n**) Suture Disc, (**o**) 1.5 mm all suture anchor

1. Antegrade suture passer (Knee Scorpion) (Arthrex, Naples, FL) (f)
2. Suture tape-2 (Arthrex, Naples, FL) (m)
3. 2-0 Fiberwire (Arthrex, Naples, FL) (l)
4. Flexible Passport Cannula (Arthrex, Naples, FL) (g)
5. ACL Jig (Acufex, Smith & Nephew, Watford, UK) (j)
6. Suture disc (ABS Button) (Arthrex, Naples, FL) (n)
7. 1.8 mm all suture anchor (Arthrex, Naples, FL) (o)
8. Suture anchor sleeve (Arthrex, Naples, FL) (a)
9. Drill bit specific for suture anchor (Arthrex, Naples, FL) (b)
10. Knot pusher (Arthrex, Naples, FL)
11. Suture cutter (Arthrex, Naples, FL)

## 11.3 Positioning (Fig. 11.2)

Leg on the operating table with a side support and bolster at the end so that the knee is in 70° of flexion. The knee is extended to about 20° flexion and a valgus force applied to do the MCL pie crusting.

V. A. Mhaskar (✉)
F7 East of Kailash, Knee & Shoulder Clinic, New Delhi, India

JMVM Sports Injury Center, Sitaram Bhartia Institute of Science & Research, New Delhi, India


V. A. Mhaskar, J. Maheshwari (eds.), *Innovative Approaches in Knee Arthroscopy*,
https://doi.org/10.1007/978-981-99-4378-4_11

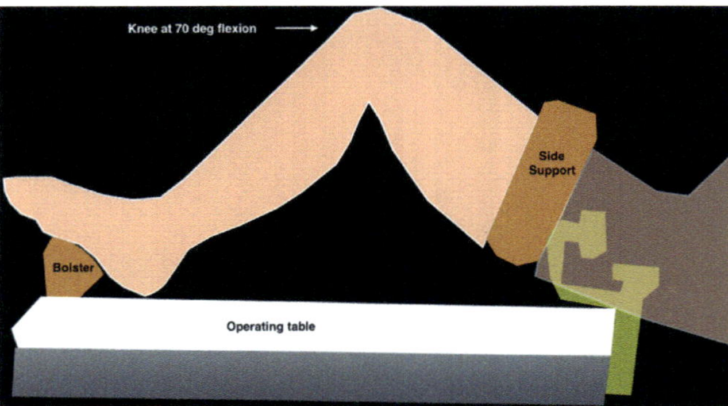


**Fig. 11.2** Illustration of the knee in 70° of flexion on the operating table with a side support and bolster at the end of the table

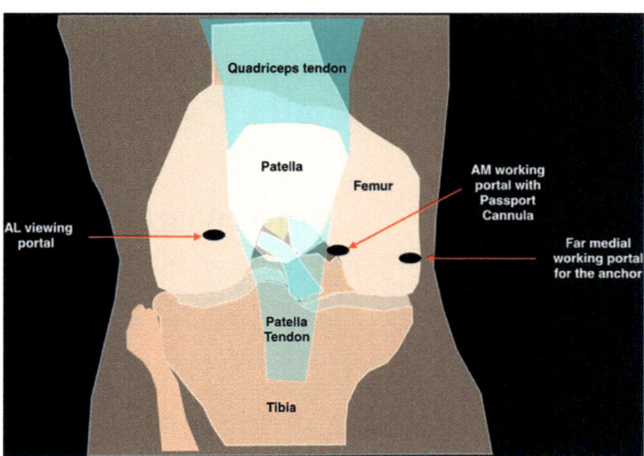


**Fig. 11.3** Illustration showing Portal A the AL portal for viewing and working during the centralisation part, Portal B the medial working portal used for viewing during the centralisation procedure, Portal C the far medial portal for applying the centralisation anchor

## 11.4 Portals (Fig. 11.3)

Portal A: Lateral viewing portal through the soft spot lateral to the patellar tendon just inferior to the inferior pole of the patella and just lateral to the patella tendon.

Portal B: Medial working portal 2 cm medial to the patellar tendon just above the medial meniscus made by introducing an 18G LP needle under vision.

Portal C: Portal is made with an 18G LP needle guidance about 1 cm above the meniscus and just posterior to the posterior border of the MCL corresponding to the body of the meniscus.

## 11.5 Surgical Steps

Step 1: The arthroscope is introduced through Portal A and the root tear visualised (Fig. 11.4a, b).

Step 2: A curette is introduced through Portal B and the Medial meniscus footprint posteriorly is curetted and prepared footprint visualised (Fig. 11.5a, b).

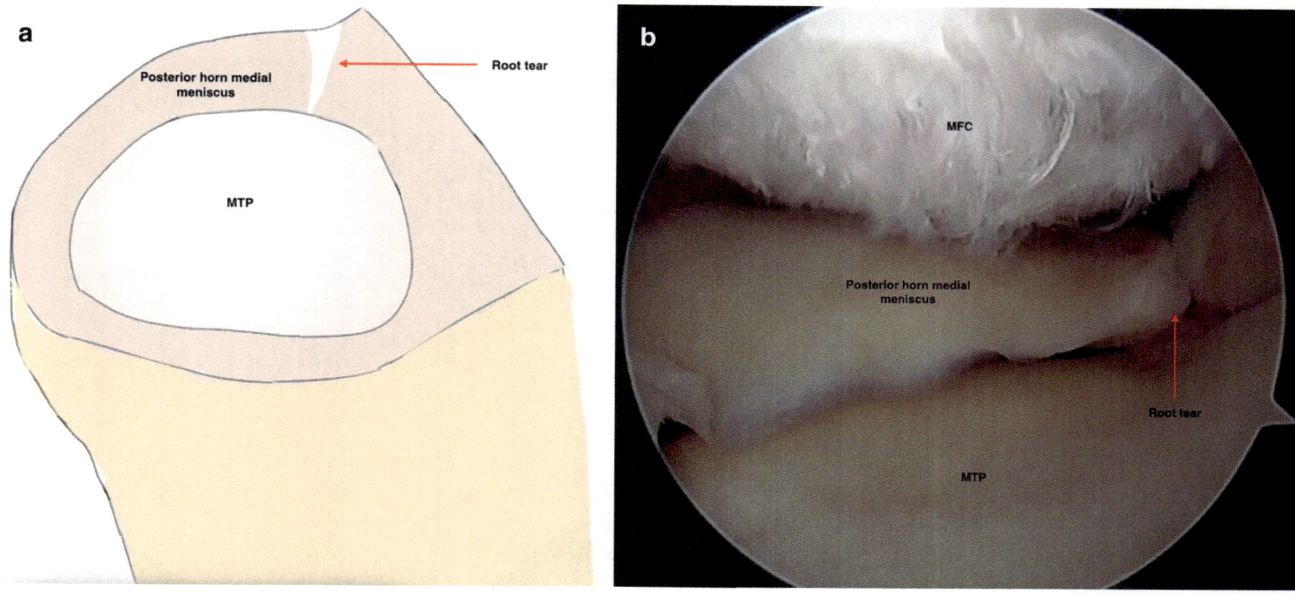


**Fig. 11.4** (**a**) Illustration of the medial meniscus root tear. (**b**) Arthroscopic image of the medial meniscus root tear viewing from the AL portal

Step 3: An ACL jig (Acufex, Smith & Nephew, Watford, UK) fixed at 60° flexion is introduced through Portal B at the centre of the footprint and the bullet applied to the anteromedial tibia and overdrilled with a guidewire (Fig. 11.6a, b).

Step 4: The guidewire is overdrilled with a 4.5 mm drill bit cannulated over it (Fig. 11.7a–c).

Step 5: A Passport cannula (Arthrex, Naples, FL) is applied through Portal B (Fig. 11.8).

Step 6: An antegrade suture passer carrying a 2-0 Fiberwire (Arthrex, Naples, FL) is passed through the cannula and bite taken through the posterior horn of the medial meniscus near the root (Fig. 11.9a–c).

Step 7: One end of the 2-0 Fiberwire is tied over one end of a Suture Tape (Arthrex, Naples, FL) to shuttle it through the meniscus (Fig. 11.10a, b).

Step 8: Same step is repeated for another Suture Tape through the posterior horn of the medial meniscus using the 2-0 Fiberwire just lateral to the first Suture Tape adjacent to the root (Fig. 11.11a, b).

Step 9: A Beath pin with a No 5 Ethibond loop (Ethicon, Raritan, NJ) is passed through the tibial tunnel from the anteromedial tibia to its opening on the meniscus root footprint (Fig. 11.12a, b).

Step 10: Deliver the loop through the cannula through Portal B using a suture manipulator (Fig. 11.13).

Step 11: The Suture tape ends in the cannula are applied to the Ethibond loop and delivered anteromedially on the tibia (Fig. 11.14a, b).

Step 12: While visualising the root arthroscopically, traction is applied to the Suture tapes that are tied over a Suture Disc on the anteromedial tibia (Fig. 11.15a, b).

Step 13: The repaired root tear is visualised and probed if stable (Fig 11.16).

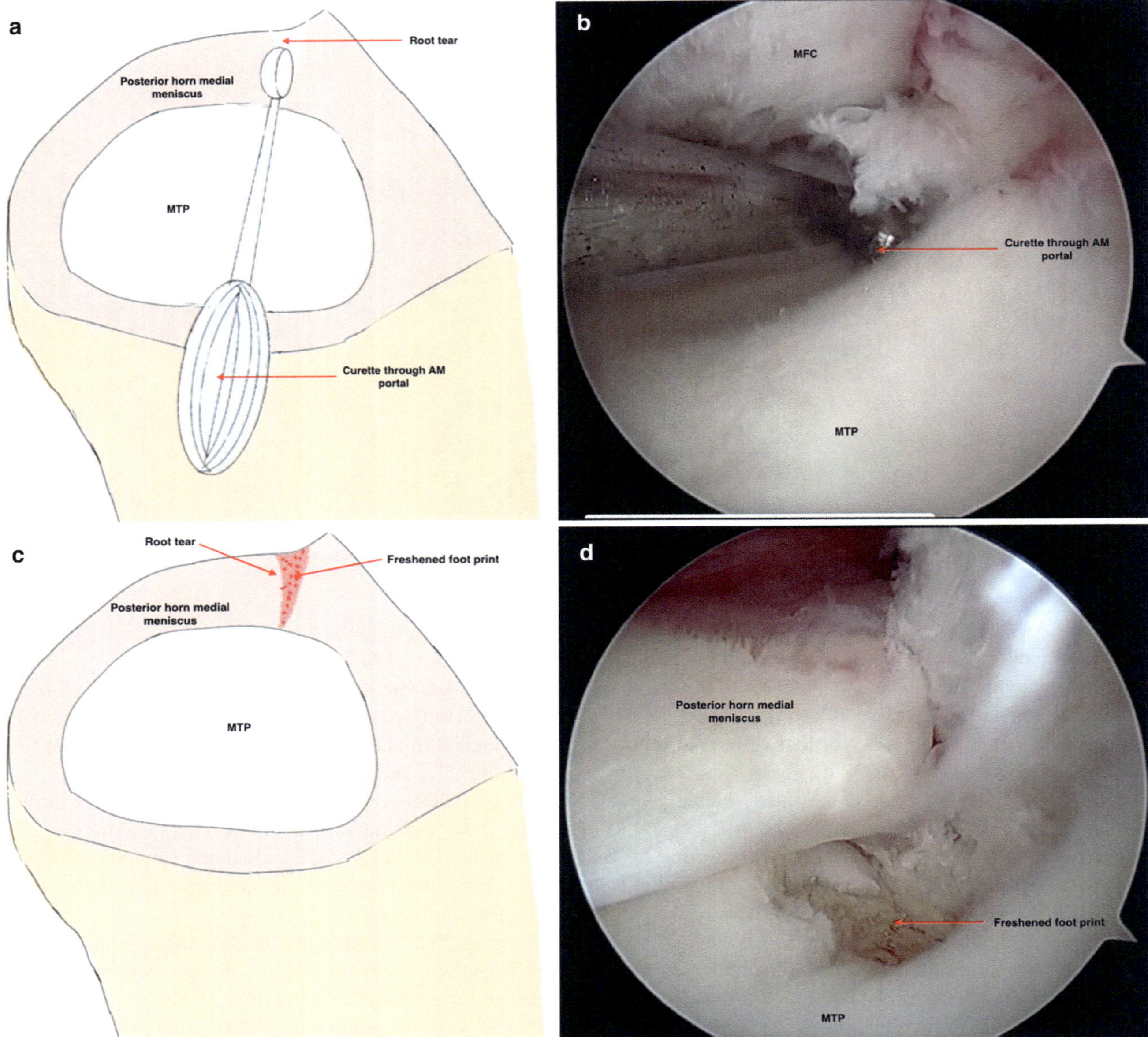


**Fig. 11.5** (**a**) Illustration of the knee showing a curette through Portal B curetting the footprint. (**b**) Arthroscopic image of the knee viewing from the AL portal showing a curette through Portal B curetting the footprint of the medial meniscus root. (**c**) Illustration showing a freshened footprint of the medial meniscus root. (**d**) Arthroscopic image of the knee viewing from the AL portal showing a freshened footprint of the medial meniscus root

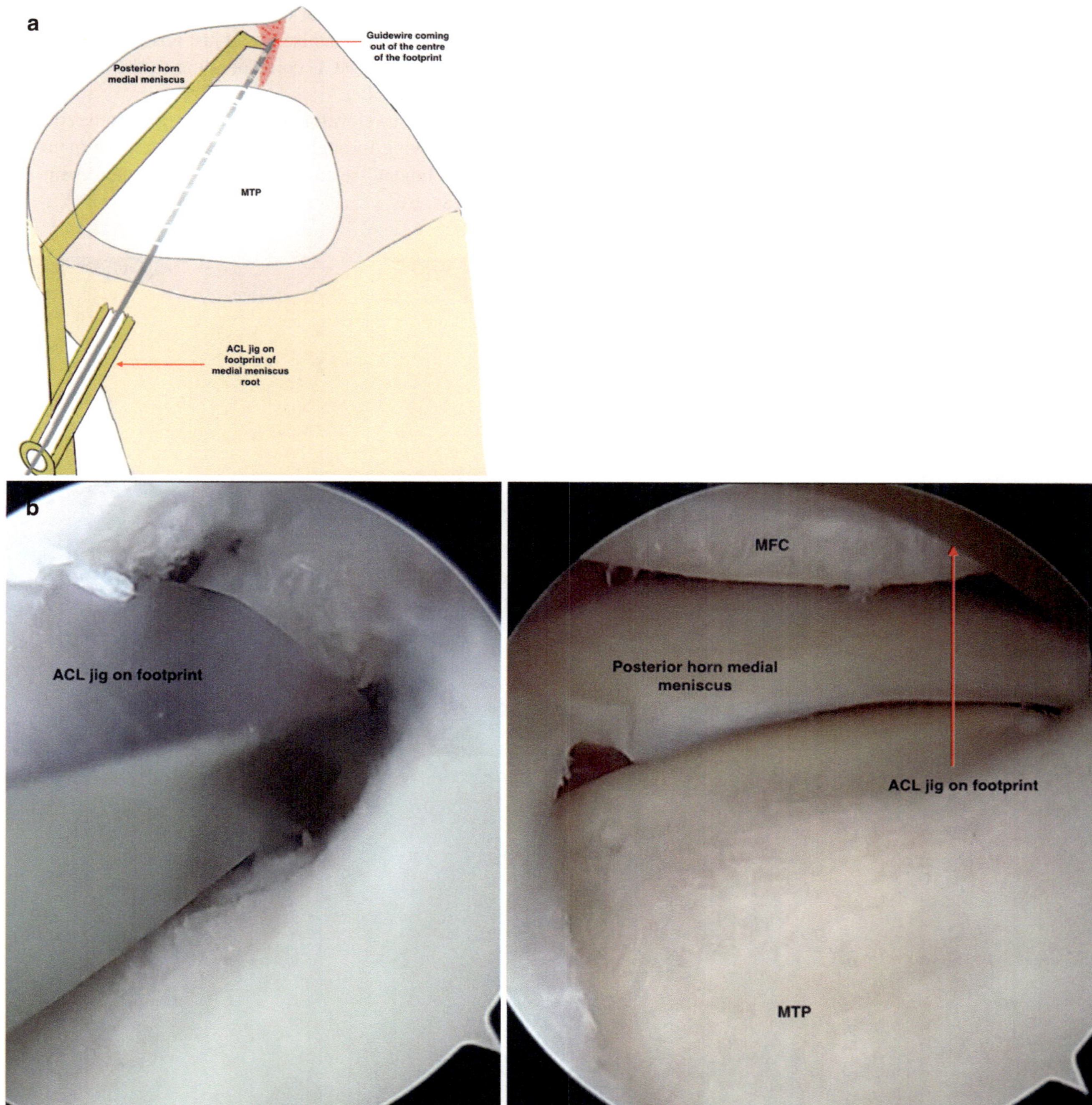


**Fig. 11.6** (**a**) Illustration of the knee showing an ACL jig through portal B applied to the footprint and set at 60° with the distal end applied to the anteromedial tibia and a guide wire drilled from the anteromedial aspect of the tibia and exiting at the centre of the footprint. (**b**) Arthroscopic image of the knee viewing from the AL portal showing two different jigs, the left being a specific jig for root repairs and the right a standard ACL elbow jig applied to the centre of the medial meniscus root footprint

## 11.6 Centralisation

This procedure is done to reduce extrusion and done before the tapes are tied over the Suture Disc on the tibia. The arthroscope is introduced through the anteromedial portal and a Passport cannula is applied to the AL portal to serve as a working portal.

Step 1: A portal is made with an 18G LP needle guidance about 1 cm above the meniscus and just posterior to the posterior border of the MCL corresponding to the body of the meniscus (Fig. 11.17).

Step 2: A tissue elevator is introduced through the AL portal while viewing through the AM Portal and the meniscotibial attachment released from under the meniscus (Fig. 11.18a, b).

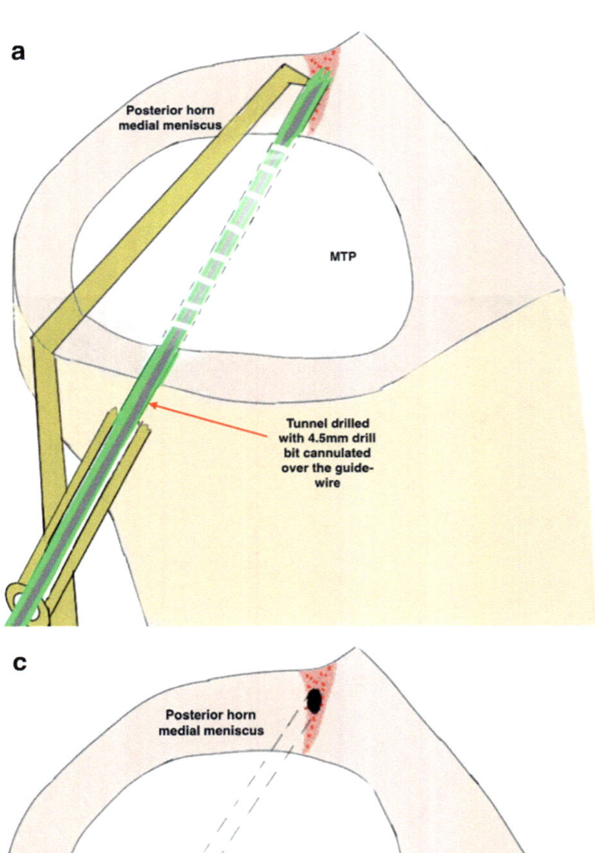


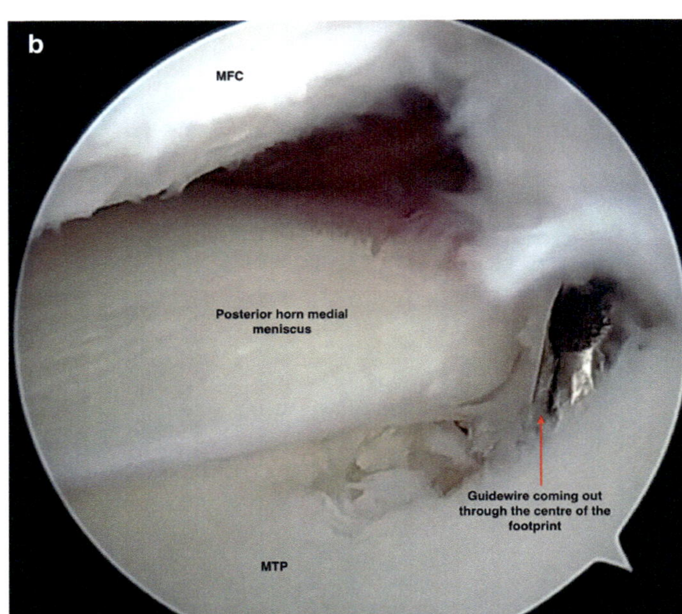


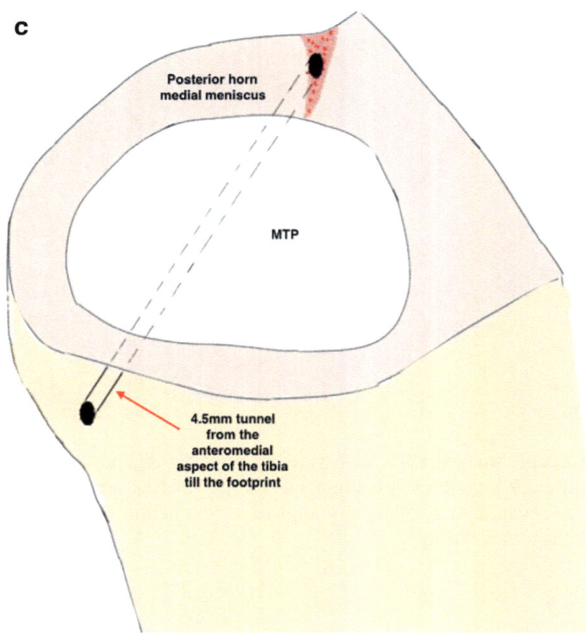


**Fig. 11.7** (**a**) Illustration showing the guidewire being overdrilled with a cannulated 4.5 mm drill bit to create the tibial tunnel from the anteromedial tibia to the medial meniscus root footprint. (**b**) Arthroscopic image of the knee viewing from the AL portal showing the tip of the guidewire while it is being overdrilled with a 4.5 mm cannulated drill bit. (**c**) Illustration of the knee showing the tibial tunnel from the anteromedial tibia to the medial meniscus root footprint

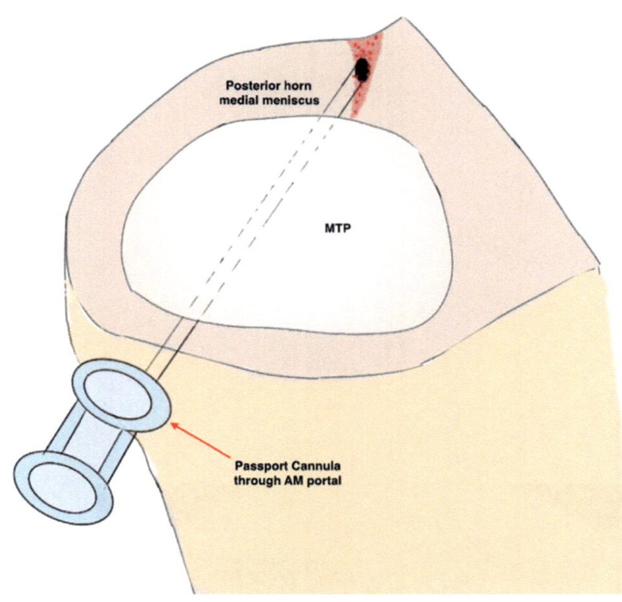


**Fig. 11.8** Illustration of the knee showing a Passport cannula applied to Portal B

Step 3: A 1.8 mm all suture anchor (Arthrex, Naples, FL) is applied to the tibia at this point just under the meniscus using a tap followed by an all suture anchor (Fig. 11.19a–d).

Step 4: One end is delivered through the cannula and loaded on the antegrade suture passer and bite taken through the meniscocapsular junction just anterior to the anchor (Fig. 11.20a–d).

Step 5: The other end is delivered through the cannula and the same step is repeated but this time bite is taken just posterior to the anchor (Fig. 11.21a, b).

Step 6: The two ends are delivered together through Portal C.

Step 7: Using a knot pusher, multiple simple knots are applied such that it reduces the extrusion (Fig. 11.22a, b).

Step 8: The two ends of the sutures are then cut (Fig. 11.23a, b).

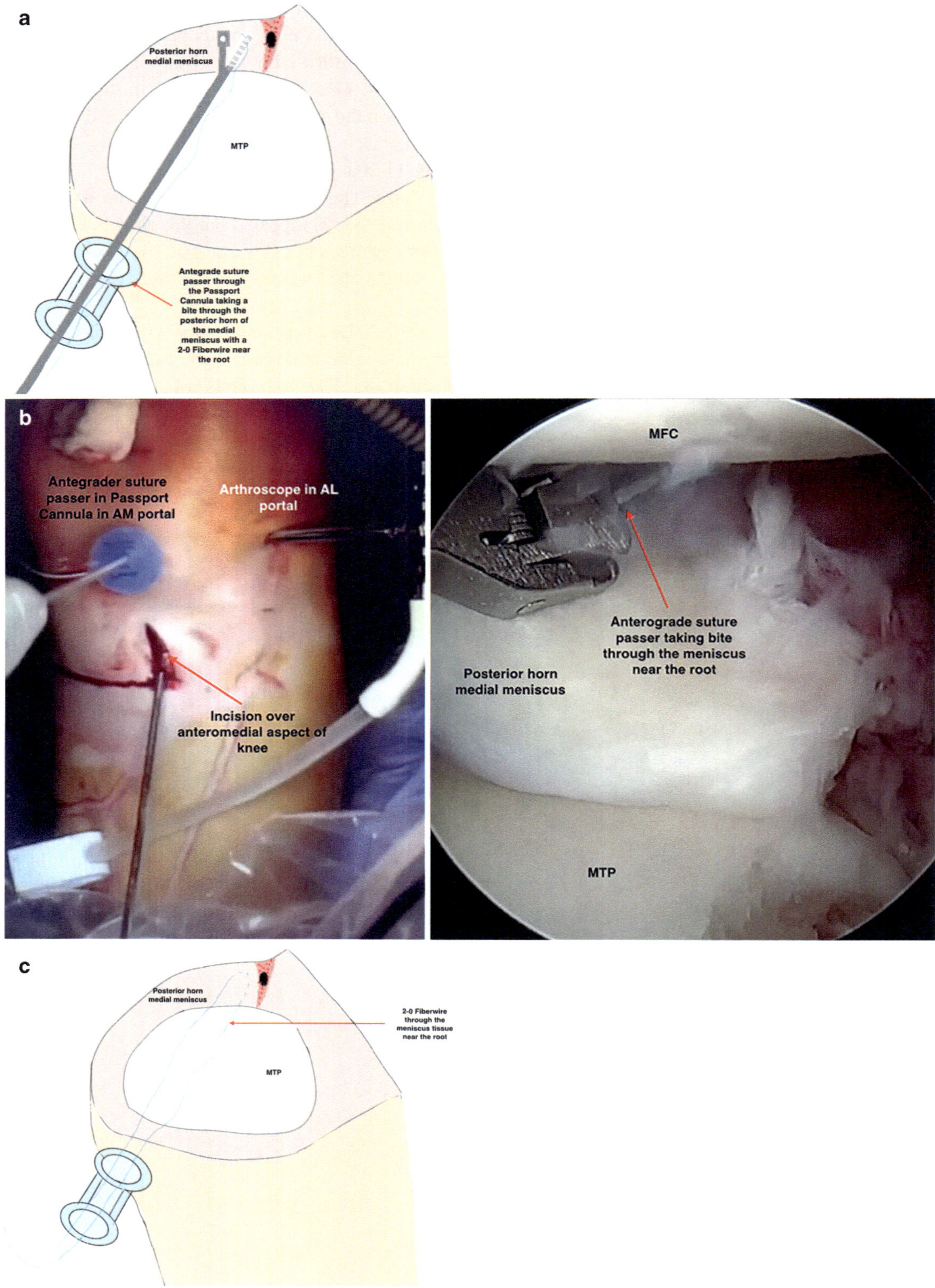


**Fig. 11.9** (**a**) Illustration of the knee showing an antegrade suture passer through Portal B taking a bite through the meniscus tissue next to the root. (**b**) External image of the knee (left) showing the antegrade suture passer through Portal B, arthroscopic image of the knee viewing from the AL portal (right) showing the antegrade suture passer taking a bite through the meniscus tissue just lateral to the root. (**c**) Illustration of the knee showing the 2-0 Fiberwire passing through the meniscus tissue just lateral to the root

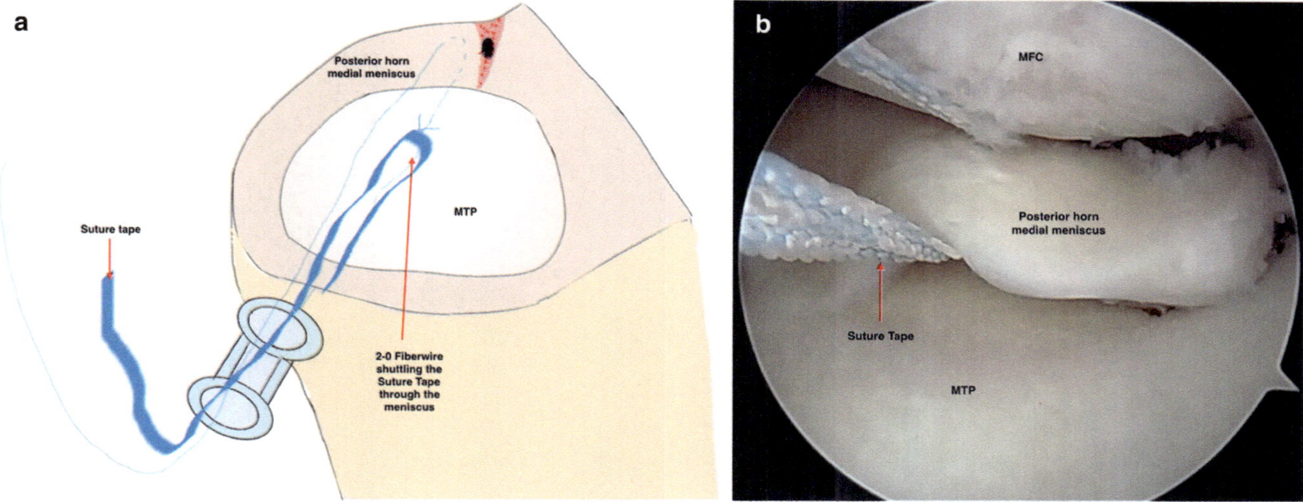


**Fig. 11.10** (**a**) Illustration of the knee showing a Suture Tape shuttled through the meniscus using the 2-0 Fiberwire. (**b**) Arthroscopic image of the knee viewing from the AL portal showing the Suture Tape passing through the meniscus just lateral to the root

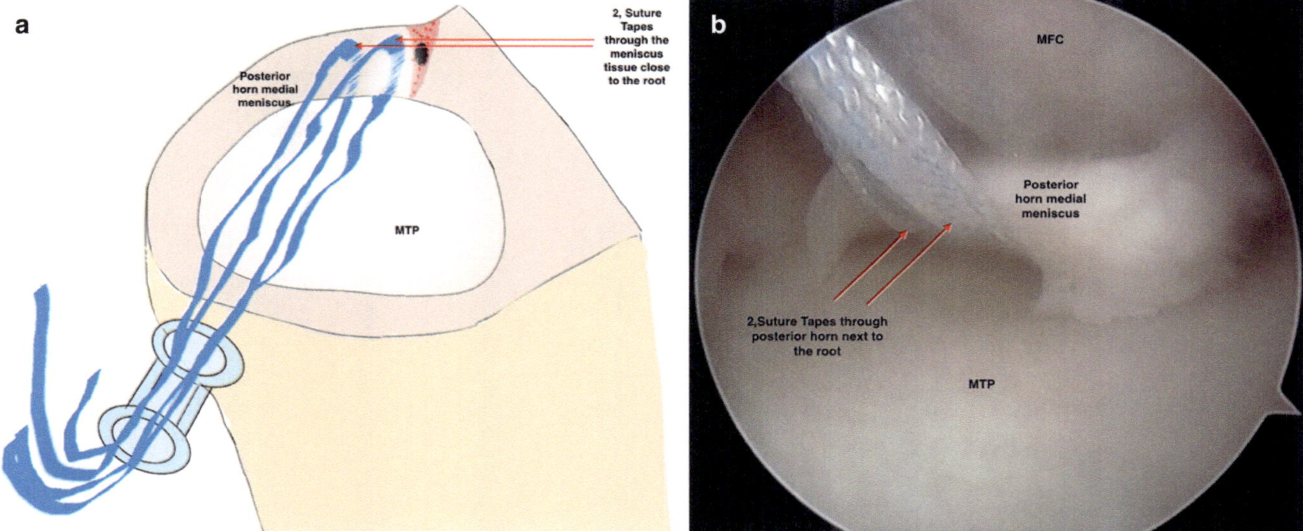


**Fig. 11.11** (**a**) Illustration of the knee showing the two suture tapes through the medial meniscus near its root. (**b**) Arthroscopic image of the knee viewing through the AL portal showing the two Suture Tapes through the medial meniscus near its root

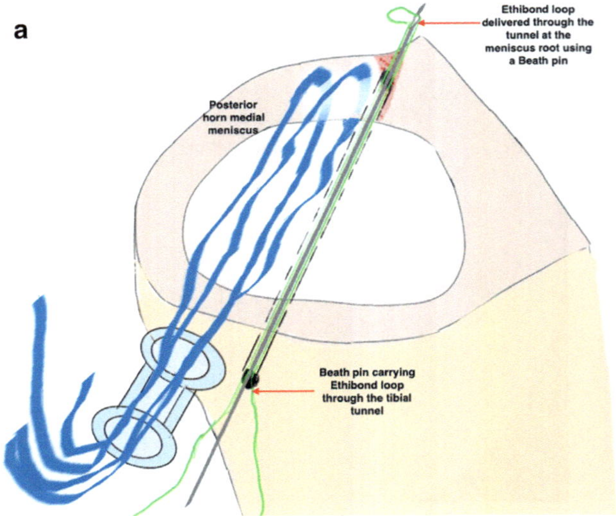


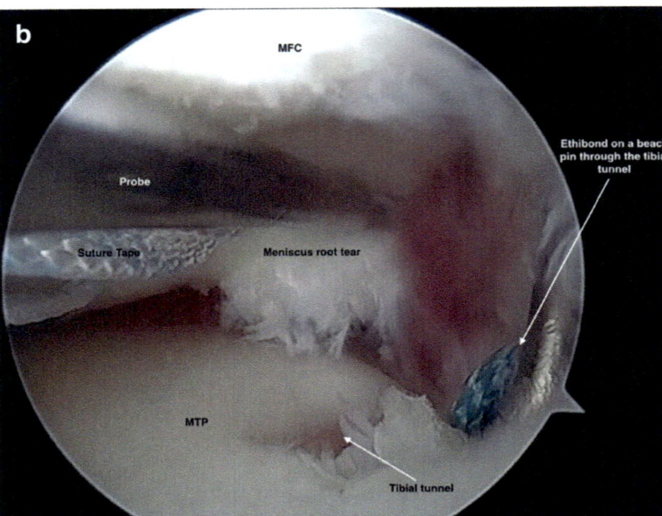


**Fig. 11.12** (**a**) Illustration of the knee showing a Beath pin with a No 5 Ethibond loop introduced through the tibial tunnel from the anteromedial aspect into the tunnel and coming out of the orifice on the medial meniscus root footprint. (**b**) Arthroscopic image of the knee viewing from the AL portal showing the Beath pin carrying the No 5 Ethibond loop coming out of the tunnel at the tunnel orifice on the footprint

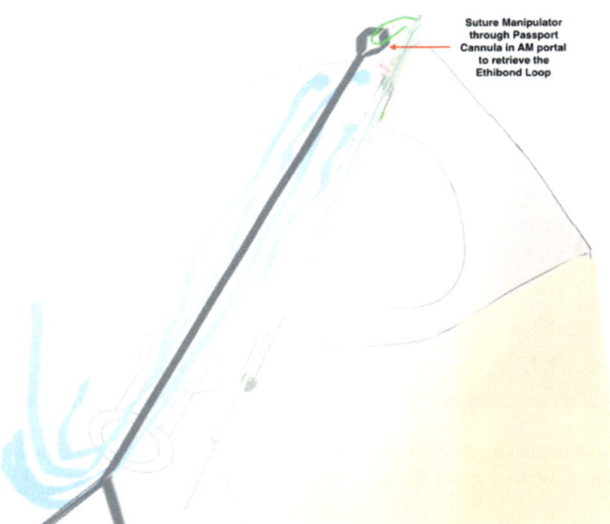


**Fig. 11.13** Illustration of the knee showing a suture manipulator from Portal B delivering the No 5 Ethibond loop through it

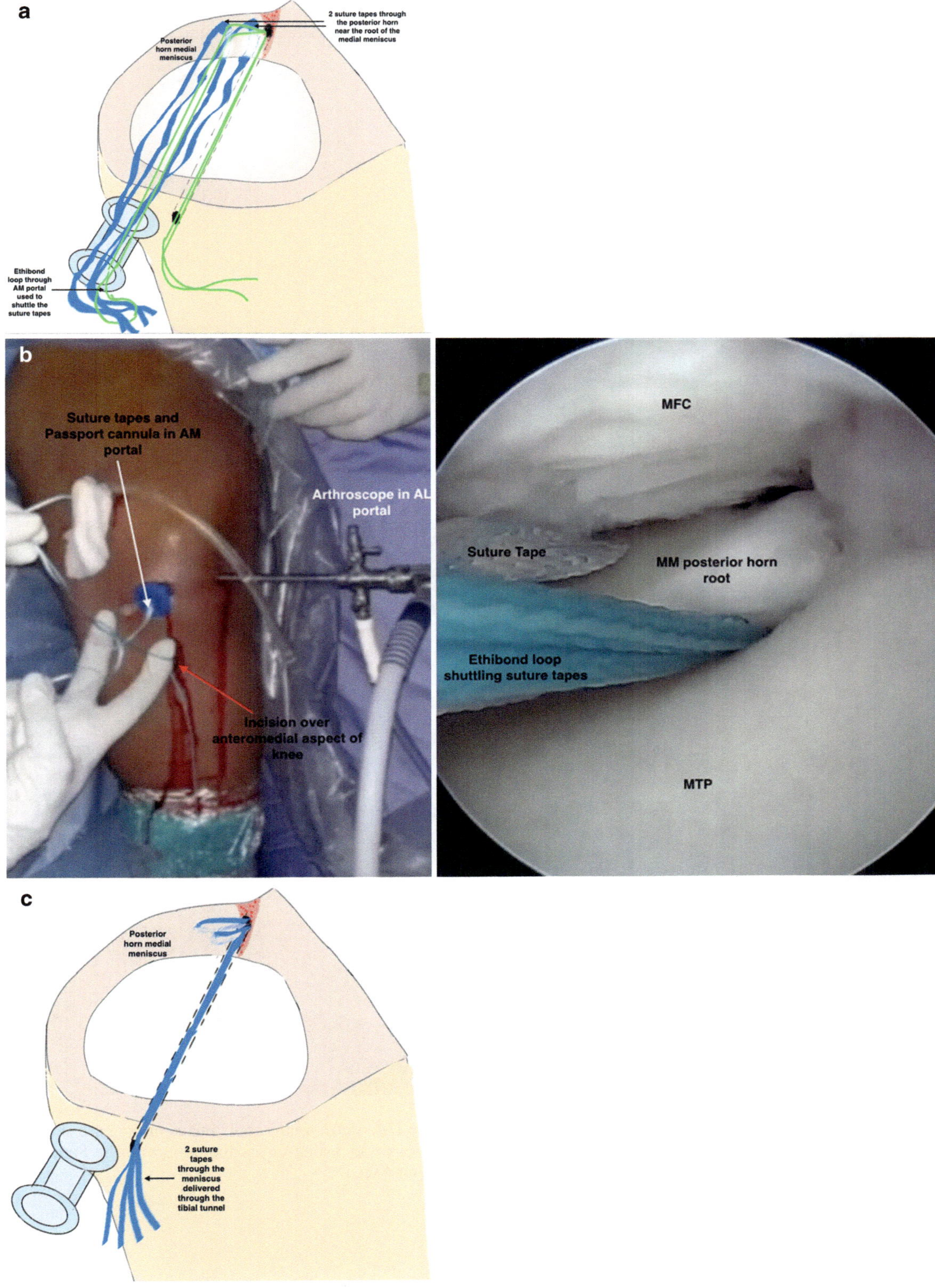


**Fig. 11.14** (**a**) Illustration of the knee showing the No 5 Ethibond loop through Portal Bused to shuttle the four ends of the Suture Tape through the tibial tunnel to the anteromedial aspect of the tibia. (**b**) External image of the knee (right) showing the four ends of the Suture Tape loaded into the Ethibond Loop. (**c**) Illustration of the knee showing the four ends of the Suture tape delivered through the tibial tunnel into the orifice on the anteromedial aspect of the knee

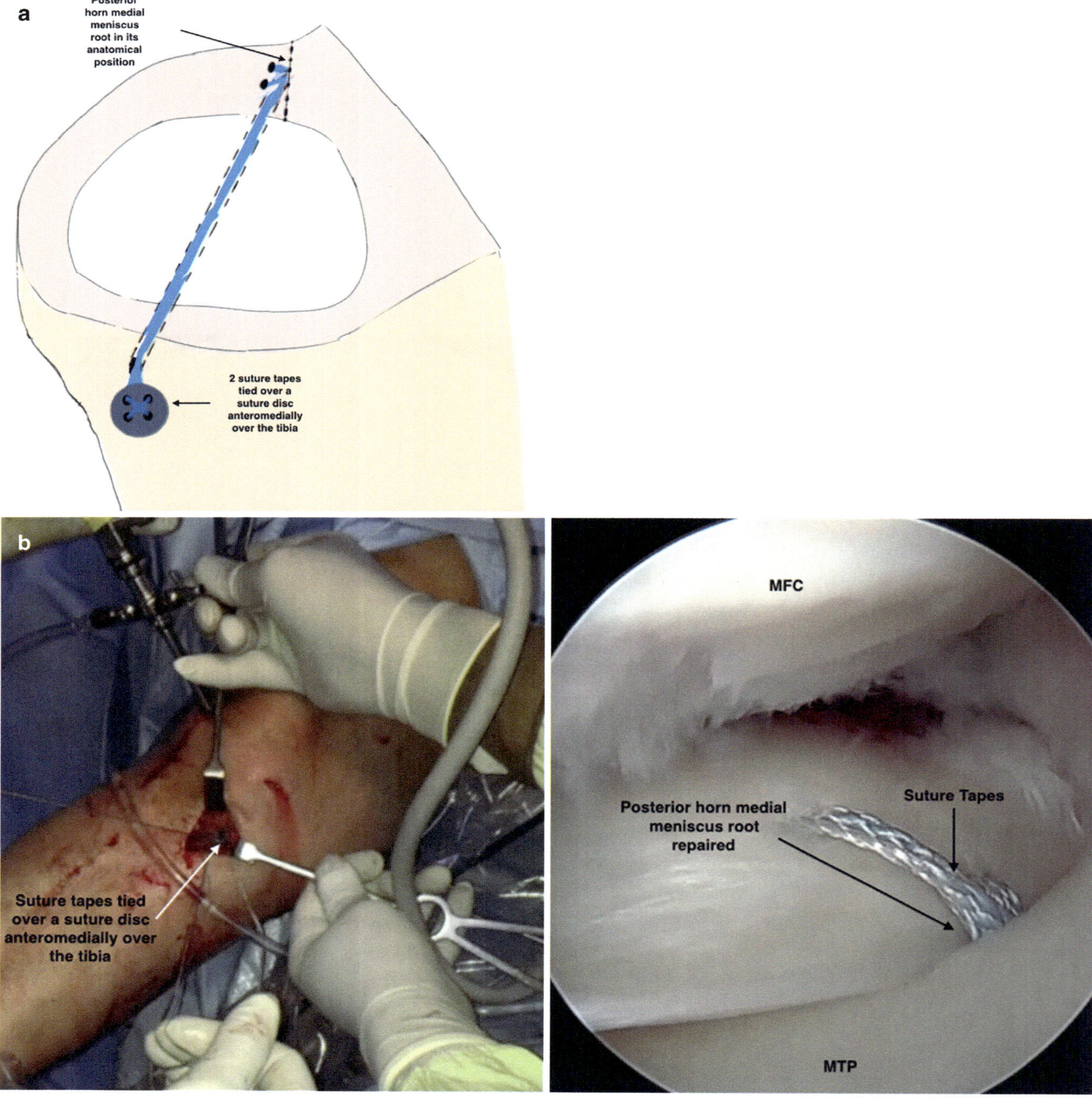


**Fig. 11.15** (**a**) Illustration of the knee showing the four ends of the Suture Tapes tied over a Suture Disc anteromedially on the tibia. (**b**) External image showing the four ends of the Suture Tape tied over the Suture Disc (left), arthroscopic image of the knee showing the medial meniscus root sitting on its footprint with the Suture Tapes passing through it seen

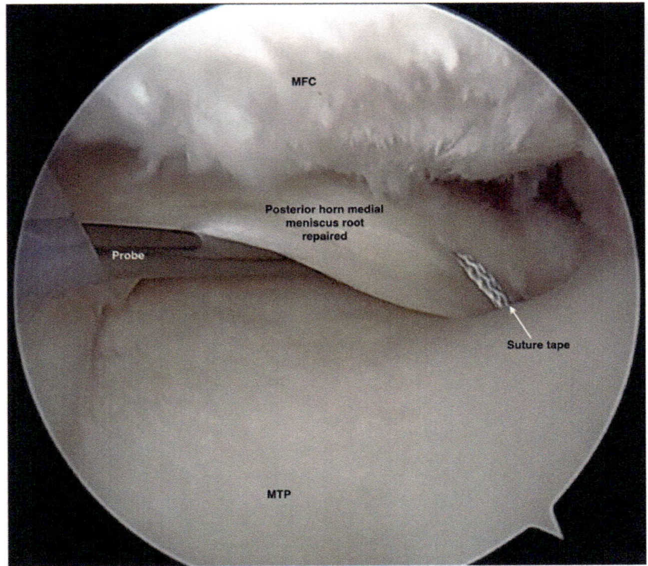


**Fig 11.16** Arthroscopic image of the knee viewing through the AL portal showing the root stabilised on its footprint and being probed to check its stability

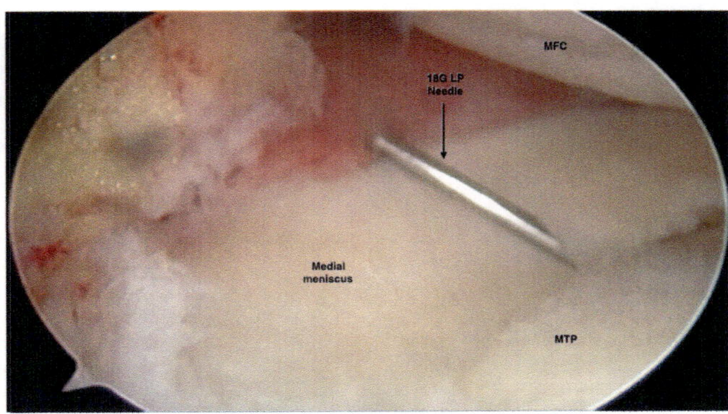


**Fig. 11.17** Arthroscopic image of the knee showing an 18G LP needle to localise the exact location of the far medial portal for the suture anchor

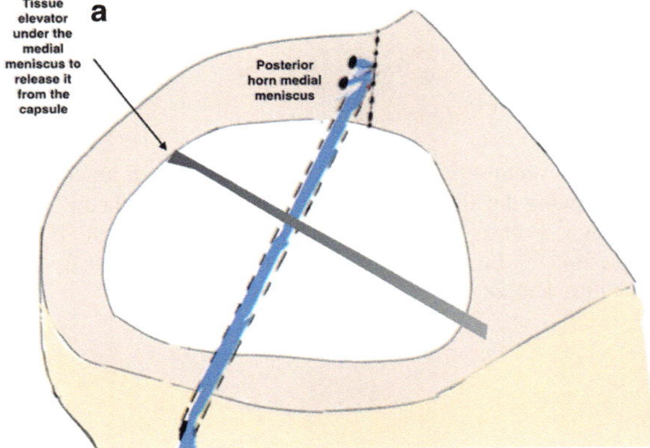


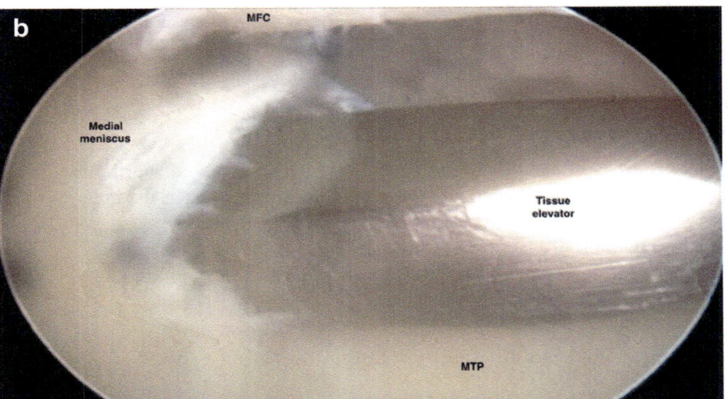


**Fig. 11.18** (**a**) Illustration of the knee showing a tissue elevator from Portal A being used to release the meniscotibial portion of the medial meniscus while viewing from Portal B. (**b**) Arthroscopic image of the knee while viewing through the AM Portal B showing a tissue elevator introduced from the AL Portal A to underneath the medial meniscus releasing its meniscotibial attachment

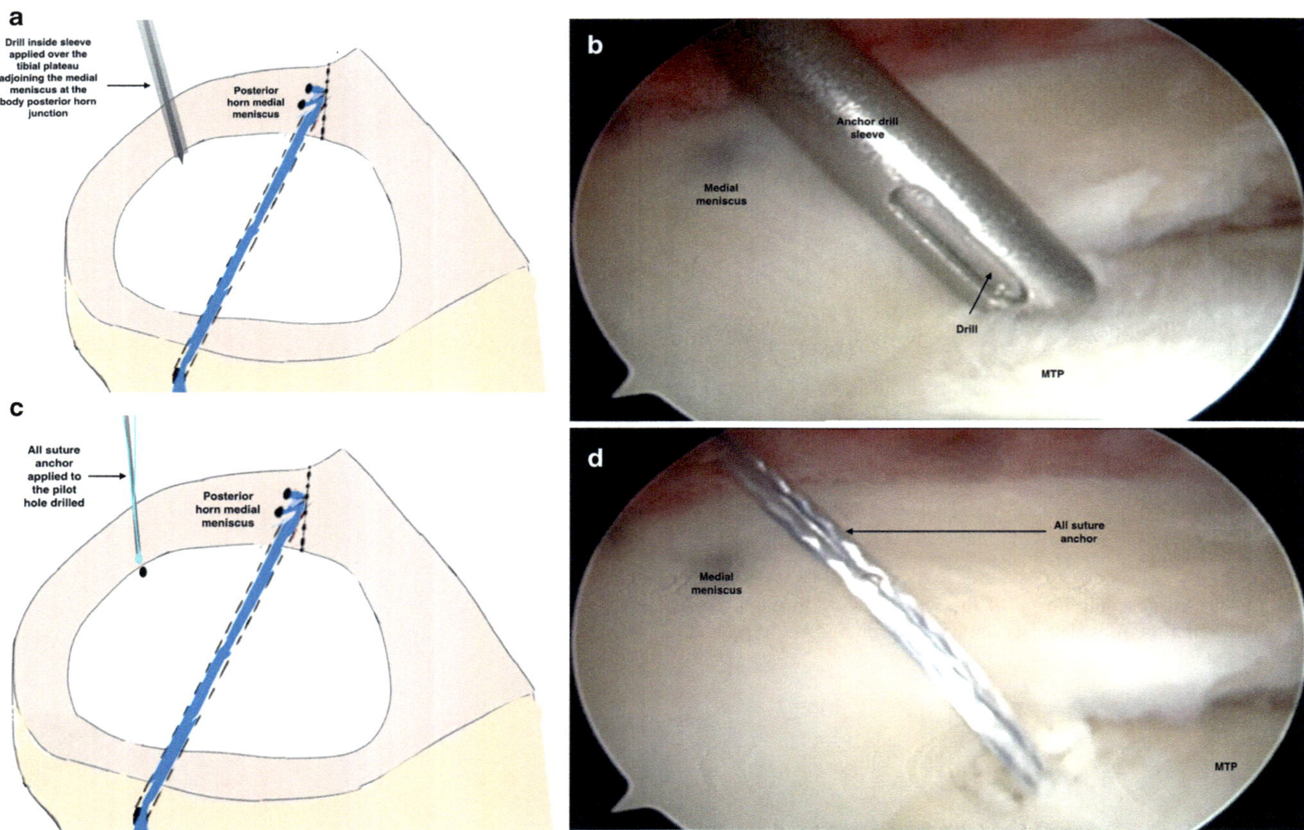


**Fig. 11.19** (**a**) Illustration of the knee showing a sleeve with a drill bit applied to the tibial plateau adjoining the medial meniscus at the body posterior horn junction. (**b**) Arthroscopic image of the knee while viewing through Portal B showing the anchor sleeve with drill bit cannulated through it from Portal C applied to the tibial plateau just adjacent and below the medial meniscus at the body and posterior horn junction. (**c**) Illustration showing the all suture anchor being applied to the pilot hole drilled through Portal C while viewing through Portal B. (**d**) Arthroscopic image of the knee while viewing through Portal B showing the all suture anchor applied to the tibial plateau

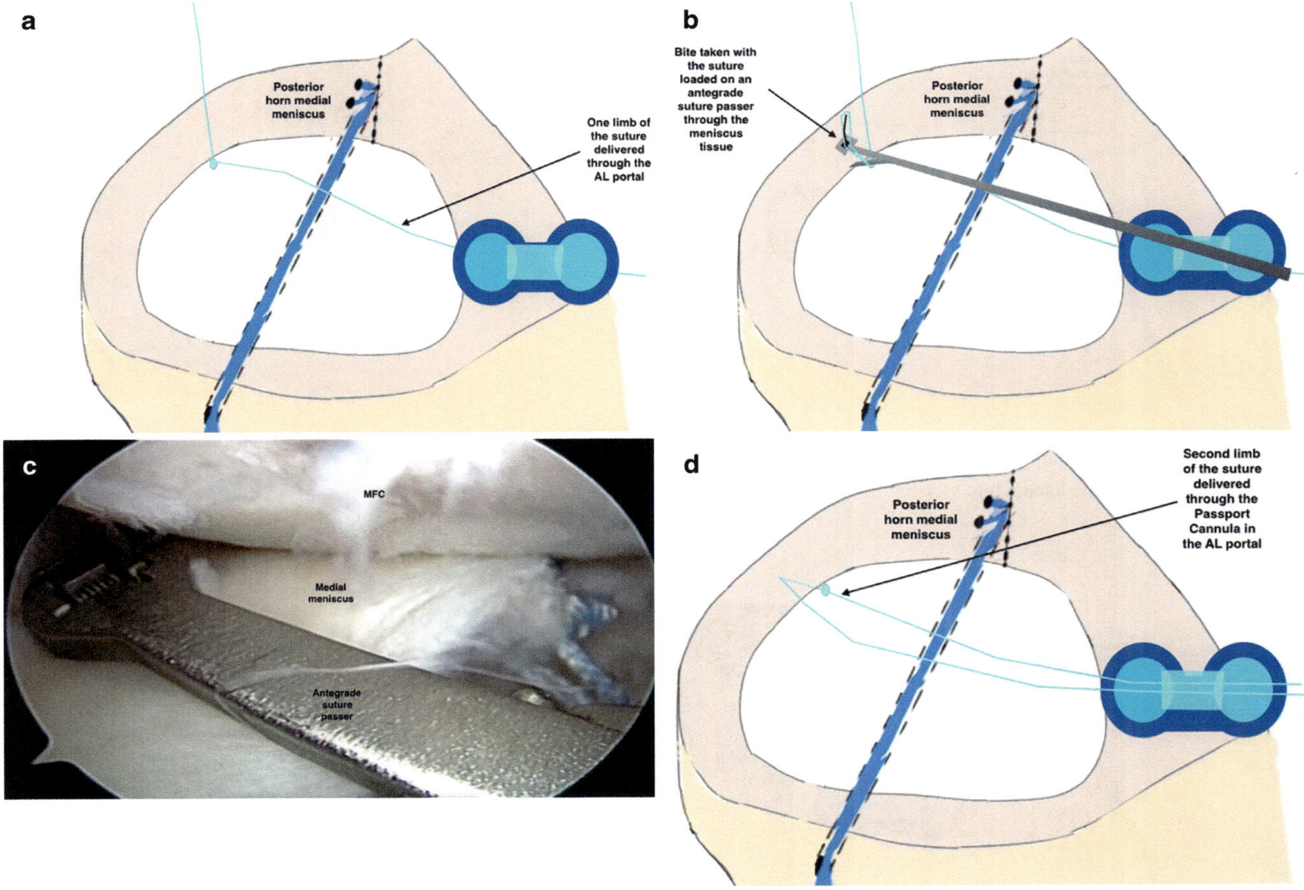

a
Posterior horn medial meniscus
One limb of the suture delivered through the AL portal

b
Bite taken with the suture loaded on an antegrade suture passer through the meniscus tissue
Posterior horn medial meniscus

c
MFC
Medial meniscus
Antegrade suture passer

d
Posterior horn medial meniscus
Second limb of the suture delivered through the Passport Cannula in the AL portal

**Fig. 11.20** (**a**) Illustration of the knee showing one arm of the suture from the suture anchor delivered into Portal A while viewing from Portal B. (**b**) Illustration of the knee viewing from Portal B and an antegrade suture passer loaded with one arm of the suture from the suture anchor taking a bite on the meniscus adjacent to the anchor. (**c**) Arthroscopic image of the knee while viewing through Portal B showing an antegrade suture passer through Portal A loaded with one arm of the suture from the all suture anchor and ready to take a bite through the medial meniscus tissue adjacent to the anchor. (**d**) Illustration of the knee showing one limb of the suture from the suture anchor passing through the meniscus adjacent to the anchor and another limb which has not passed through the meniscus tissue through Portal A

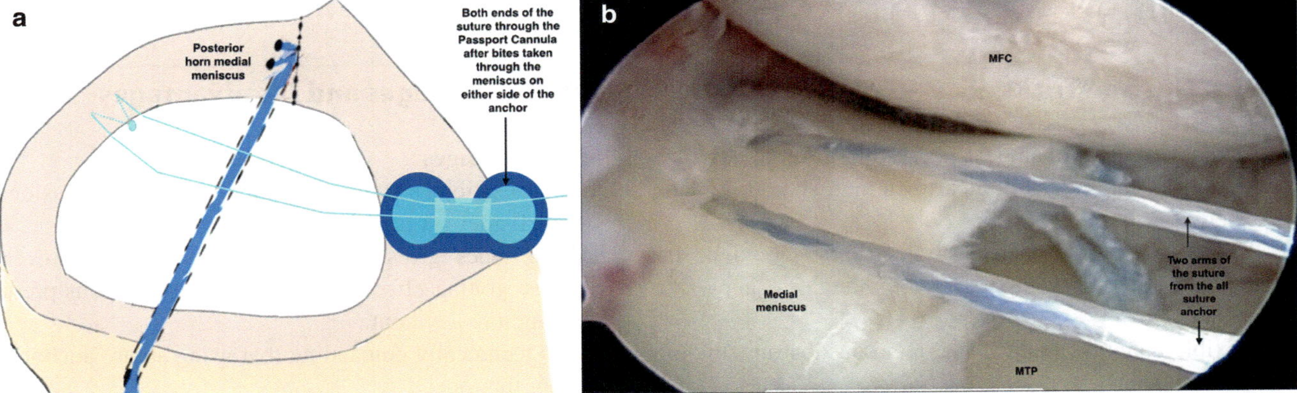


**Fig. 11.21** (**a**) Illustration of the knee while viewing through Portal B showing the two limbs of the suture from the suture anchor passing through the meniscus adjacent to the anchor on either side and delivered through Portal A. (**b**) Arthroscopic image of the knee while viewing through Portal B showing two limbs of the suture from the suture anchor passing through the medial meniscus adjacent to the all suture anchor and on either side

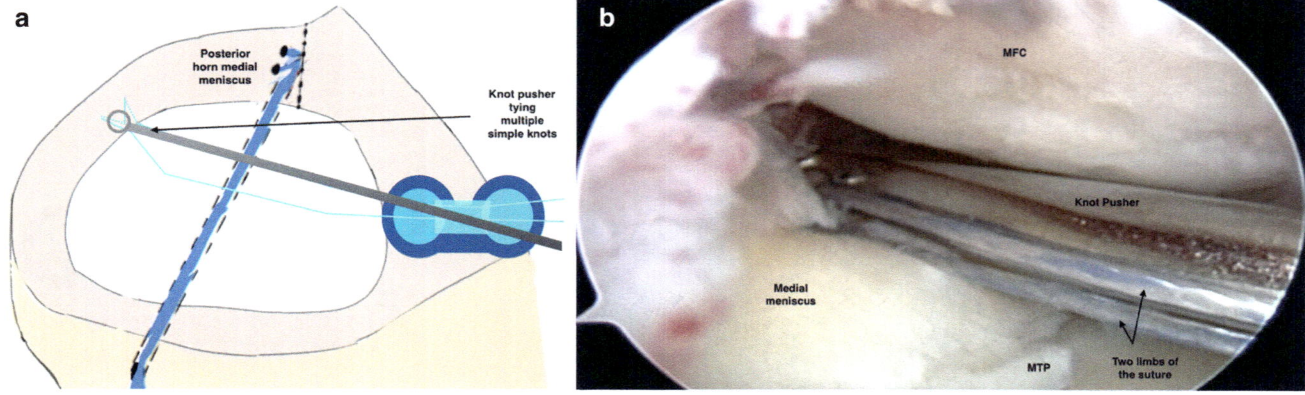


**Fig. 11.22** (**a**) Illustration of the knee while viewing through Portal B showing a knot pusher through Portal A tying multiple simple knots. (**b**) Arthroscopic image of the knee while viewing through Portal B showing a knot pusher through Portal A tying multiple simple knots to secure the meniscus to the anchor

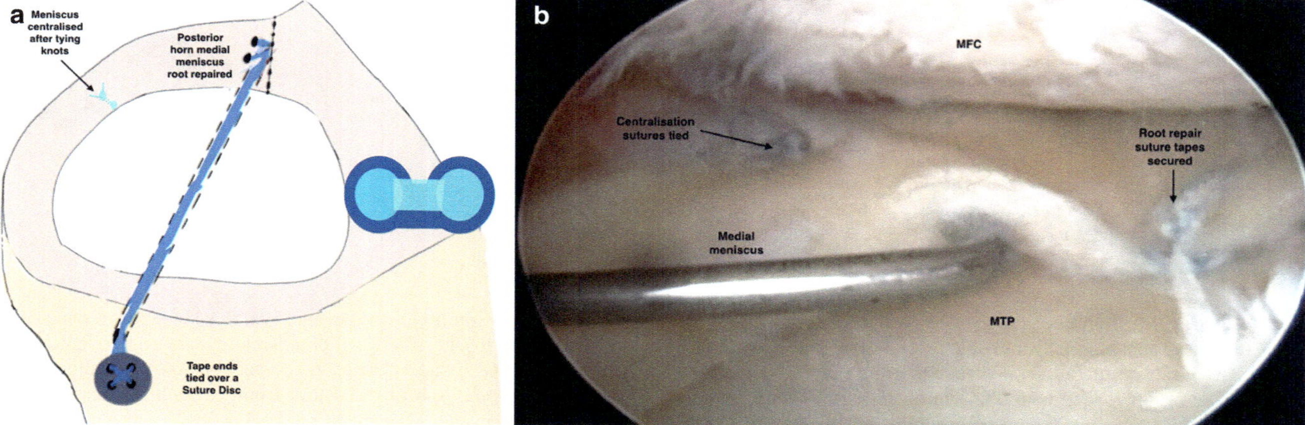


**Fig. 11.23** (**a**) Illustration of the knee while viewing through Portal B showing the centralisation sutures tied and Suture tapes tied over the anteromedial aspect of the tibia, repairing the root and centralising the meniscus. (**b**) Arthroscopic image of the knee viewing through Portal B showing the repaired and centralised medial meniscus being probed and found to be stable

## 11.7 Tips and Tricks

1. Medial collateral ligament pie crusting gives more space to work in the medial compartment and should be done wherever required.
2. The portal for the centralisation anchor should be far medial and slightly high to get the angle to apply the anchor.
3. Flexible cannulas help in manipulating instrumentation intra-articularly.

## 11.8 Advantages and Disadvantages

**Advantages**

1. Centralisation ensures reduction of meniscus extrusion at Time 0 after surgery.
2. Using tapes gives uniform compression and prevents cheese grating effect of sutures on the meniscus predisposing it to a cut out.
3. Less technically demanding that using suture anchors to repair the root.

**Disadvantages**

1. The knot security of tapes is less than sutures and knots can loosen over a period of time.

## References

1. Allaire R, Muriuki M, Gilbertson L, Harner CD. Biomechanical consequences of a tear of the posterior root of the medial meniscus. J Bone Joint Surg Am. 2008;90(9):1922–31.
2. Jung YH, Choi NH, Oh JS, Victoroff BN. All-Inside repair for a root tear of the medial meniscus using a suture anchor. Am J Sports Med. 2012;40(6):1406–11.
3. Kim YM, Rhee KJ, Lee JK, Hwang DS, Yang JY, Kim SJ. Arthroscopic pullout repair of a complete radial tear of the tibial attachment site of the medial meniscus posterior horn. Arthroscopy. 2006;22(7):e1–4.
4. Mochizuki Y, Kawahara K, Samejima Y, Kaneko T, Ikegami H, Musha Y. Short-term results and surgical technique of arthroscopic centralization as an augmentation for medial meniscus extrusion caused by medial meniscus posterior root tear. Eur J Orthop Surg Traumatol. 2021;31(6):1235–41.

# Two Portal RAMP Repair Using an Antegrade Suture Passer

# 12

Sheetal Gupta and Anmol Sharma

## 12.1 Introduction

First described by Strobel in 1980s, ramp lesions are defined as longitudinal peripheral tear of the posterior horn of medial meniscus which can be meniscocapsular or meniscosynovial. Ramp lesions are commonly associated with ACL deficiency with an incidence of 9–17%. Longer delay in ACL reconstruction increases the incidence of ramp lesion. Ramp possesses diagnostic dilemma and is commonly described as "Hidden Lesion" which is associated with pain, instability, and dysfunction of knee. Thaunat et al. classified ramp Lesions into five types.

## 12.2 Special Equipments Required (Fig. 12.1)

1. Arthroscopic Cannula
2. Knee Scorpion/suture passer
3. Knot pusher
4. Flexible cannula (passport cannula)
5. Spinal needle
6. No. 2-0 Fiberwire (multistrand, long chain ultra-high molecular weight polyethylene core braided with polyester)
7. Switching rod

S. Gupta (✉) · A. Sharma
Galaxy Knee & Shoulder Hospital, Bhopal, Madhya Pradesh, India


V. A. Mhaskar, J. Maheshwari (eds.), *Innovative Approaches in Knee Arthroscopy*,
https://doi.org/10.1007/978-981-99-4378-4_12

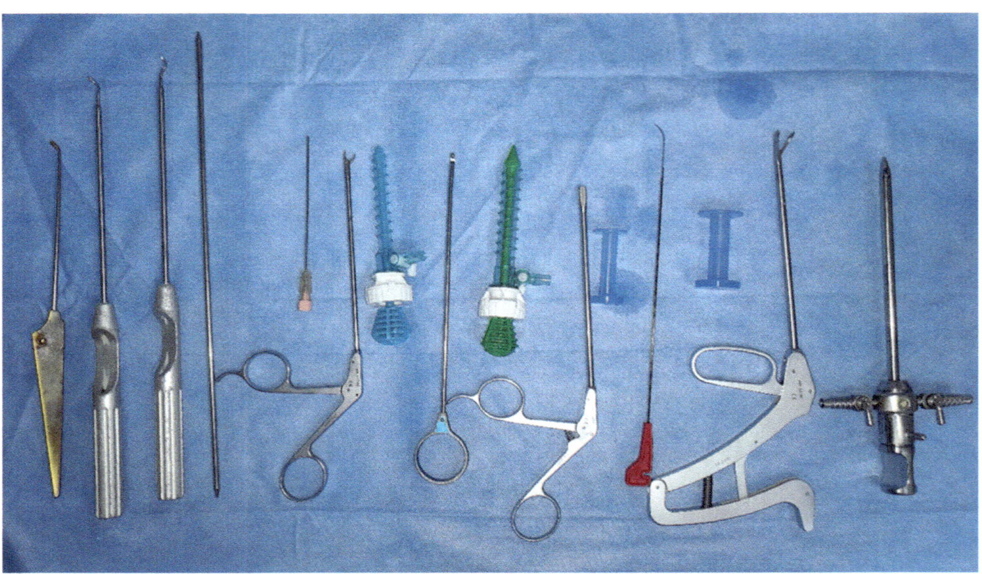

**Fig. 12.1** Instruments used in ramp repair

## 12.3 Positioning

Under spinal anaesthesia, the patient is positioned supine on the operating table with the knee in 90° of flexion at the edge of the table on the affected side in order to allow full range of motion and adequate exposure to back of the knee (Fig. 12.2). In this position the neurovascular bundle falls posteriorly. A thigh support is placed just proximal to the knee at mid-thigh level. The tourniquet is placed high on the thigh.

### 12.3.1 Draping

The operative site is prepared with an aseptic sterile technique. Draping is done in the standard way in order to expose distal 1/3rd of thigh and proximal 1/3rd of leg (Fig. 12.3). The lower limb is exsanguinated and the tourniquet is inflated.

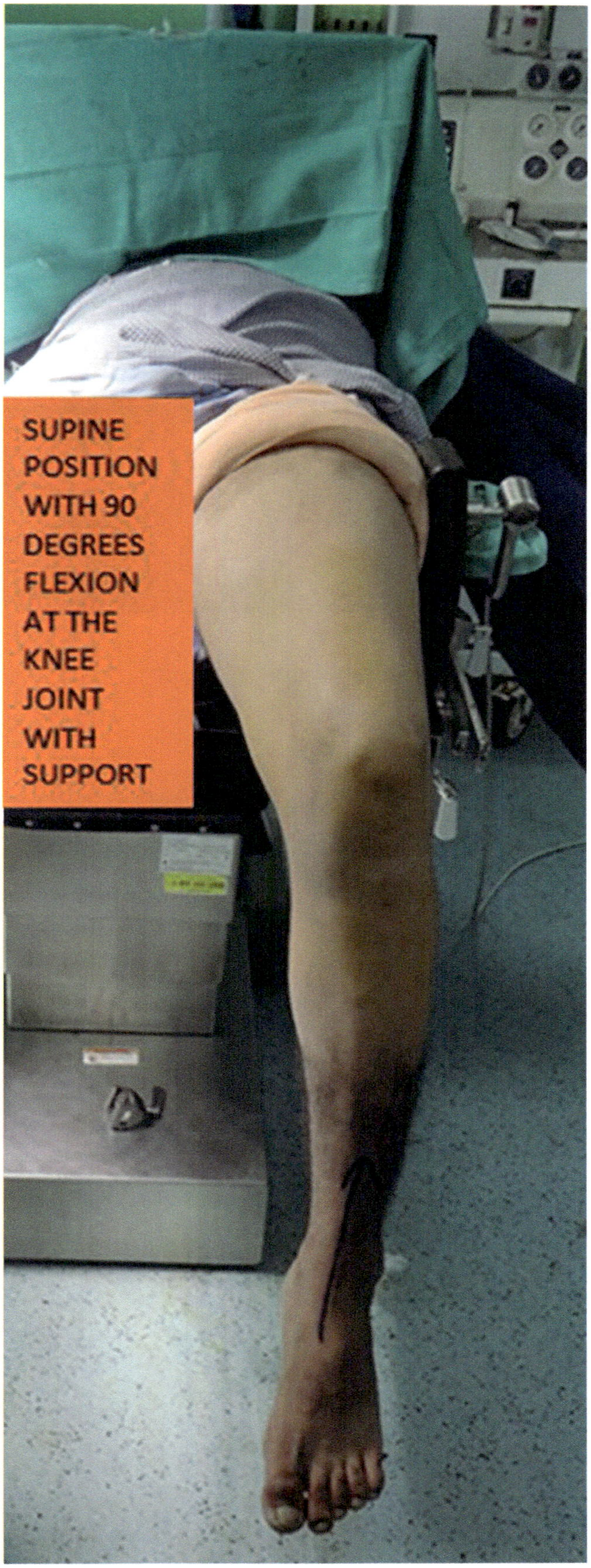

SUPINE POSITION WITH 90 DEGREES FLEXION AT THE KNEE JOINT WITH SUPPORT

**Fig. 12.2** Positioning of the patient

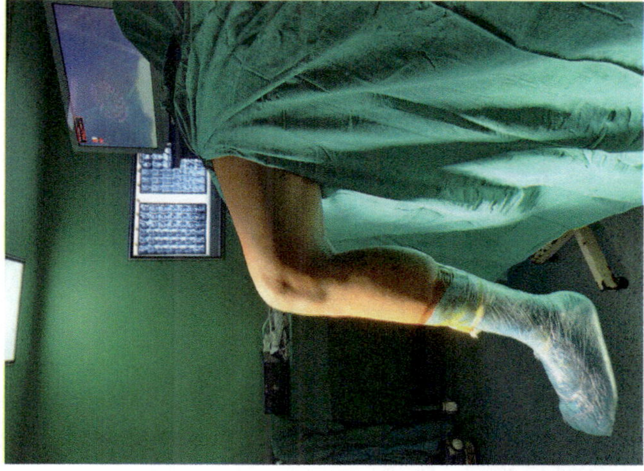

**Fig. 12.3** Draping of the limb

## 12.4 Portals

Standard anterolateral portal: Placed 1 cm above the joint line and just next to the patellar tendon in a palpable soft spot.

Standard anteromedial portal: Placed 1 cm above the joint line and 1 cm medial to the patellar tendon in a palpable soft spot.

Low posteromedial portal (PM portal): Just above the joint line.

High posteromedial portal: 4 cm above the joint line.

## 12.5 Surgical Steps

Step 1: A standard anterolateral portal is made 1 cm above the joint line and just next to the patellar tendon in a palpable soft spot. It is used as a viewing portal for arthroscopic evaluation of anterior, lateral, medial, and posteromedial compartment.

Step 2: A second anteromedial portal is made 1 cm above the joint line and 1 cm medial to the patellar tendon in a palpable soft spot. The placement of anteromedial portal can be confirmed with a spinal needle using the arthroscope. This portal is used as a working portal in the anterior compartment through which instruments are passed.

Step 3: A diagnostic arthroscopy is performed first. We look for ACL tear, any associated meniscal tear, and the meniscal mobility.

For identification of RAMP lesion from anterior compartment, a 30-degree arthroscope (AL portal) is passed between the medial wall of intercondylar notch and the PCL with the knee slightly flexed in valgus (Gillquist manoeuvre). An 18 G spinal needle or probe is passed outside in from low PM portal using help of transillumination (Fig. 12.4a). From the

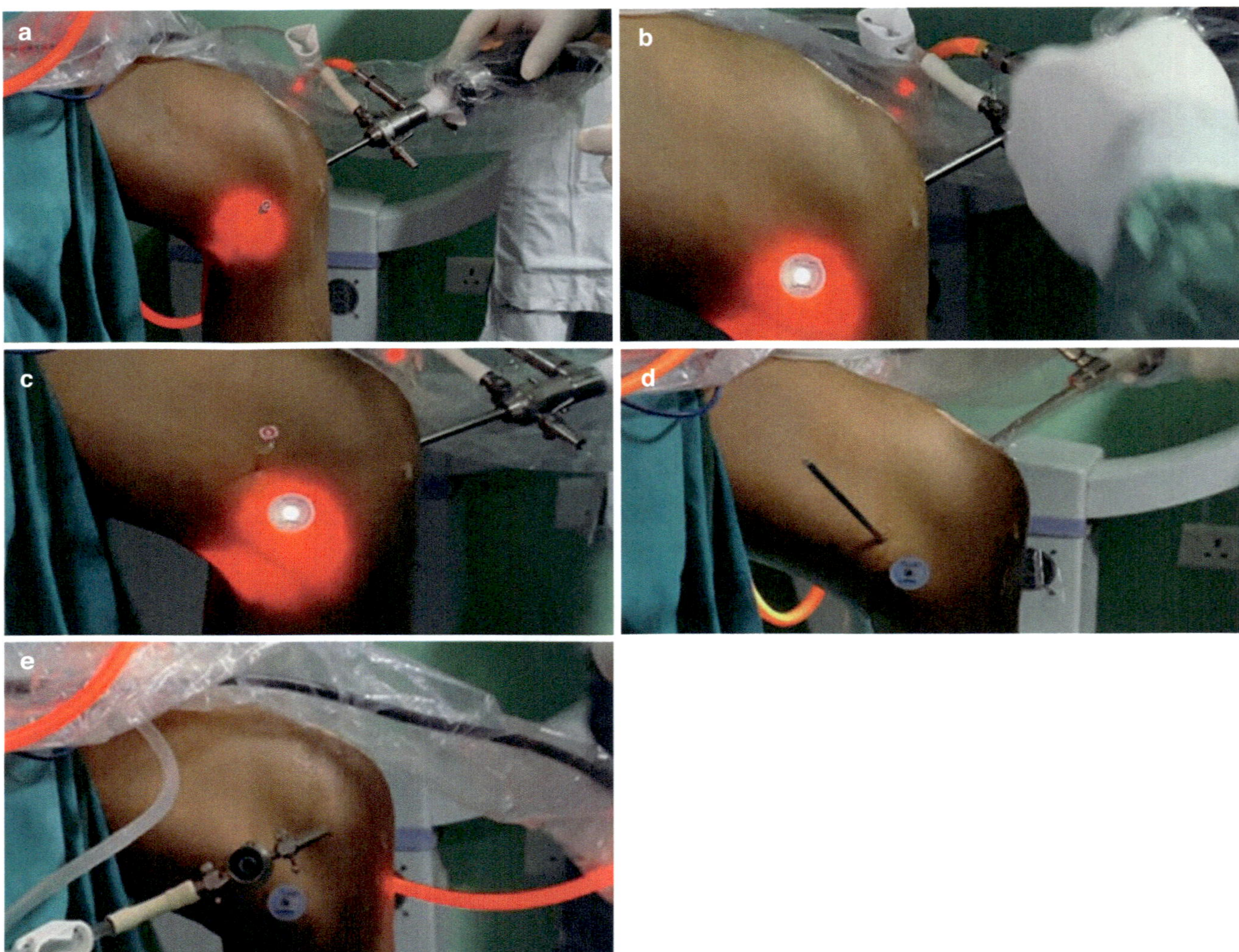


**Fig. 12.4** (**a**) Spinal needle for low posteromedial portal using transillumination technique and doing needle test at the same time. (**b**) Passport cannula through low PM Portal. (**c**) Spinal needle for high PM Portal. (**d**) switching stick through high PM portal for shifting scope for visualisation port. (**e**) Arthroscopic sheath through high PM portal

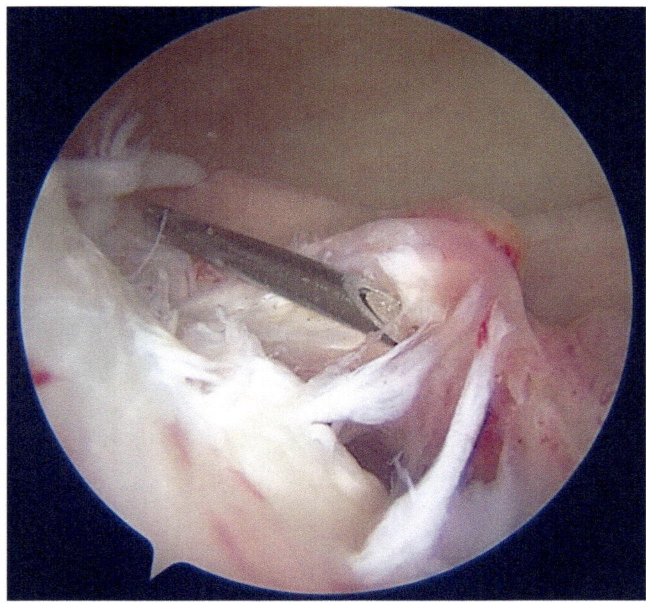

**Fig. 12.5** 18 G spinal needle passed under direct vision for assessing the meniscocapsular junction of medial meniscus

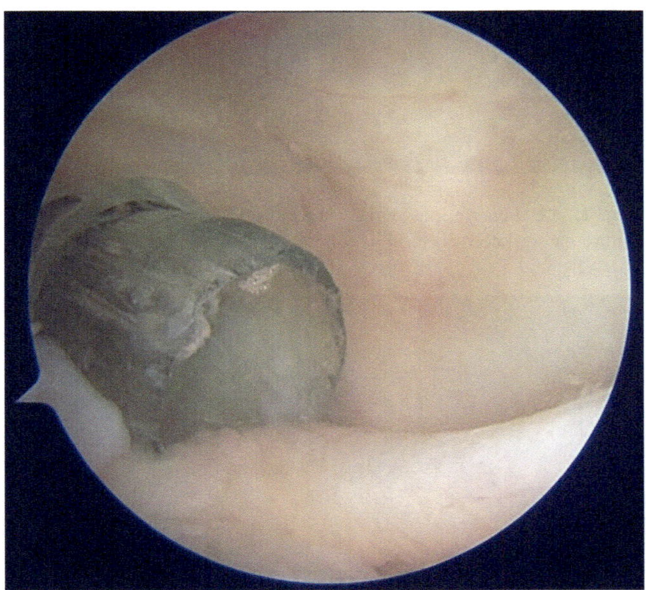

**Fig. 12.6** An 8 mm arthroscopic cannula/passport through the low posteromedial portal for instrumentation

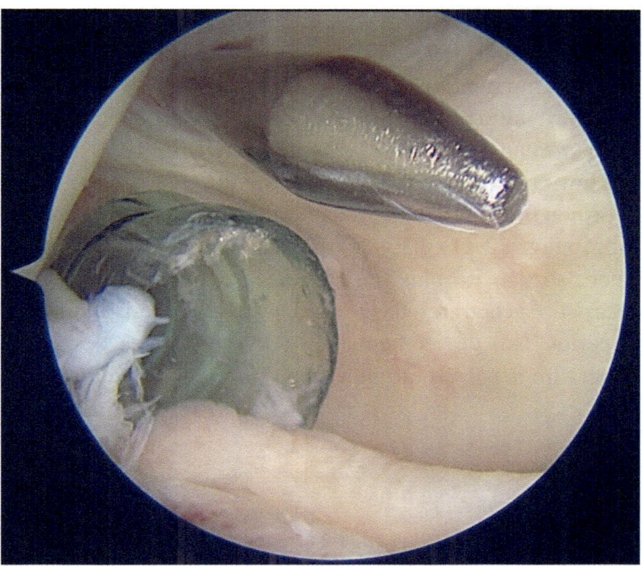

**Fig. 12.7** Switching rod through the high posteromedial portal

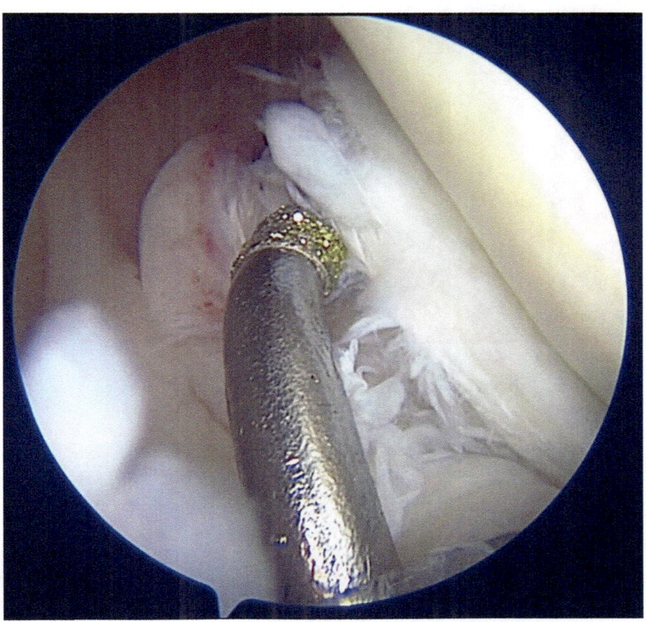

**Fig. 12.8** Rasping of the RAMP lesion

posteromedial aspect of knee, just above the joint line, posterior horn of medial meniscus and meniscocapsular junction is assessed. Tear at meniscocapsular junction, palpable via needle or probe confirms ramp lesion (Fig. 12.5).

Step 4: Once the diagnosis of RAMP lesion is confirmed, two posteromedial portals are made. A low posteromedial portal is made just above the joint line by transillumination technique in order to avoid neurovascular structures. An 18 G spinal needle is passed followed by portal creation with a no. 11 blade scalpel and a haemostat under direct vision. An 8 mm arthroscopic cannula or passport cannula is then placed for ease of instrumentation through this portal (Figs. 12.4b and 12.6).

Step 5: After the confirmation of diagnosis, a high posteromedial portal is made in the same manner 4 cm above the joint line (Fig. 12.4c). A switching rod is then passed (Figs. 12.4d and 12.7) and the arthroscope is switched to high posteromedial portal (Fig. 12.4e). We use all inside suture technique for repair of the RAMP lesion.

Step 6: The edges of the tear are abraded with the help of a shaver or meniscal rasp to stimulate the healing response (Fig. 12.8).

Step 7: As the RAMP is a longitudinal tear, there are two portions: anterior (meniscal side) and posterior (capsular side). Ramp repair is basically approximating these two surfaces. A suture passer/knee scorpion is introduced, loaded with one end of no. 2-0 Fiberwire suture (Fig. 12.9), through the low posteromedial portal via cannula (Fig. 12.10). Using scorpion first bite is taken on anterior aspect of tear (Meniscal side) (Fig. 12.11). The scorpion suture passer is manipulated, so that it holds the substance of meniscus well and sharp tip penetrates the medial meniscus from inferior to superior. This device being self-retrieving suture device 2-0 Fiberwire is passed through meniscus and retrieved via posteromedial portal. 2-0 Fiberwire is removed from scorpion. Other end of 2-0 Fiberwire is now mounted on to scorpion again to take bite of posterior aspect of tear.

The Knee Scorpion is introduced through low PM cannula and this time bite is taken on posterior aspect (capsular side) of tear (Fig. 12.12). Ensure good tissue bite from capsular side also, this step passes suture through capsular side and is retrieved out through PM cannula. Now both the

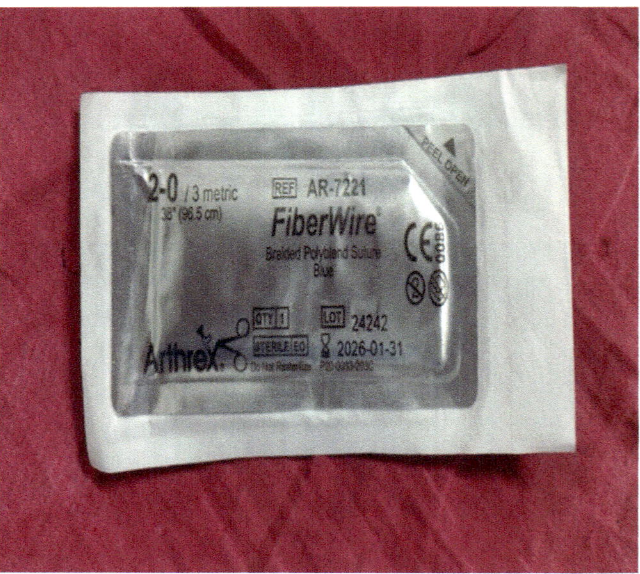


**Fig. 12.9** Fiberwire used for repairing RAMP lesion

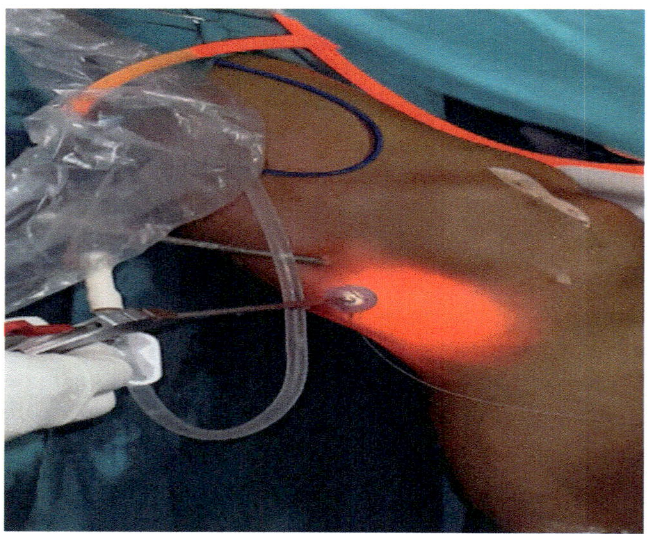

**Fig. 12.10** Fiberwire mounted on scorpion passed through low PM Portal

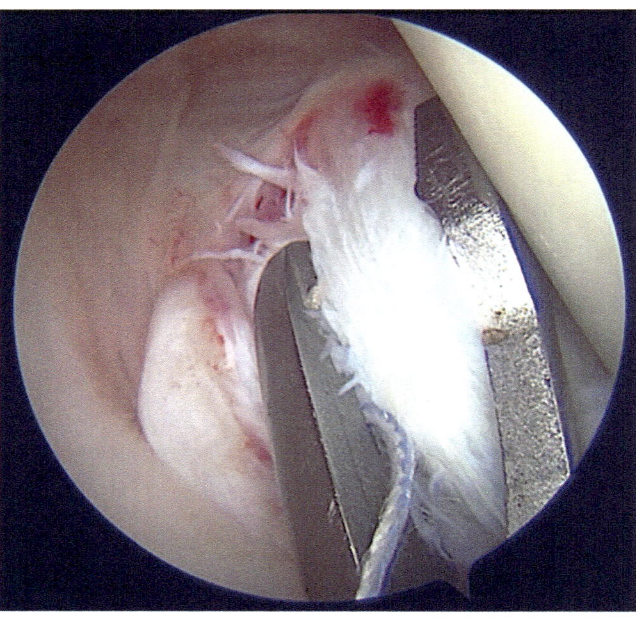

**Fig. 12.11** Penetration of the anterior side of tear with the help of suture passer/knee scorpion

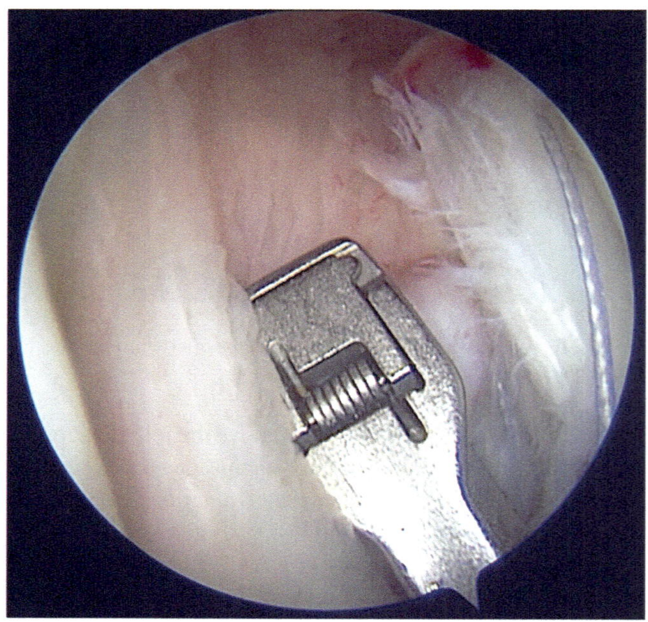

**Fig. 12.12** Penetration of the posterior side of tear with the help of suture passer/knee scorpion

sutures are ready and already passed though both leafs (meniscus side and capsular side). Confirm that there is no entanglement of sutures (can verify by passing knot pusher in suture). Now we are ready for knot tying. We prefer to use nonsliding multiple half hitches so cheese grating effect on capsule can be avoided (Figs. 12.13 and 12.14).

Three to four simple knots are applied with the help of knot pusher under direct view.

Step 8: This maneuverer was repeated as per the length of tear up to the root attachment. One knot was inserted per 5–6 mm of tear (Fig. 12.15).

After RAMP lesion repair, the other repair/reconstruction procedures are performed.

### 12.5.1 Postoperative Rehabilitation

From the next day, quadriceps tightening, ankle pumping, hip rotation exercises is advised. Toe touch weight bearing and passive range of motion up to 45° is permitted in the first 2 weeks. From 2nd to 4th week, 0–90° of motion with partial weight bearing is allowed. After 6 weeks, full weight wearing and range of motion is allowed. Return to sports activity is permitted from 8 to 9 months.

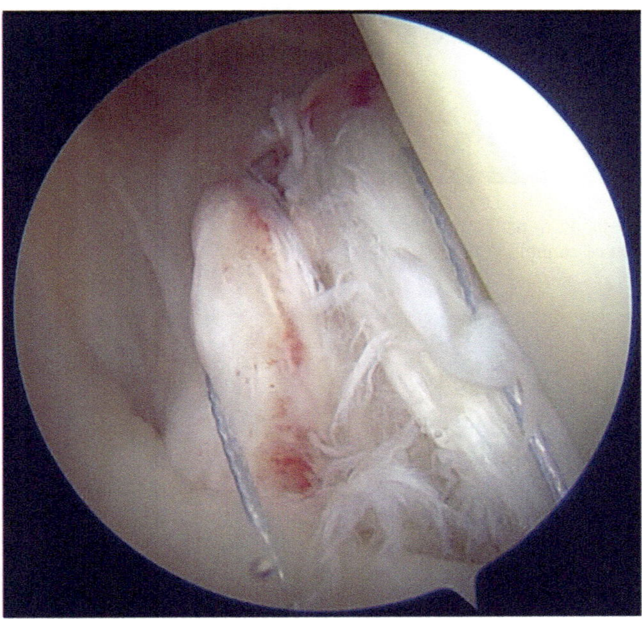

**Fig. 12.13** Both the suture ends taken out through low PM portal

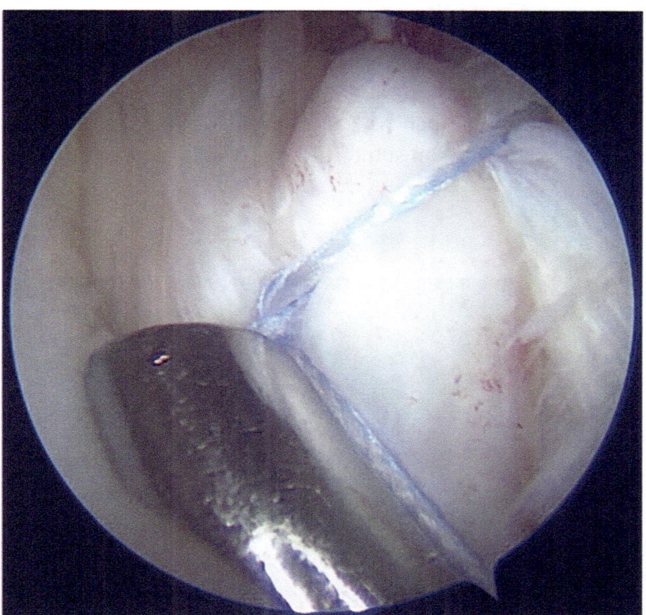

**Fig. 12.14** Simple knot is applied with the help of knot pusher

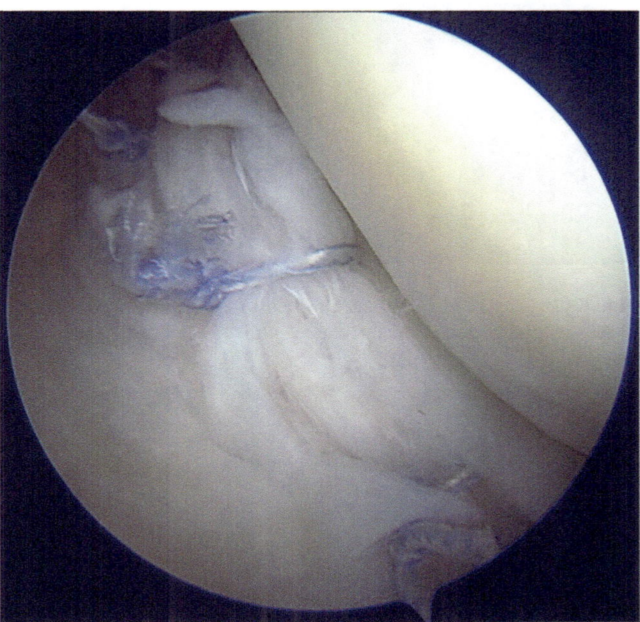

**Fig. 12.15** The repair procedure is repeated as per the length of tear and final repair is confirmed with the help of probe

### 12.5.2 Variation

- If passing suture through the tear is not possible with the knee scorpion, then we can use shuttle suture lasso. Here, we use no. 1 nylon suture/Ethilon which is passed into the tear with the help of lasso suture passer/suture hook. Initial surgical steps for this variation remains same (Fig. 12.16).
- Bite is taken from both edges of ramp lesion and Ethilon is retrieved from high PM Portal and 2-0 Fiberwire is tied and relayed through lesion. Now both suture ends are retrieved from low PM Portal and knot tying done (Figs. 12.17, 12.18, 12.19, 12.20, and 12.21).

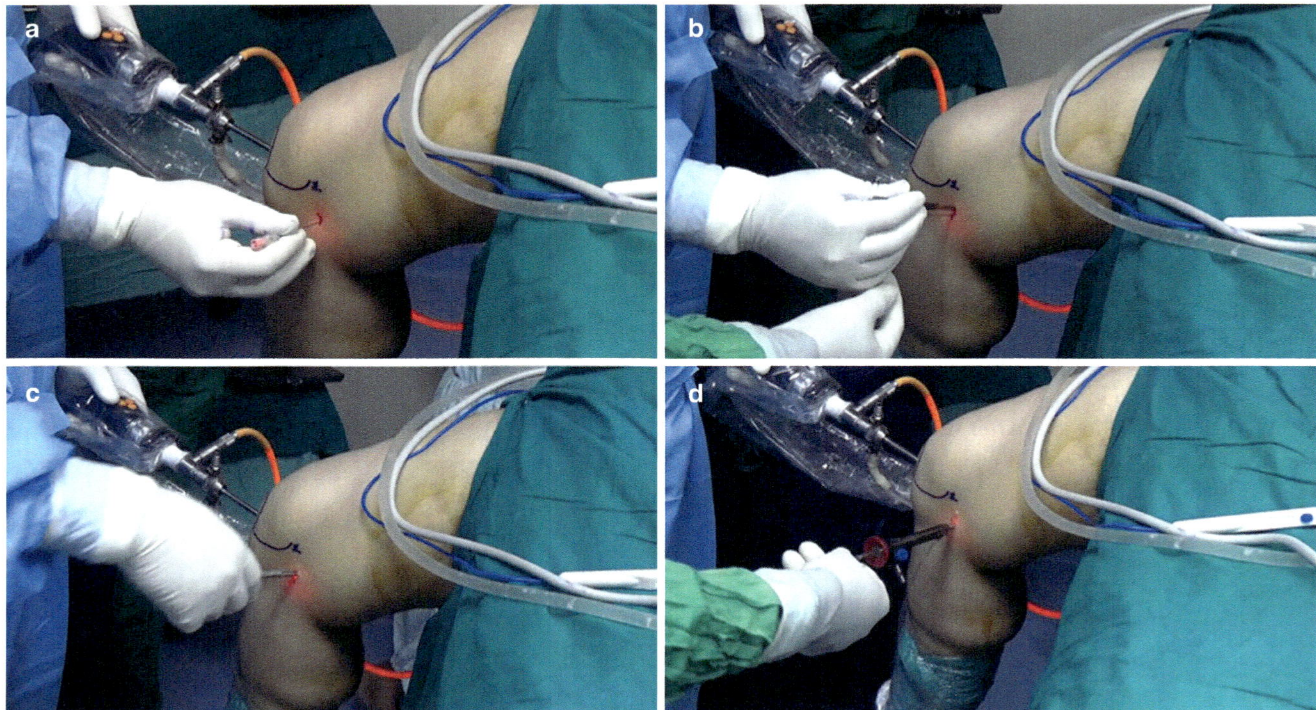

**Fig. 12.16** (**a**) 18 G spinal needle used to create low posteromedial portal using transillumination technique, (**b**) no. 11 scalpel to create low posteromedial portal, (**c**) haemostat to further widen the portal, (**d**) placement of cannula with the help of switching rod

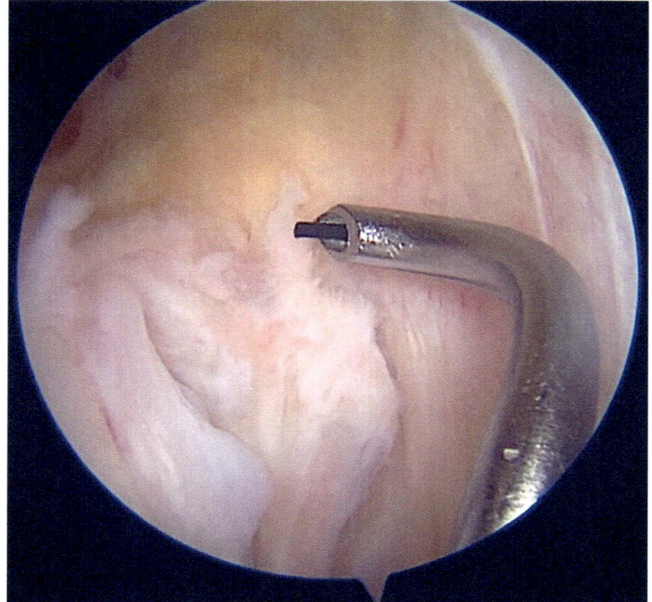

**Fig. 12.17** Suture passer with Ethilon 1 NO

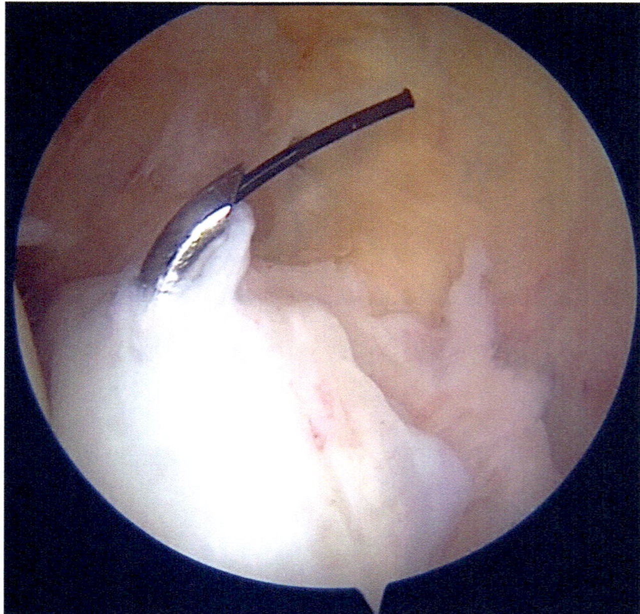

**Fig. 12.18** Bite taken from a part of meniscal tear

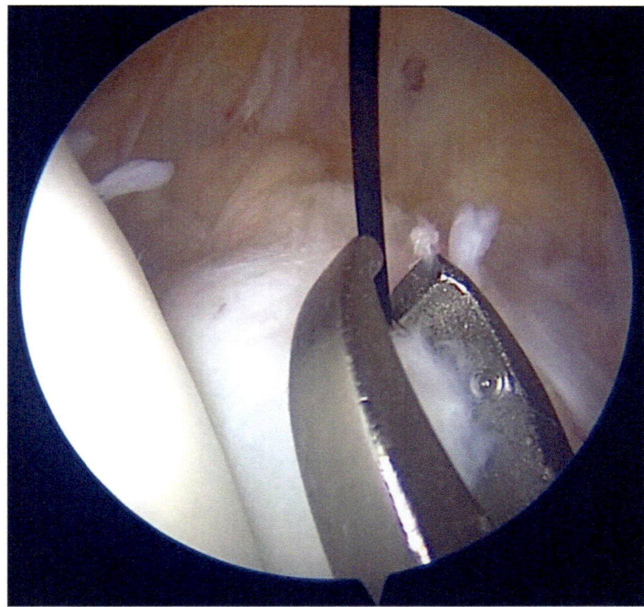

**Fig. 12.19** Ethilon used as a shuttle to pass the suture with the help of suture manipulator

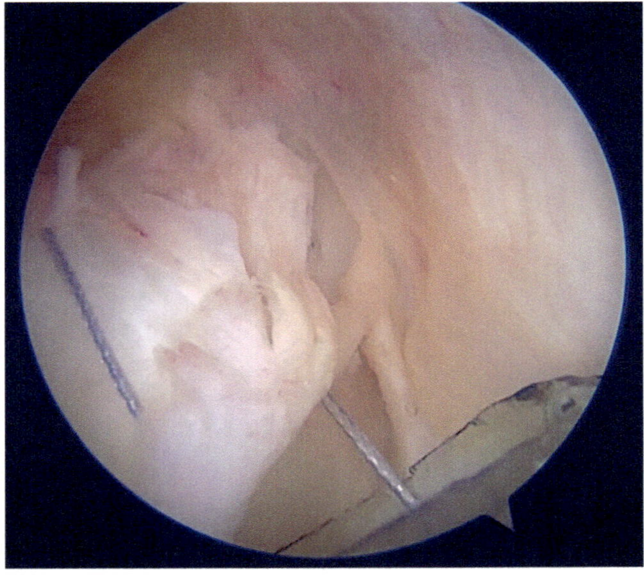

**Fig. 12.20** Both the suture ends taken out through working cannula

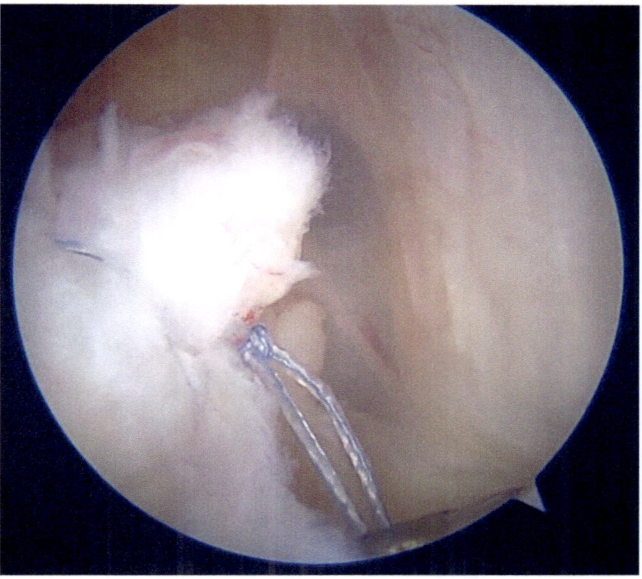

**Fig. 12.21** Knot tied and final repair done with the help of knot pusher

## 12.6 Advantages and Disadvantages

**Advantages**

- Easy application
- Quick, less time consuming
- Reproducible
- Performed under direct vision
- Less chances of injury to posterior structures
- Less associated morbidity
- Use of posteromedial portals allows better visualisation of the extent of the tear, hidden lesions, better manoeuvring, and repair.
- Repair of ramp lesion in conjunction with ACL reconstruction yields good functional outcome as biological factors are released during reaming.
- High healing rates
- Strong repair construct

**Disadvantages**

- Risk of cartilage injury in tight medial compartment to the posterior aspect of femoral condyles.
- Demands experience, skill, and instruments.
- May require medial release.
- Failure to heal or inappropriate rehabilitation can lead to changes in knee biomechanics.

# Part IV

# ACL

# 13 Arthroscopic Primary ACL Repair

Vikram Arun Mhaskar

## 13.1 Introduction

Anterior cruciate ligament (ACL) tears that are Sherman's Type I or II [1] are amenable to repair. This is possible as these tears are femoral avulsion tears with most of the stump intact. The aim is to reattach the stump to the femoral footprint as anatomically as possible with least tension. This technique described is familiar as the same principles of doing an ACL reconstruction like drilling a femoral tunnel and using an adjustable suspensory device to reattach the stump are used here.

## 13.2 Specialised Equipment (Fig. 13.1)

1. Knee Scorpion (Arthrex, Naples, FL) (f).
2. 2–0, Fiberwire-1 (Arthrex, Naples, FL) (j)
3. Suture tape-1 (Arthrex, Naples, FL) (k).
4. Passport Cannula (Arthrex, Naples, FL).
5. ACL jig (Acufex, Smith and Nephew, Watford, UK) (g).
6. Bone awl (Acufex, Smith and Nephew, Watford, UK) (a).
7. Mallet (b).
8. 4.5 mm drill bit (Acufex, Smith and Nephew, Watford, UK) (d)
9. Guidewire (Arthrex, Naples, FL) (c).
10. 2, Ethibond loops No 5 (Ethicon, Raritan, NJ) (e)
11. Tightrope RT button (Arthrex, Naples, FL).
12. ABS button (Arthrex, Naples, FL) (l).
13. Knot Pusher (Arthrex, Naples, FL) (i).

V. A. Mhaskar (✉)
F7 East of Kailash, Knee & Shoulder Clinic, New Delhi, India

JMVM Sports Injury Center, Sitaram Bhartia Institute of Science & Research, New Delhi, India


V. A. Mhaskar, J. Maheshwari (eds.), *Innovative Approaches in Knee Arthroscopy*,
https://doi.org/10.1007/978-981-99-4378-4_13

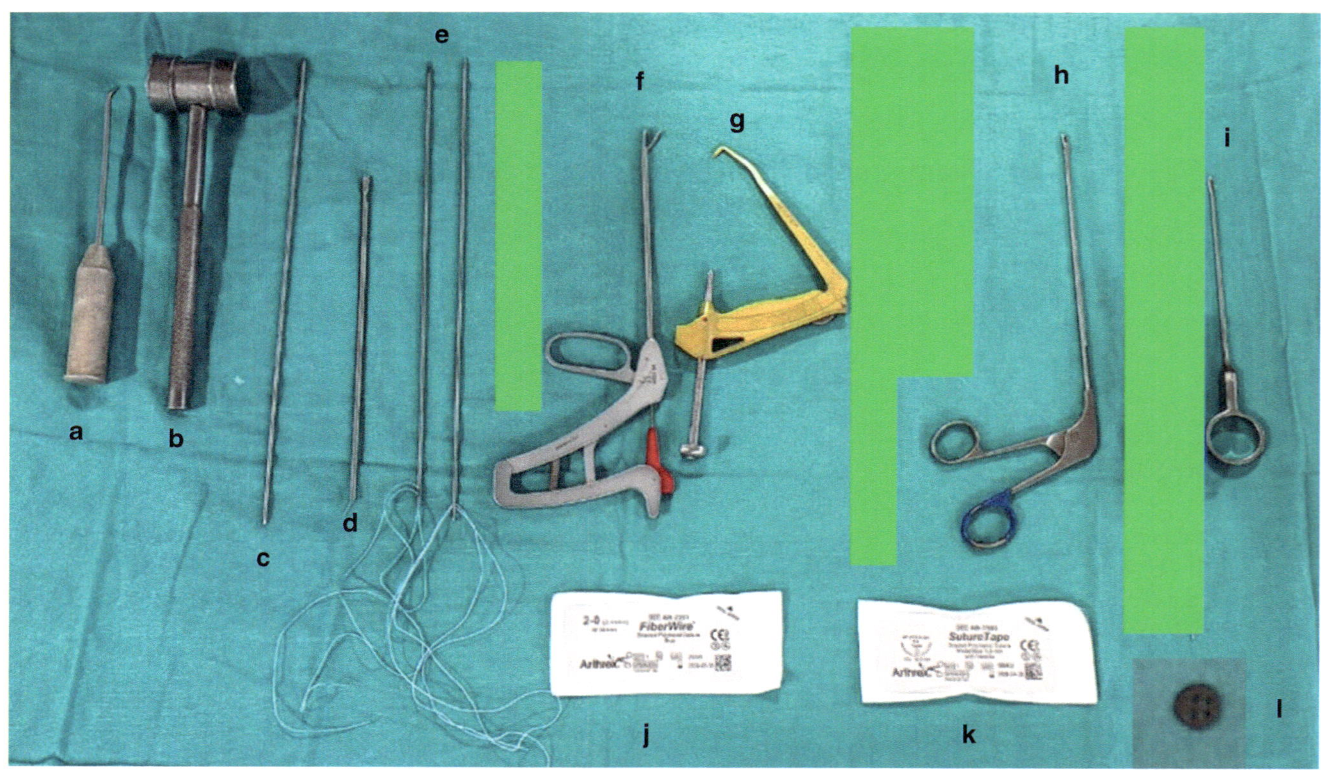


**Fig. 13.1** Image showing equipment used for doing a primary ACL reconstruction. (**a**) Bone awl, (**b**) mallet, (**c**) guidewire, (**d**) 4.5 mm drill bit, (**e**) 2, Beath pins with Ethibond loops, (**f**) Knee Scorpion, (**g**) ACL tibial jig, (**h**) arthroscopic grasper, (**i**) knot pusher, (**j**) 2–0 Fiberwire, (**k**) Suture Tape, (**l**) ABS button

## 13.3 Positioning (Fig. 13.2)

The patient is positioned supine on an operating table with a side support and a bolster at the foot end, keeping the knee in 70° flexion.

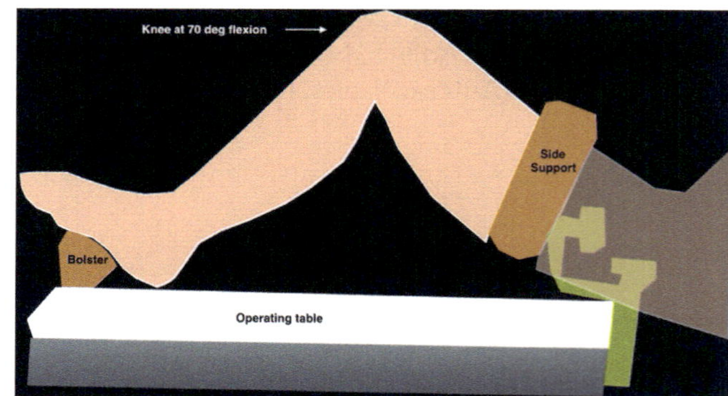


**Fig. 13.2** Illustration of knee in 70° flexion with a side support and bolster at the end of the table

## 13.4 Portals (Fig. 13.3)

Anterolateral viewing portal is a vertical portal made just adjacent to the patellar tendon at the level of the inferior pole of the patella.

Low far medial horizontal working portal is made medial to the patellar tendon and just above the medial meniscus under vision by introducing an 18G LP needle, such that when instruments are introduced, they do not scuff the cartilage over the medial femoral condyle. This portal is used to drill the femoral tunnel.

High anteromedial vertical working portal just medial to the patellar tendon that is used for the Passport cannula to stitch the ACL stump.

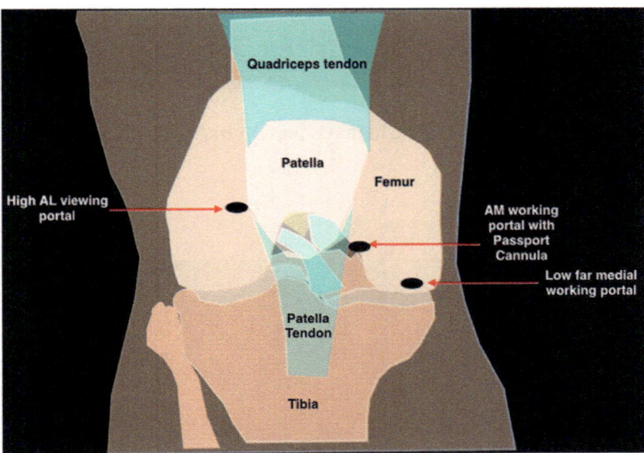


**Fig. 13.3** Illustration of the anterior aspect of the knee showing the position of the high AL viewing portal, AM working portal with Passport Cannula and low far medial portal

## 13.5 Surgical Steps

Step 1: The arthroscope is introduced through the AL portal and the ACL visualised (Fig. 13.4a, b).

Step 2: The far medial portal is made under vision and a probe introduced to palpate the ACL stump and see if the stump can be coapted to the femoral footprint with adequate tissue (Fig. 13.5a, b).

Step 3: A radiofrequency (RF) (Stryker, Kalamazoo, MI) device is introduced through the far medial portal and used to identify the femoral footprint of the ACL by gradually clearing tissue on the lateral side of the notch adjoining the ACL footprint (Fig. 13.6a, b, c).

Step 4: A bone awl is then introduced through the far medial portal and multiple trephinations about 1 mm deep are made in the footprint (Fig. 13.7a, b, c, d).

Step 5: The centre of the footprint is marked with a Beath pin, the knee flexed to 100° flexion and the pin is tapped into the bone using a mallet (Fig. 13.8a, b, c).

Step 6: Keeping the knee in 100° flexion a 4.5 mm drill bit is introduced over the Beath pin through the far medial portal and the footprint drilled till the far cortex is breached (Fig. 13.9a, b).

Step 7: The length of the tunnel is measured by introducing a depth gauge through the far medial portal and into the femoral tunnel (Fig. 13.10a, b, c).

Step 8: A Beath pin carrying a No 5 Ethibond (Ethicon, Raritan, NJ) loop is then introduced through the drill hole with the knee still in 100° flexion. The Beath pin goes beyond the far cortex and pierces the skin on the lateral aspect of the thigh, an incision is made over the Beath pin about 2 cm in length and dissected down to the bone using an artery forceps and pulled out. It carries with it two ends of the Ethibond loop that are

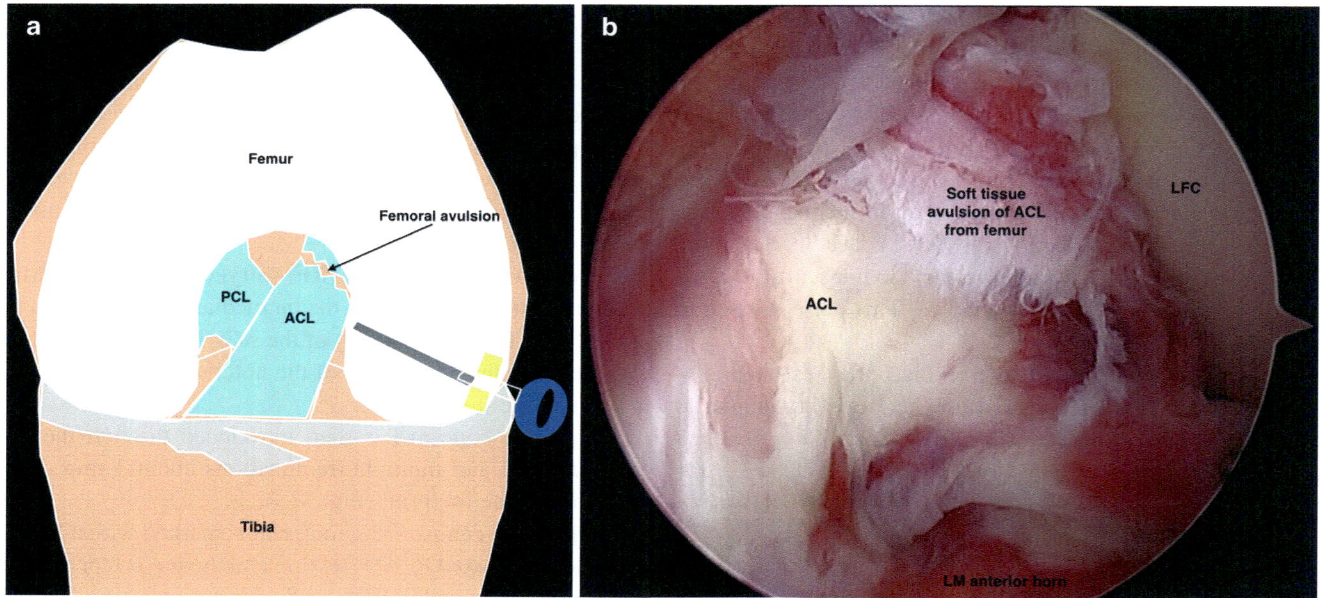


**Fig. 13.4** (**a**) Illustration of the knee showing a femoral avulsion ACL tear while viewing through the high AL portal. (**b**) Arthroscopic picture of the ACL stump avulsed from the femur

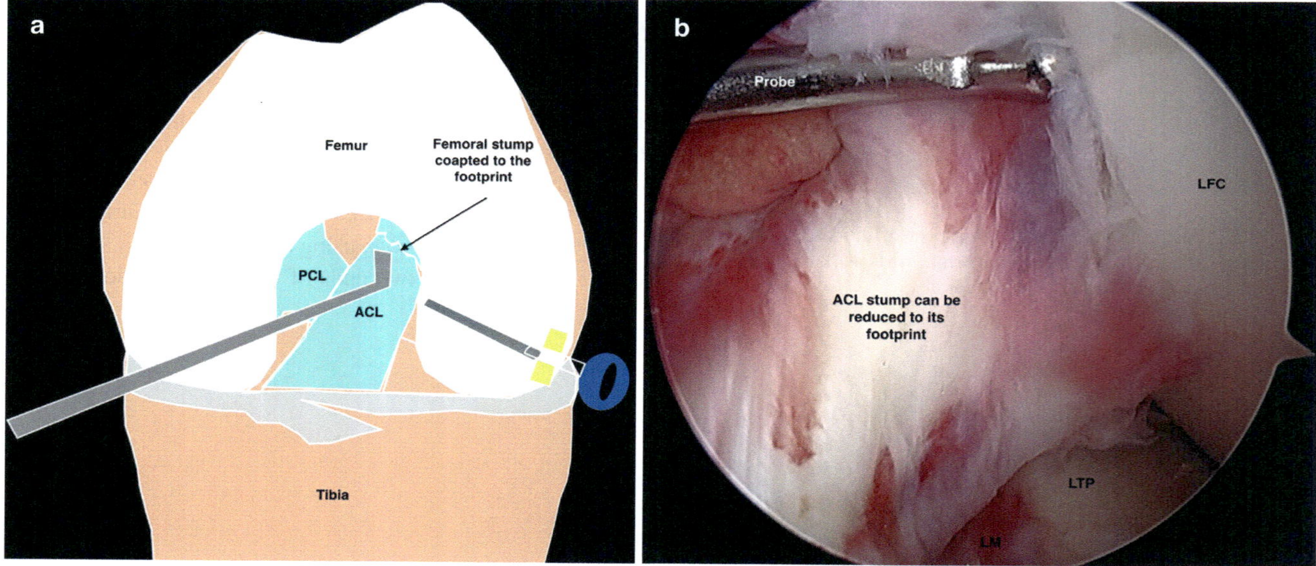


**Fig. 13.5** (**a**) Illustration of the knee showing a probe coapting the femoral stump to its footprint. (**b**) Arthroscopic picture of the ACL stump being coapted to the femoral footprint

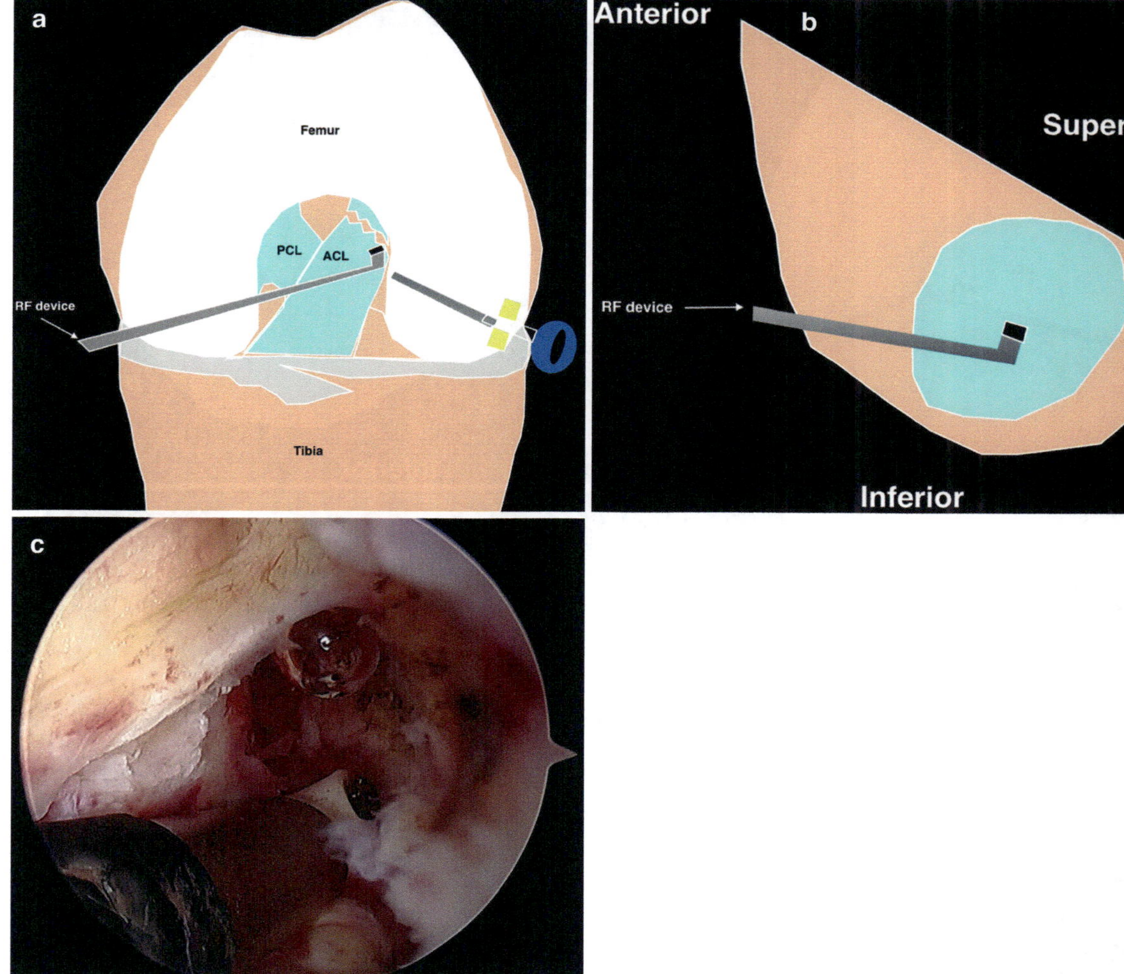


**Fig. 13.6** (**a**) Illustration of the knee showing radiofrequency (RF) device cleaning the femoral footprint in the lateral aspect of the notch. (**b**) Illustration of the lateral aspect of the notch showing RF device cleaning the femoral footprint. (**c**) Arthroscopic image of the notch showing the RF device cleaning the femoral footprint

delivered out of the lateral cortex and the loop is made to just project outside the drill hole at the footprint (Fig. 13.11a, b).

Step 9: Still keeping the knee in 100° flexion, another Beath pin carrying a different coloured suture loop is again introduced through the far medial portal, into the femoral tunnel and delivered through the lateral aspect of the thigh. While introducing this pin it is important to make sure it does not go through the previous suture. This can be facilitated by first delivering the loop out of the medial portal pulling both the loop end and free ends of this suture in tension while introducing the second Beath pin.

The two Ethibond loops are then identified (Fig. 13.12a, b).

Step 10: A high anteromedial portal is then made at the level of the anterolateral portal but on the medial side just adjacent to the patella tendon at the level of the inferior pole of the patella and a Passport cannula (Arthrex, Naples, Fl) is introduced through it using an artery forceps (Fig. 13.13).

Step 11: A Knee Scorpion device loaded with a 2–0 Fiberwire (Arthrex, Naples, FL) is introduced through the Passport cannula and the upper 1/3 of the ACL stump is held in its jaws and needle deployed to pass the 2–0 Fiberwire through the substance of the ACL (Fig. 13.14a, b, c, d).

Step 12: One end of the Fiberwire is tied over one end of the suture tape and the other end of the Fiberwire pulled to shuttle the Suture Tape (Arthrex, Naples, FL) through the substance of the ACL (Fig. 13.15a, b, c).

Step 13: The Knee Scorpion is again loaded with the 2–0 Fiberwire and introduced through the Passport cannula to take a bite proximal to the previous bite. Opposite ends of the suture tape and Fiberwire are identified and the Fiberwire is used to shuttle the suture tape through the ACL as described

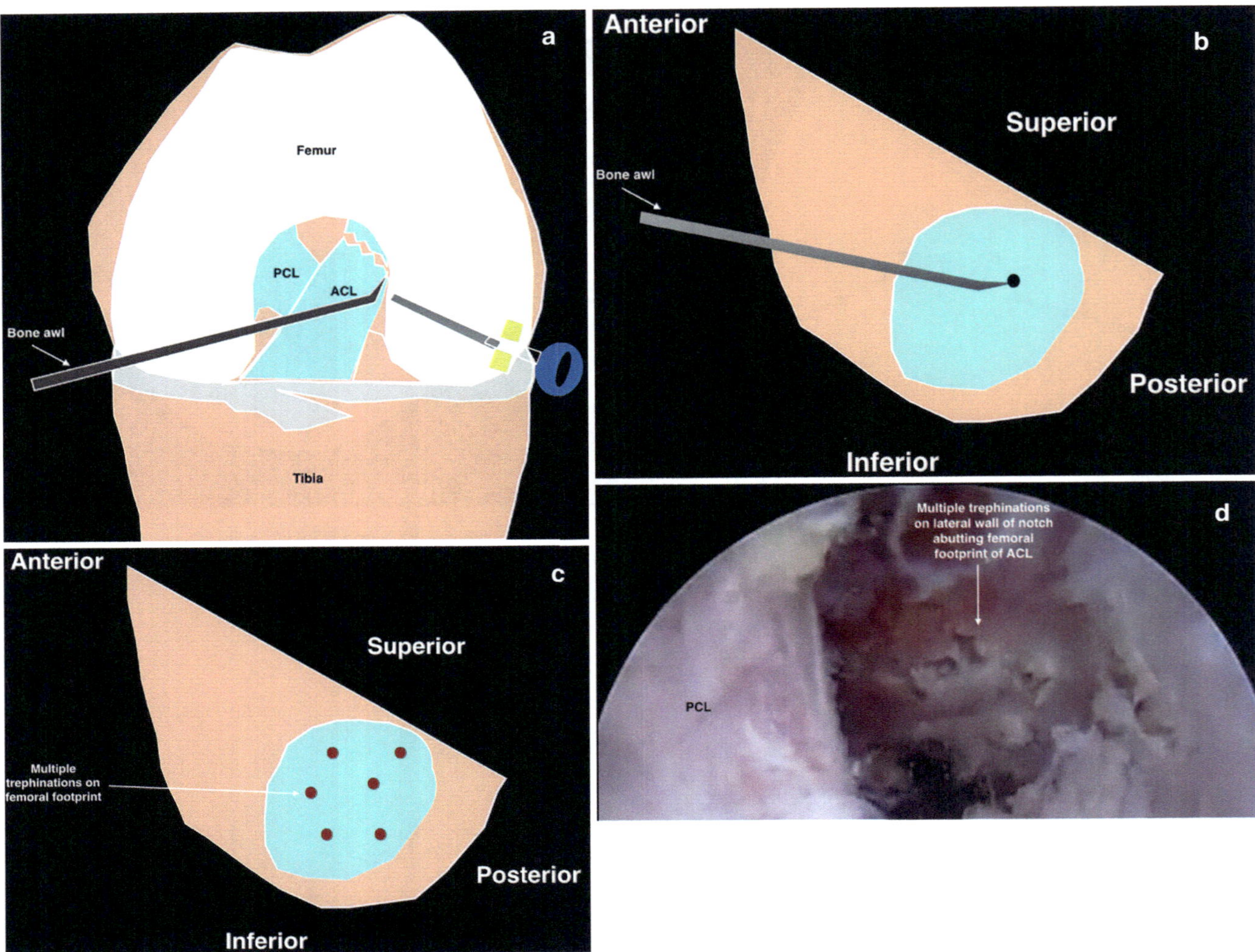


**Fig. 13.7** (**a**) Illustration of the knee showing a bone awl introduced into the notch to make multiple trephinations in the lateral aspect of the notch. (**b**) Illustration of the lateral aspect of the notch showing the bone awl making a trephination into the lateral aspect of the notch. (**c**) Illustration of the lateral aspect of the notch showing multiple trephinations around the femoral footprint. (**d**) Arthroscopic picture of the lateral aspect of the notch showing multiple trephinations on the femoral footprint

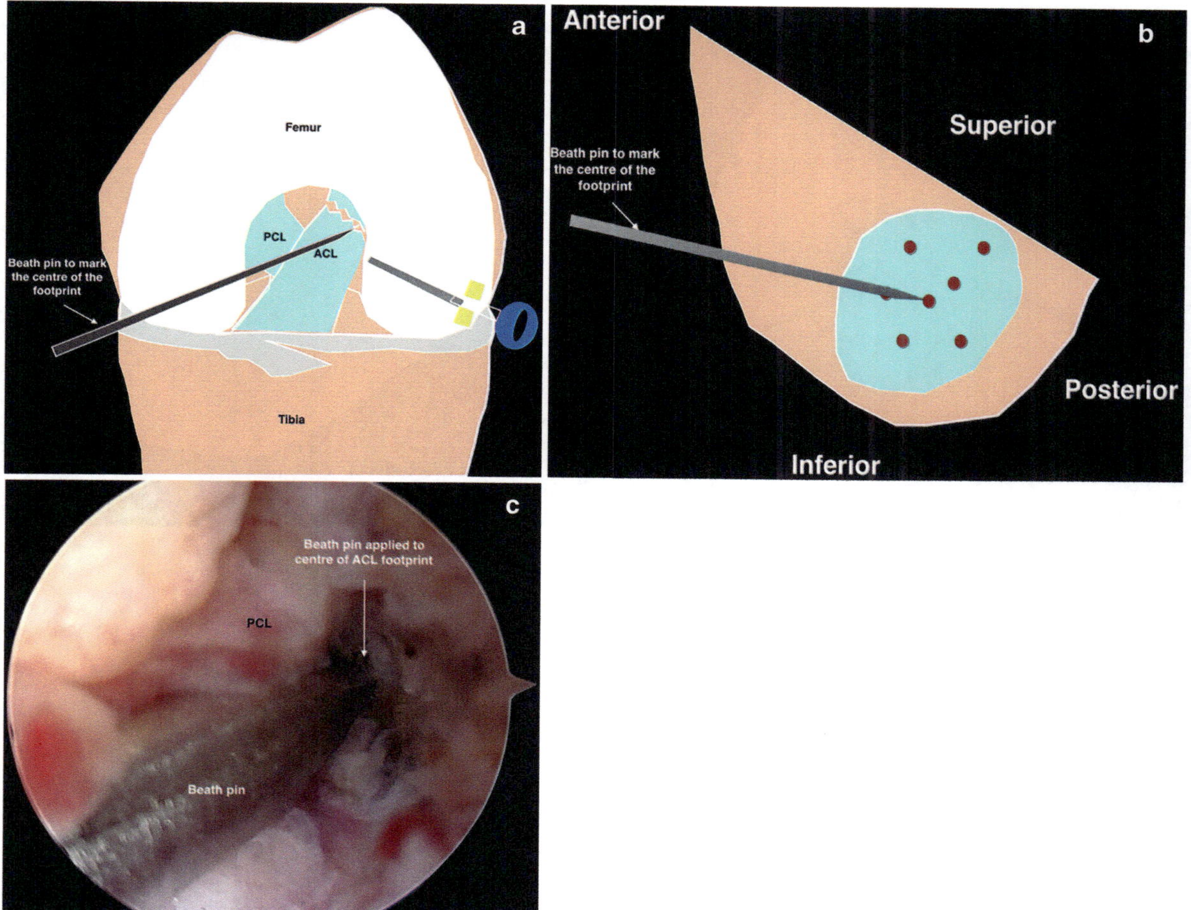


**Fig. 13.8** (**a**) Illustration of the knee showing a Beath pin applied to the centre of the femoral footprint. (**b**) Illustration of the lateral aspect of the notch showing beath pin at the centre of the femoral footprint. (**c**) Arthroscopic image of the lateral aspect of the notch showing the beath pin at the centre of the femoral footprint

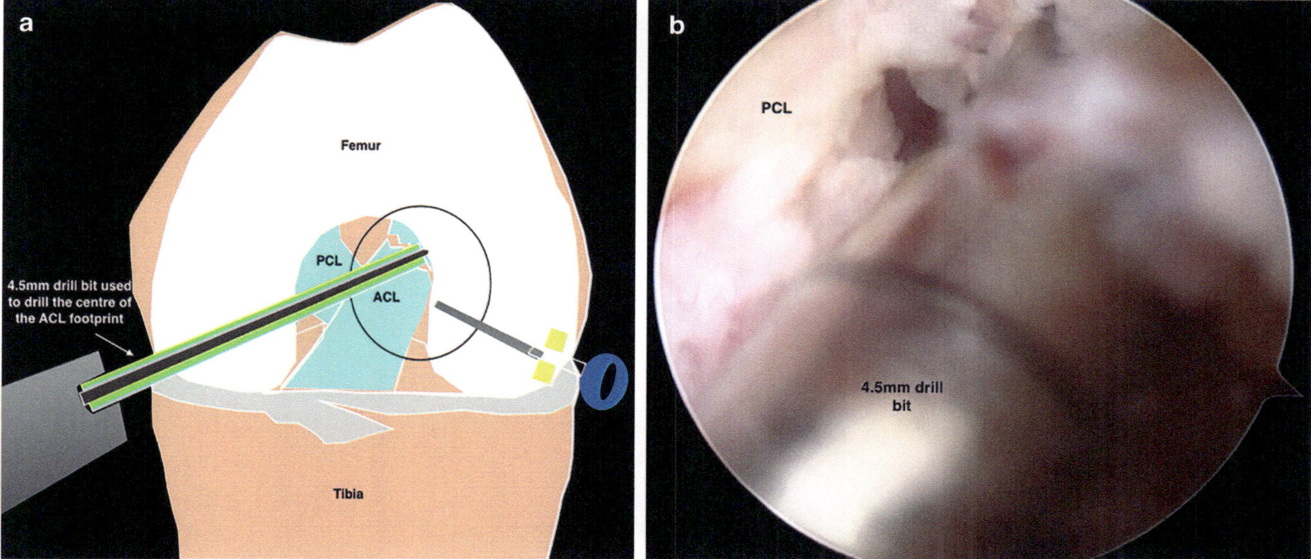


**Fig. 13.9** (**a**) Illustration of the knee showing the centre of the femoral footprint with a 4.5 mm drill bit. (**b**) Arthroscopic picture of the knee showing a 4.5 mm drill bit at the centre of the femoral footprint in the lateral aspect of the notch

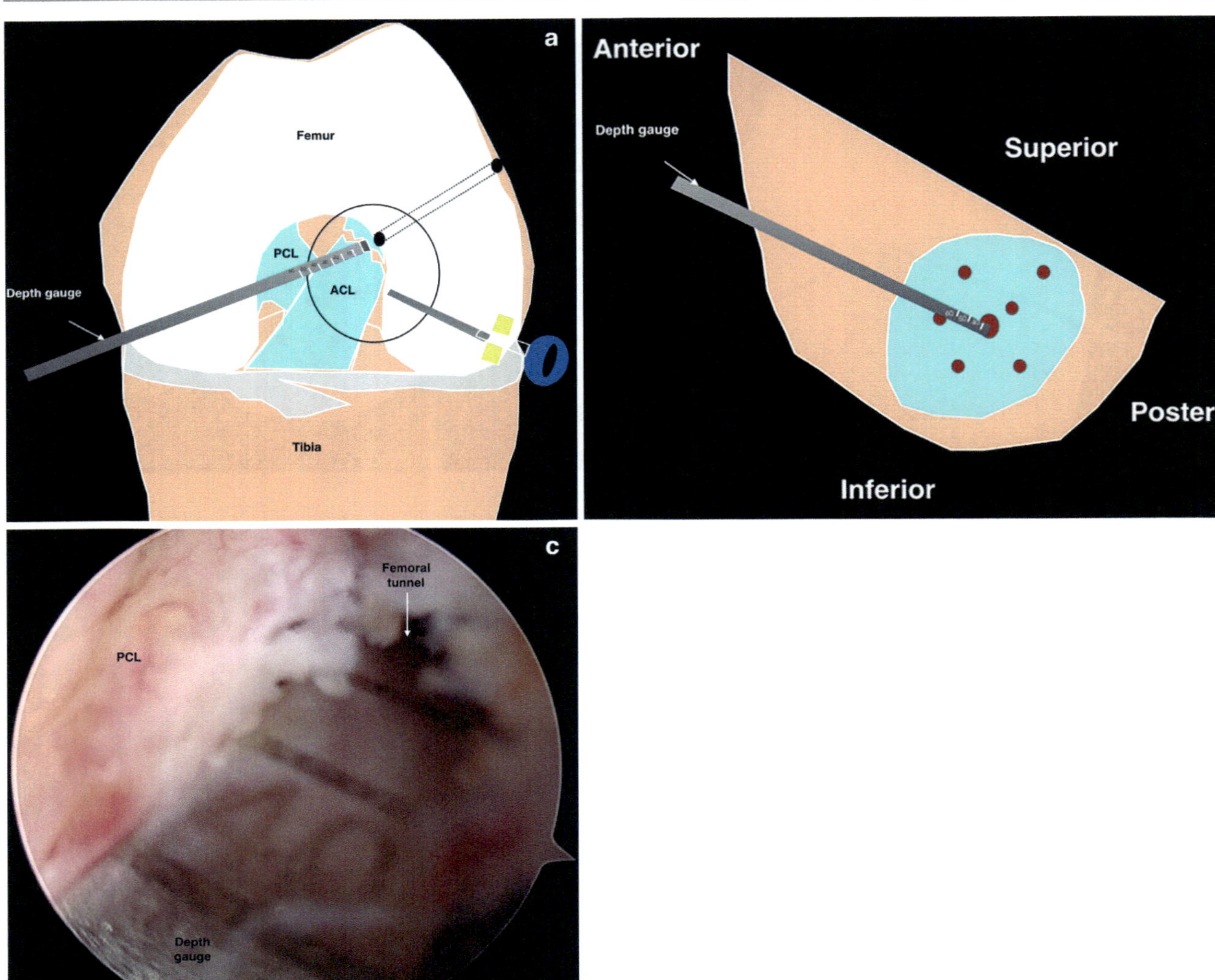


**Fig. 13.10** (**a**) Illustration of the knee showing a depth gauge being introduced into the femoral tunnel. (**b**) Illustration of the lateral aspect of the notch showing a depth gauge measuring the length of the femoral tunnel. (**c**) Arthroscopic image of the knee showing a depth gauge measuring the femoral tunnel length

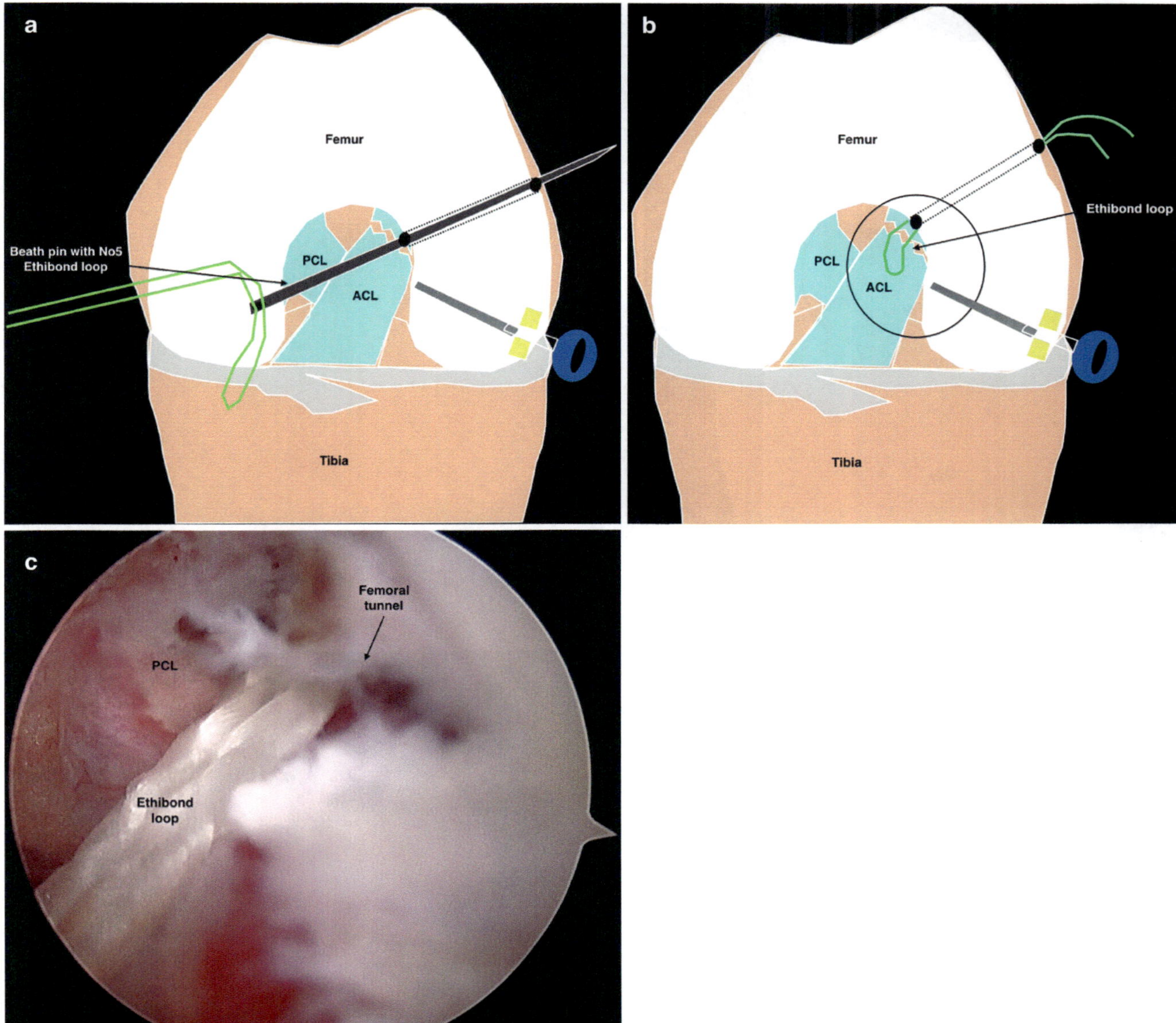


**Fig. 13.11** (**a**) Illustration of the knee showing a Beath pin carrying a No 5 Ethibond loop being passed through the femoral tunnel. (**b**) Illustration of the knee showing an Ethibond loop at the orifice of the femoral tunnel. (**c**) Arthroscopic image of the knee showing an Ethibond loop at the orifice of the femoral tunnel

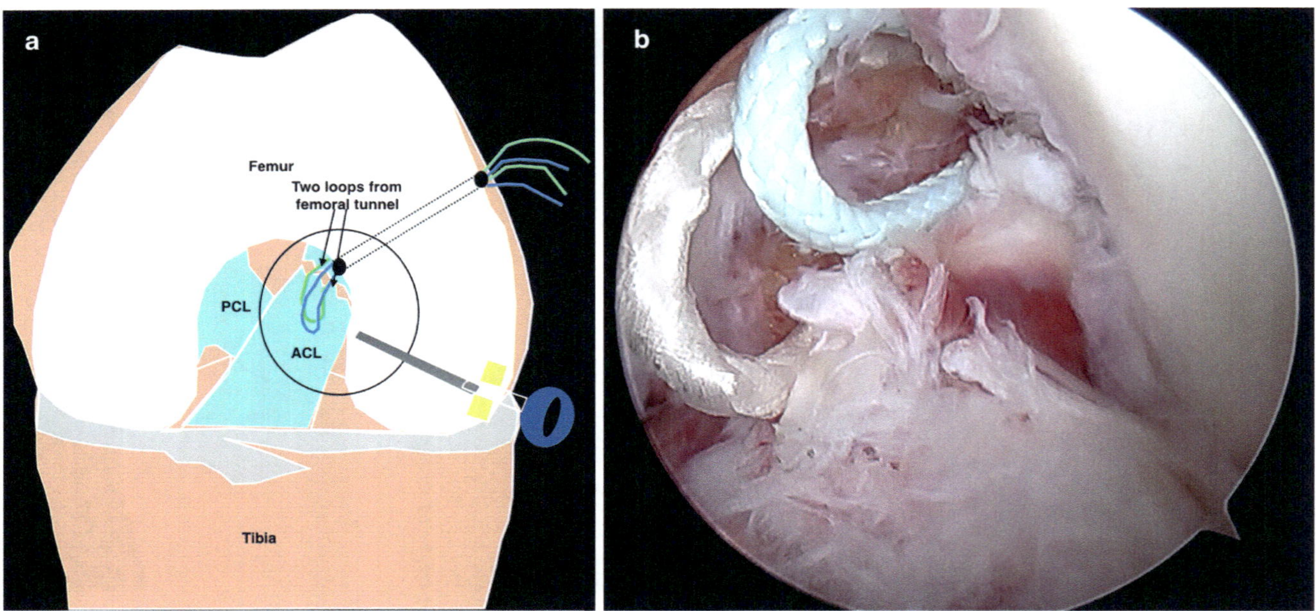


**Fig. 13.12** (**a**) Illustration of the knee showing 2 Ethibond loops at the femoral tunnel orifice. (**b**) Arthroscopic image of the lateral aspect of the notch showing two Ethibond loops at the femoral tunnel orifice

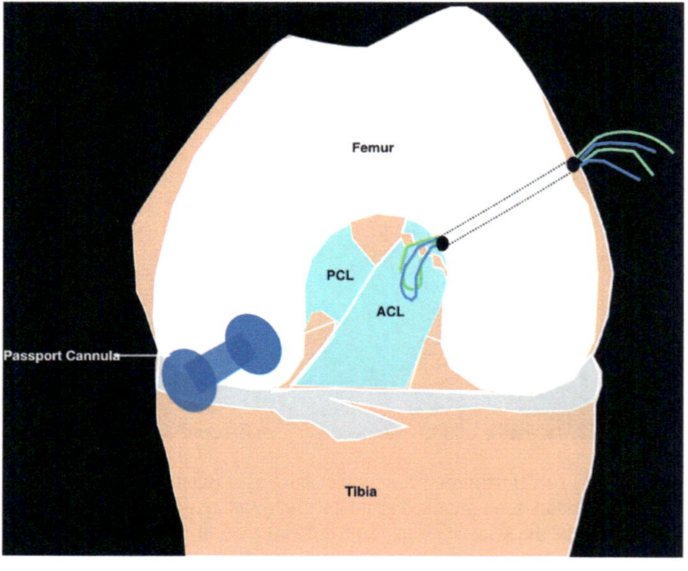


**Fig. 13.13** Illustration of the knee showing a Passport cannula through the anteromedial portal

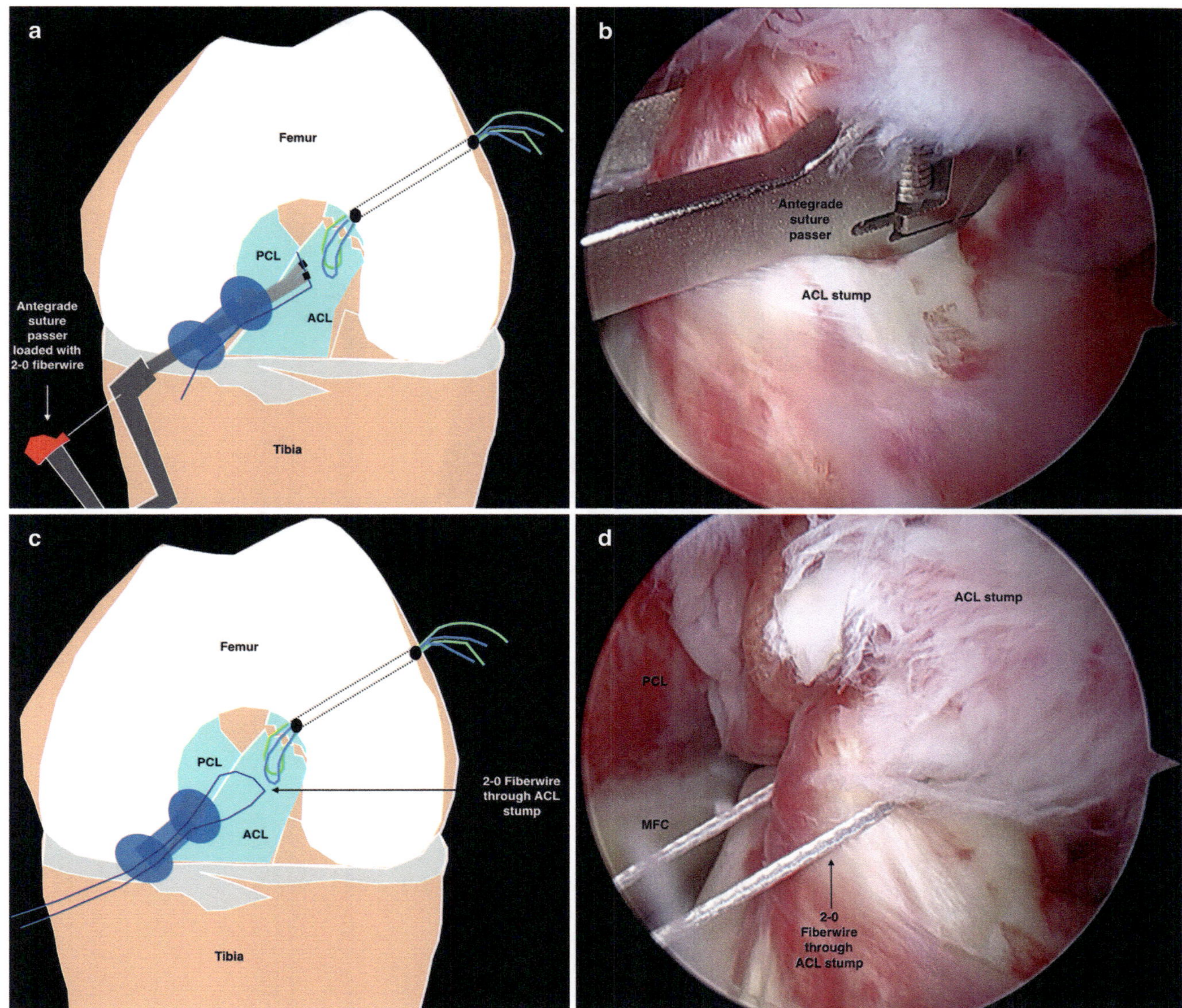


**Fig. 13.14** (**a**) Illustration of the knee showing antegrade suture passer through Passport cannula taking a bite through the ACL stump using a 2–0 Fiberwire. (**b**) Arthroscopic image of the knee showing the antegrade suture passer taking a bite through the ACL stump using a 2–0 Fiberwire. (**c**) Illustration of the knee showing a 2–0 Fiberwire through the ACL stump. (**d**) Arthroscopic image of the knee showing a 2–0 Fiberwire through the ACL stump

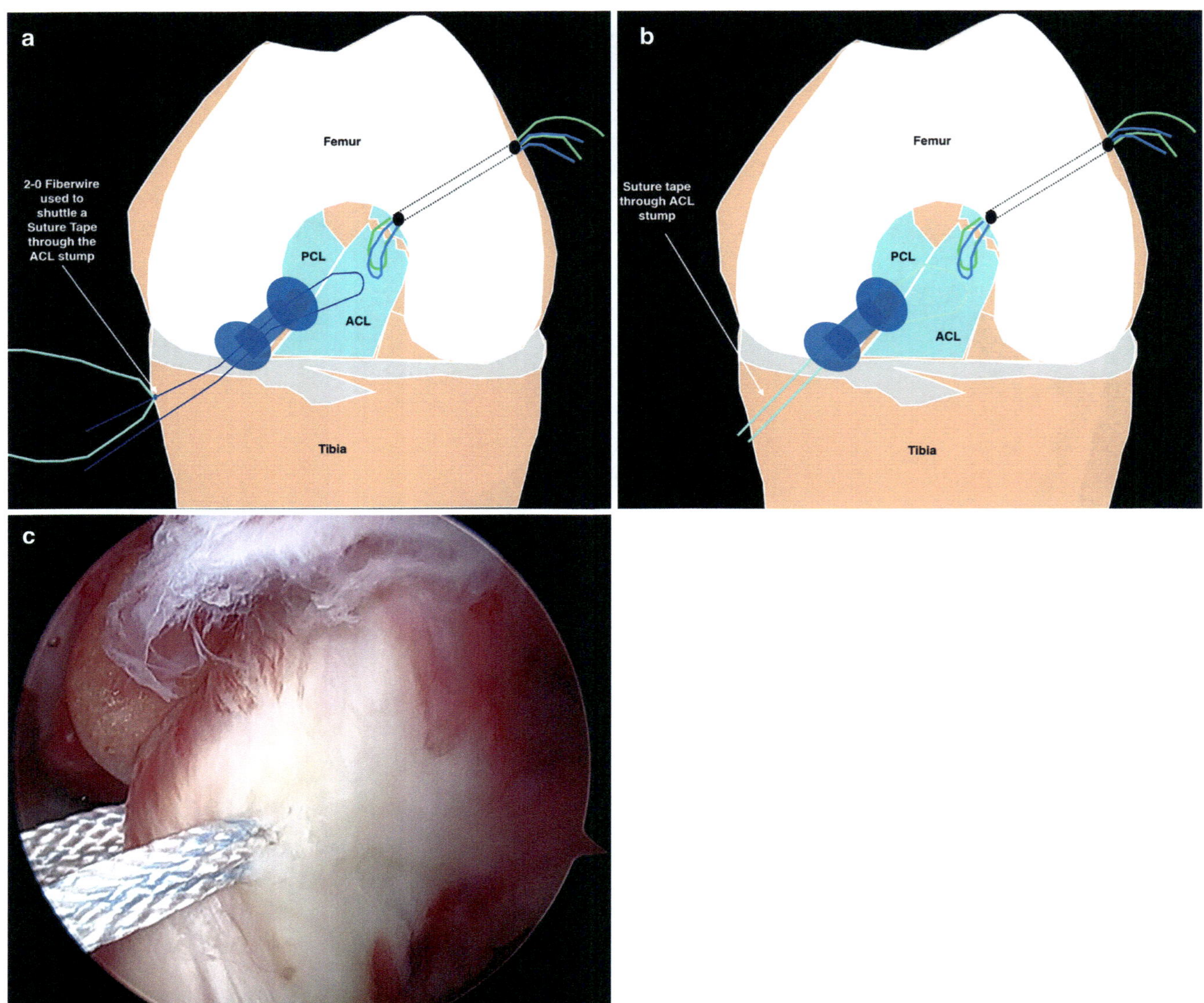


**Fig. 13.15** (**a**) Illustration of knee showing one limb of the 2–0 Fiberwire tied to one of the limbs of the Suture Tape. (**b**) Illustration of the knee showing the Suture Tape shuttled through the ACL stump. (**c**) Arthroscopic image of the knee showing Suture Tape passing through the ACL stump

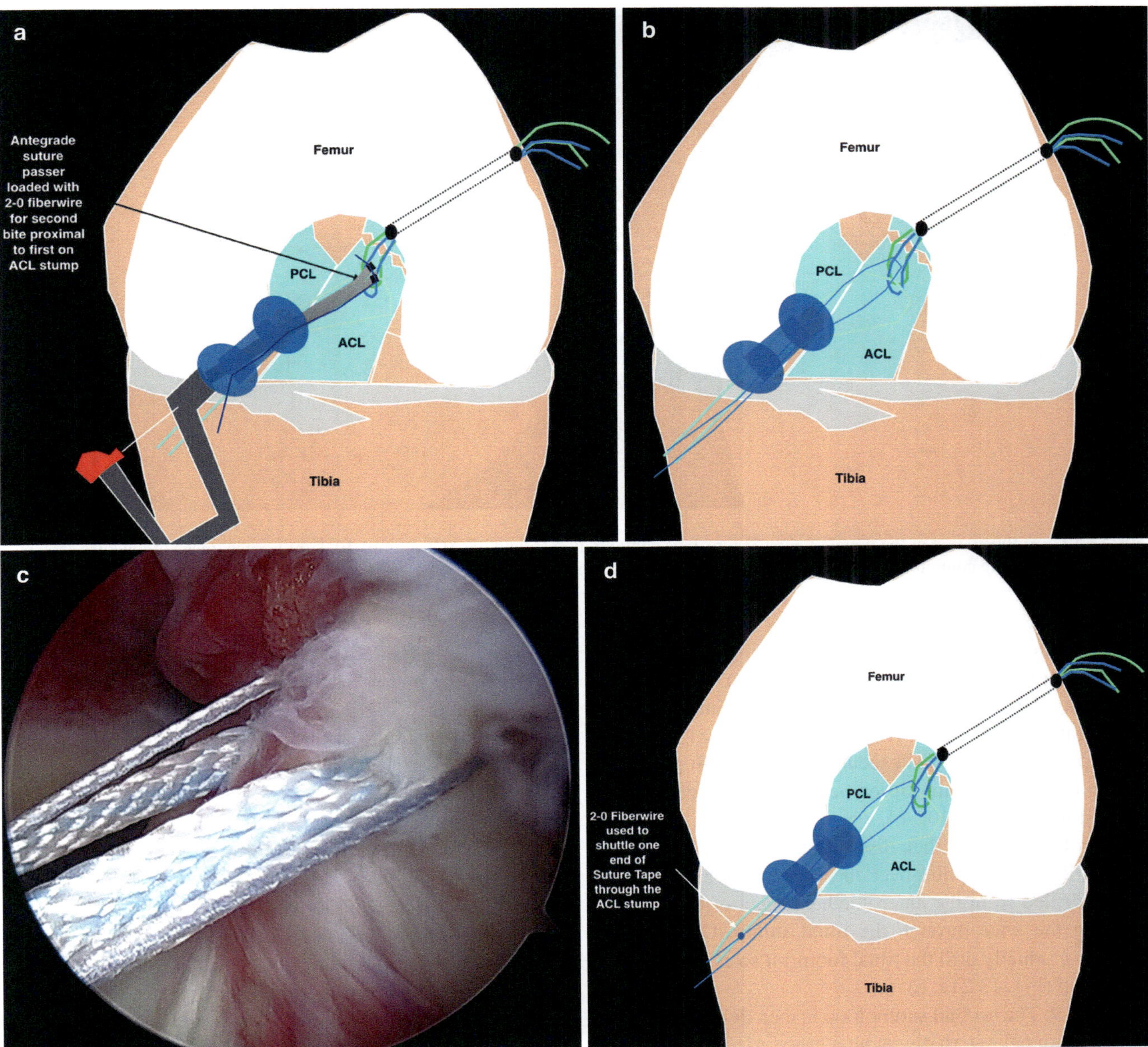


**Fig. 13.16** (**a**) Illustration of the knee showing the Antegrade suture passer taking a bite with a 2–0 Fiberwire just proximal to where the Suture Tape is passing in the ACL stump. (**b**) Illustration of the knee showing the 2–0 Fiberwire passing proximal to the Suture Tape through the ACL stump. (**c**) Arthroscopic image of knee showing 2–0 Fiberwire passing through the ACL stump above the Suture Tape. (**d**) Illustration of the knee showing one end of the 2–0 Fiberwire being tied over the opposite end of the Suture Tape to be shuttled through the ACL stump again to form one limb of the Figure of '8' suture configuration around the ACL stump

in the previous step. This makes one arm of the figure of '8' configuration of the suture tape around the ACL (Fig. 13.16a, b, c, d).

Step 14: The Knee Scorpion is again introduced through the Passport cannula to take a bite proximal to the previous bite, and the Suture Tape is shuttled through the ACL to form a figure of '8' suture configuration around the ACL (Fig. 13.17a, b).

Step 15: One Ethibond loop is delivered through the Passport cannula and the two ends of the Suture Tape are introduced into the loop and the two ends of the loop on the lateral aspect of the thigh are pulled to shuttle the Suture Tape out of the lateral cortex (Fig. 13.18a, b, c, d).

Step 16: An ACL jig set at 70° is introduced through the far medial portal and the tip centred on the centre of the ACL tibial stump and the bullet secured on the anteromedial

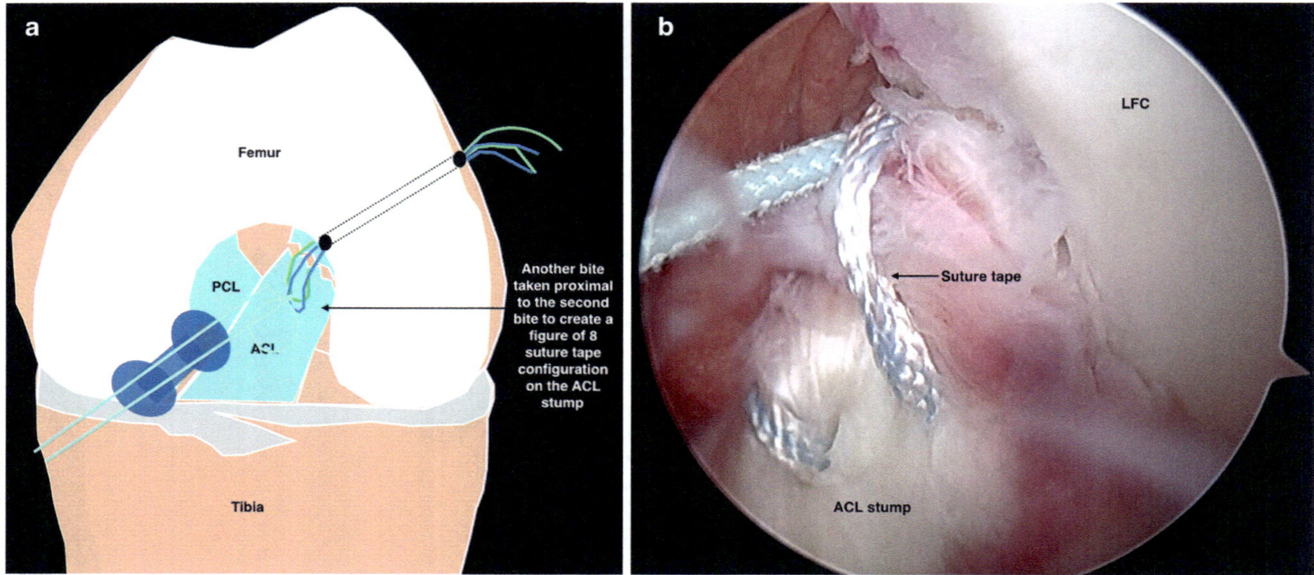


**Fig. 13.17** (**a**) Illustration of the figure of eight Suture Tape configuration around the ACL stump. (**b**) Arthroscopic image of the knee showing a figure of eight suture configuration of the Suture Tape around the ACL stump

aspect of the tibia. This is done by making an incision of 3 cm where the tip of the bullet enters the skin and then advancing the bullet to the anteromedial tibia and securing it by the ratchet mechanism (Fig. 13.19a, b).

Step 17: The jig is held securely and a Beath pin drilled through it such that the tip comes out of the centre of the tibial stump (Fig. 13.20a, b).

Step 18: The jig is then disengaged and a 4.5 mm cannulated drill bit is applied over the Beath pins and the tibial tunnel drilled from the anteromedial aspect of the tibia and entering the knee through the tibial stump. Care must be taken to gradually drill the tibial footprint so as not to disrupt the stump (Fig. 13.21a, b).

Step 19: The second suture loop is then delivered through the tibial tunnel externally using a grasper (Fig. 13.22a, b).

Step 20: The tightrope button and loop system are opened. The loop is lengthened to about 100 mm. The length of the tibial tunnel is marked on the elongated loop measuring from the tip of the button backwards. Mark another point 5 mm proximal to this (Fig. 13.23).

Step 21: A suture tape is applied through the loop like a graft and the traction sutures are put into the Ethibond loop (Fig. 13.24).

Step 22: The two ends of the Ethibond loop are then pulled to shuttle the traction sutures of the Tightrope RT out of the lateral cortex (Fig. 13.25a, b, c).

Step 23: The traction sutures (all 4) are then pulled gradually so that the button passes intra-articularly, then through the tunnel to the lateral cortex. One knows observing the marking on the loop crosses the lateral cortex. Once the button crosses the lateral cortex, a downward traction force will not pull the button out (Fig. 13.26a, b).

Step 24: Once the button has flipped, the white milking sutures are alternately pulled continuously to pull the suture

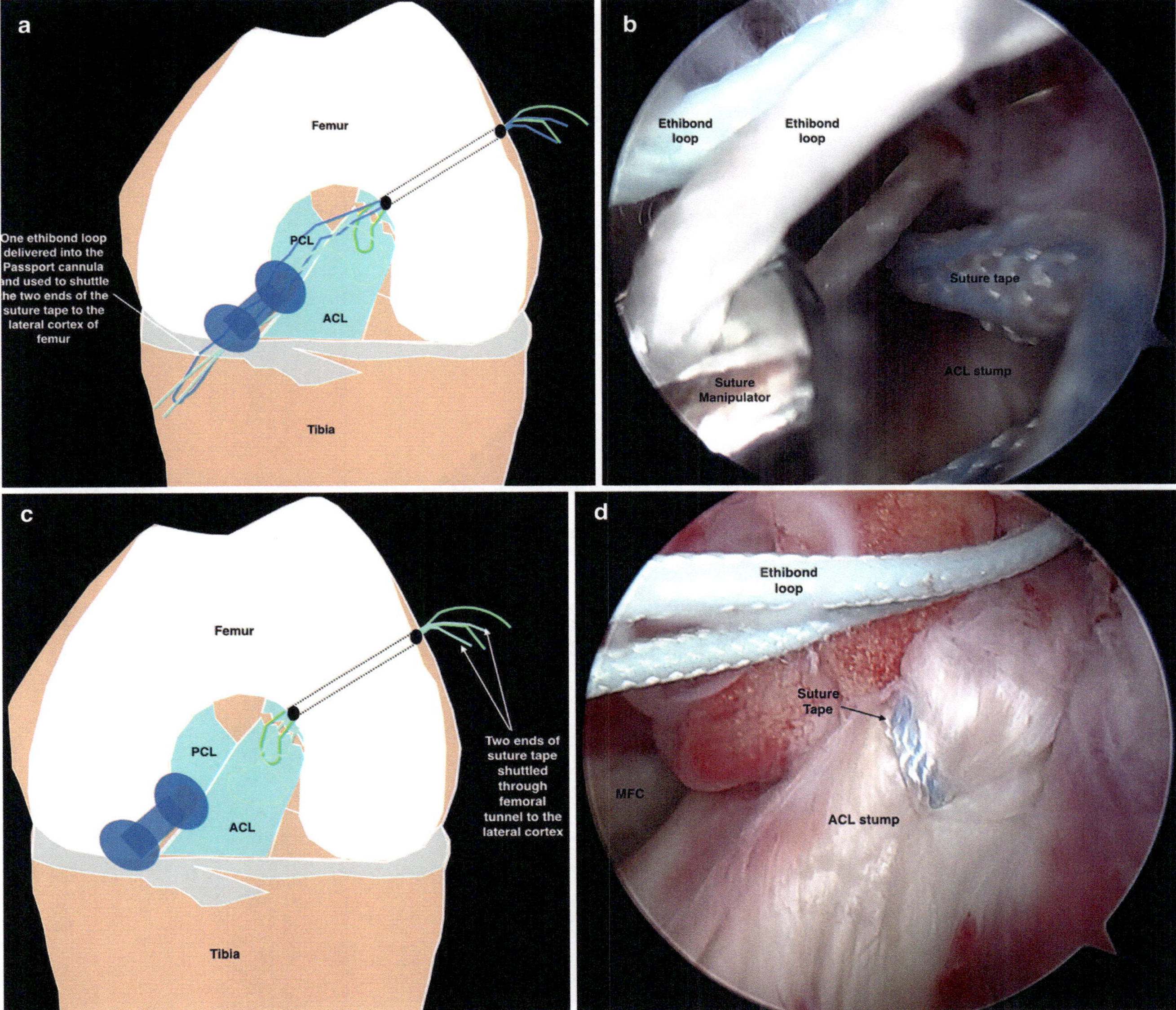


**Fig. 13.18** (**a**) Illustration of the knee showing one Ethibond loop delivered through the Passport cannula to shuttle the two ends of the Suture Tape. (**b**) Arthroscopic image of the knee showing one Ethibond loop being held with a suture manipulator to deliver it through the Passport cannula. (**c**) Illustration of the knee showing two ends of the Suture Tape shuttled through the femoral tunnel to the lateral femoral cortex. (**d**) Arthroscopic image of the knee showing the figure of eight suture configuration of the Suture Tape on the ACL stump after the two ends of the Suture Tape were shuttled through the femoral tunnel to the lateral cortex of the femur

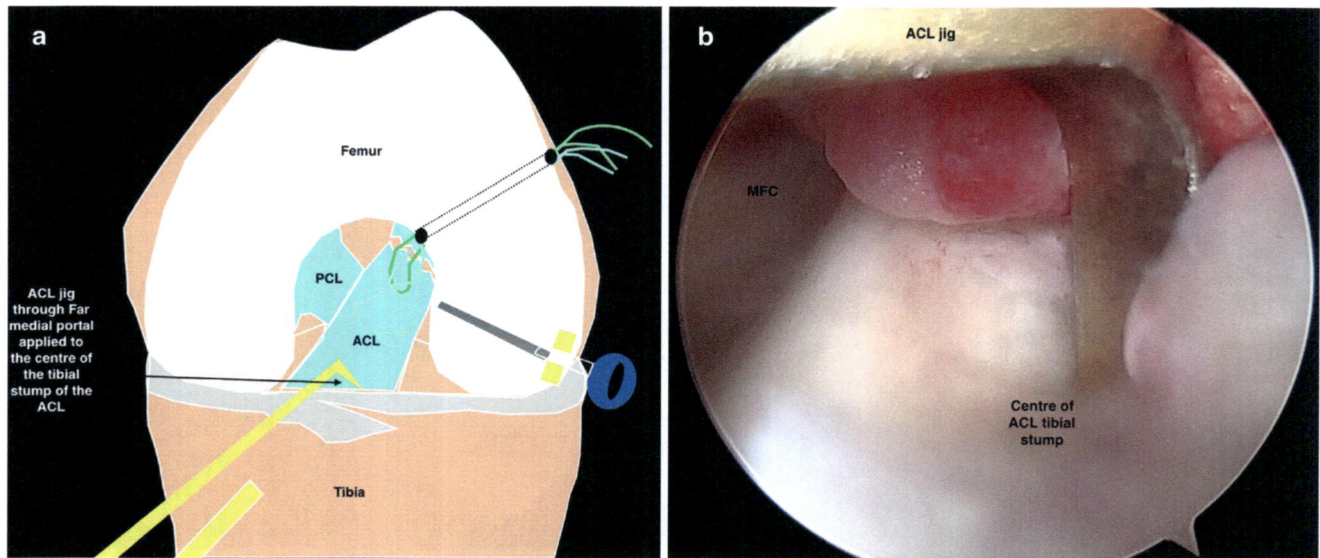


**Fig. 13.19** (**a**) Illustration of the knee showing ACL jig applied to the centre of the tibial stump. (**b**) Arthroscopic image of the knee showing the ACL jig at the centre of the tibial stump

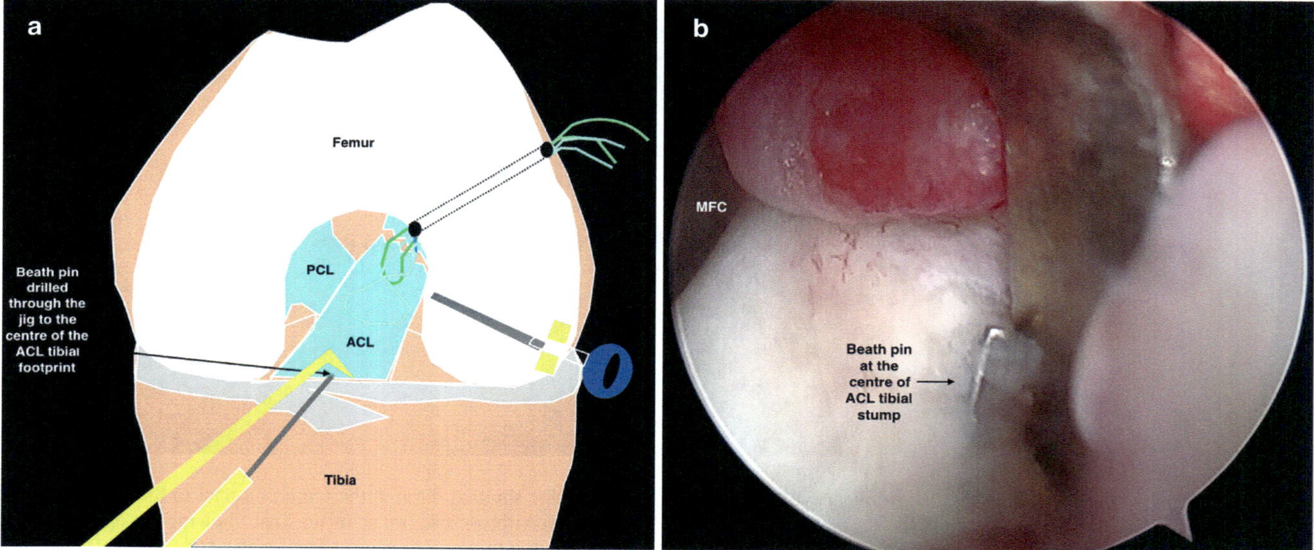


**Fig. 13.20** (**a**) Illustration of the knee showing the Beath pin drilled to the centre of the tibial stump through the ACL jig fixed at 70°. (**b**) Arthroscopic image of the knee showing the Beath pin at the centre of the tibial stump through the ACL jig

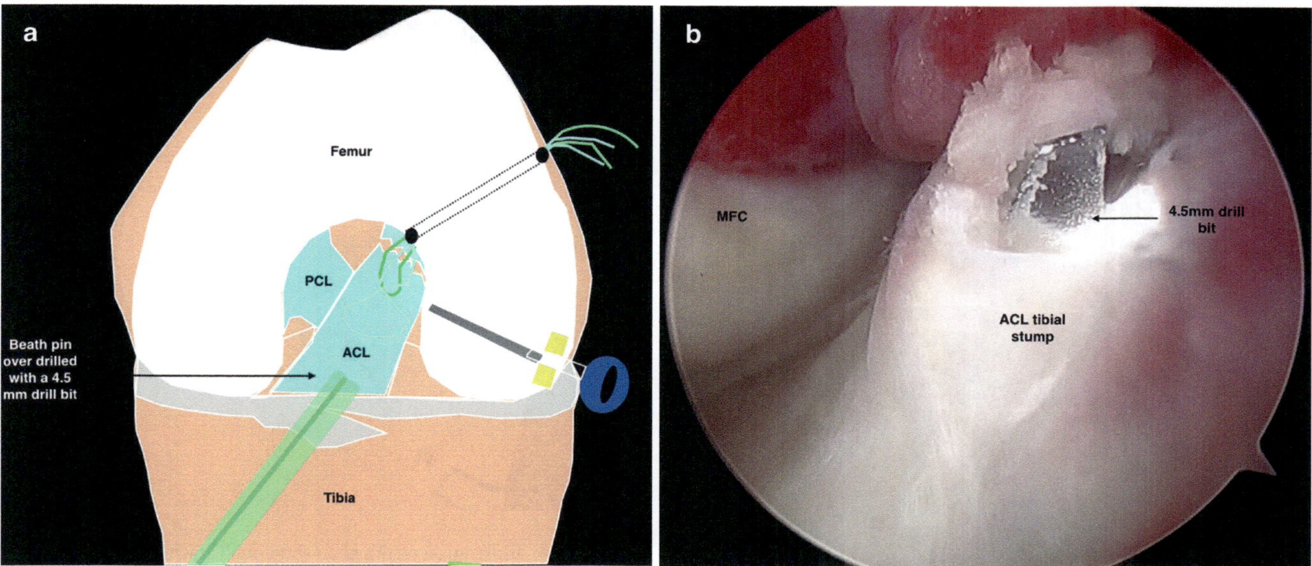


**Fig. 13.21** (**a**) Illustration of the knee showing a 4.5 mm drill bit passing through the centre of the ACL stump over the Beath pin. (**b**) Arthroscopic image of the knee showing a 4.5 mm drill bit coming out at the centre of the ACL stump

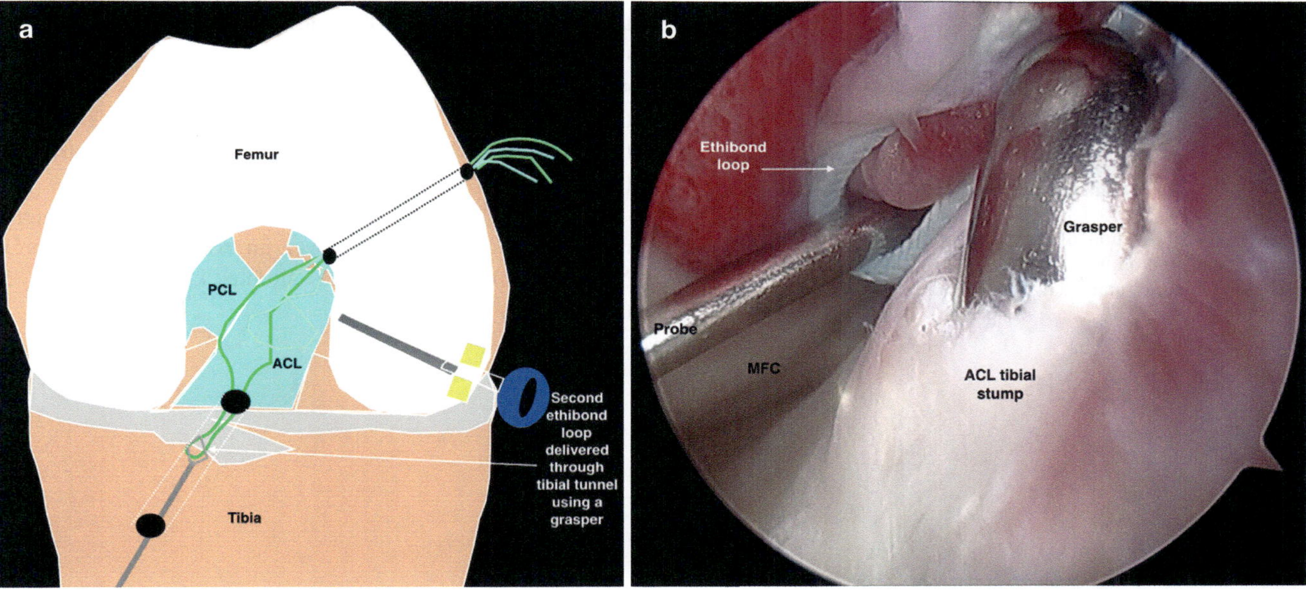


**Fig. 13.22** (**a**) Illustration of the knee showing the second Ethibond loop delivered through the tibial tunnel. (**b**) Arthroscopic image of a grasper coming out of the ACL tibial tunnel to grasp the second Ethibond loop to be delivered through the tibial tunnel orifice on the anteromedial aspect of the tibia

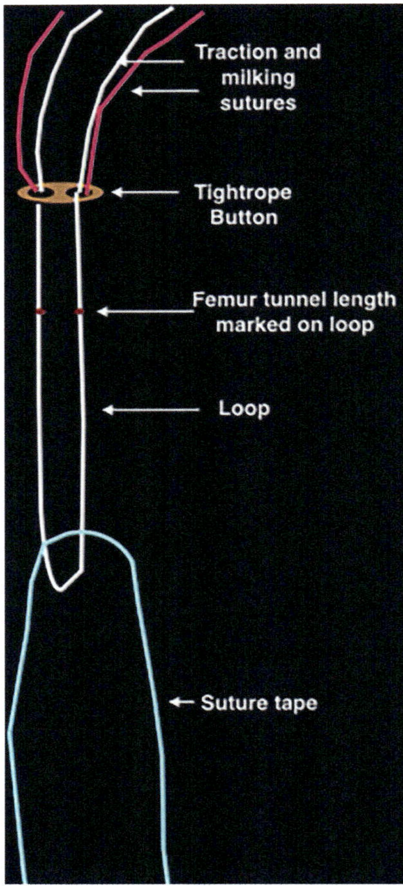


**Fig. 13.23** Illustration of the Tightrope construct consisting of the Tightrope RT button with loop made long and marked from the button end of the femoral tunnel length and suture tape through the loop to act an internal brace

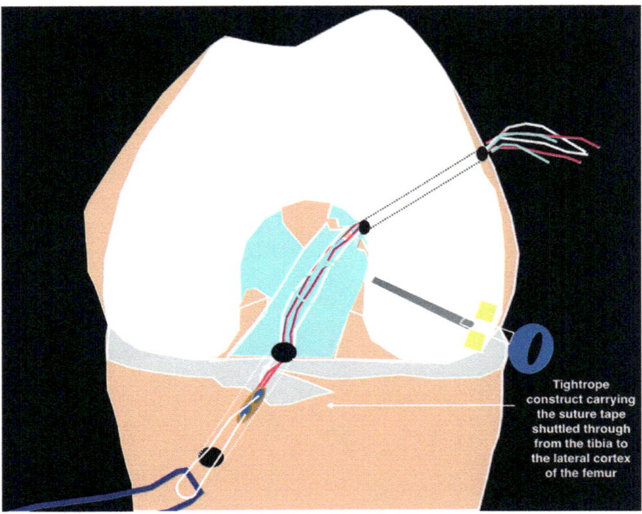


**Fig. 13.24** Illustration of the knee showing Tightrope RT traction and milking sutures passed into the Ethibond loop coming out of the tibial tunnel

tape intra-articularly and up the femoral tunnel. While doing this a constant downward traction force is applied on the suture tapes distally to make sure the button does not go pass the lateral cortex and into the IT band. This can happen as there is no differential drilling like an ACL reconstruction (Fig. 13.27a, b, c).

Step 25: The two ends of the Suture Tape on the antero-medial tibia are then tied over an ABS button (Arthrex, Naples, FL) with multiple simple knots (at least 5) (Fig. 13.28).

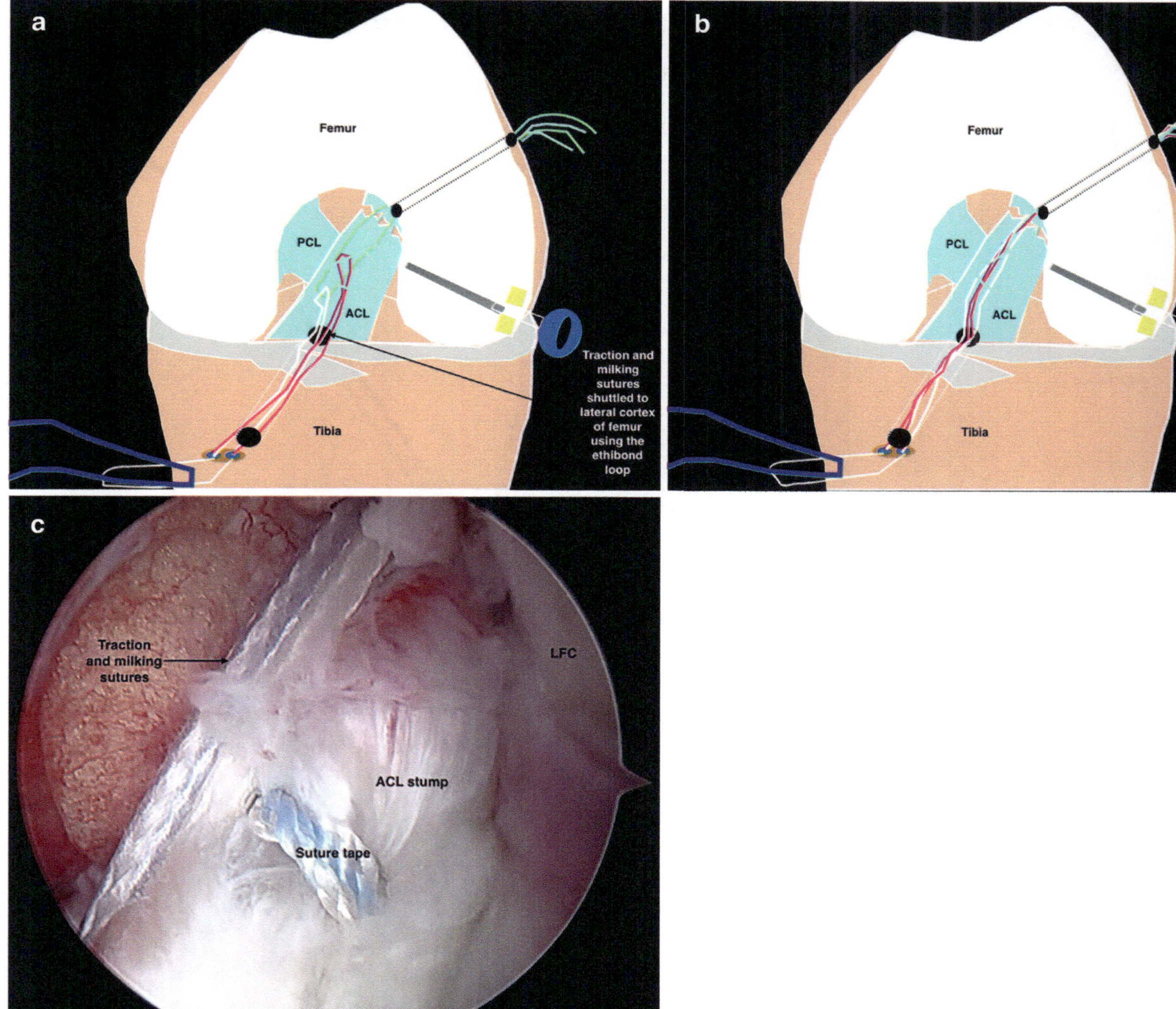


**Fig. 13.25** (**a**) Illustration of the knee showing the traction and milking sutures being shuttled to the lateral cortex of the femur with the Ethibond loop. (**b**) Illustration of the knee showing the traction and milking sutures of the Tightrope RT coming out through the femoral tunnel at the lateral femoral cortex. (**c**) Arthroscopic image of the knee showing the traction and milking sutures intra-articularly lying parallel to the ACL stump after being shuttled through the femoral tunnel to the lateral femoral cortex

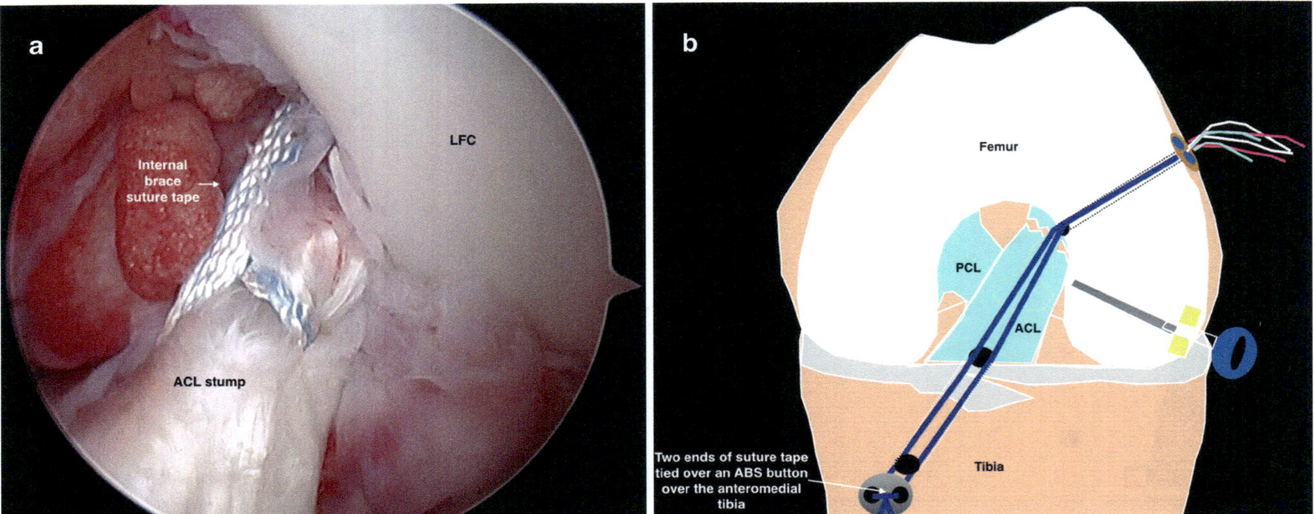


**Fig. 13.26** (**a**) Illustration of the knee showing the Tightrope RT button being shuttled to the lateral cortex of the femur from the tibial tunnel through the femoral tunnel to the lateral cortex of the femur by pulling both the traction and milking sutures together. (**b**) Arthroscopic image of the Tightrope RT button passing through the knee and parallel to the ACL stump

Step 26: The two ends of the suture tapes used to stitch the ACL stump are tied with the milking white sutures over the Tightrope button on the bone using a knot pusher. At least 5 throws are done using both ends of the sutures tape and milking sutures together (Fig. 13.29).

Step 27: The Knot ends are cut on the anteromedial tibia and lateral cortex of femur and the repaired ACL construct is visualised (Fig. 13.30a, b).

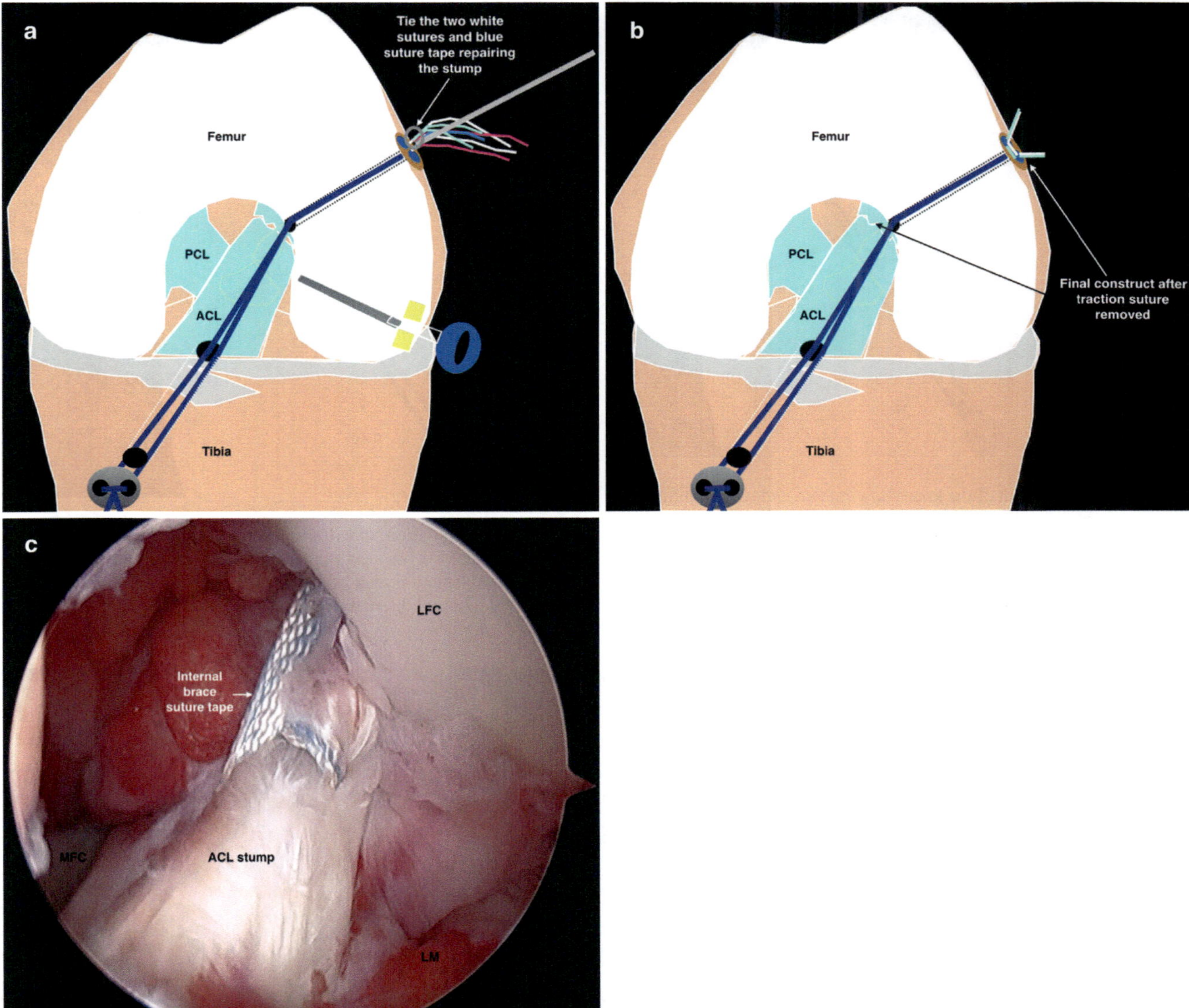


**Fig. 13.27** (**a**) Illustration of the knee showing the milking sutures being pulled alternately to shuttle the suture tape through the tibial tunnel into the joint. (**b**) Illustration of the knee showing the suture tape passing from the tibial tunnel, intra-articularly and through the femoral tunnel. (**c**) Arthroscopic image of the knee showing the ACL stump with suture tape around it and the internal brace parallel to the stump

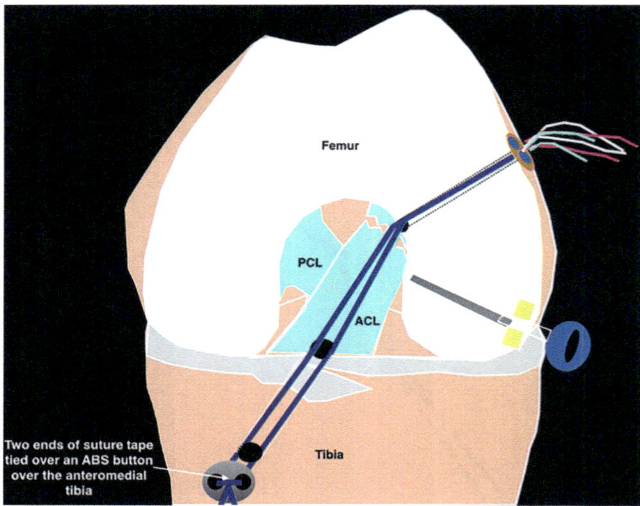


**Fig. 13.28** Illustration of the knee showing two ends of the suture tape coming out of the tibial tunnel that is part of the internal brace tied over an ABS button

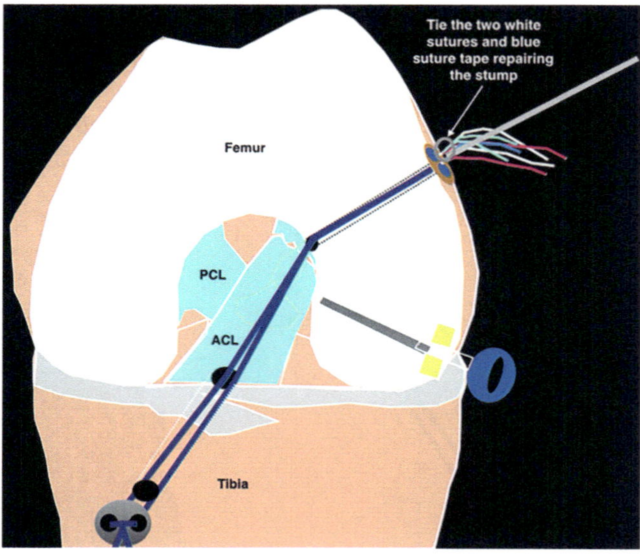


**Fig. 13.29** Illustration showing two ends of the suture tape used to repair the stump being tied to the two milking sutures using a knot pusher on the lateral cortex of the femur after making an incision corresponding to it and dissecting down to the bone

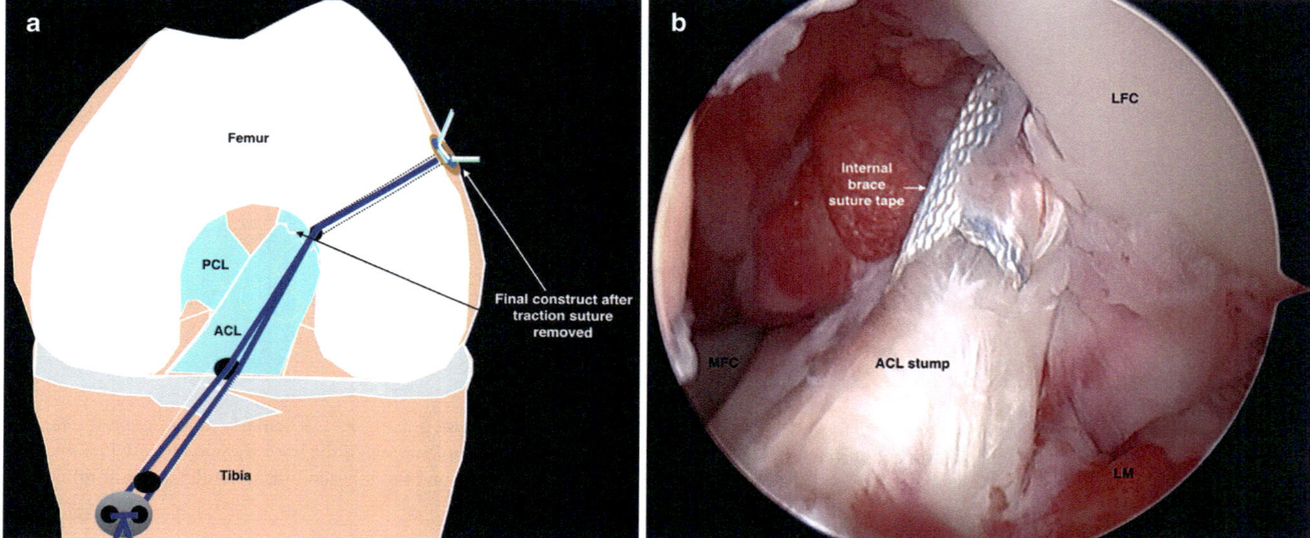


**Fig. 13.30** (**a**) Illustration of the knee showing the final construct of the repaired ACL and internal brace. (**b**) Arthroscopic image of the knee showing the repaired ACL stump and internal brace system

## 13.6 Tips and Tricks

1. The bites through the ACL stump should be through the full thickness of the ACL.
2. While pulling one loop to shuttle the repair sutures, use a probe to pull the other loop through the second working portal.
3. While shuttling the Tightrope RT button across the tunnel to the lateral cortex watch the marking on the suture so that it effectively flips on the lateral cortex of the femur.
4. Use an RF probe to clear the footprint so that the stump does not get destroyed.

## 13.7 Advantages and Disadvantages

### 13.7.1 Advantages

1. Preserves the native ACL.
2. The technique of drilling the femoral and tibial tunnels as well as passing the internal brace is similar to a standard ACL reconstruction using a Tightrope RT.
3. The sutures used to repair the ACL are delivered through the same tunnel through which the Tightrope RT button passes. This repairs the graft in line with its fibres and does not cause twisting of the ACL fibres that may happen when a suture anchor is used to repair it to the femoral footprint.
4. The Tightrope RT button serves as a post to tie the suture tapes used to repair the ACL.
5. The internal brace protects the repaired ACL till it heals providing additional support.

### 13.7.2 Disadvantages

1. Technically demanding in comparison to an ACL reconstruction.
2. Possible Bungee effect of the sutures used to repair the ACL in the tunnel.
3. Literature supporting ACL primary repair is promising but long term studies are scarce.

## Reference

1. Sherman MF, Lieber L, Bonamo JR, Podesta L, Reiter I. The long ter follow up of primary anterior cruciate ligament repair. Defining a rationale for augmentation. Am J Sports Med. 1991;19:243–55.

# Arthroscopic ACL Stump Repair with Reconstruction

# 14

Vikram Arun Mhaskar

## 14.1 Introduction

Anterior cruciate ligament (ACL) tears may occur with a part of the stump intact. This stump may be avulsed from the femur or lax. It however is vascular and contains proprioceptive nerve fibres. Preserving the stump by retensioning it or fixing it to the femur apart from reconstructing the ACL with a graft has distinctive potential advantages of better structural support and vascularisation of the graft as well as preserving proprioception.

## 14.2 Specialised Equipment (Fig. 14.1)

1. Knee Scorpion (Arthrex, Naples, FL) (h).
2. 2–0, Fiberwire-1 (Arthrex, Naples, FL)
3. Suture tape-1 (Arthrex, Naples, FL).
4. Passport Cannula (Arthrex, Naples, Fl).
5. ACL jig (Acufex, Smith and Nephew, Watford, UK) (i).
6. Bone awl (Acufex, Smith and Nephew, Watford, UK) (a).
7. 4.5 mm drill bit (Arthrex, Naples, FL) (d)
8. 6, 7, 8, 9, 10 mm flower drill bit (Arthrex, Naples, FL) (g)
9. 6, 7, 8, 9, 10 full drill bits (Arthrex, Naples, FL) (k)
10. Guidewire (Arthrex, Naples, FL) (j).
11. 2, Ethibond loops No 5 (Ethicon, Raritan, NJ)
12. Tightrope RT button (Arthrex, Naples, FL).
13. PEEK screw 7, 8, 9, 10, 11 mm (Arthrex, Naples, FL).
14. Screwdriver specific for screw (Arthrex, Naples, FL) (m).
15. Shaver with Tip (Stryker, Kalamazoo, MI).
16. Radiofrequency Device (Stryker, Kalamazoo, MI).
17. Knot Pusher (n).

V. A. Mhaskar (✉)
F7 East of Kailash, Knee & Shoulder Clinic, New Delhi, India

JMVM Sports Injury Center, Sitaram Bhartia Institute of Science & Research, New Delhi, India


V. A. Mhaskar, J. Maheshwari (eds.), *Innovative Approaches in Knee Arthroscopy*,
https://doi.org/10.1007/978-981-99-4378-4_14

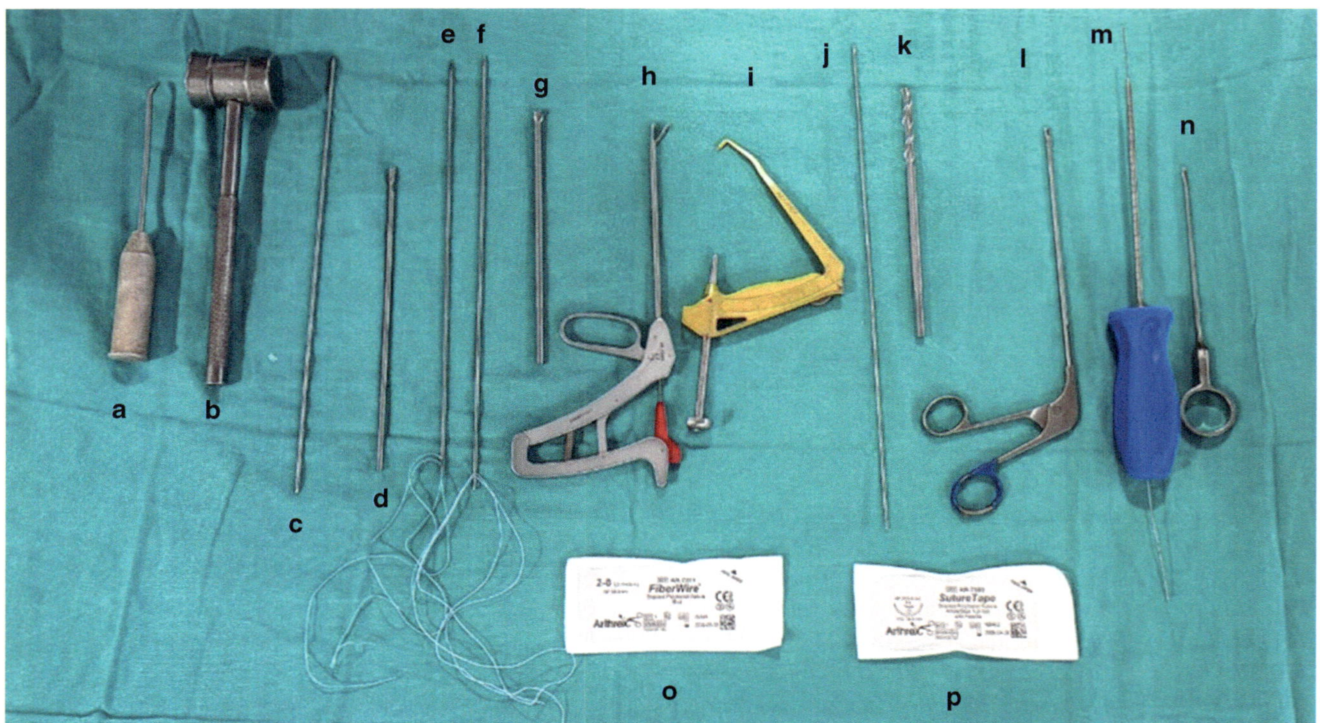


**Fig. 14.1** (**a**) Bone awl, (**b**) Mallet, (**c**) Beath pin, (**d**) 4.5 mm drill bit, (**e**, **f**) Beath pin with No 5 Ethibond loop, (**g**) Graft size femoral drill bit, (**h**) Knee Scorpion, (**i**) ACL Tibial guide, (**j**) Guidewire, (**k**) Graft size tibial drill bit, (**l**) Suture manipulator, (**m**) Guidewire with Screw Driver, (**n**) Knot pusher

## 14.3 Positioning (Fig. 14.2)

The patient is positioned supine on an operating table with a side support and a bolster at the foot end, keeping the knee in 70° flexion.

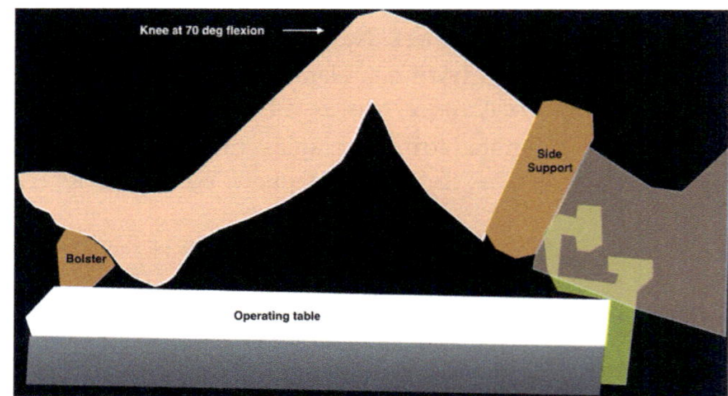


**Fig. 14.2** Knee positioned on the operating table at 70° flexion with side support and bolster at the end of the table

## 14.4 Portals (Fig. 14.3)

Anterolateral viewing portal (AL) is a vertical portal made just adjacent to the patellar tendon at the level of the inferior pole of the patella.

Low far medial horizontal working portal (AM) is made medial to the patellar tendon and just above the medial meniscus under vision by introducing an 18G LP needle, such that when instruments are introduced they do not scuff

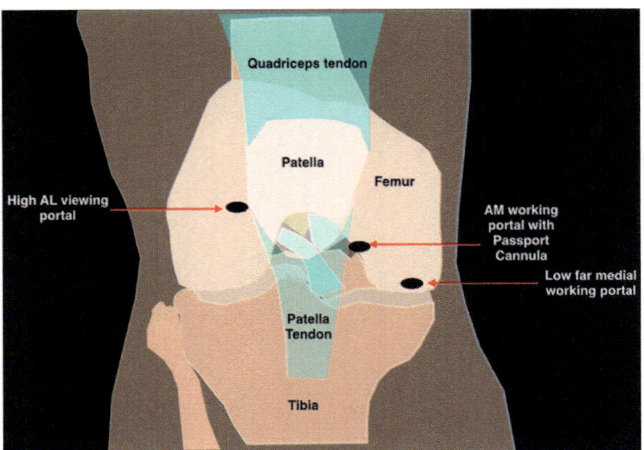


**Fig. 14.3** Illustration of the anterior aspect of the knee showing the position of the high AL viewing portal, AM working portal with Passport Cannula, and low far medial portal

the cartilage over the medial femoral condyle. This portal is used to drill the femoral tunnel.

High anteromedial (high AM) vertical working portal just medial to the patellar tendon that is used for the Passport cannula to stitch the ACL stump.

## 14.5 Surgical Steps

Step 1: The arthroscope is introduced through the AL portal and the ACL visualised (Fig. 14.4a, b).

Step 2: A radiofrequency (RF) device (Stryker, Kalamazoo, MI) is introduced through the far medial portal and used to identify the femoral footprint of the ACL by gradually clearing tissue on the lateral side of the notch adjoining the ACL footprint (Fig. 14.5a, b).

Step 3: A bone awl is then introduced through the far medial portal and the centre of the footprint is marked by tapping the bone awl (Fig. 14.6a, b).

Step 4: The centre of the footprint is marked with a Beath pin, the knee flexed to 100° flexion, and the pin is tapped into the bone using a mallet (Fig. 14.7a, b).

Step 5: Keeping the knee in 100° flexion a 4.5 mm drill bit is introduced over the Beath pin through the far medial portal and the footprint drilled till the far cortex is breached (Fig. 14.8).

Step 6: The length of the tunnel is measured by introducing a depth gauge through the far medial portal and into the femoral tunnel (Fig. 14.9a, b).

Step 7: A Beath pin is then applied through the tunnel and overdrilled with a graft sized drill bit through the far medial portal till 20 mm (Fig. 14.10a, b).

Step 8: A Beath pin carrying a No 5 Ethibond loop (Ethicon, Raritan, NJ) is then introduced through the drill hole with the knee still in 100° flexion. The Beath pin goes beyond the far cortex and pierces the skin on the lateral aspect of the thigh, an incision is made over the Beath pin about 2 cm and dissected down to the bone using an artery forceps and pulled out. It carries with it two ends of the Ethibond loop that are delivered out of the lateral cortex and the loop is made to just project outside the drill hole at the footprint (Fig. 14.11a, b).

Step 9: Still keeping the knee in 100° flexion, another Beath pin carrying a different coloured suture loop is again introduced through the far medial portal, into the femoral tunnel, and delivered through the lateral aspect of the thigh. While introducing this pin it is important to make sure it does not go through the previous suture. This can be facilitated by first delivering the loop out of the medial portal pulling both the loop end and free ends of this suture in tension while introducing the second Beath pin.

The two Ethibond loops are then identified (Fig. 14.12a, b, c).

Step 10: A high anteromedial portal is then made at the level of the anterolateral portal but on the medial side just adjacent to the patella tendon at the level of the inferior pole of the patella and a Passport cannula is introduced through it using an artery forceps (Fig. 14.13).

Step 11: A Knee Scorpion (Arthrex, Naples, FL) device loaded with a 2–0 Fiberwire (Arthrex, Naples, FL) is introduced through the Passport cannula and the upper 1/3 of the ACL stump is held in its jaws and needle deployed to pass the 2–0 Fiberwire through the substance of the ACL (Fig. 14.14a, b, c).

Step 12: One end of the Fiberwire is tied over one end of s suture tape and the other end of the Fiberwire pulled to shuttle the Suture Tape (Arthrex, Naples, FL) through the substance of the ACL (Fig. 14.15a, b).

Step 13: The Knee Scorpion is again loaded with the 2–0 Fiberwire and introduced through the Passport cannula to take a bite proximal to the previous bite. Opposite ends of the suture tape and Fiberwire are identified and the Fiberwire is used to shuttle the suture tape through the ACL as described in the previous step. This makes one arm of the figure of '8' configuration of the suture tape around the ACL (Fig. 14.16a, b, c, d).

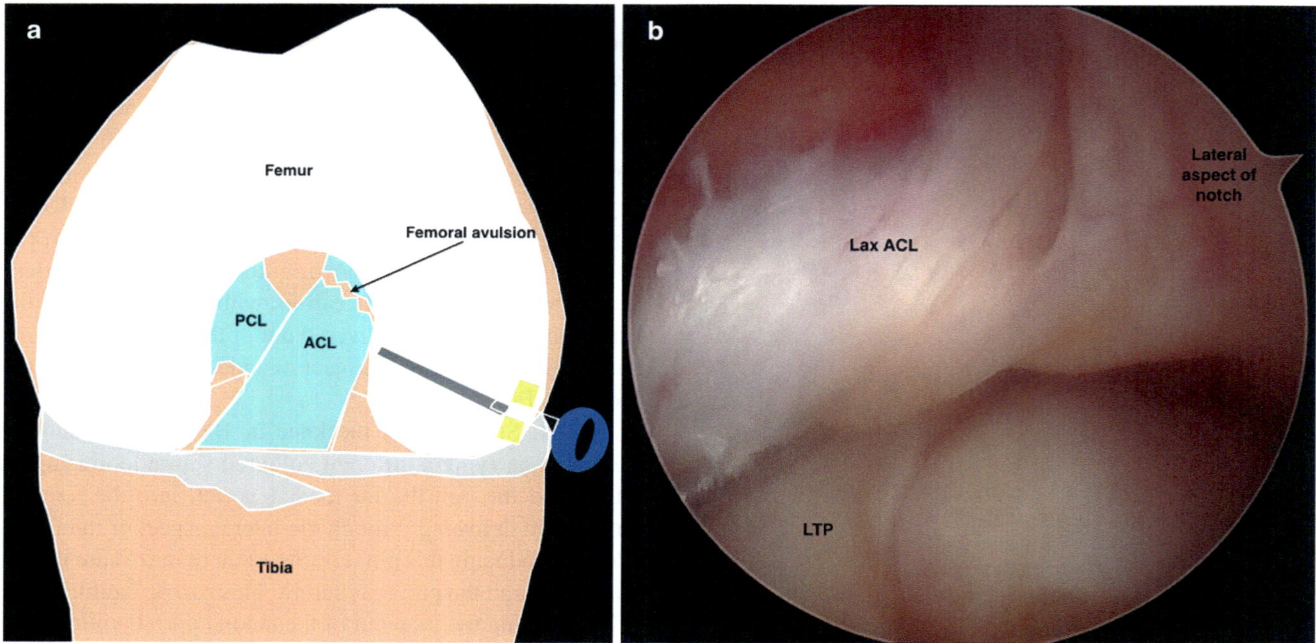


**Fig. 14.4** (**a**) Illustration of the knee showing a femoral avulsion ACL tear while viewing through the high AL portal. (**b**) Arthroscopic picture of the ACL stump avulsed from the femur

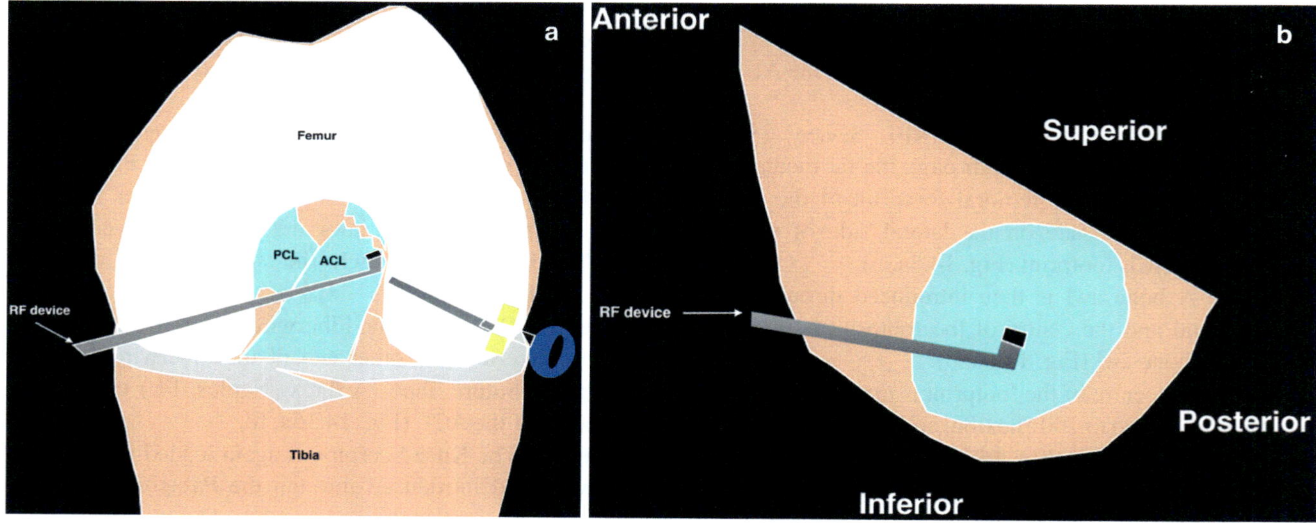


**Fig. 14.5** (**a**) Illustration of the knee showing radiofrequency (RF) device cleaning the femoral footprint in the lateral aspect of the notch. (**b**) Illustration of the lateral aspect of the notch showing RF device cleaning the femoral footprint

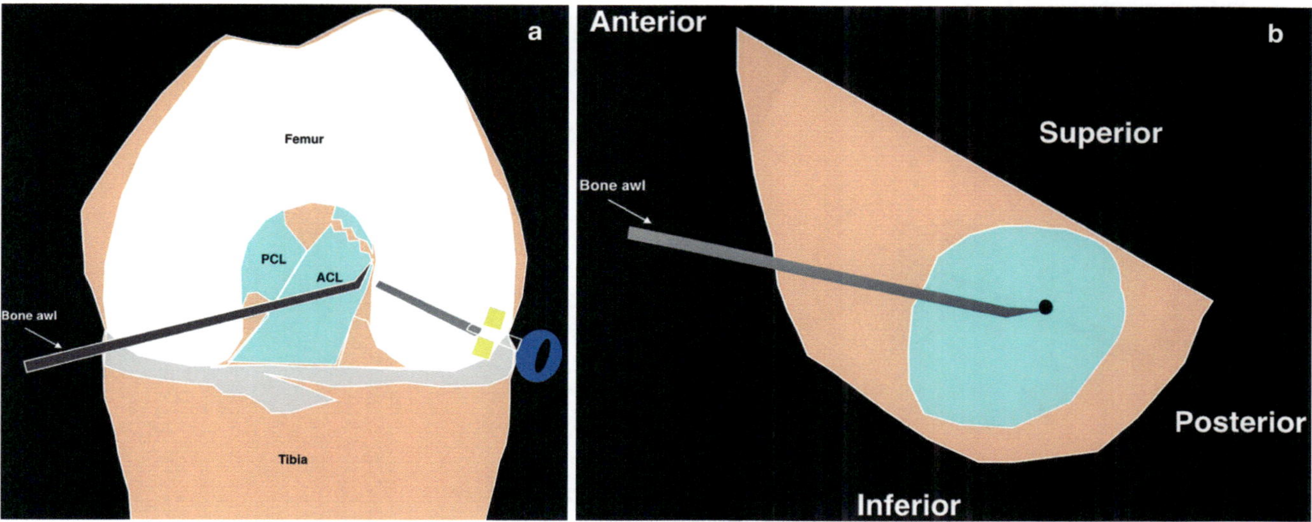


**Fig. 14.6** (**a**) Illustration of the knee showing a bone awl introduced into the notch to make multiple trephinations in the lateral aspect of the notch. (**b**) Illustration of the lateral aspect of the notch showing the bone awl making a trephination into the lateral aspect of the notch

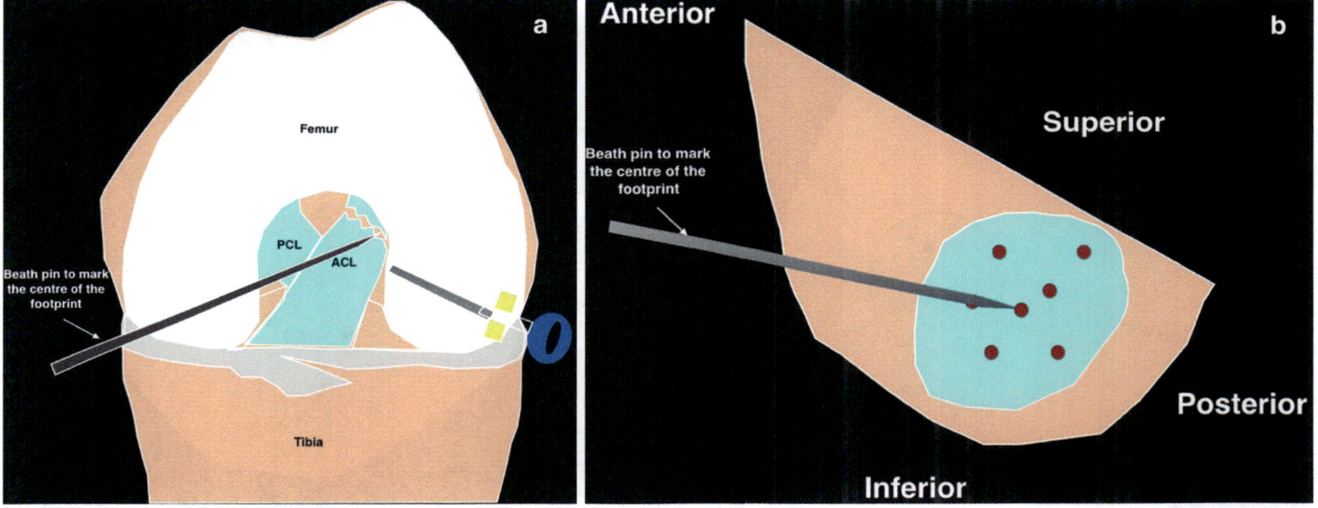


**Fig. 14.7** (**a**) Illustration of the knee showing a Beath pin applied to the centre of the femoral footprint. (**b**) Illustration of the lateral aspect of the notch showing Beath pin at the centre of the femoral footprint

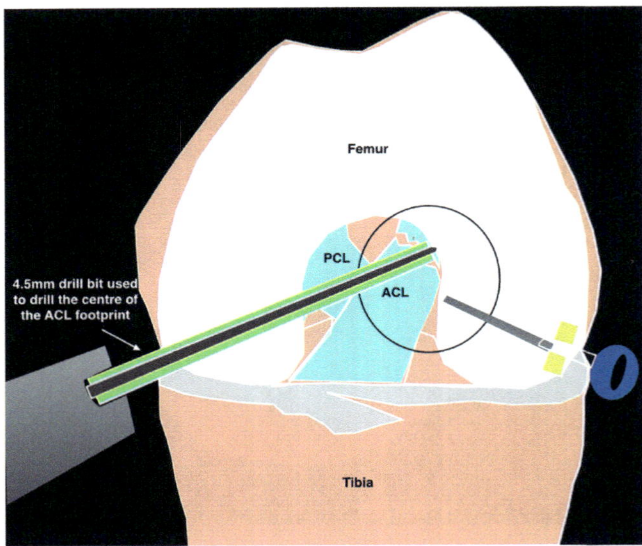


**Fig. 14.8** Illustration of the knee showing the centre of the femoral footprint with a 4.5 mm drill bit

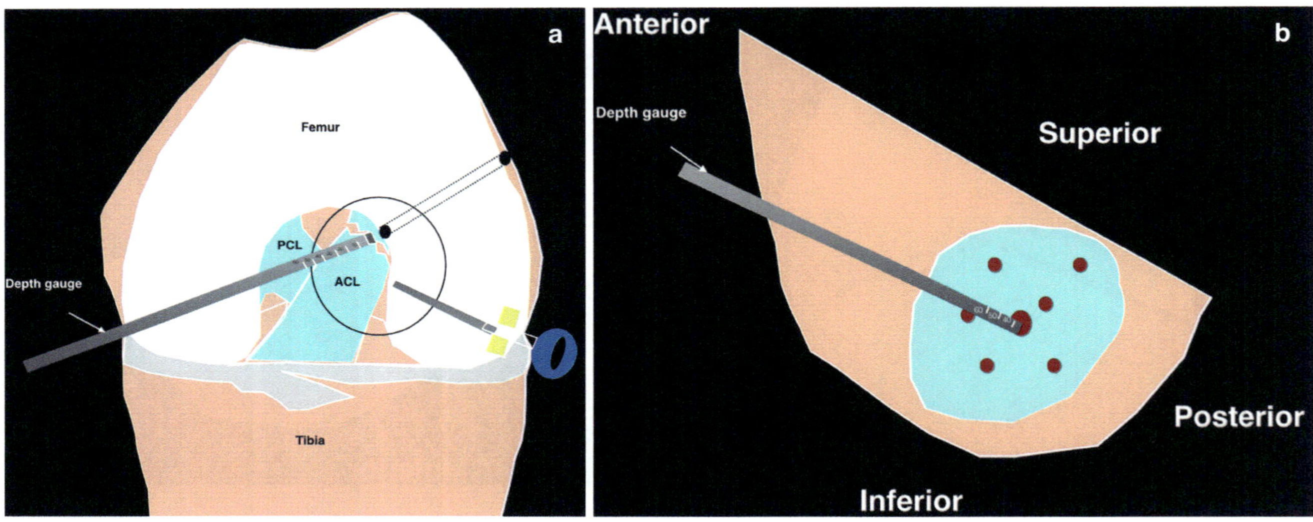


**Fig. 14.9** (**a**) Illustration of the knee showing a depth gauge being introduced into the femoral tunnel. (**b**) Illustration of the lateral aspect of the notch showing a depth gauge measuring the length of the femoral tunnel

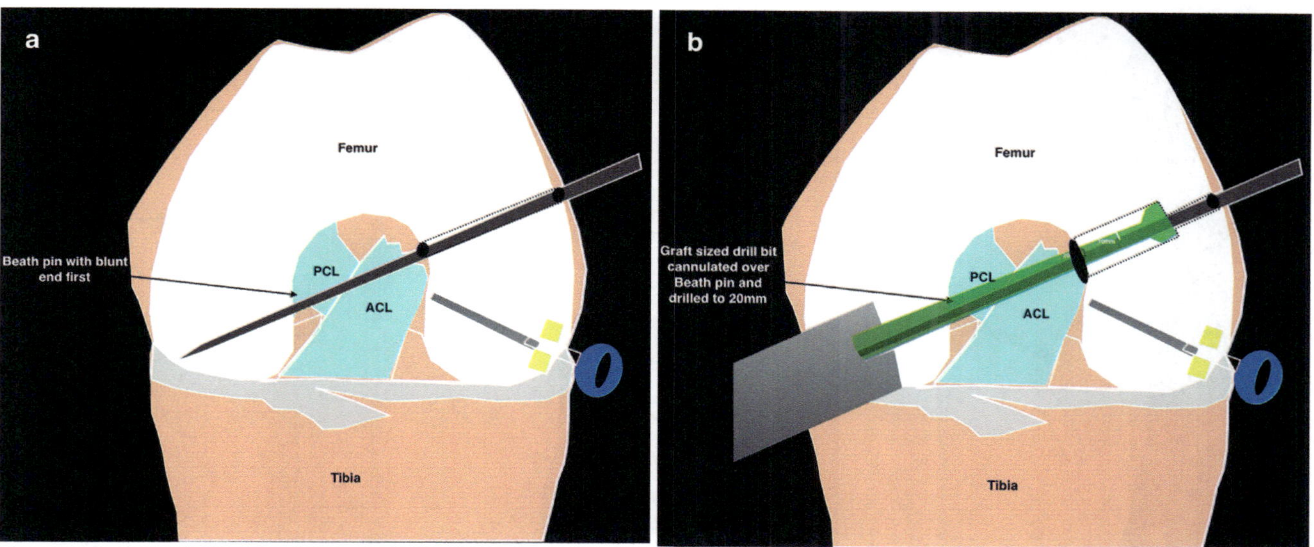


**Fig. 14.10** (**a**) Illustration of the knee showing a Beath pin inserted upside down through the femoral tunnel. (**b**) Illustration of the knee showing the graft sized drill bit cannulated over the Beath pin and drilled to 20 mm

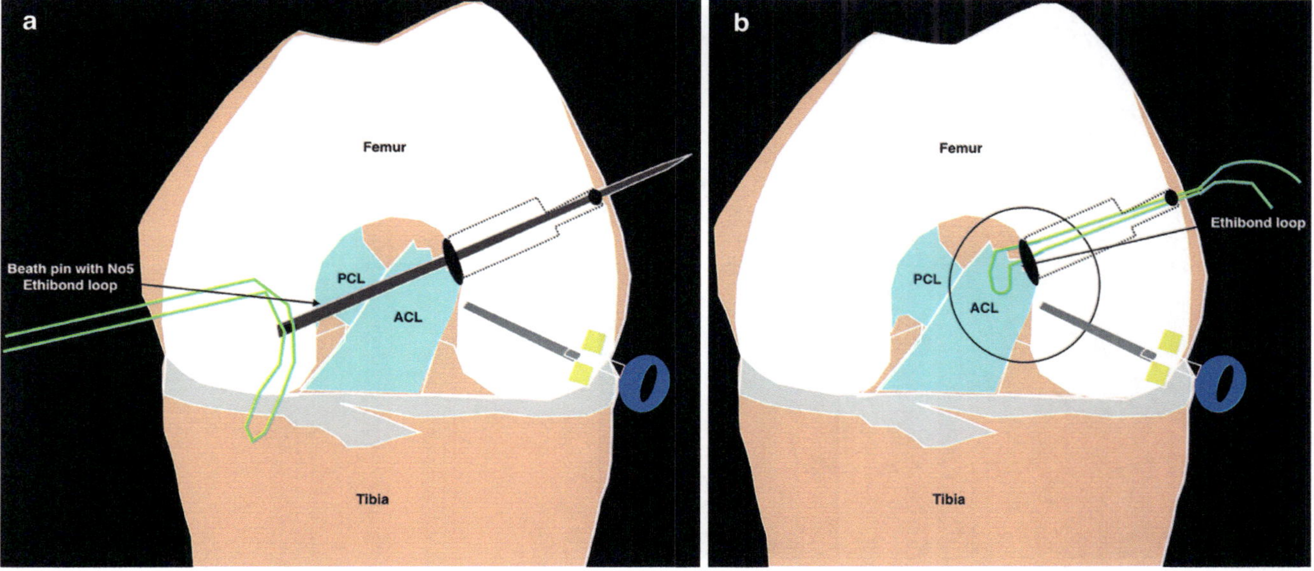


**Fig. 14.11** (**a**) Illustration of the knee showing a Beath pin carrying a No 5 Ethibond loop being passed through the femoral tunnel. (**b**) Illustration of the knee showing an Ethibond loop at the orifice of the femoral tunnel

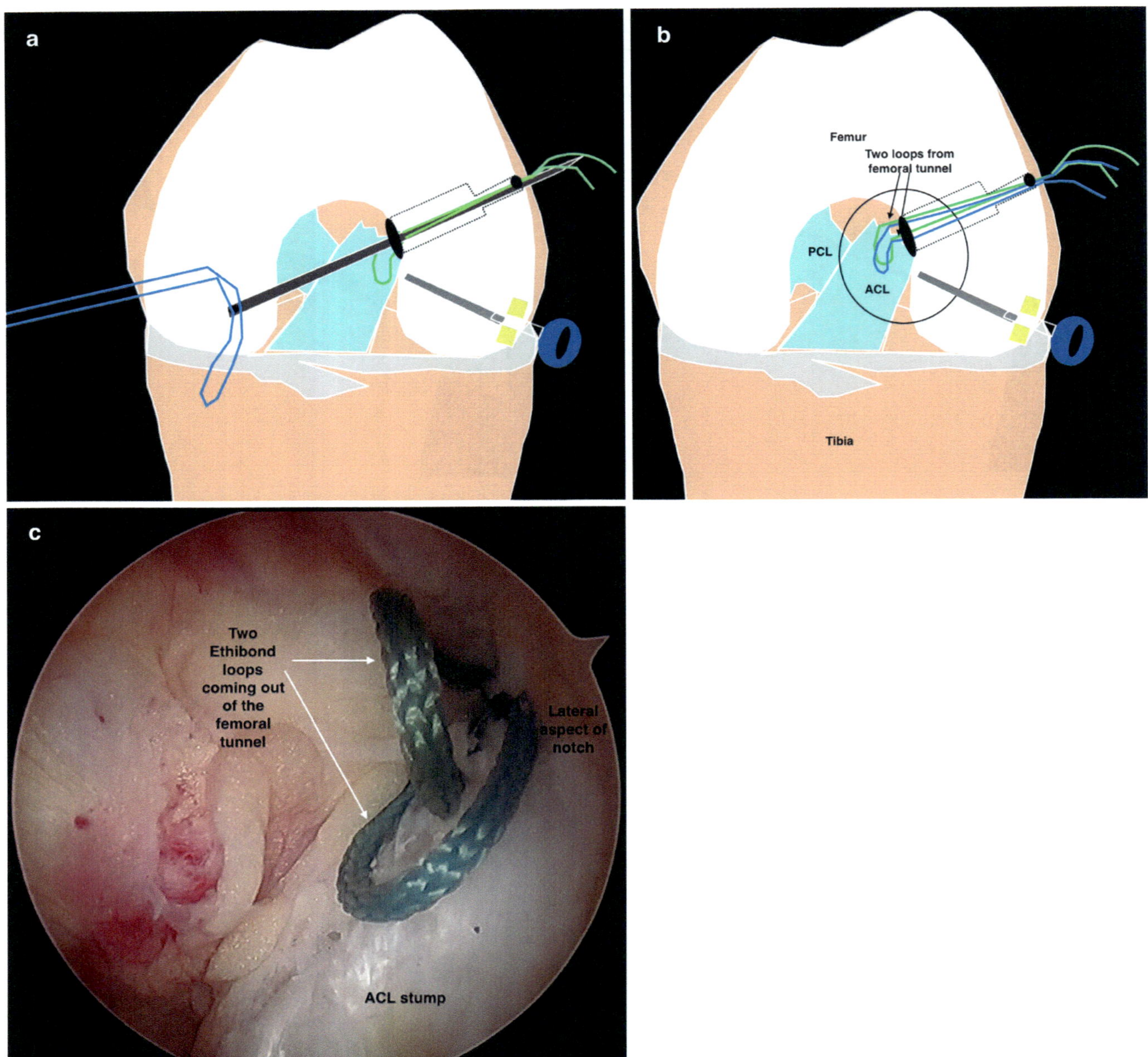


**Fig. 14.12** (**a**) Illustration of the knee showing second Ethibond loop passed through femoral tunnel. (**b**) Illustration of the knee showing two Ethibond loops at femoral tunnel orifice. (**c**) Arthroscopic image of the knee showing two Ethibond loops at the femoral tunnel orifice

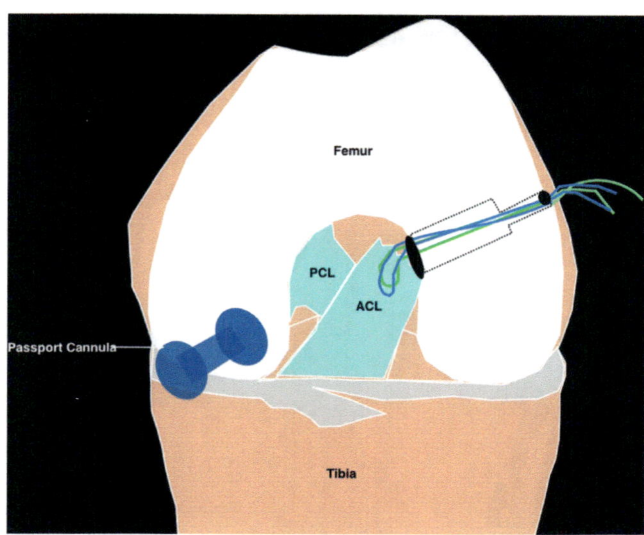


**Fig. 14.13** Illustration of the knee showing a Passport cannula (Arthrex, Naples, FL) through the anteromedial portal

Step 14: The Knee Scorpion is again introduced through the Passport cannula to take a bite proximal to the previous bite, and the Suture Tape is shuttled through the ACL to form a figure of '8' suture configuration around the ACL (Fig. 14.17a, b).

Step 15: One Ethibond loop is delivered through the Passport cannula and the two ends of the Suture Tape are introduced into the loop and the two ends of the loop on the lateral aspect of the thigh are pulled to shuttle the Suture Tape out of the lateral cortex (Fig. 14.18a, b, c).

Step 16: An ACL jig set at 70° is introduced through the far medial portal and the tip centred on the centre of the ACL tibial stump and the bullet secured on the anteromedial aspect of the tibia. This is done by making a 3 cm vertical incision where the tip of the bullet enters the skin and then advancing the bullet to the anteromedial tibia and securing it by the ratchet mechanism (Fig. 14.19).

Step 17: The jig is held securely and a Beath pin drilled through it such that the tip comes out of the centre of the tibial stump (Fig. 14.20).

Step 18: The jig is then disengaged and a Graft diameter cannulated drill bit is applied over the Beath pins and the tibial tunnel drilled from the anteromedial aspect of the tibia and entering the knee through the tibial stump. Care must be taken to gradually drill the tibial footprint so as not to disrupt the stump (Fig. 14.21).

Step 19: The second suture loop is then delivered through the tibial tunnel externally using a grasper (Fig. 14.22a, b).

Step 20: The Tightrope button (Arthrex, Naples, FL) and loop system are opened. The loop lengthened to about 100 mm. The length of the tibial tunnel is marked on the elongated loop measuring from the tip of the button backwards. Mark another point 5 mm proximal to this.

Step 21: A graft is applied through the Tightrope RT loop and the traction sutures are put into the Ethibond loop (Fig. 14.23).

Step 22: The two ends of the Ethibond loop are then pulled to shuttle the traction sutures of the Tightrope RT out of the lateral cortex (Fig. 14.24).

Step 23: While viewing through the far medial portal, the traction sutures (all 4) are then pulled gradually so

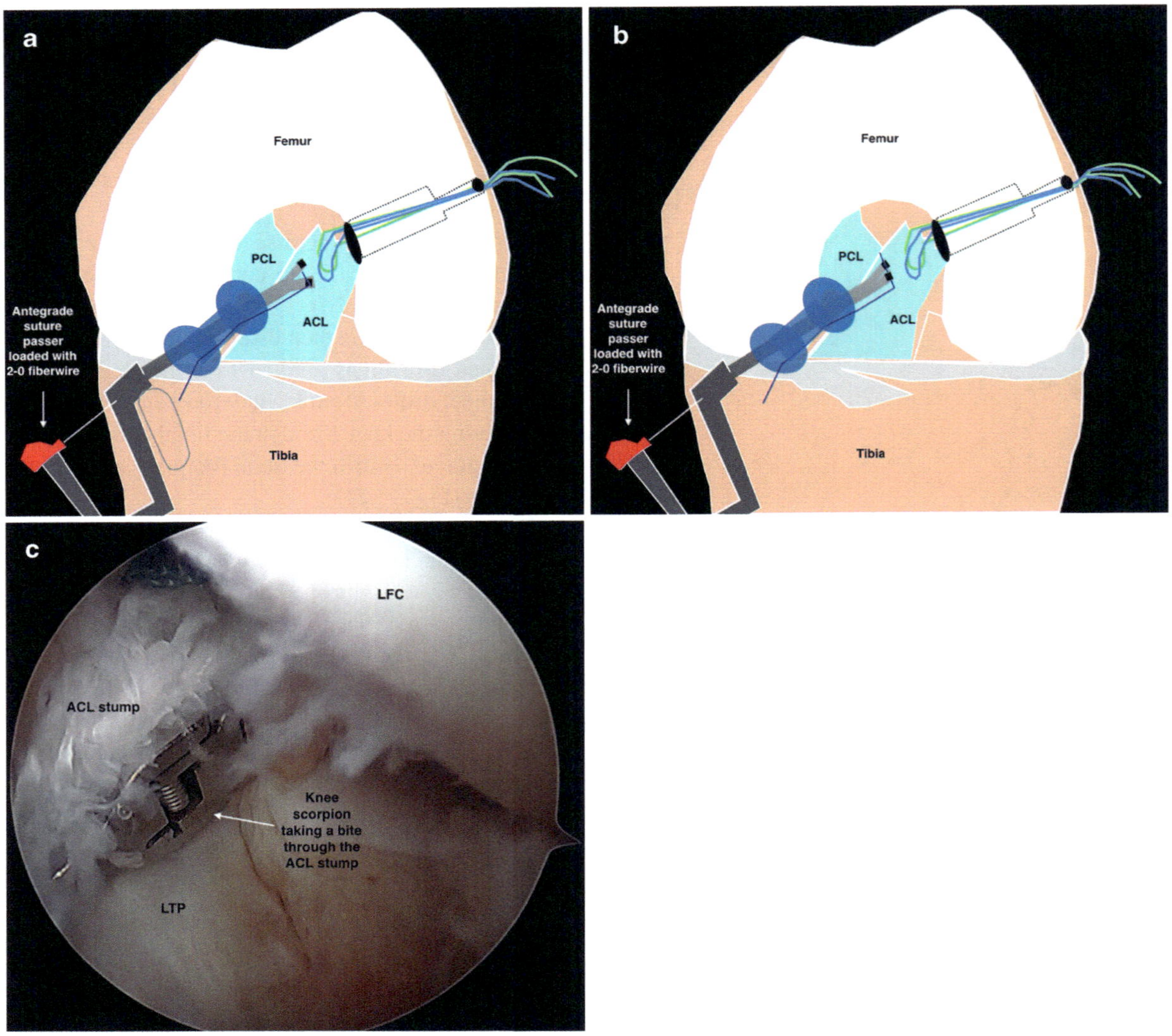

**Fig. 14.14** (**a**) Illustration of the knee showing Antegrade suture passer through Passport cannula taking a bite through the ACL stump using a 2–0 Fiberwire. (**b**) Illustration of the knee showing a 2–0 Fiberwire through the ACL stump. (**c**) Arthroscopic image of the knee showing a 2–0 Fiberwire through the ACL stump

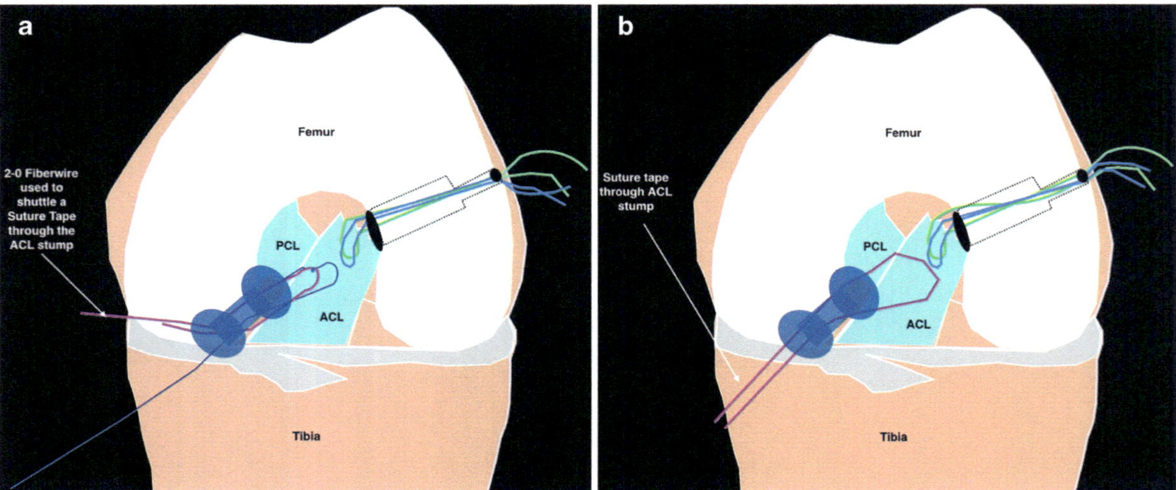


**Fig. 14.15** (**a**) Illustration of knee showing one limb of the 2–0 Fiberwire tied to one of the Suture Tape. (**b**) Illustration of the knee showing the Suture Tape shuttled through the ACL stump

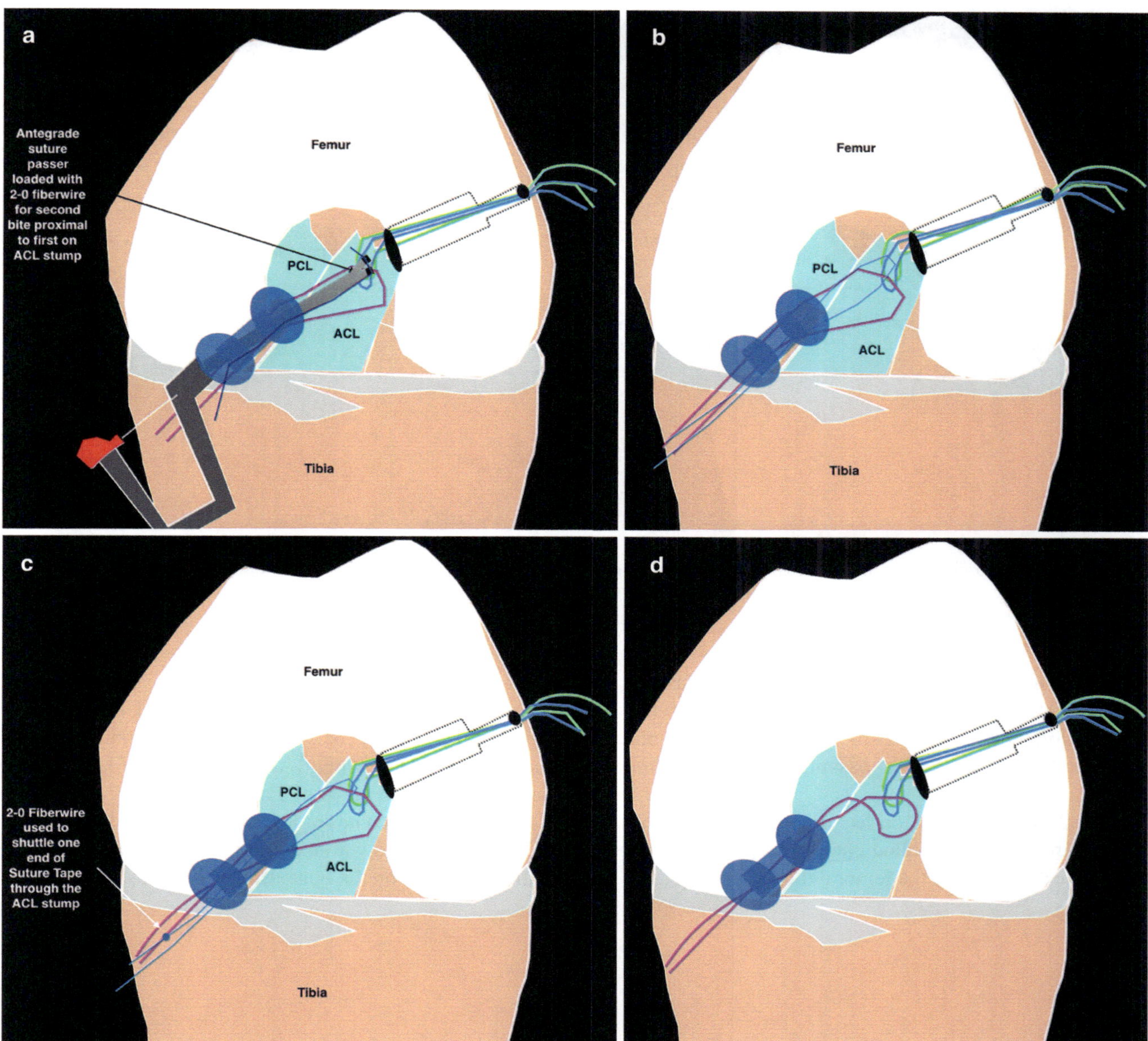


**Fig. 14.16** (**a**) Illustration of the knee showing the antegrade suture passer taking a bite with a 2–0 Fiberwire just proximal to where the Suture Tape is passing in the ACL stump. (**b**) Illustration of the knee showing the 2–0 Fiberwire passing proximal to the Suture Tape through the ACL stump. (**c**) Arthroscopic image of knee showing 2–0 Fiberwire passing through the ACL stump above the Suture Tape. (**d**) Illustration of the knee showing one end of the 2–0 Fiberwire being tied over the opposite end of the Suture Tape to be shuttled through the ACL stump again to form one limb of the Figure of '8' suture configuration around the ACL stump

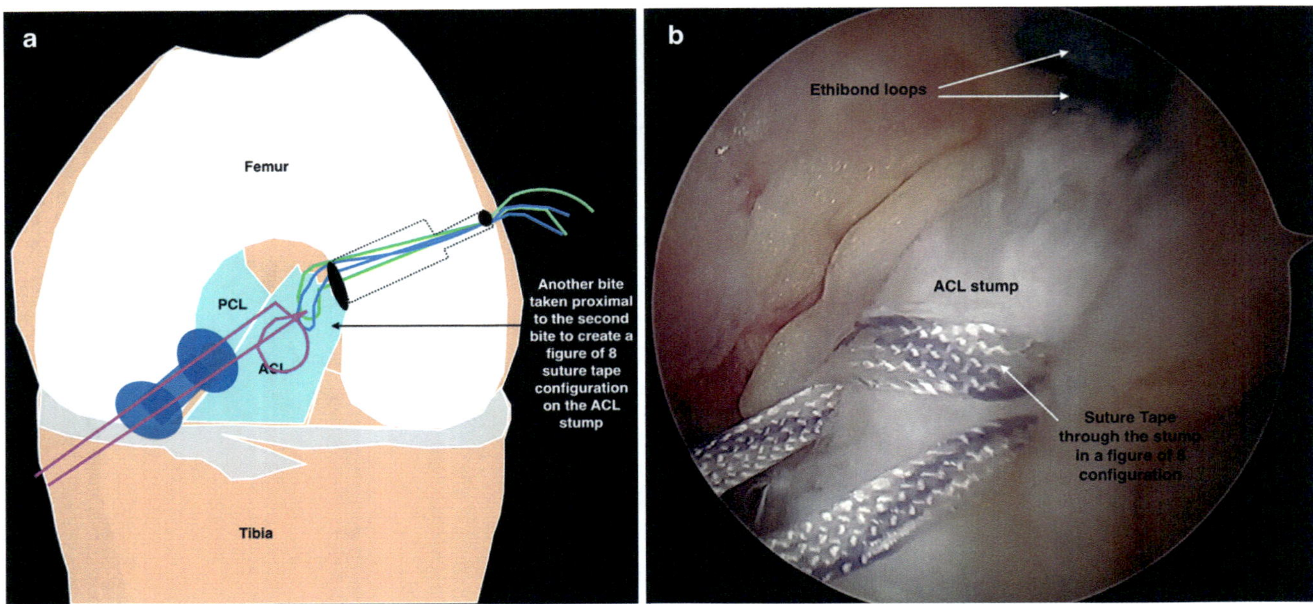


**Fig. 14.17** (**a**) Illustration of the figure of eight Suture Tape configuration around the ACL stump. (**b**) Arthroscopic image of the knee showing a figure of eight suture configuration of the Suture Tape around the ACL stump

that the button passes intra-articularly, then through the tunnel to the lateral cortex. One knows observing the marking on the loop crosses the lateral cortex and observing the button flip after passing across the femoral tunnel.

Step 24: Once the button has flipped, the white milking sutures are alternately pulled continuously to pull the graft intra-articularly and up the femoral tunnel.

Step 25: While applying a traction on the sutures coming out of the graft coming out of the tibial tunnel, the guidewire is passed posterior to the graft through the tibial tunnel and fixed with a PEEK screw (Arthrex, Naples, FL) 1 mm in diameter more than the graft diameter.

Step 26: The two ends of the suture tapes used to stitch the ACL stump are tied with the milking white sutures over the Tightrope button on the bone using a knot pusher. At least 5

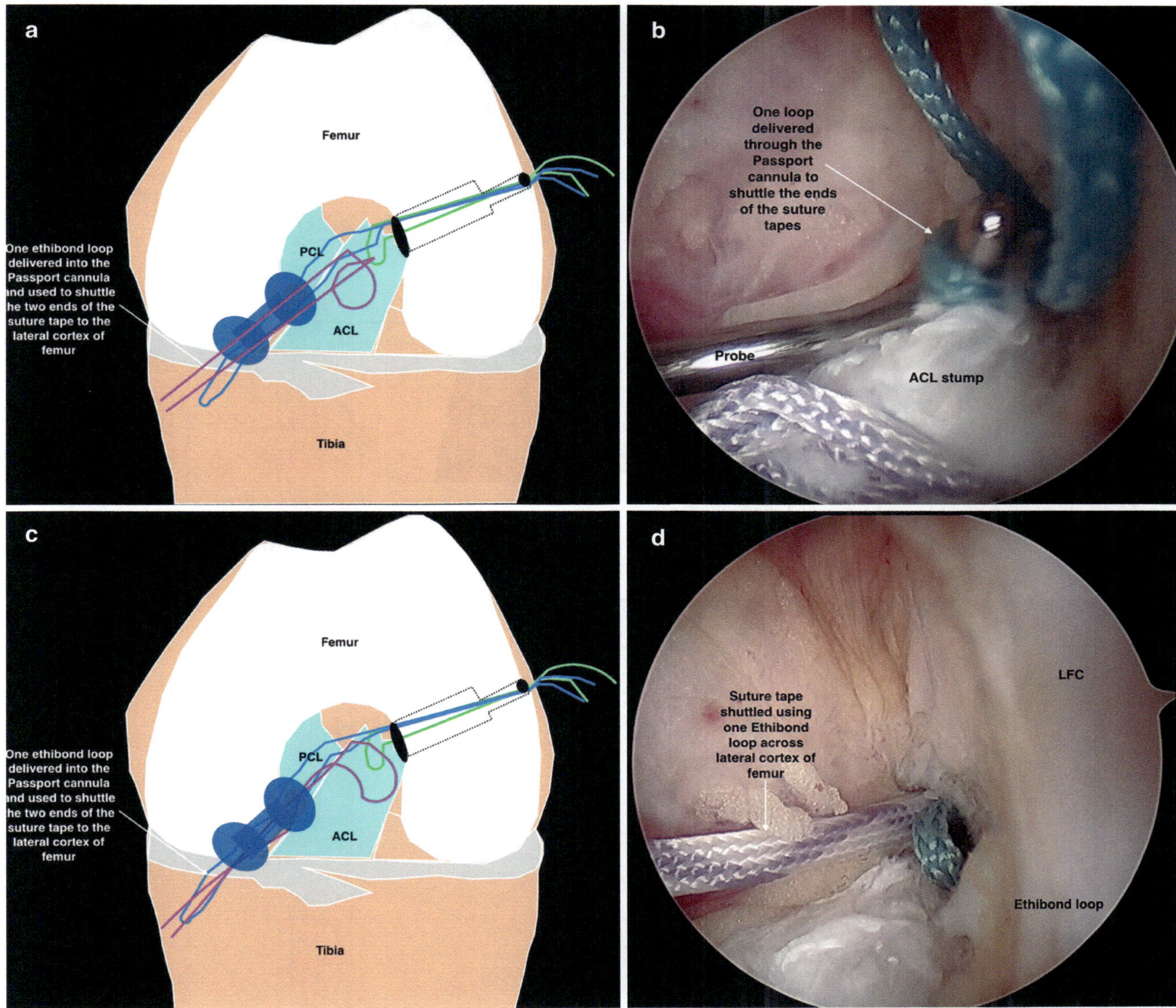


**Fig. 14.18** (**a**) Illustration of the knee showing one Ethibond loop delivered through the Passport cannula to shuttle the two ends of the Suture Tape. (**b**) Arthroscopic image of the knee showing one Ethibond loop being held with a probe to deliver it through the Passport cannula. (**c**) Illustration of the knee showing two ends of the Suture Tape shuttled through the femoral tunnel to the lateral femoral cortex. (**d**) Arthroscopic image of the knee showing two ends of the suture tape around the ACL stump being shuttled across the femoral tunnel to the lateral cortex of the femur. (**e**) Illustration of the knee showing the two ends of the suture tape shuttled across the lateral cortex of the femur

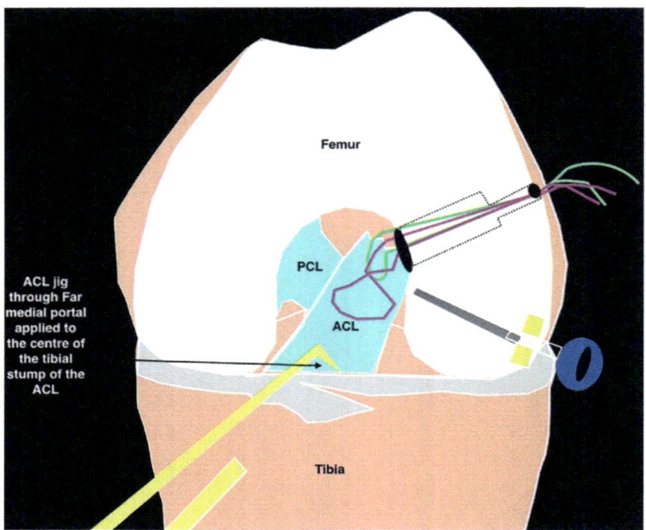


**Fig. 14.19** Illustration of the knee showing ACL jig applied to the centre of the tibial stump

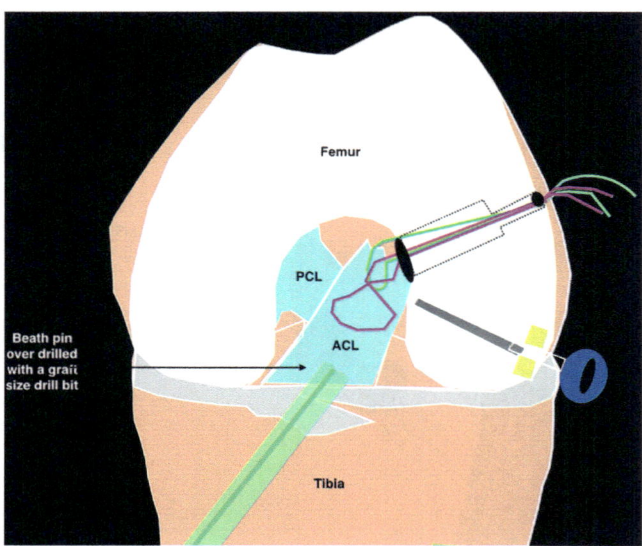


**Fig. 14.21** Illustration of the knee showing a graft size drill bit passing through the centre of the ACL stump over the Beath pin

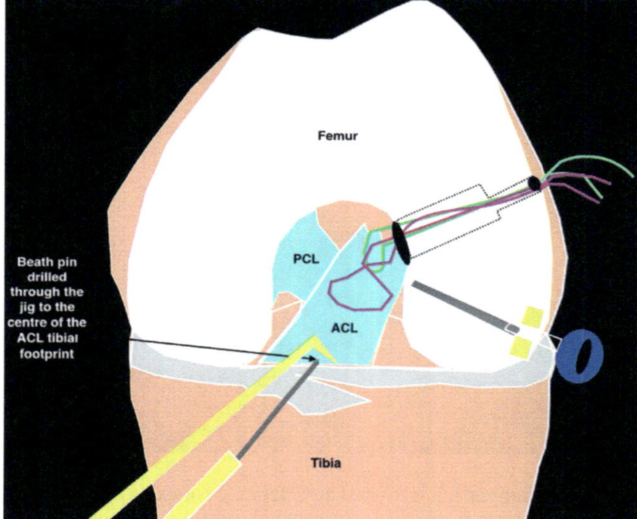


**Fig. 14.20** Illustration of the knee showing the Beath pin drilled to the centre of the tibial stump through the ACL jig fixed at 70°

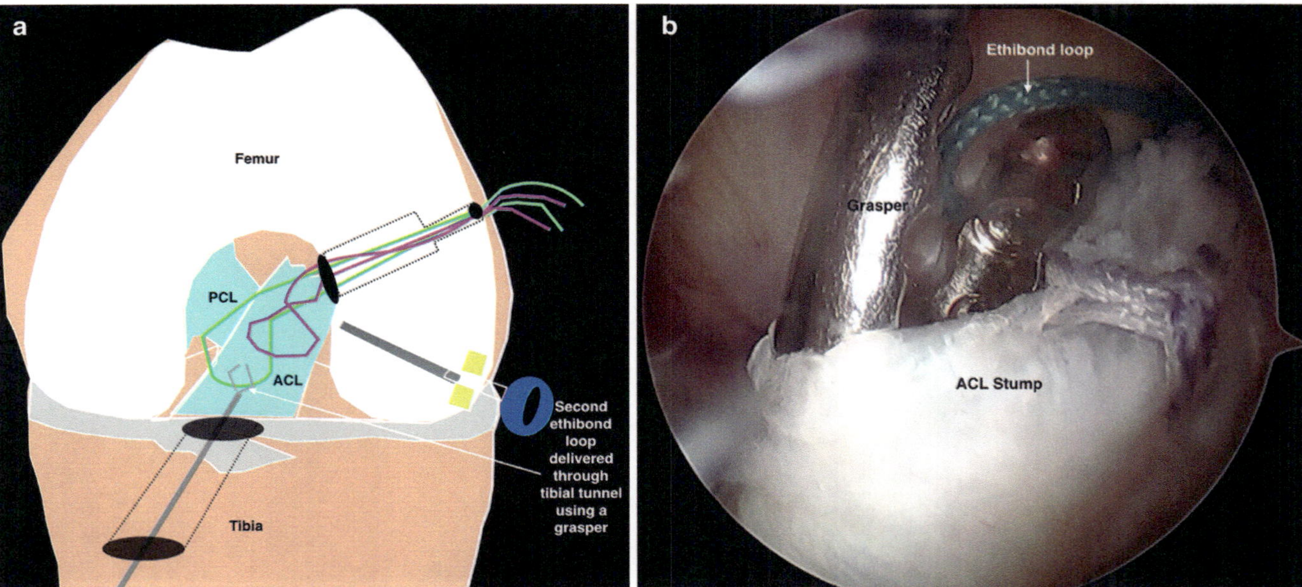


**Fig. 14.22** (**a**) Illustration of the knee showing the second Ethibond loop delivered through the tibial tunnel. (**b**) Arthroscopic image of a grasper coming out of the ACL tibial tunnel to grasp the second Ethibond loop to be delivered through the tibial tunnel orifice on the anteromedial aspect of the tibia

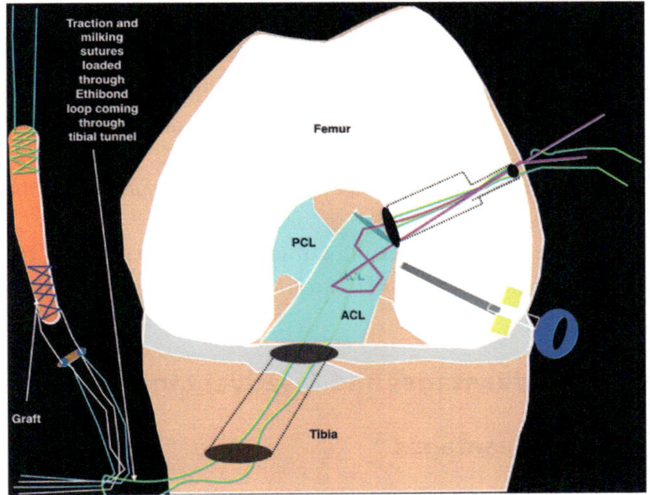


**Fig. 14.23** Illustration of the knee showing Tightrope RT traction and milking sutures passed into the Ethibond loop coming out of the tibial tunnel

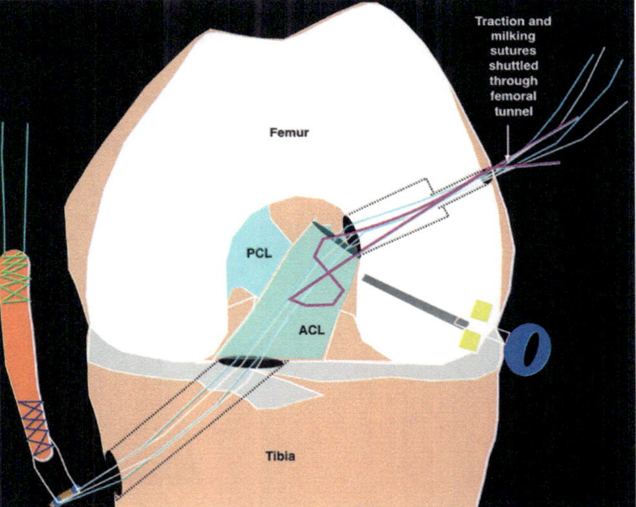


**Fig. 14.24** Illustration of the knee showing the traction and milking sutures being shuttled to the lateral cortex of the femur

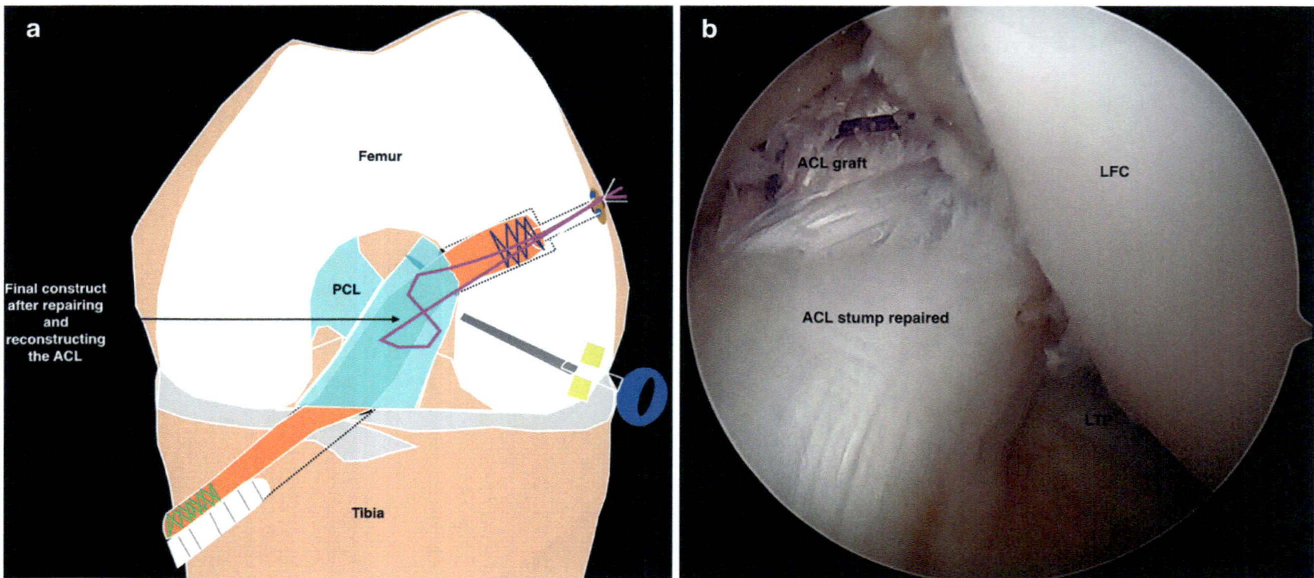


**Fig. 14.26** (**a**) Illustration of the knee showing the final construct of the repaired ACL stump and reconstructed ACL. (**b**) Arthroscopic image of the knee showing the repaired ACL stump and reconstructed ACL

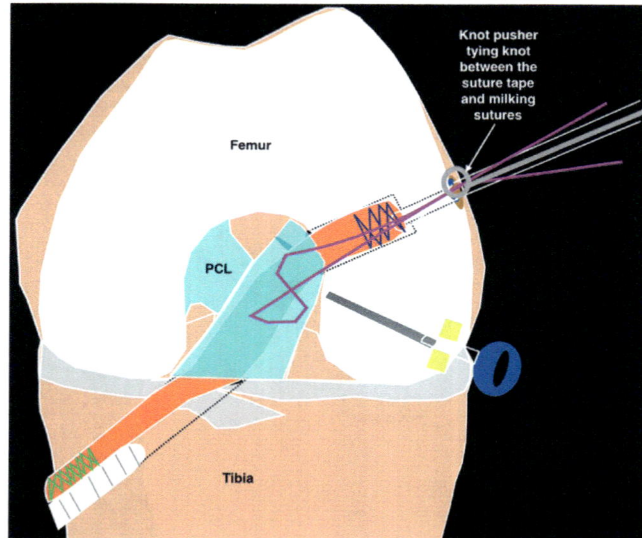


**Fig. 14.25** Illustration showing two ends of the suture tape used to repair the stump being tied to the two milking sutures using a knot pusher on the lateral cortex of the femur after making an incision corresponding to it and dissecting down to the bone

throws are done using both ends of the sutures tape and milking sutures together (Fig. 14.25).

Step 27: The Knot ends are cut on the anteromedial tibia and lateral cortex of femur and the repaired ACL construct is visualised (Fig. 14.26a, b).

## 14.6 Tips and Tricks

1. Take a bite through the full thickness of the ACL stump so that the suture does not cut out.
2. The shuttling suture for the ACL graft should be held with a probe while the other loop is shuttling the repair sutures so that it does not pull out.
3. Use a knot pusher to tie knots of the repair suture with the milking suture.
4. Tie the repair sutures only after the graft is fixed on the tibia so that the post (Tightrope Button) is stable.

## 14.7 Advantages and Disadvantages

### 14.7.1 Advantages

1. Preserves the native ACL.
2. The sutures used to repair the ACL are delivered through the same tunnel through which the Tightrope RT button passes. This repairs the graft in line with its fibres and does not cause twisting of the ACL fibres that may happen when a suture anchor is used to repair it to the femoral footprint.

3. The Tightrope RT button serves as a post to tie the suture tapes used to repair the ACL.
4. Vascularity of the stump and proprioceptive fibres of the native ACL are preserved.

### 14.7.2 Disadvantages

1. Technically demanding in comparison to a standard ACL reconstruction.
2. Impingement if the notch is overstuffed and tunnels are not in the right position.

# 15 Stump Preservation ACL Reconstruction

Vikram Arun Mhaskar

## 15.1 Introduction

Tears of the anterior cruciate ligament (ACL) can be mid-substance or at either end of their attachment on the femur or tibia. Preserving the native ligament along with reconstructing it gives the added advantage of more structural stability, vascularity, and proprioception. However this is not at the cost of impingement. The key aspects of this technique are to preserve the stump while drilling through it, making sure the graft comes through the centre of the stump and at the end of the procedure there is no impingement of the graft in the notch.

## 15.2 Specialized Equipment (Fig. 15.1)

1. Beath pin (c, h, e).
2. 4.5 mm drill bit (Arthrex, Naples, FL) (d)
3. 6, 7, 8, 9, 10 mm flower drill bits (Arthrex, Naples, FL) (f)
4. 6, 7, 8, 9, 10 mm full drill bits (Arthrex, Naples, FL) (i)
5. No 5 Ethibond (Ethicon, Raritan, NJ) (e).
6. Graft preparation board (Arthrex, Naples, FL).
7. Bird Beak arthroscopic grasper (Smith and Nephew, Watford, UK).
8. Arthroscopic bone awl (a).

V. A. Mhaskar (✉)
F7 East of Kailash, Knee & Shoulder Clinic, New Delhi, India

JMVM Sports Injury Center, Sitaram Bhartia Institute of Science & Research, New Delhi, India


V. A. Mhaskar, J. Maheshwari (eds.), *Innovative Approaches in Knee Arthroscopy*,
https://doi.org/10.1007/978-981-99-4378-4_15

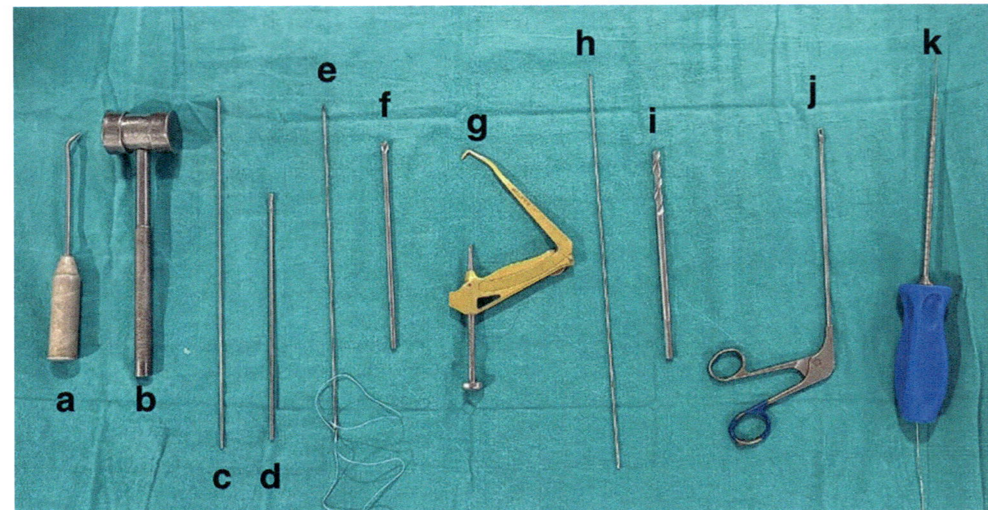


**Fig. 15.1** (**a**) Bone Awl, (**b**) Mallet, (**c**) Beath Pin, (**d**) 4.5 mm drill bit, (**e**) Beth pin with No 5 Ethibond, (**f**) Graft size femoral drill bit, (**g**) ACL tibial jig, (**h**) Beath pin, (**i**) Graft size tibial drill bit, (**j**) Suture Manipulator, (**k**) Guidewire with screwdriver

## 15.3 Positioning (Fig. 15.2)

Supine on an operating table with a side support and knee at 70° flexion with a bolster on the operating bed.

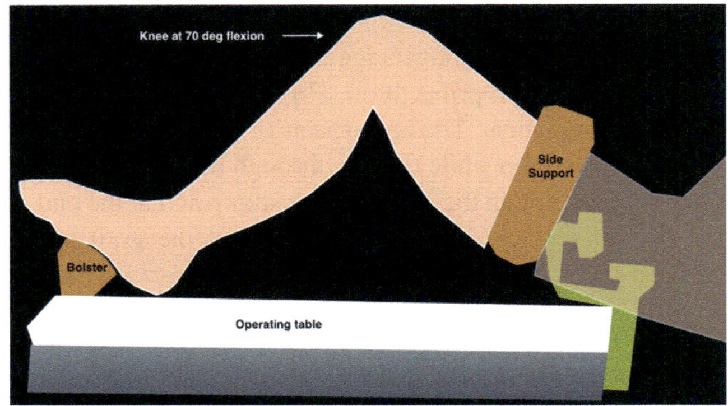


**Fig. 15.2** Knee in 70° flexion on the operating table with a side support and bolster on the operating table

## 15.4 Portals (Fig. 15.3)

1. High vertical AL portal just abutting the patellar tendon at the level of the inferior pole of the patella.
2. Low horizontal medial portal just above the medial meniscus body.

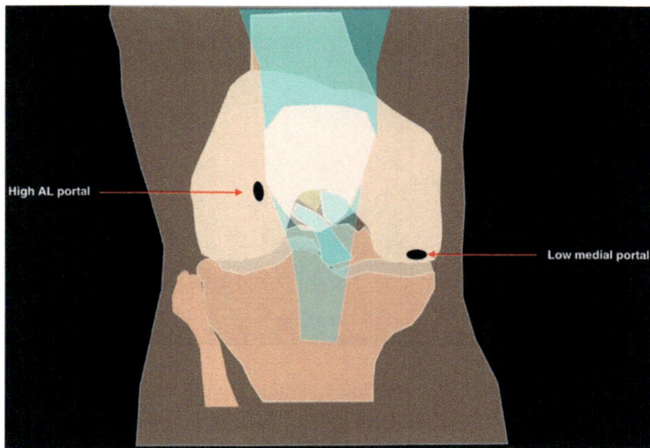


**Fig. 15.3** Illustration of the knee showing a high anterolateral viewing portal just above the inferior pole of the patella abutting the patella

## 15.5 Surgical Steps

Step 1: A diagnostic arthroscopy is done and the torn ACL is identified (Fig. 15.4a, b).

Step 2: The semitendinosus and gracilis grafts are harvested and prepared into a 4, 5, 6 tailed graft according to the length of the tendon harvested. The diameter is measured for both the tibial and femoral ends. It is fitted with a Tightrope RT button on the femoral end.

Step 3: While viewing from the AL portal a bone awl is used to mark the centre of the ACL femoral footprint on the lateral aspect of the notch. The landmarks used are the resident's ridge, just above the line dividing the lateral aspect of the notch into a superior and inferior portion (Fig. 15.5a, b, c).

Step 4: The tip of the Beath pin is applied to the mark and flexed to 110° flexion and tapped into the bone (Fig. 15.6a, b).

Step 5: Keeping the knee in 110° flexion, a 4.5 mm drill bit is introduced over the Beath pin and drilled into the footprint till it crosses the opposite cortex (Fig. 15.7a, b).

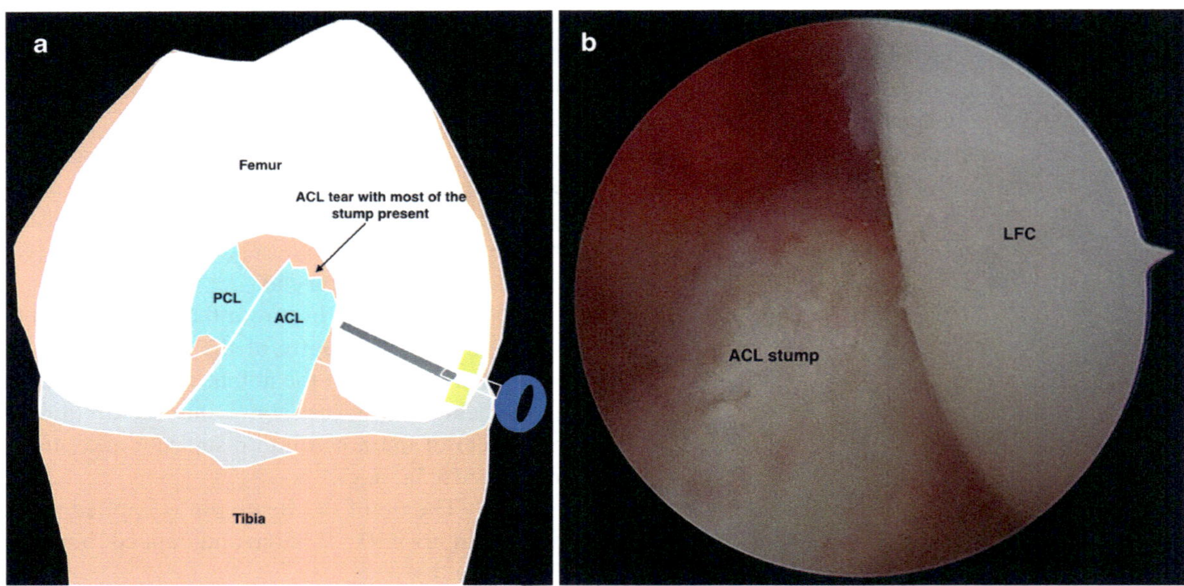


**Fig. 15.4** (**a**) Illustration of the knee showing an ACL tear from the femoral end with most of the stump intact while viewing from the AL portal. (**b**) Arthroscopic image of the knee while viewing from the AL portal showing a torn ACL from the femoral end with most of the stump intact

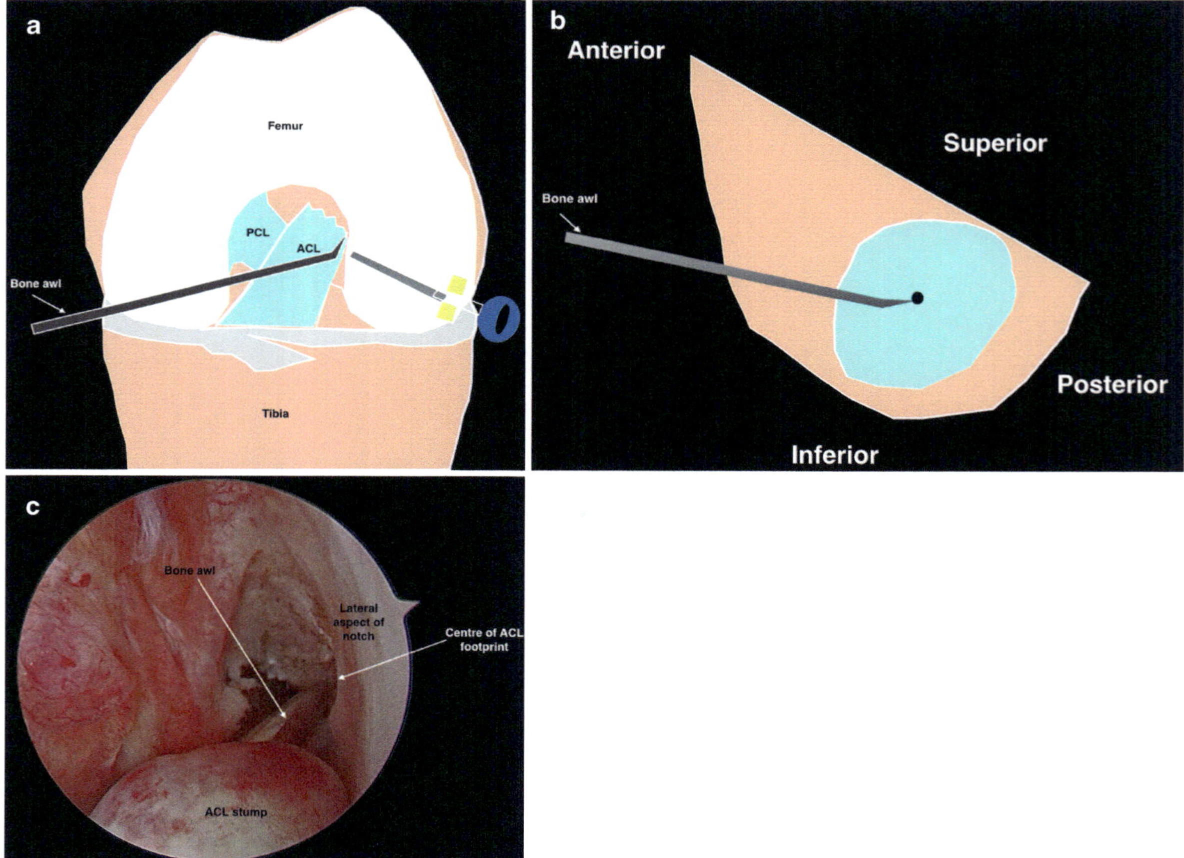


**Fig. 15.5** (**a**) Illustration of the knee showing a bone awl introduced through the medial portal used to mark the centre of the ACL footprint on the lateral aspect of the notch. (**b**) Illustration of the lateral aspect of the notch showing the ACL footprint in blue and the bone awl marking the centre of it. (**c**) Arthroscopic image of the knee showing the bone awl marking the centre of the ACL footprint on the lateral aspect of the notch while viewing from the AL portal

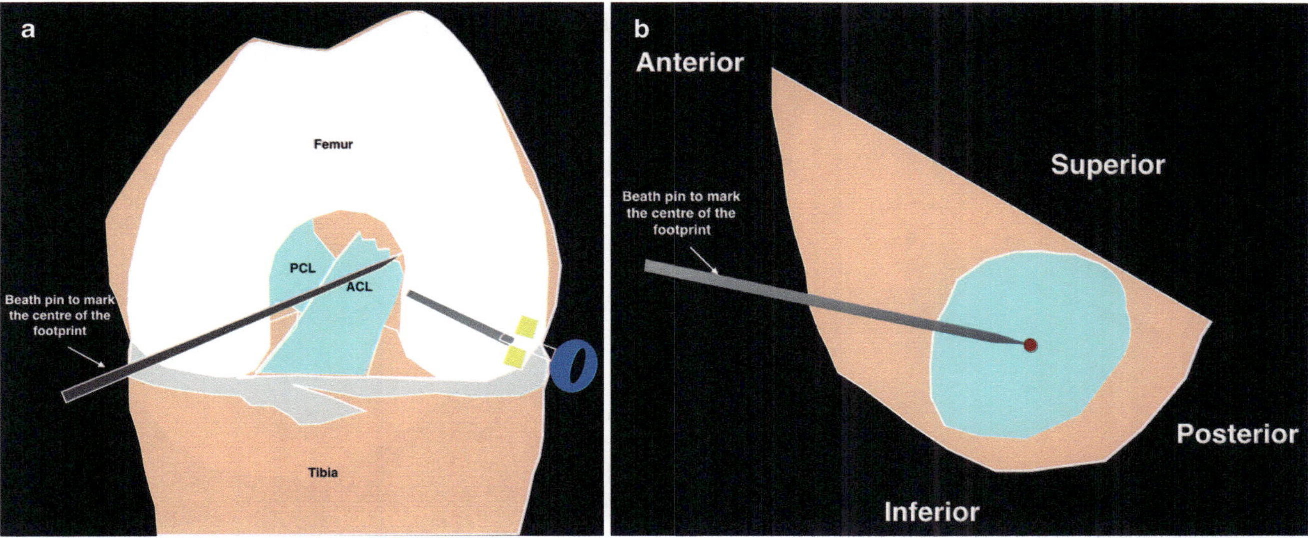


**Fig. 15.6** (**a**) Illustration of the knee showing a Beath pin placed and tapped into the mark made by the bone awl. (**b**) Illustration of the lateral aspect of the notch showing the ACL footprint and a Beath pin placed and tapped into the mark left by the bone awl

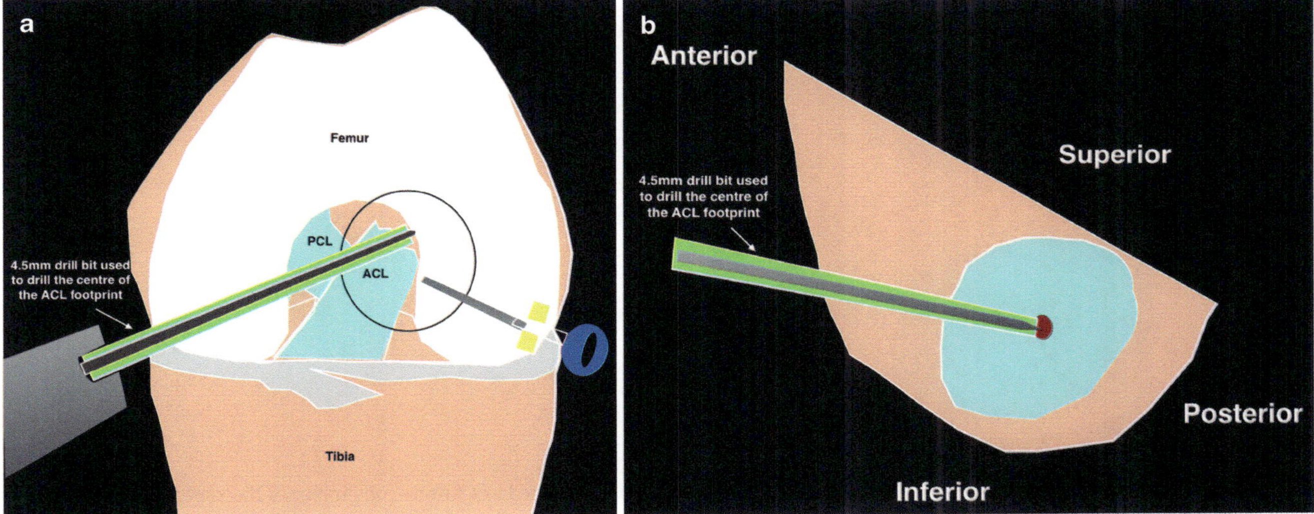


**Fig. 15.7** (**a**) Illustration of the knee showing a 4.5 mm drill bit cannulated over the Beath pin with the knee in 110° of flexion to drill the femoral tunnel beyond the opposite cortex. (**b**) Illustration of the lateral aspect of the notch showing the 4.5 mm drill bit cannulated over the Beath pin to drill the femoral tunnel across the opposite cortex

Step 6: The depth of the tunnel is measured by introducing a depth gauge through the medial portal (Fig. 15.8a, b, c).

Step 7: A Beath pin is then reversed and introduced into the femoral tunnel from the medial portal (Fig. 15.9).

Step 8: The femoral tunnel is then overdrilled with the graft sized drill bit for 20 mm by cannulating it over the Beath pin through the medial portal (Fig. 15.10a, b).

Step 9: A Beath pin with a No 5 Ethibond loop is introduced through the medial portal to shuttle the loop through the tunnel such that the loop end is at the orifice of the tunnel in the joint and two ends are delivered outside the lateral cortex (Fig. 15.11a, b, c).

Step 10: The ACL jig is set to 55° and is introduced through the medial portal and the tip applied to the centre of the ACL tibial stump and the bullet applied to the tibia anteromedially through the wound used for the graft harvest.

Step 11: A guide wire is drilled through the jig to exit through the centre of the ACL tibial stump at the elbow of the jig (Fig. 15.12a, b).

Step 12: A graft diameter full drill bit is then cannulated over the guidewire and the tibial tunnel drilled, the drill exits the centre of the stump such that it does a samba in the joint. The drilling should then be stopped (Fig. 15.13a, b).

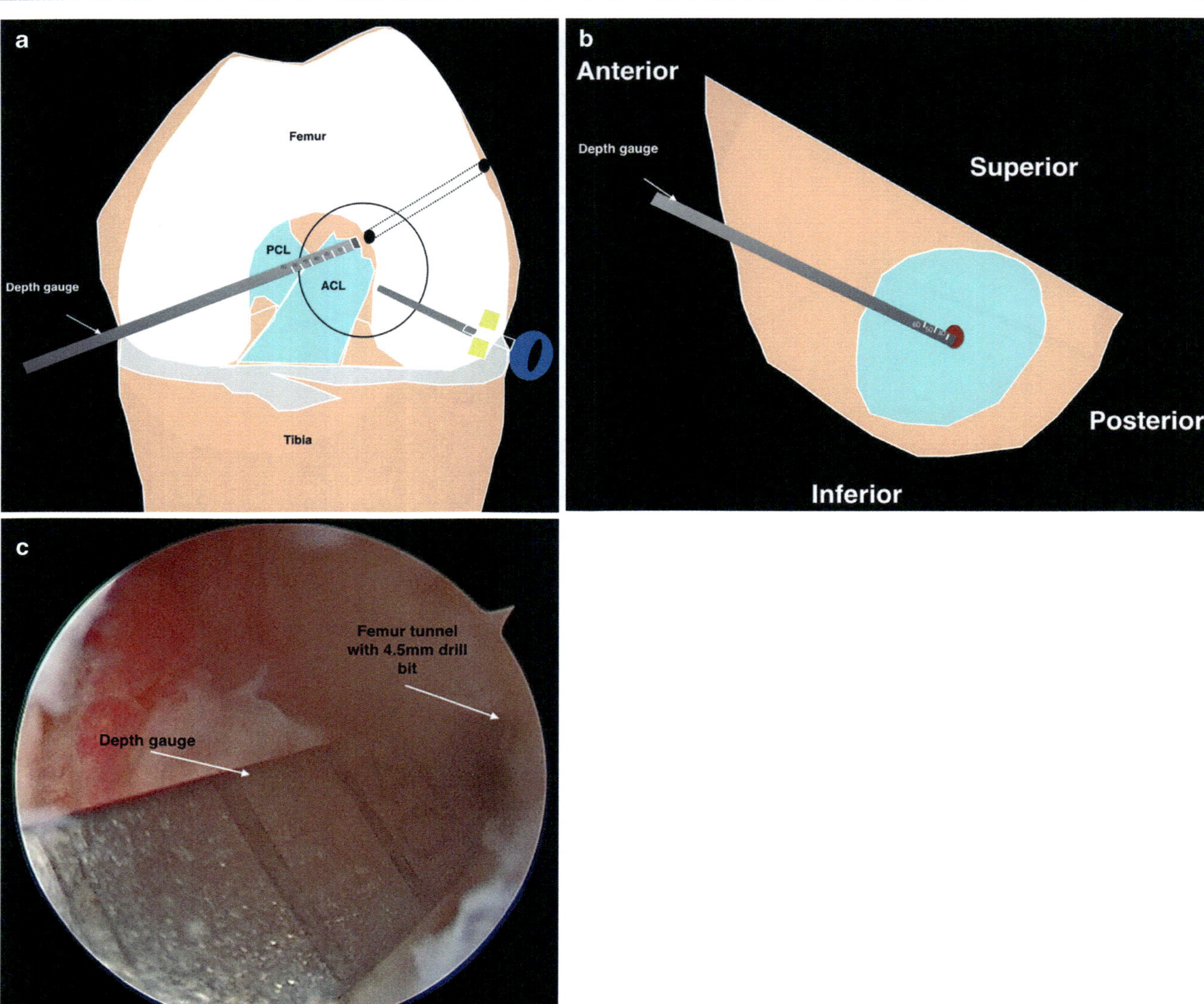


**Fig. 15.8** (**a**) Illustration of the knee showing a depth gauge introduced through the medial portal to measure the depth of the femoral tunnel. (**b**) Illustration of the lateral aspect of the notch showing a depth gauge introduced through the medial portal measuring the length of the femoral tunnel. (**c**) Arthroscopy image of the knee while viewing from the AL portal showing the depth gauge introduced through the medial portal measuring the depth of the femoral tunnel

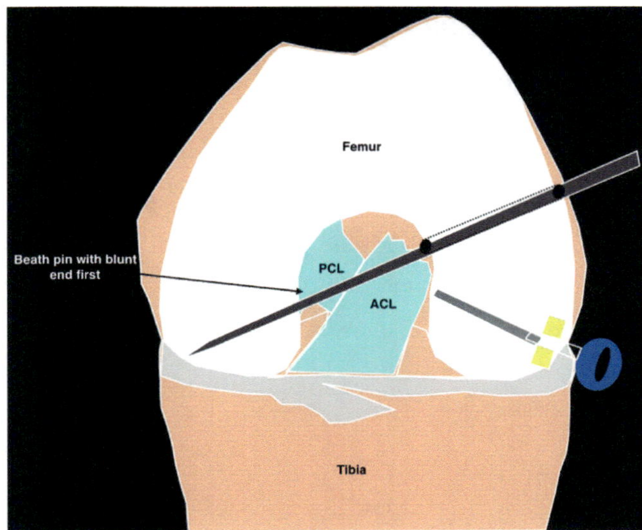


**Fig. 15.9** Illustration of the knee showing a Beath pin introduced through the femoral tunnel with the blunt end first while viewing from the AL portal

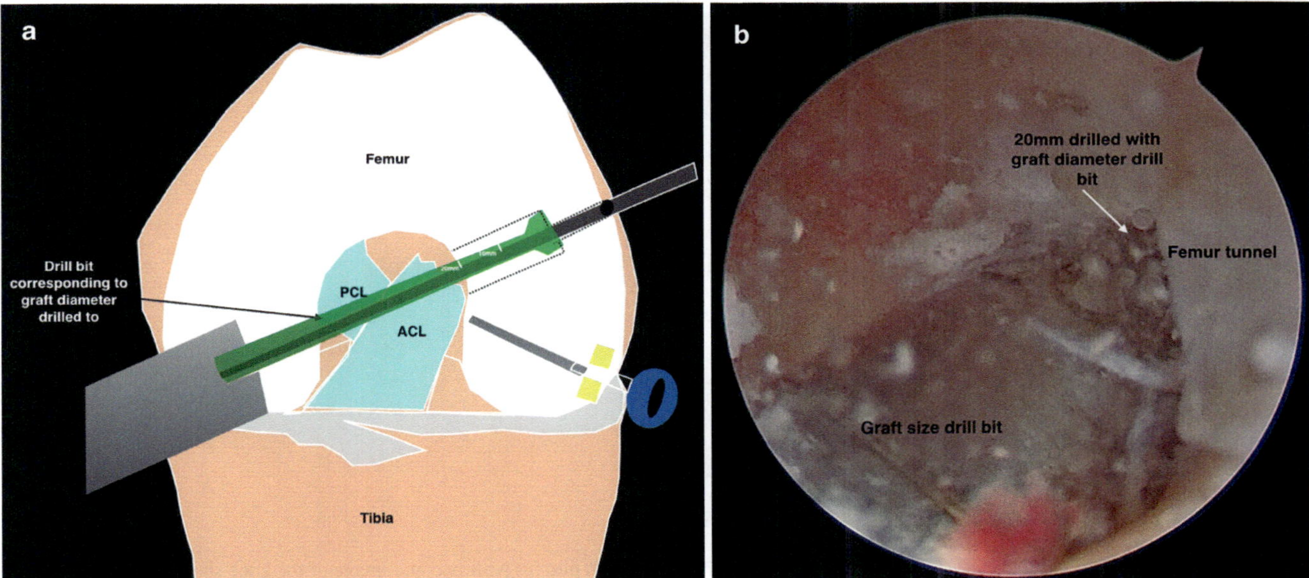


**Fig. 15.10** (**a**) Illustration of the knee showing the graft size drill bit cannulated over the Beath pin and drilling the femoral tunnel till 20 mm while viewing through the AL portal. (**b**) Arthroscopic image of the knee showing the graft size dill bit cannulated over the Beath pin drilling the femoral tunnel till 20 mm while viewing through the AL portal

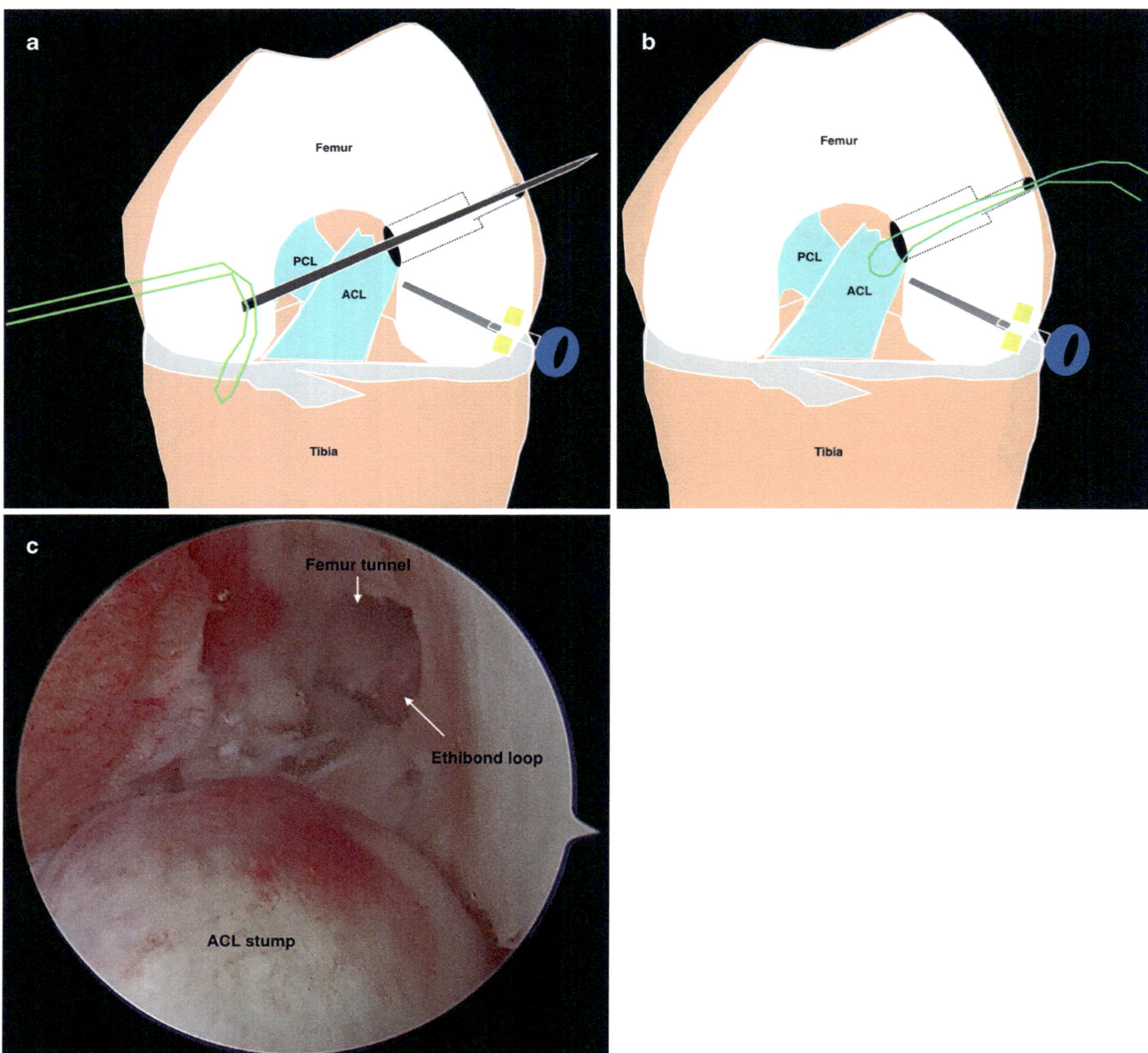


**Fig. 15.11** (**a**) Illustration of the knee showing a Beath pin carrying a No 5 Ethibond loop at its end introduced through the medial portal into the femoral tunnel. (**b**) Illustration of the knee showing the Ethibond loop at the orifice of the femoral tunnel after it is shuttled using the Beath pin. (**c**) Arthroscopic image of the knee showing the femoral tunnel with the Ethibond loop at its orifice while viewing through the AL portal

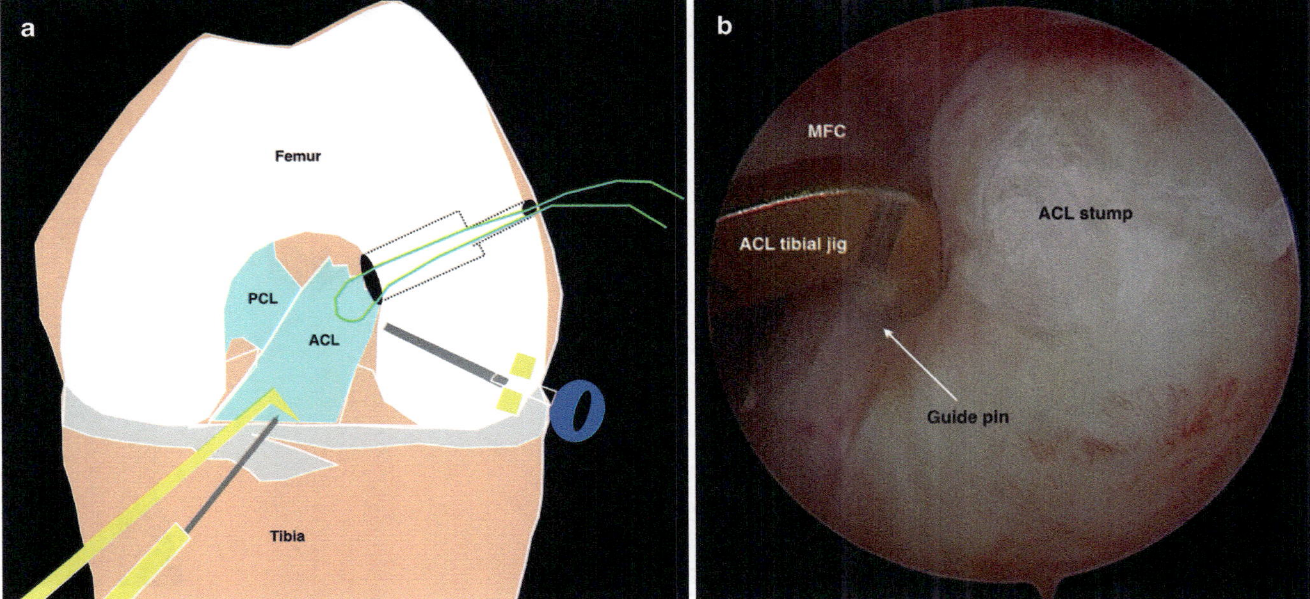


**Fig. 15.12** (**a**) Illustration of the knee showing the ACL jig through the medial portal placed at the centre of the ACL stump on the tibia and drilled with a guidewire that has come out at the centre of the stump while viewing from the AL portal. (**b**) Arthroscopic image of the knee showing the ACL jig at the centre of the ACL tibial stump with the guidewire coming out at the elbow of the jig while viewing through the AL portal

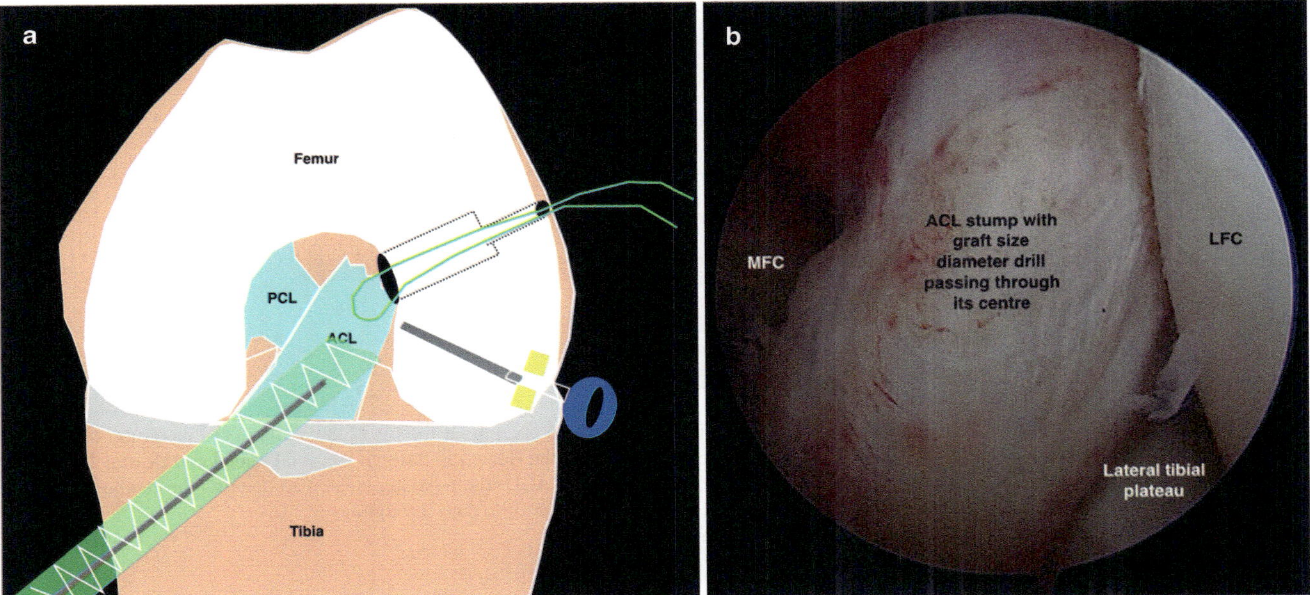


**Fig. 15.13** (**a**) Illustration of the knee showing the guidewire coming out the centre of the ACL tibial stump being overdrilled with the graft size drill bit cannulated over it and the drill bit coming out through the centre of the stump. (**b**) Arthroscopic image of the knee showing the ACL stump and drill bit that is passing through its centre while viewing through the AL portal

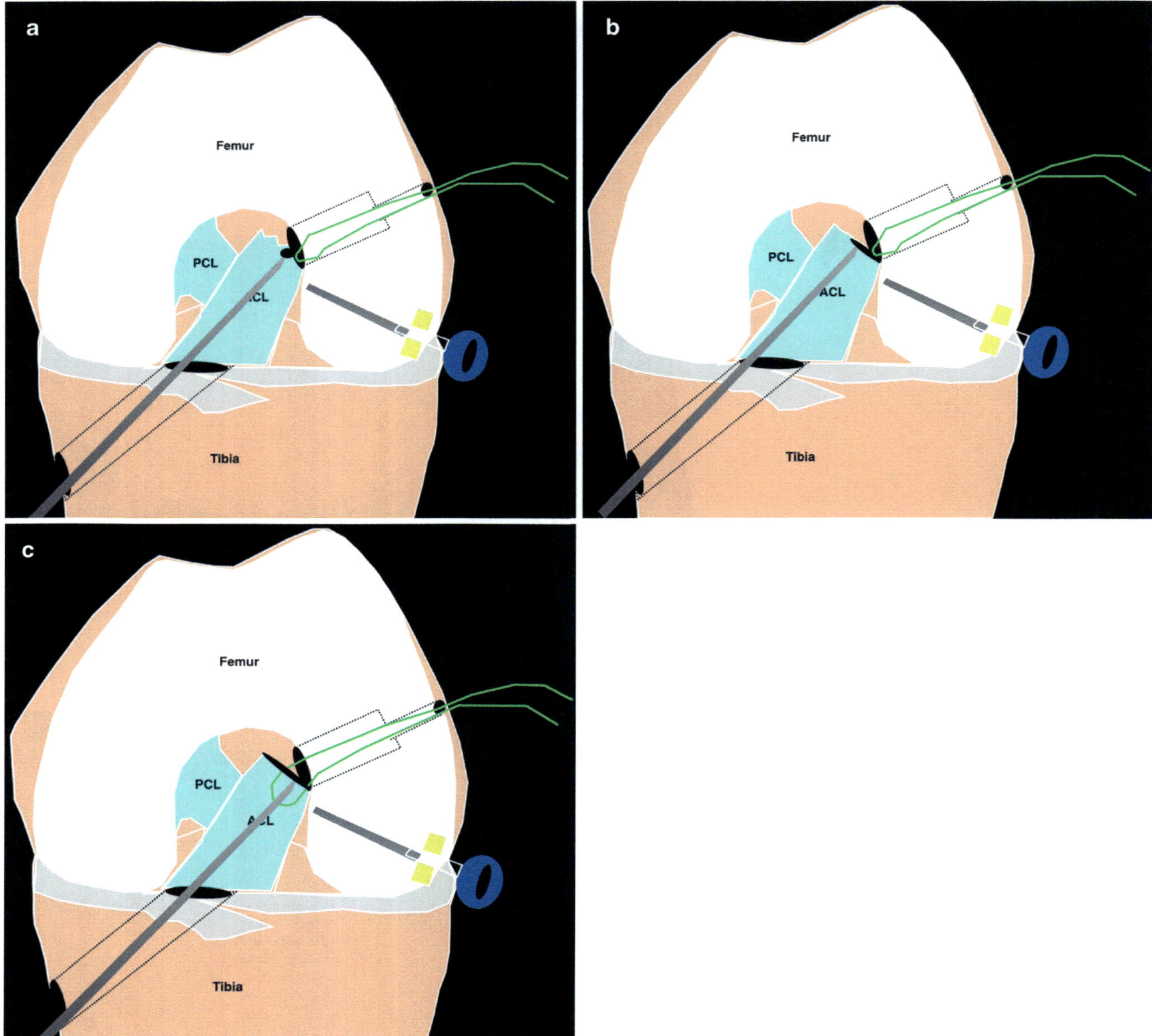


**Fig. 15.14** (**a**) Illustration of the knee showing a Beath pin introduced through the tibial tunnel and the ACL tibial stump till it exits at the tip of the stump while viewing through the AL portal. (**b**) Illustration of the knee showing the Beath pin introduced through the tibial tunnel and out of the tip of the ACL stump a little more medial to its first exit so as to widen the opening at the tip of the stump. (**c**) Illustration of the knee showing the Beath pin through the tibial tunnel and exiting through the tip of the ACL stump having created an opening throughout its apex to allow the graft to pass through it

Step 13: A Beath pin is then introduced through the tibial tunnel through the stump till its apex and with slow to and fro movements, to create an opening in its apex to allow the graft to pass through (Fig. 15.14a, b, c).

Step 14: A Bird beak grasper is then introduced through the tibial tunnel from the anteromedial aspect of the tibia and passes through the centre of the stump and exits from where a space was made. It is used to grasp the Ethibond loop that is pulled down the tibial tunnel to shuttle the graft (Fig. 15.15a, b).

Step15: The sutures attached to the Tightrope construct are first shuttled outside the lateral cortex, and the graft is milked up the tibial tunnel into the femoral tunnel, passing through the stump till 20 mm in the femur tunnel.

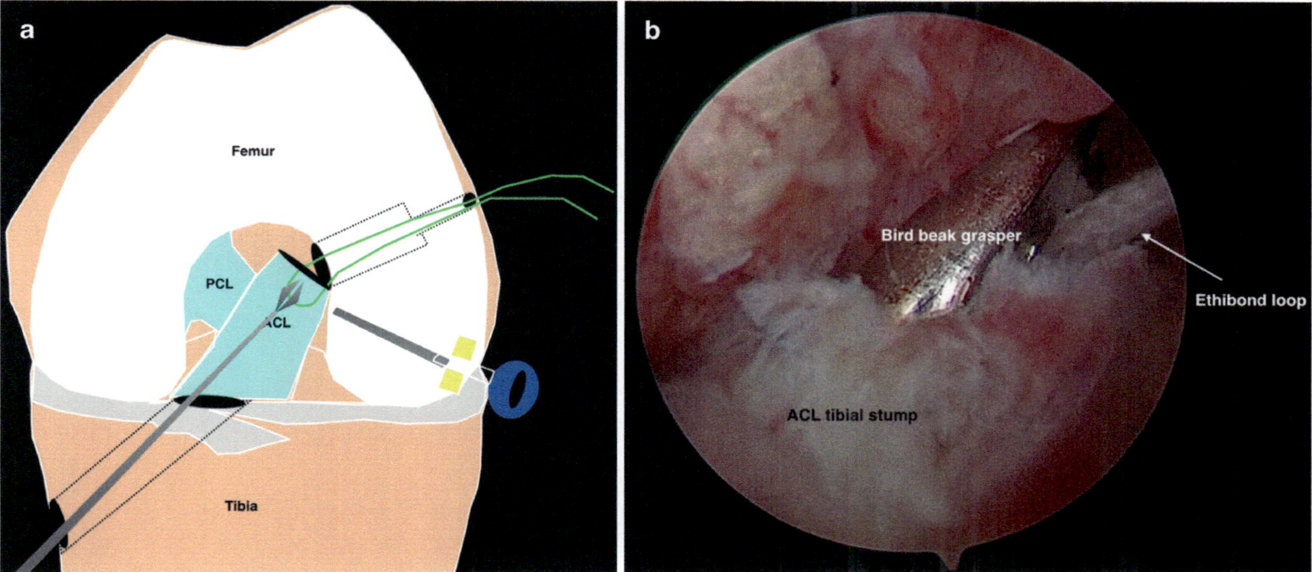


**Fig. 15.15** (**a**) Illustration of the knee showing a Bird beak grasper introduced through the tibial tunnel into the centre of the ACL stump through the opening created on the tip of the ACL stump to pull the Ethibond loop at the femoral tunnel orifice down the tibial tunnel. (**b**) Arthroscopic image of the knee showing a Bird beak grasper introduced through the tibial tunnel and the centre of the ACL tibial stump grasping the Ethibond loop to be brought down the tibial tunnel

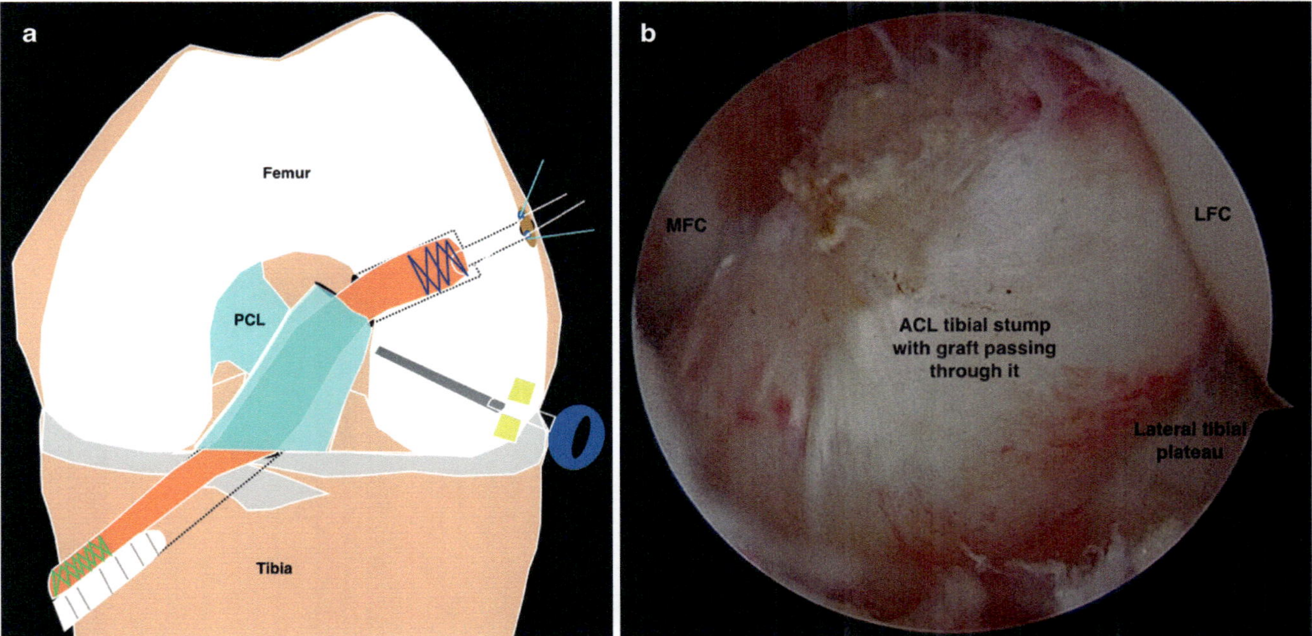


**Fig. 15.16** (**a**) Illustration of the knee showing the final graft construct passing through the ACL stump, fixed with a Tightrope RT on the femur and an interference screw on the tibia. (**b**) Arthroscopic image of the knee showing the intact ACL tibial stump after the graft is passed through it

The loop is premarked with the total length of the femur tunnel and 20 mm is marked on the femoral end of the graft to be sure that adequate graft goes into the tunnel and to counter check if the button has flipped (Fig. 15.16a, b).

## 15.6 Tips and Tricks

1. Using a Bird Beak grasper can help dilate the tip of the stump at the femoral end and also retrieve the Ethibond loop through the stump and tibial tunnel.

2. At the end of the graft fixation at the tibial end check for impingement and a notchplasty may be required.

## 15.7 Advantages and Disadvantages

### 15.7.1 Advantages

1. Possibly improved vascularity.
2. Better structural support.
3. Preserved proprioception.

### 15.7.2 Disadvantages

1. Technically demanding.
2. Can cause impingement of the graft on the notch roof.

# Arthroscopic Bony ACL Femoral Avulsion Fixation

# 16

Vikram Arun Mhaskar

## 16.1 Introduction

Bony femoral avulsions of the anterior cruciate ligament (ACL) are uncommon. The ACL can be repaired in these cases and this provides an opportunity for better healing as bone-to-bone contact happens. Repair of the ligament requires a secure fixation technique that does not twist the ligament. We describe a technique to fix a bony avulsion using suture tapes that are passed through the ACL stump in a figure of '8' configuration and fixed on the lateral femoral cortex with a suture disc after drilling through the femoral footprint with a 4.5 mm drill bit.

## 16.2 Specialized Equipment (Fig. 16.1)

1. Knee Scorpion (Arthrex, Naples, Fl).
2. 2–0 Fiberwire (Arthrex, Naples, Fl)
3. Suture Tape (Arthrex, Naples, Fl).
4. Passport Cannula (Arthrex, Naples, Fl).
5. Probe (Smith and Nephew, Watford, UK).
6. Shaver with tip (Stryker, Kalamazoo, MI).
7. Radiofrequency device (Stryker, Kalamazoo, MI).
8. Suture Disc (ABS Button) (Arthrex, Naples, Fl).

V. A. Mhaskar (✉)
F7 East of Kailash, Knee & Shoulder Clinic, New Delhi, India

JMVM Sports Injury Center, Sitaram Bhartia Institute of Science & Research, New Delhi, India


V. A. Mhaskar, J. Maheshwari (eds.), *Innovative Approaches in Knee Arthroscopy*,
https://doi.org/10.1007/978-981-99-4378-4_16

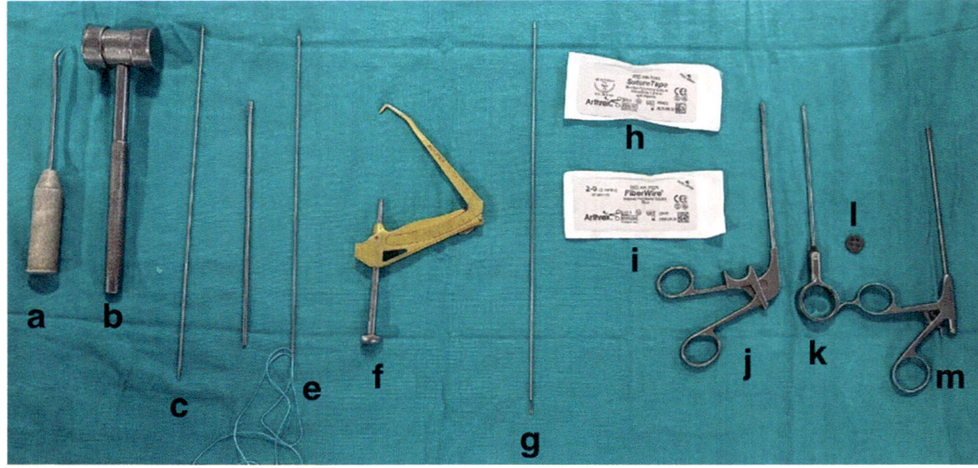


**Fig. 16.1** (**a**) Bone awl, (**b**) Mallet, (**c**) Beath Pin, (**d**) 4.5 mm drill bit, (**e**) Beath Pin with No5 Ethibond loop, (**f**) ACL tibial jig, (**g**) Guidewire, (**h**) Suture Tape, (**i**) 2–0 Fiberwire, (**j**) Arthroscopic grasper, (**k**) Knot pusher, (**l**) Suture Disc, (**m**) Arthroscopic knot cutter

## 16.3 Positioning (Fig. 16.2)

Knee is positioned at 70° flexion with a side support and bolster on the table.

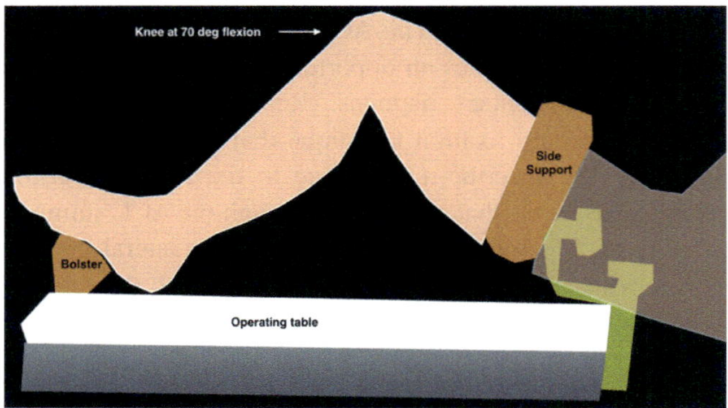


**Fig. 16.2** Illustration of the position of the knee in 70° flexion with a side support and bolster at the end of the table

## 16.4 Portals (Fig. 16.3)

1. High anterolateral (AL) viewing portal A just lateral to the patellar tendon at the level of the inferior pole of the patella.
2. Low medial working portal B just above the medial meniscus made with LP needle such that it reaches the femoral footprint without touching the lateral femoral condyle.
3. High anteromedial (AM) working portal C just medial to the medial border of the patellar tendon at the level of the inferior pole of the patella.

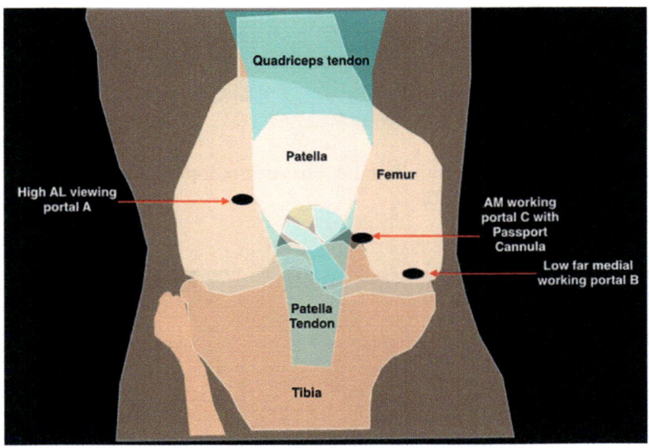


**Fig. 16.3** Illustration of the knee showing Portal A: High AL portal, Portal B: low far medial portal and Portal C: AM working portal

## 16.5 Surgical Technique

Step 1: The ACL stump with bony avulsion is visualized with the arthroscope in Portal A (Fig. 16.4a, b).

Step 2: A probe is introduced through Portal B to co-apt the ACL avulsion to the femoral footprint while viewing through Portal A (Fig. 16.5a, b).

Step 3: A Radiofrequency device (Stryker, Kalamazoo, MI) (RF) is introduced through Portal B to clear the femoral footprint while viewing through Portal A (Fig. 16.6).

Step 4: A Beath pin is then introduced through Portal B and tapped into the centre of the ACL femoral footprint while viewing through Portal A (Fig. 16.7a, b, c).

Step 5: A 4.5 mm drill bit is cannulated over the Beath pin and the femoral tunnel is drilled across the lateral cortex (Fig. 16.8a, b, c).

Step 6: A depth gauge is introduced through Portal B to measure the length of the femoral tunnel while viewing through Portal A (Fig. 16.9a, b).

Step 7: A Beath pin with a Ethibond loop (Ethicon, Rariton, NJ) is then introduced through Portal B across the femoral tunnel so that the loop just projects out of the femoral tunnel intra articularly and the two ends are coming out of the lateral cortex of the femur and out of the skin (Fig. 16.10a, b, c).

Step 8: A Passport cannula is introduced through Portal C (Fig. 16.11).

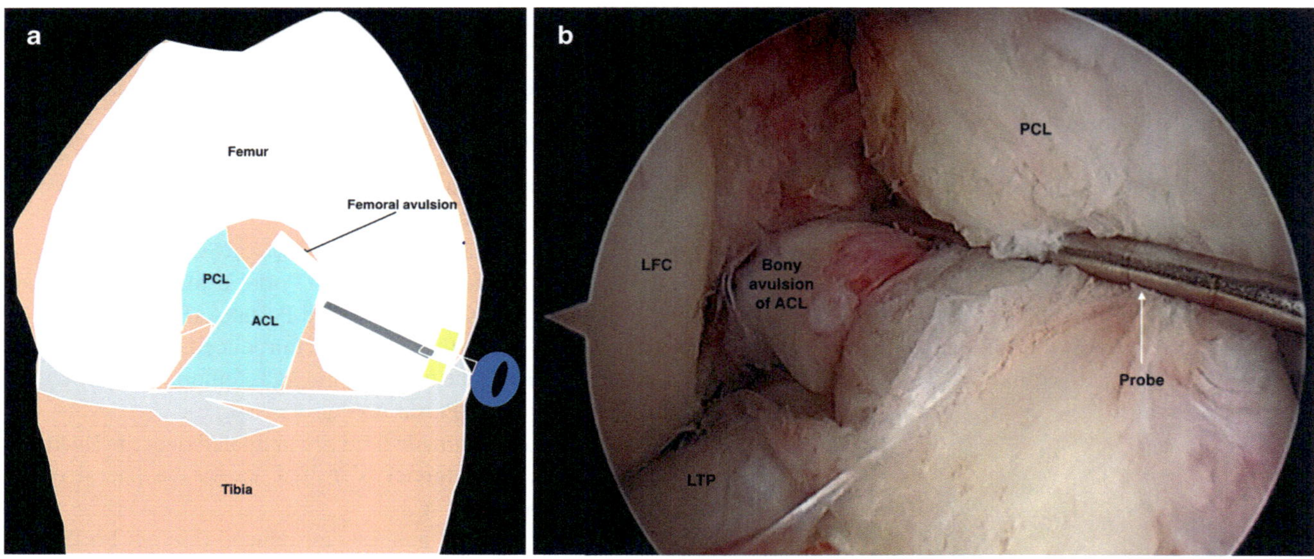


**Fig. 16.4** (**a**) Illustration of the knee showing the ACL bony femoral avulsion while viewing from Portal A. (**b**) Arthroscopic image of the knee viewing through Portal A showing the bony femoral avulsion while being probed through Portal B

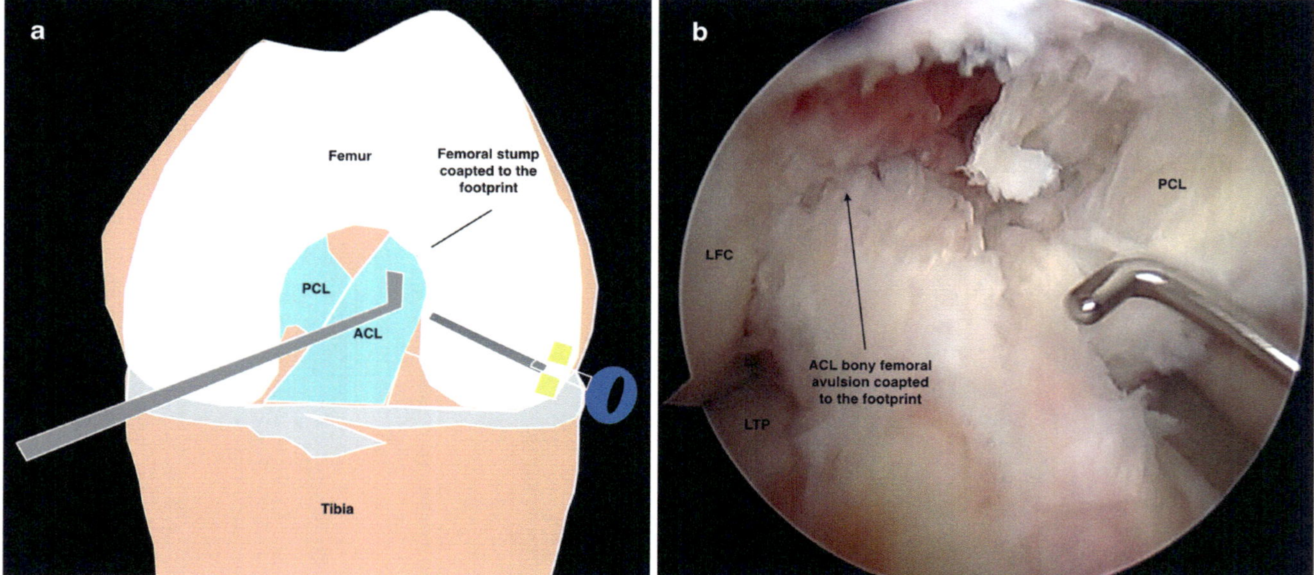


**Fig. 16.5** (**a**) Illustration of the knee showing the probe through Portal B co-apting the avulsed ACL to its footprint while viewing through Portal A. (**b**) Arthroscopic image of the knee while viewing through Portal A showing the ACL stump anatomically reduced to its femoral footprint using a probe from Portal B

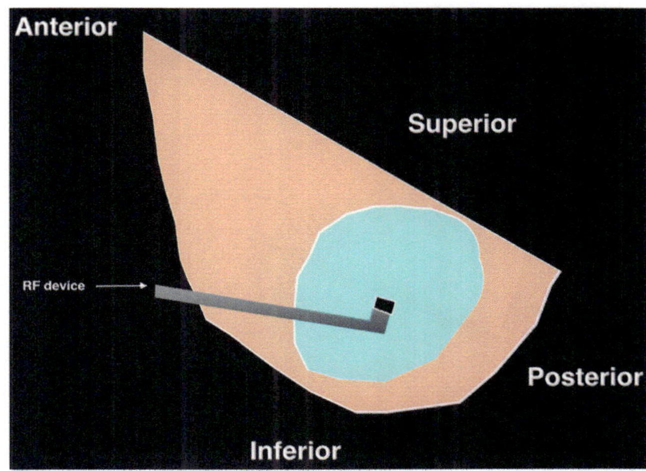


**Fig. 16.6** Illustration of the knee showing a RF device through Portal B while viewing through Portal A

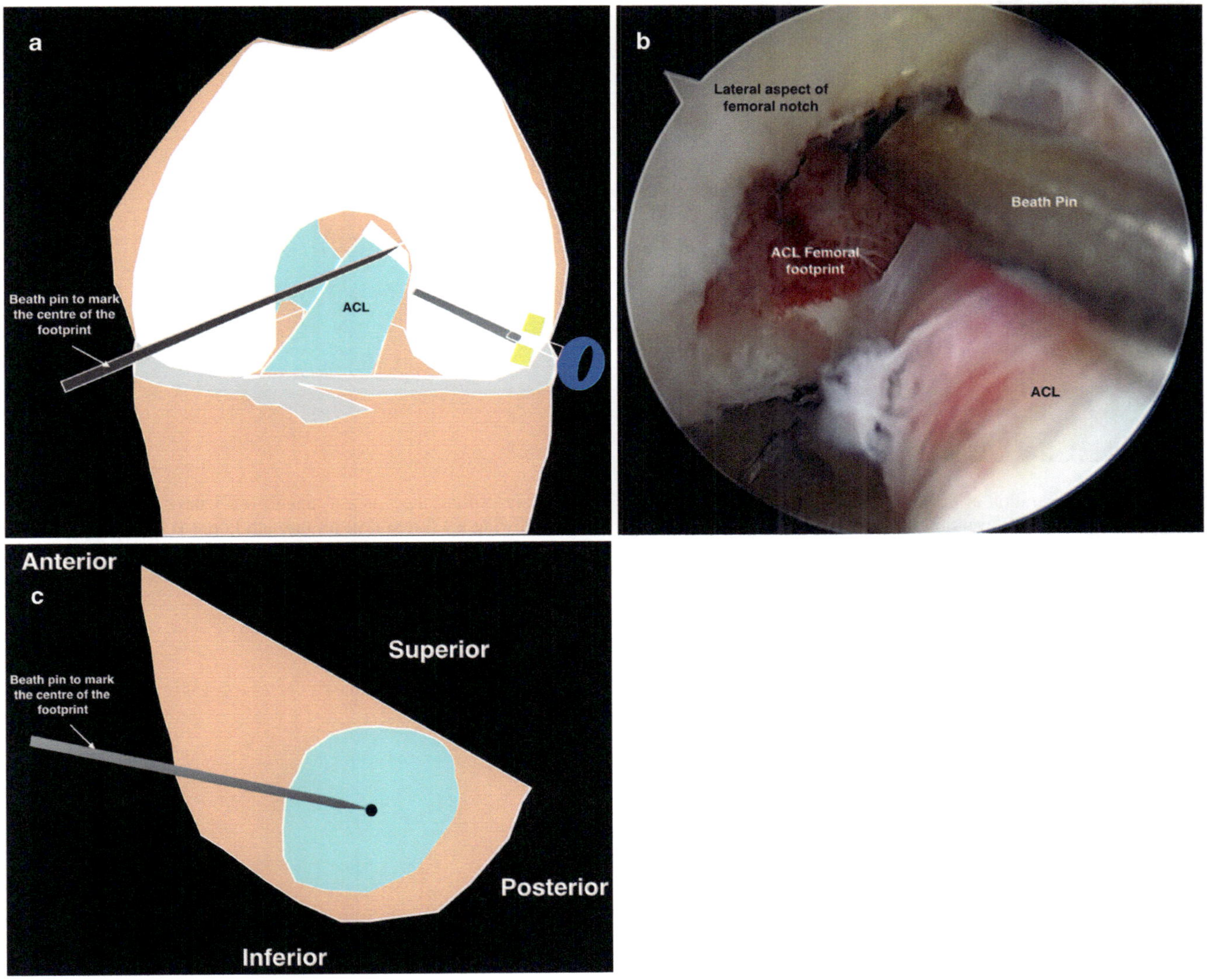

**Fig. 16.7** (**a**) Illustration of the knee viewing from Portal A showing a Beath pin through Portal C tapped into the centre of the ACL femoral footprint. (**b**) Arthroscopic image of knee while viewing through Portal A showing the Beath pin through Portal B applied to the centre of the femoral footprint. (**c**) Illustration of the knee showing a Beath pin through Portal B applied to the centre of the femoral footprint while viewing through Portal A

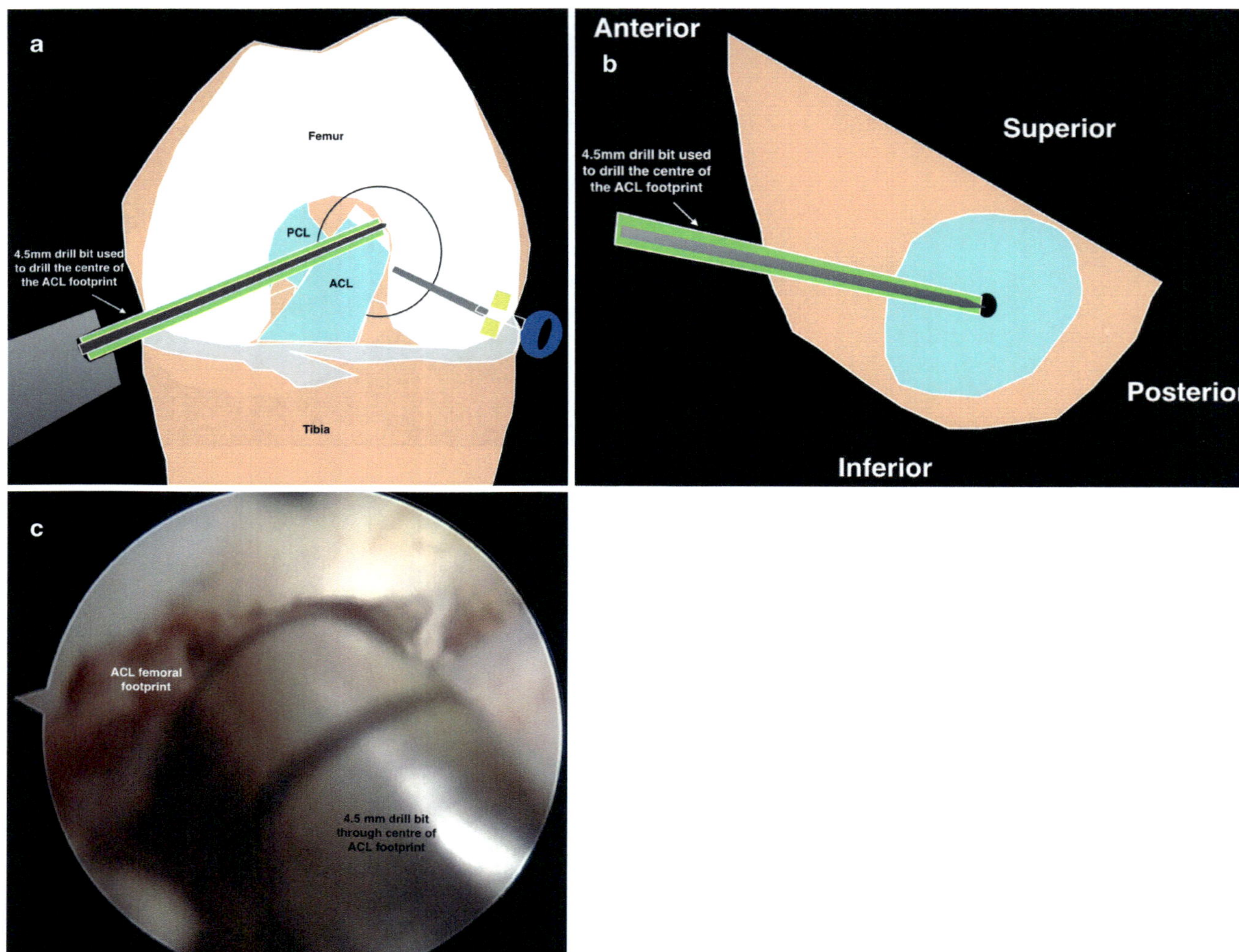


**Fig. 16.8** (**a**) Illustration of the knee showing a 4.5 mm drill bit cannulated through Portal B over the Beath pin tapped into the centre of the footprint while viewing through Portal A. (**b**) Illustration of the lateral aspect of the notch showing the 4.5 mm drill bit cannulated over the Beath pin drilling the femoral tunnel. (**c**) Arthroscopic image of the knee showing a 4.5 mm drill bit through Portal B drilling the femoral tunnel while viewing through Portal A

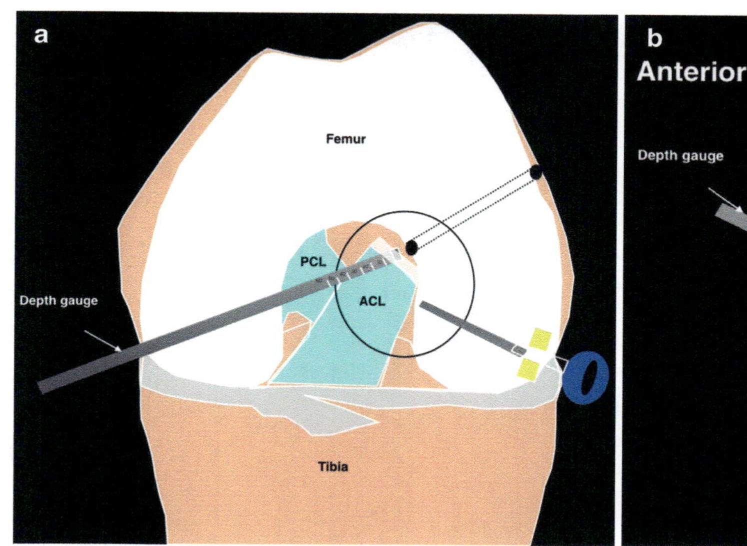


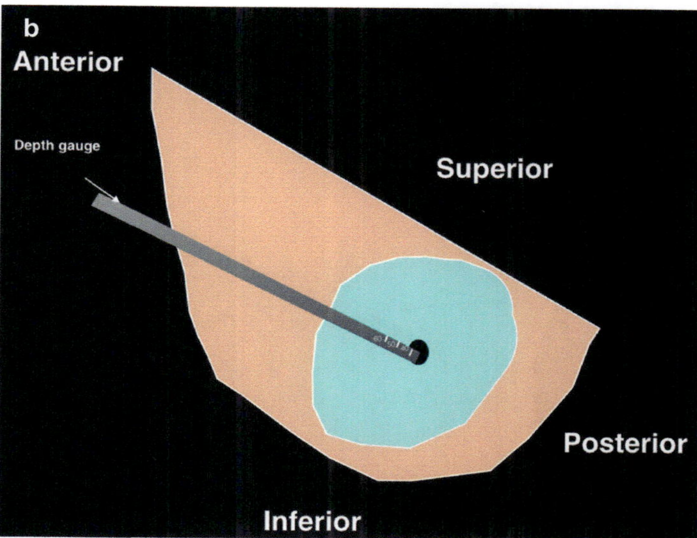


**Fig. 16.9** (**a**) Illustration of the knee showing a depth gauge introduced through Portal B measuring the femoral tunnel length while viewing through Portal A. (**b**) Illustration of the lateral aspect of the notch showing a depth gauge introduced through Portal B while viewing through Portal A measuring the femoral tunnel

Step 9: A Knee Scorpion loaded with a 2–0 Fiberwire (Arthrex, Naples, Fl) is introduced through the Passport Cannula to take a bite through the substance of the ACL close to the avulsed fragment (Fig. 16.12a, b).

Step 10: The 2–0 Fiberwire is seen passing through the ACL stump (Fig. 16.13a, b).

Step 11: The 2–0 Fiberwire is tied around a Suture Tape (Arthrex, Naples, Fl) to shuttle it through the ACL (Fig. 16.14a, b, c, d).

Step 12: The Knee Scorpion loaded with the 2–0 Fiberwire is introduced through Portal C and a bite is taken through the tip of the fragment (Fig. 16.15a, b).

Step 13: One end of the suture tape is tied over the end of the 2–0 Fiberwire opposite to it, to shuttle that end of the Suture Tape to form one end of the Figure of '8' configuration (Fig. 16.16a, b).

Step 14: The Knee Scorpion loaded with the 2–0 Fiberwire is introduced through Portal C and a bite is taken through the tip of the fragment to be used to shuttle the other end of the Suture tape to form a Figure of '8' configuration around the ACL stump (Fig. 16.17a, b).

Step 15: The Ethibond loop is delivered through Portal C using a Suture manipulator to shuttle the two ends of the Suture Tape across the lateral cortex of the femur and out of the skin (Fig. 16.18a, b).

Step 16: A small incision about 1 cm is made in the skin just next to the Suture Tape and the ends delivered through the incision and using artery forceps, dissected to the bone on the lateral cortex of the femur (Fig. 16.19).

Step 17: The two ends of the Suture Tape are then applied over two eyes on the suture disc and the disc pushed to the lateral cortex of the femur with a knot pusher and multiple simple knots (5) tied with the two ends of the Suture Tape over the suture disc using a knot pusher (Fig. 16.20).

Step 18: The ACL avulsion is reduced and secured over its footprint (Fig. 16.21a, b).

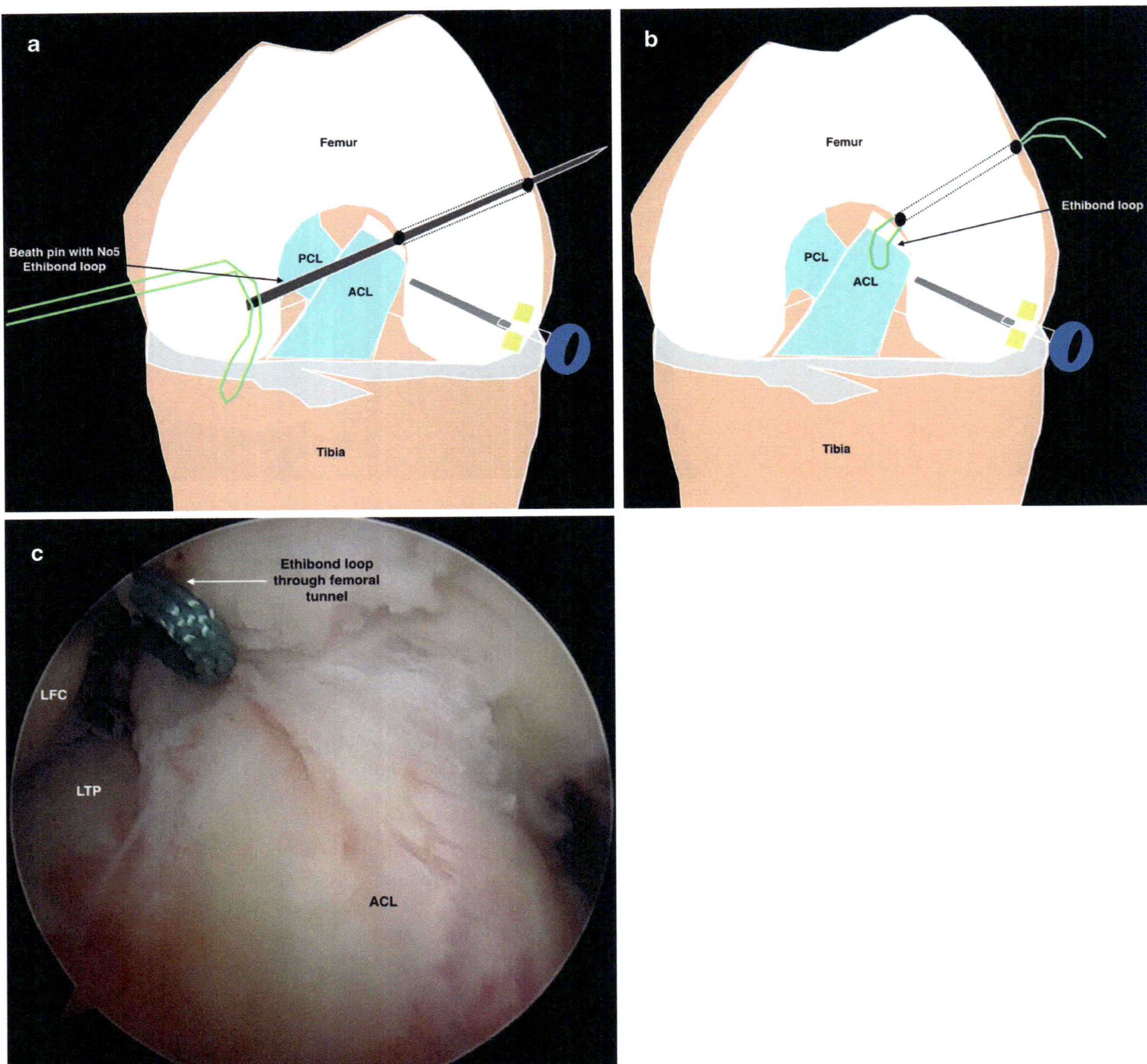


**Fig. 16.10** (**a**) Illustration of the knee showing a Beath pin carrying an Ethibond loop introduced through Portal B into the femoral tunnel while viewing through Portal A. (**b**) Illustration of the knee showing the Ethibond loop at the femoral tunnel orifice. (**c**) Arthroscopic image of the knee showing the Ethibond loop at the femoral tunnel orifice while viewing through Portal A

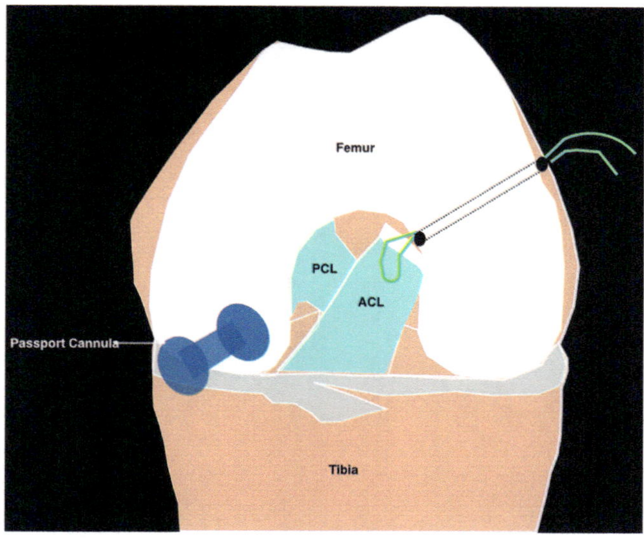


**Fig. 16.11** Illustration of the knee showing a Passport (Arthrex, Naples, Fl) cannula through Portal C

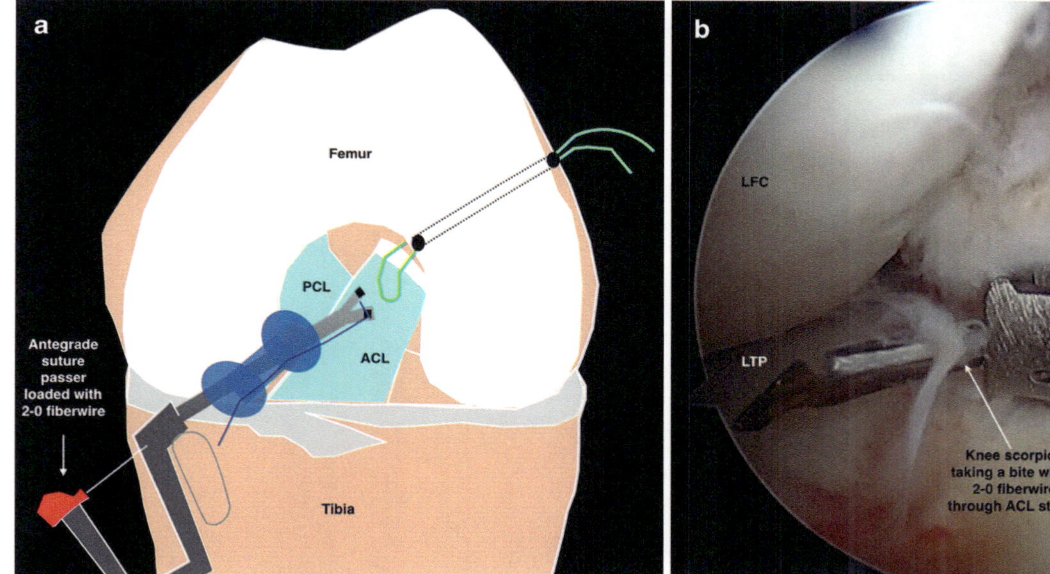


**Fig. 16.12** (**a**) Illustration of the knee showing a Knee Scorpion (Arthrex, Naples, Fl) through Portal C taking a bite with a 2–0 Fiberwire through the ACL stump while viewing through Portal A. (**b**) Arthroscopic image of the knee showing a Knee Scorpion through Portal C taking a bite with a 2–0 Fiberwire through the ACL stump while viewing through Portal A

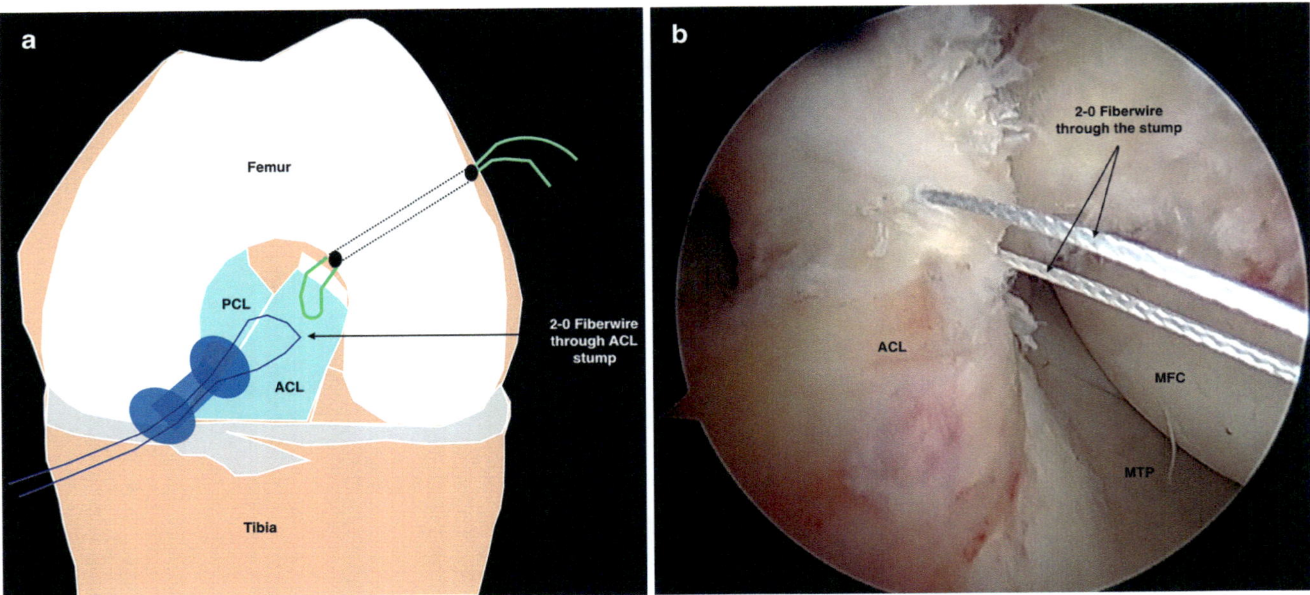


**Fig. 16.13** (**a**) Illustration of the knee showing a 2–0 Fiberwire passing through the ACL stump while viewing through Portal A. (**b**) Arthroscopic image of the knee showing the ACL stump with a 2–0 Fiberwire passing through it while viewing through Portal A

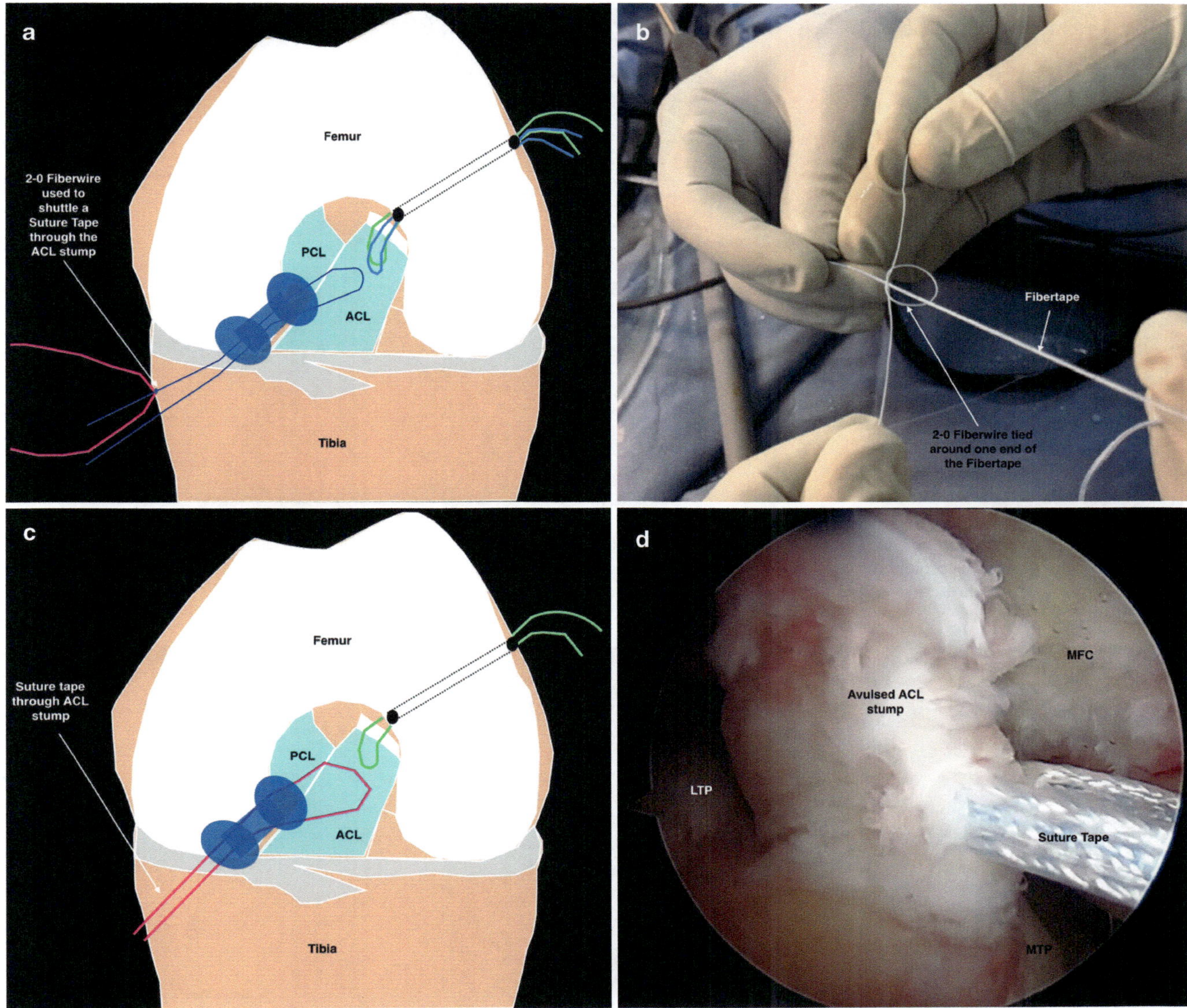


**Fig. 16.14** (**a**) Illustration of the knee showing the two ends of 2–0 Fiberwire through the ACL stump, with one end tied over a Suture tape to shuttle it through the ACL stump while viewing through Portal A. (**b**) Image showing one end of the 2–0 Fiberwire being tied over one end of the Suture Tape. (**c**) Illustration of the knee showing the Suture Tape passing through the ACL stump with its two ends through Portal C. (**d**) Arthroscopic image showing the Suture Tape through the ACL stump while viewing through Portal A

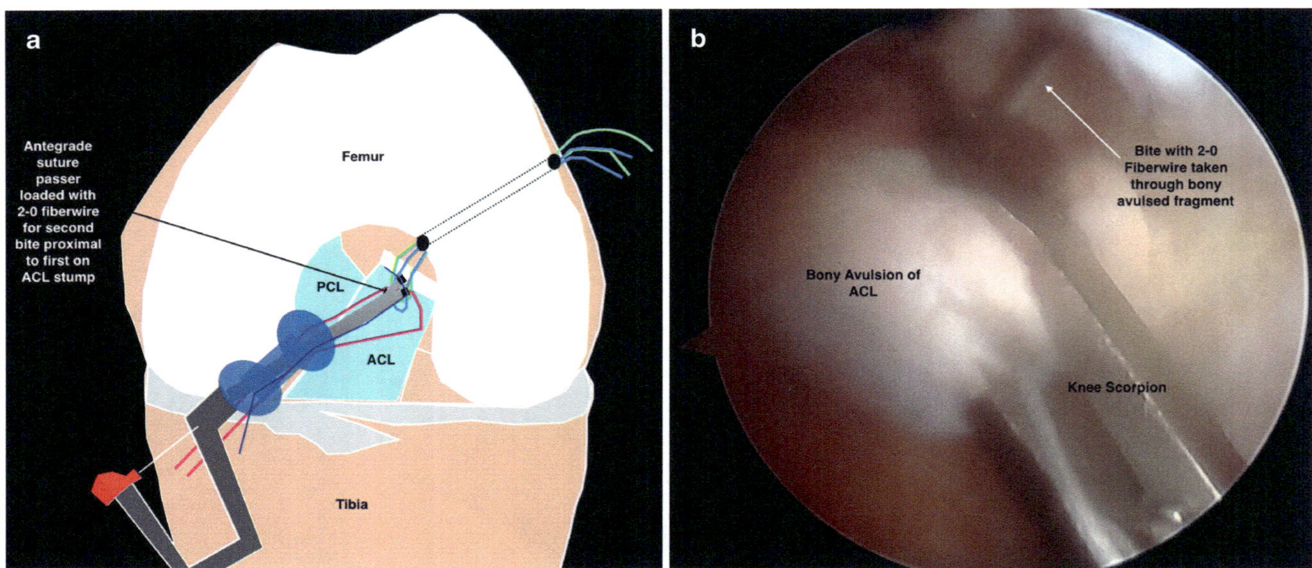


**Fig. 16.15** (**a**) Illustration of the knee showing a bite taken with a 2–0 Fiberwire using a Knee Scorpion through Portal C while viewing through Portal A. (**b**) Arthroscopic image of the knee showing a bite being taken at the tip of the ACL avulsed fragment with a Knee Scorpion using a 2–0 Fiberwire through Portal C while viewing through Portal A

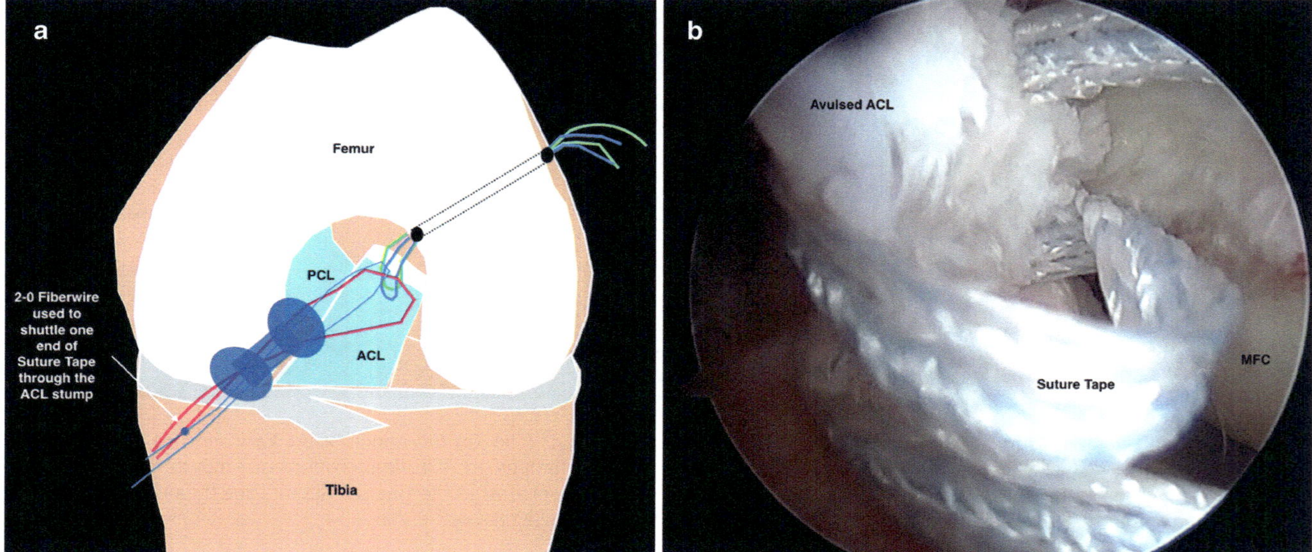


**Fig. 16.16** (**a**) Illustration of the knee showing a Suture Tape through the ACL stump and a 2–0 Fiberwire through the avulsed fragment whose one end is tied to one end of the Suture Tape to shuttle it through. (**b**) Arthroscopic image of the knee showing the Suture tape encircling the ACL stump forming one limb of the Figure of '8' configuration while viewing through Portal A

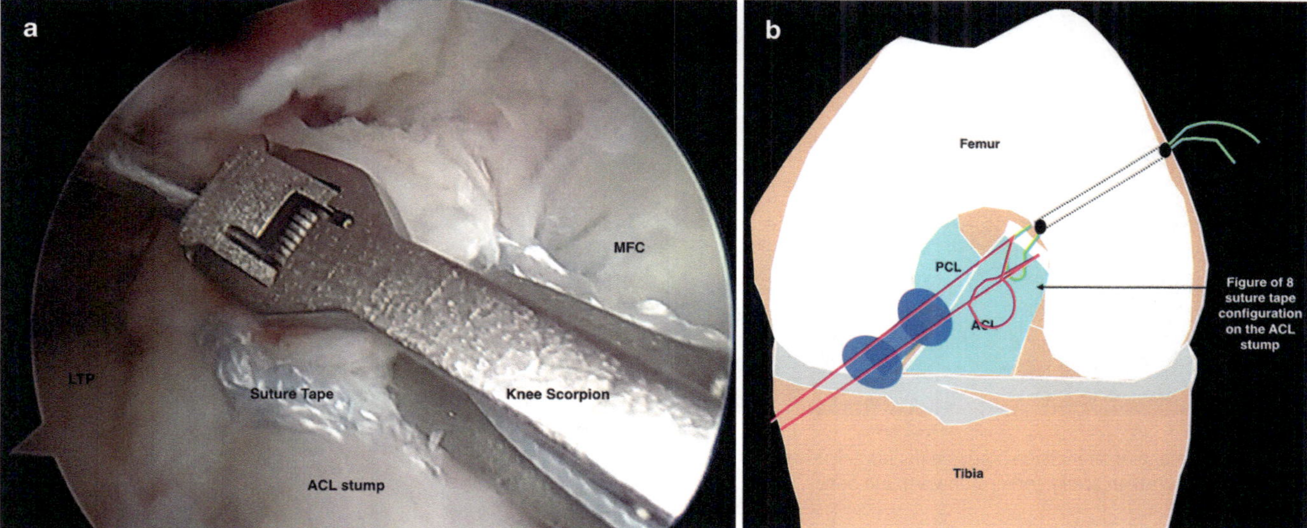


**Fig. 16.17** (**a**) Arthroscopic image showing a Knee Scorpion through Portal C taking a bite through the ACL avulsed fragment with a 2–0 Fiberwire while viewing through Portal A. (**b**) Illustration of the knee showing the suture tape in a Figure of '8' configuration around the ACL stump while viewing through Portal A

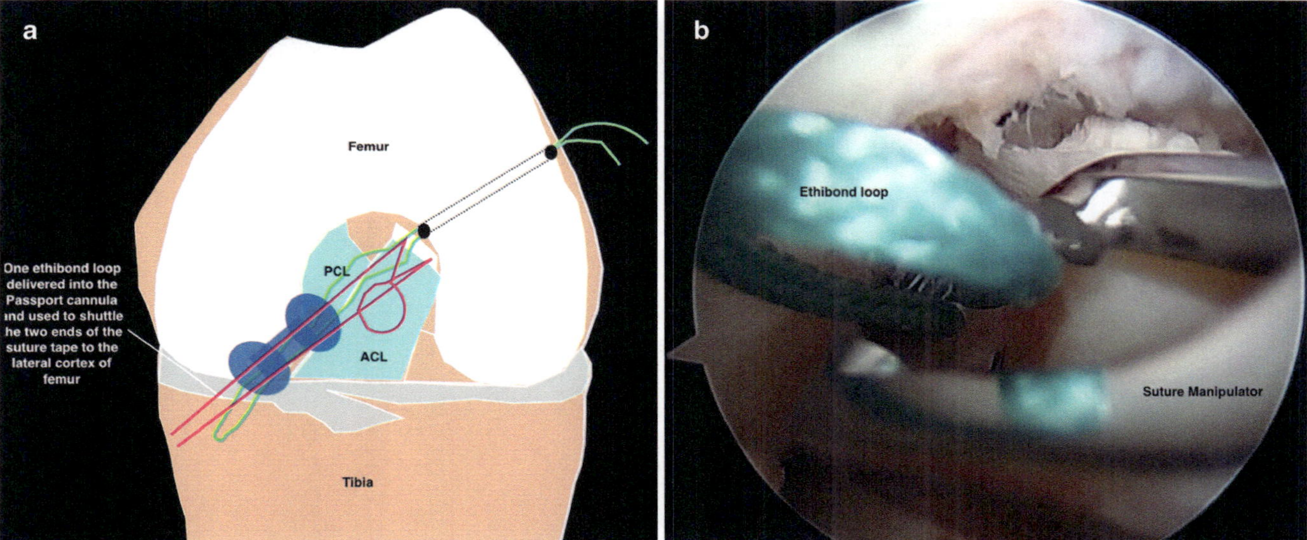


**Fig. 16.18** (**a**) Illustration of the knee showing the Ethibond loop and two end ends of the Suture tape in Passport Cannula in Portal C while viewing through Portal A. (**b**) Arthroscopic image of the knee showing a Suture manipulator through Portal C holding the Ethibond loop while viewing through Portal A

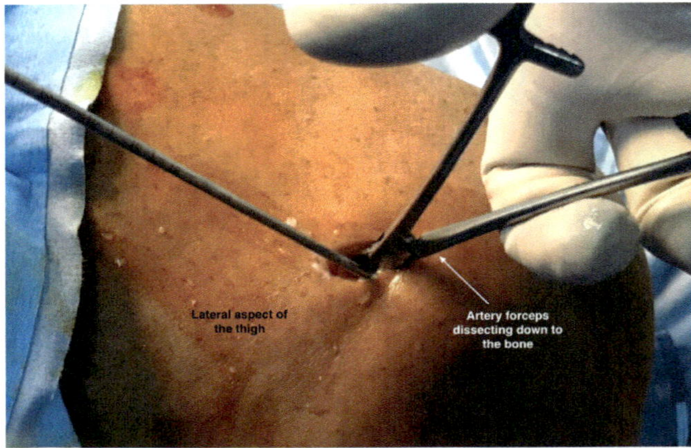


Fig. 16.19 Image of an incision made on the lateral side of the thigh to dissect tissues with an artery forceps down to the bone

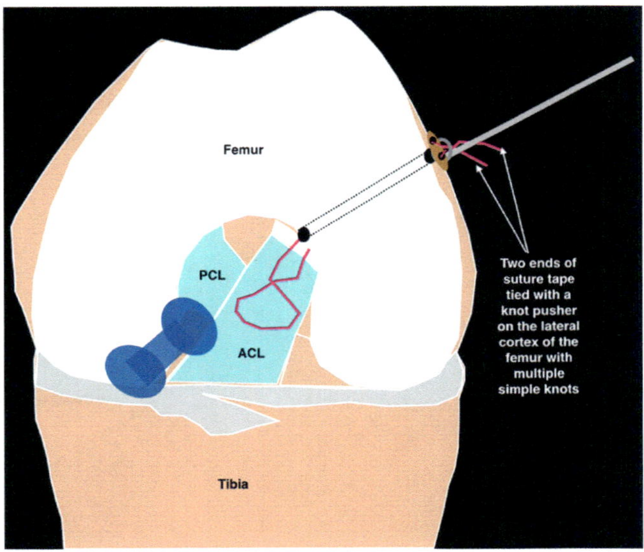


Fig. 16.20 Illustration of the knee showing two ends of the Suture Tape through the eyes of the suture disc being tied over the suture disc over the lateral cortex of the femur using a knot pusher

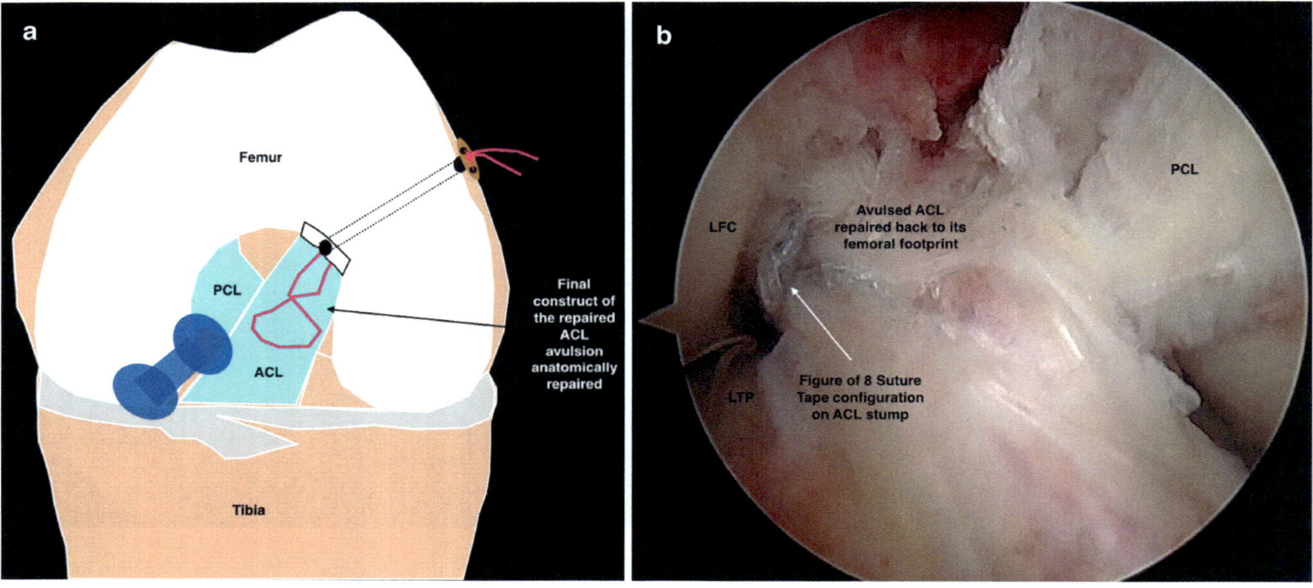


Fig. 16.21 (a) Illustration of the knee showing the reduced and fixed ACL avulsion and the two ends of the Suture Tape tied over the suture disc on the lateral cortex of the femur. (b) Arthroscopic image of the knee showing the repaired ACL avulsion while viewing through Portal A

## 16.6 Technical Tips

1. Take a bite through the full thickness of the ACL stump so that the suture does not cut out.
2. Tie the Suture tape with a simple knot using the 2–0 Fiberwire such that only 1 cm of the Suture Tape is beyond the knot.
3. Make an incision on the lateral aspect of the thigh with a No 11 blade at the point where the shaft of the Beath pin can be felt sub-cutaneously under the skin. Use the blade to cut the IT band deeper in the same direction and artery forceps is used to dilate the cut till it can feel the femur bone. Then deliver the ends of the suture loop through the skin. This helps in not having a soft tissue bridge in between the knot and so that the knot sits on the bone directly.
4. Using a knot pusher to tie the knots on the lateral aspect of the femur make sure the knot sits on the bone.

## 16.7 Advantages and Disadvantages

### 16.7.1 Advantages

1. Preserves the native ACL and proprioception.
2. Preserves the direction of the fibres of the ACL.
3. Cost effective.

### 16.7.2 Disadvantages

1. Technically demanding.
2. Requirement of specialized equipment for passing sutures and the tape through the ACL.
3. The sutures can potentially not be tied tight enough if not adequately pushed to the button while tying them.
4. Potential Bungee effect of the suture tape.

# 17 Arthroscopic ACL Avulsion: Mini Tightrope Technique

Vikram Arun Mhaskar

## 17.1 Introduction

Tibial avulsions of the anterior cruciate ligament (ACL) can be treated by open or arthroscopic fixation. Arthroscopic fixation techniques have the advantages of being less invasive, less painful, and have equivalent results. Bony avulsions have a good capacity to heal and thus should be fixed. We describe a technique of fixing larger tibial avulsions arthroscopically using an adjustable suspensory device. The advantage of this technique is that uniform pressure is applied over the fragment with the button that is flat. The loop has a Chinese knot configuration that approximates the two buttons when its two ends are sequentially pulled by reducing the length of the loop to facilitate the fixation. The technique is fast, accurate, and stable.

## 17.2 Specialised Equipment

1. ACL jig (Acufex, Smith and Nephew, Watford, UK).
2. 3.2 drill bit (Arthrex, Naples, Fl).
3. Guidewire (Arthrex, Naples, Fl).
4. Plastic sleeve to be applied to the ACL jig (Arthrex, Naples, Fl).
5. Probe (Smith and Nephew, Watford, UK).
6. Shaver with tip (Stryker, Kalamazoo, MI).
7. Radiofrequency device (Stryker, Kalamazoo, MI).
8. Mini Tightrope (Arthrex, Naples, Fl).
9. ABS Button (Arthrex, Naples, Fl).

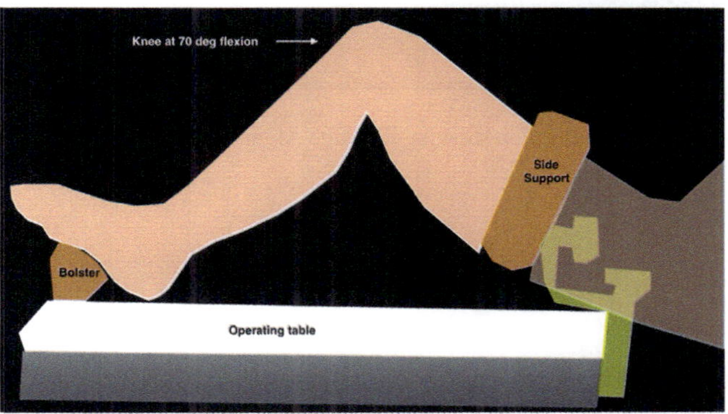


**Fig. 17.1** Illustration showing the knee in 70° flexion with a side support and bolster at the end of the table

## 17.3 Positioning (Fig. 17.1)

Knee bent to 70° flexion with a side support and bolster at the end of the operating table.

## 17.4 Portals (Fig. 17.2)

Portal A: High vertical anterolateral (AL) viewing portal just lateral to the patellar tendon 1 cm above the level of the inferior pole of the patella.

Portal B: Horizontal Medial portal (AM) just medial to the patellar tendon in the soft spot.

V. A. Mhaskar (✉)
F7 East of Kailash, Knee & Shoulder Clinic, New Delhi, India

JMVM Sports Injury Center, Sitaram Bhartia Institute of Science & Research, New Delhi, India


V. A. Mhaskar, J. Maheshwari (eds.), *Innovative Approaches in Knee Arthroscopy*,
https://doi.org/10.1007/978-981-99-4378-4_17

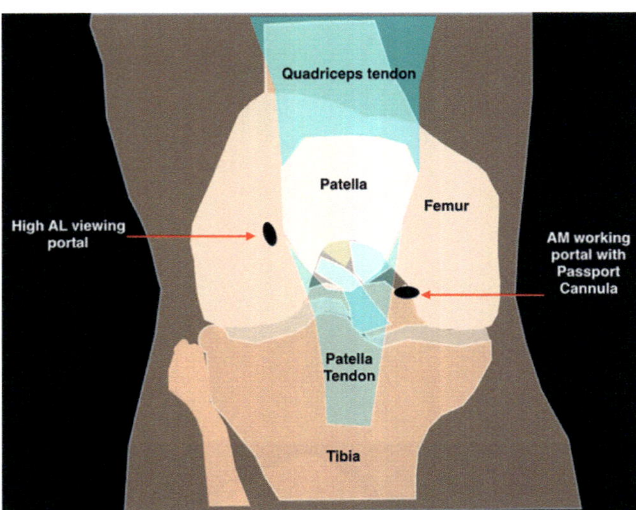


**Fig. 17.2** Illustration showing the High AL and AM portal used in the technique

## 17.5 Surgical Technique

Step 1: The avulsed ACL is visualized with the arthroscope in Portal A (Fig. 17.3a, b).

Step 2: Reduction of the avulsion to its footprint is attempted using a probe (Fig. 17.4a, b, c).

Step 3: A shaver is introduced through Portal B and the footprint cleared of fibrous tissue. If the avulsion is not reducible, the intermeniscal ligament is cut using the shaver (Fig. 17.5a, b).

Step 4: A 'K' wire is introduced through the skin superomedially and drilled into the avulsed fragment to temporarily fix it (Fig. 17.6a, b).

Step 5: The ACL jig set at 55° is introduced through Portal B and applied to the centre of the fragment and the bullet fixed to the anteromedial tibia after incising the skin at the point where the bullet with ratchet touches the skin (Fig. 17.7a, b).

Step 6: The red sleeve is applied into the bullet and guidewire drilled from the anteromedial tibia into the fragment (Fig. 17.8a, b).

Step 7: The jig is taken out keeping the guidewire in position.

Step 8: A 3.2 mm cannulated drill bit is applied over the guidewire and the fragment drilled from the anteromedial tibia (Fig. 17.9a, b).

Step 9: The Mini Tightrope (Arthrex, Naples, Fl) assembly on a handle is introduced through the tibial tunnel (Fig. 17.10).

Step 10: The assembly with the button is advanced till the button exits the fragment (Fig. 17.11).

Step 11: A probe is introduced through Portal B to flip the button (Fig. 17.12a, b, c).

Step 12: An ABS button (Arthrex, Naples, Fl) is applied to the loop just external to the tibial tunnel (Fig. 17.13).

Step 13: The two ends of the loop are alternately pulled to tighten the loop and make the button compress the fragment anatomically. The final stabilized fragment is visualized with the button compressing the fragment after an additional simple knot is tied over the button anteromedially on the tibia (Fig. 17.14a, b, c).

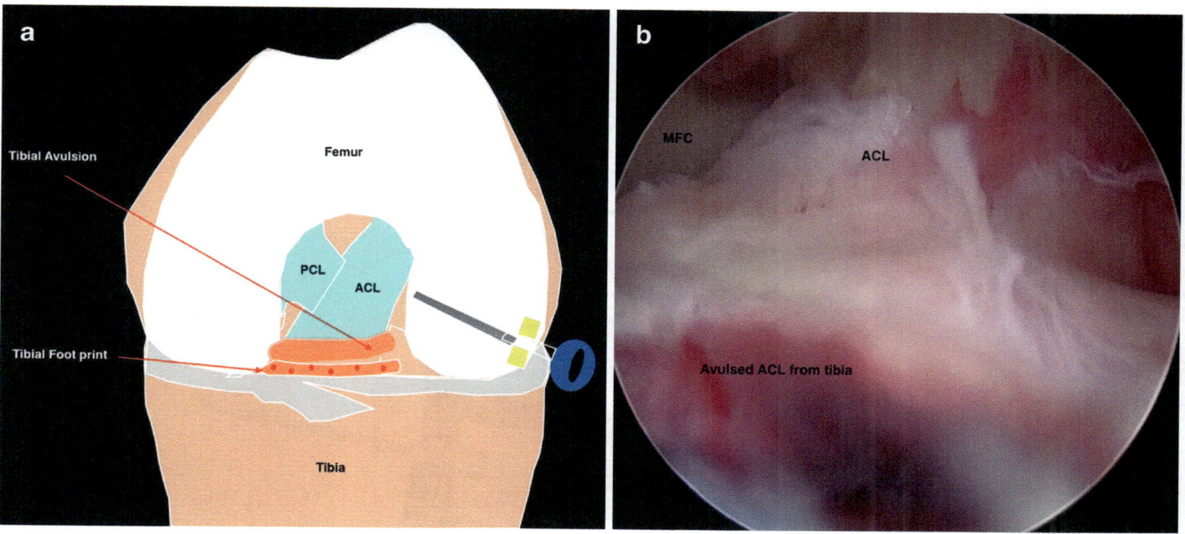


**Fig. 17.3** (**a**) Illustration of the knee with the arthroscope in Portal A showing the bony ACL avulsion from the tibia. (**b**) Arthroscopic image of the knee with the arthroscope in Portal A showing the bony ACL avulsion

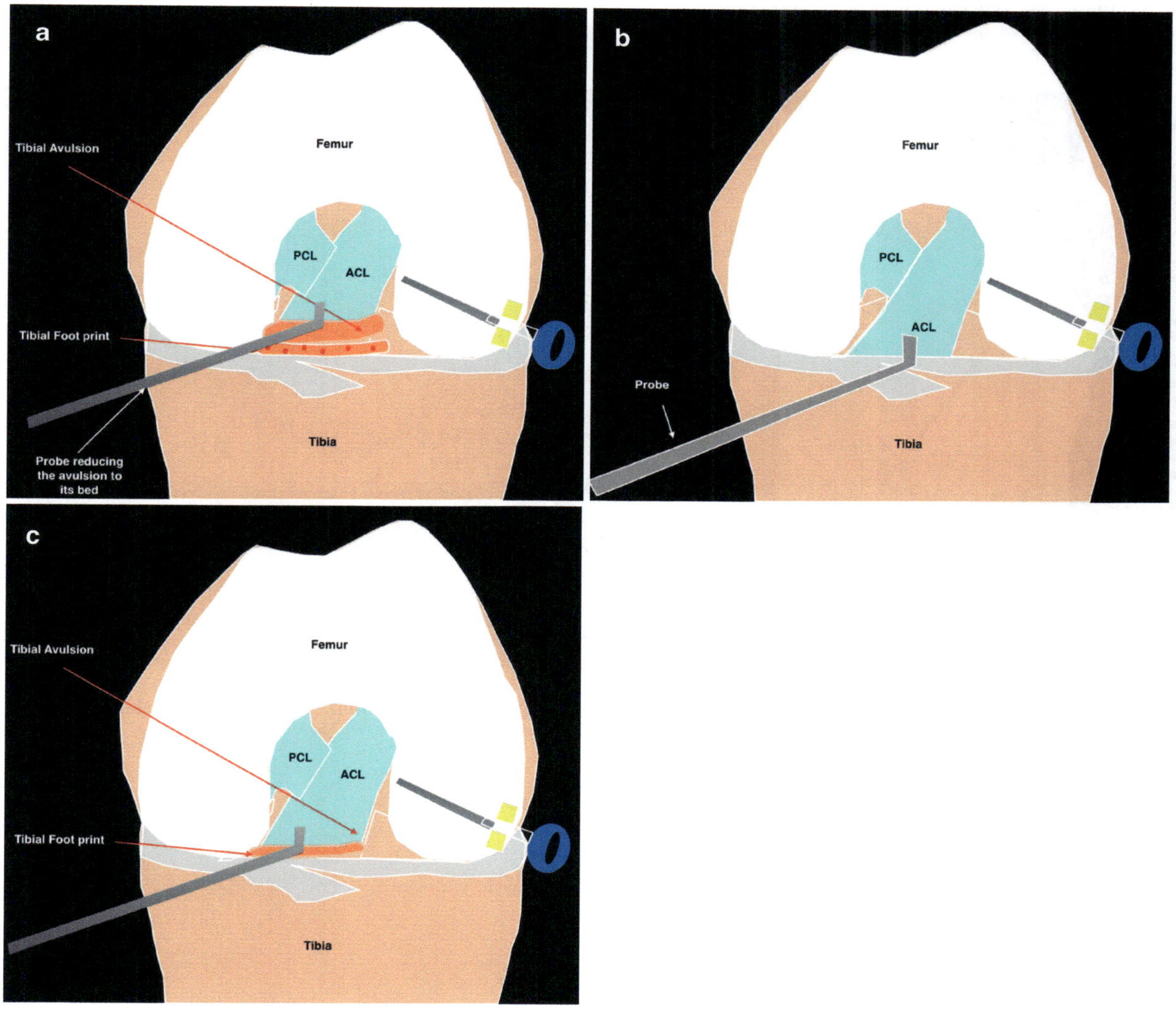

**Fig. 17.4** (**a**) Illustration of the knee with the scope through Portal A showing a probe through Portal B reducing the avulsion to its footprint on the tibia. (**b**) Illustration of the knee while viewing through Portal A showing the probe reducing the ACL avulsion anatomically. (**c**) Illustration of the knee while viewing through Portal A showing the probe through Portal B not being able to reduce the fragment anatomically because the intermeniscal ligament is interposed between the footprint and the avulsed fragment

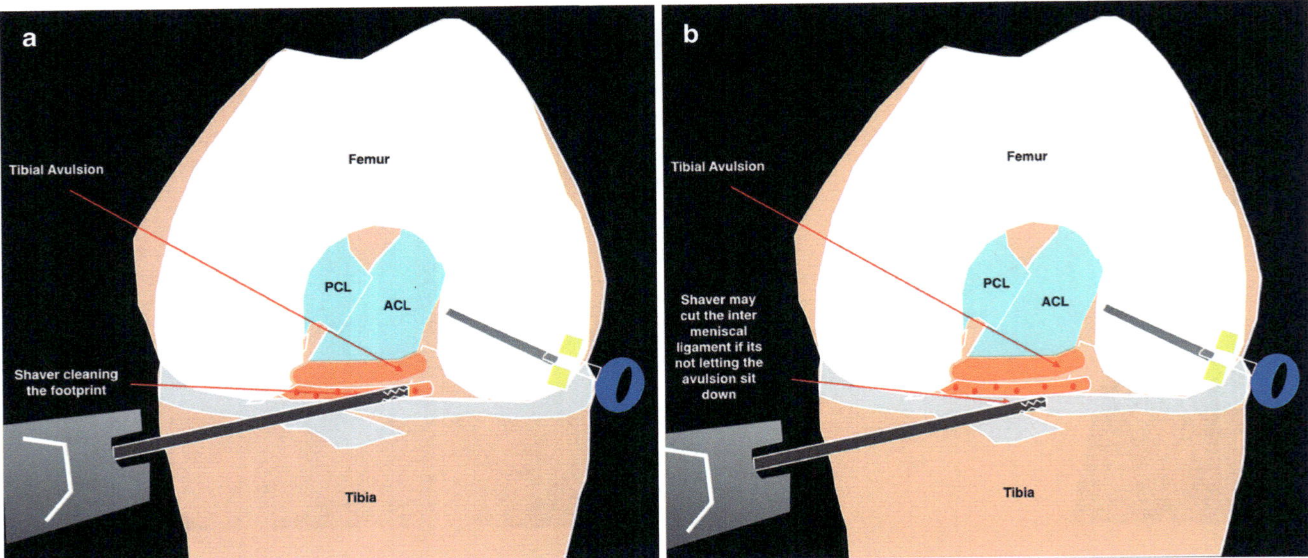


**Fig. 17.5** (**a**) Illustration of the knee while viewing through Portal A showing a shaver introduced through Portal B cleaning the footprint of the ACL. (**b**) Illustration of the knee with the scope in Portal A showing the shaver through Portal B cutting the intermeniscal ligament if it is interposed between the avulsed fragment and its footprint

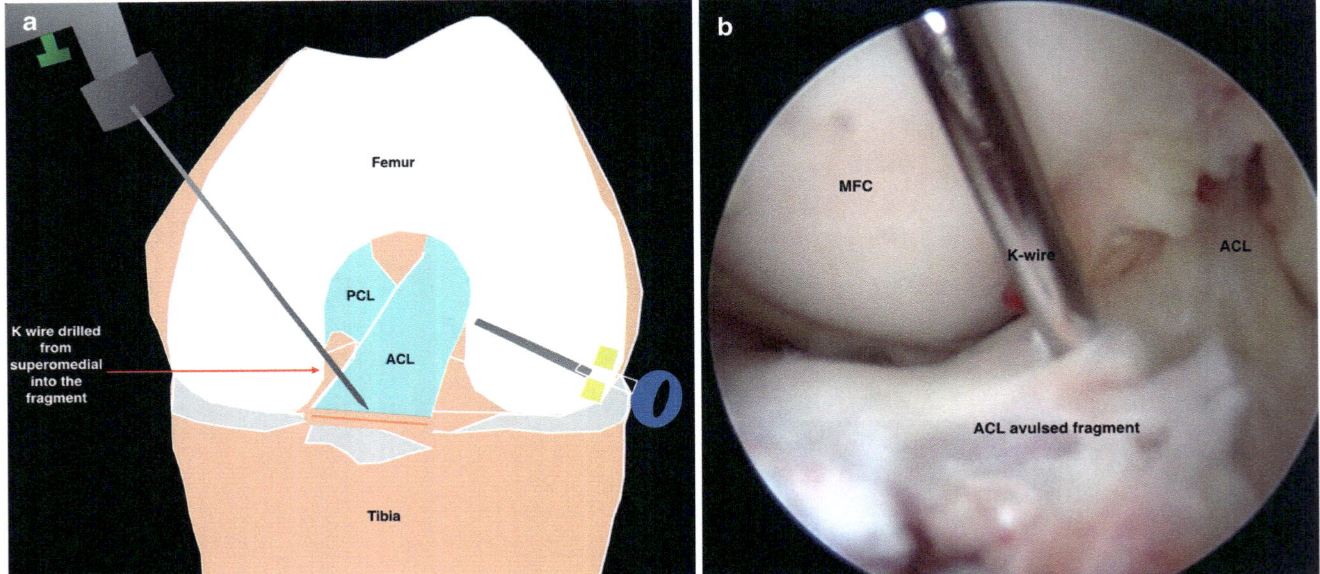


**Fig. 17.6** (**a**) Illustration of the knee while viewing through Portal A showing a 'K' wire introduced from the superomedial aspect and drilled into the fragment to reduce it temporarily anatomically. (**b**) Arthroscopic image of the knee with the scope through Portal A, a 'K' wire through the avulsed ACL

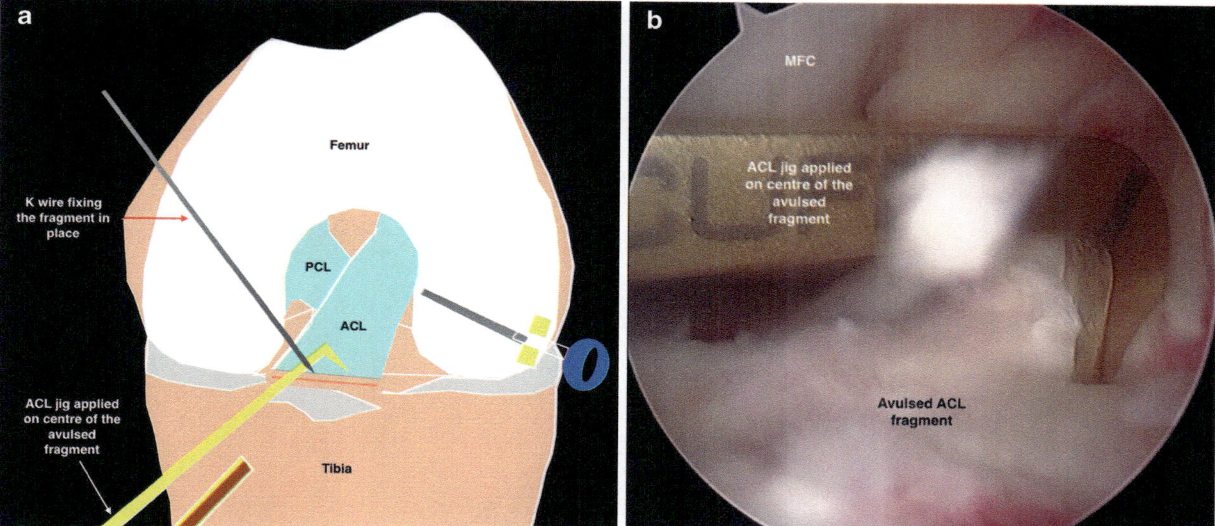


**Fig. 17.7** (**a**) Illustration of the knee with the scope through Portal A showing the ACL jig placed at the centre of the avulsed fragment with the bullet against the anteromedial aspect of the tibia with the sleeve through the bullet. (**b**) Arthroscopic image of the knee while viewing from Portal A showing the ACL jig from Portal B on the avulsed fragment

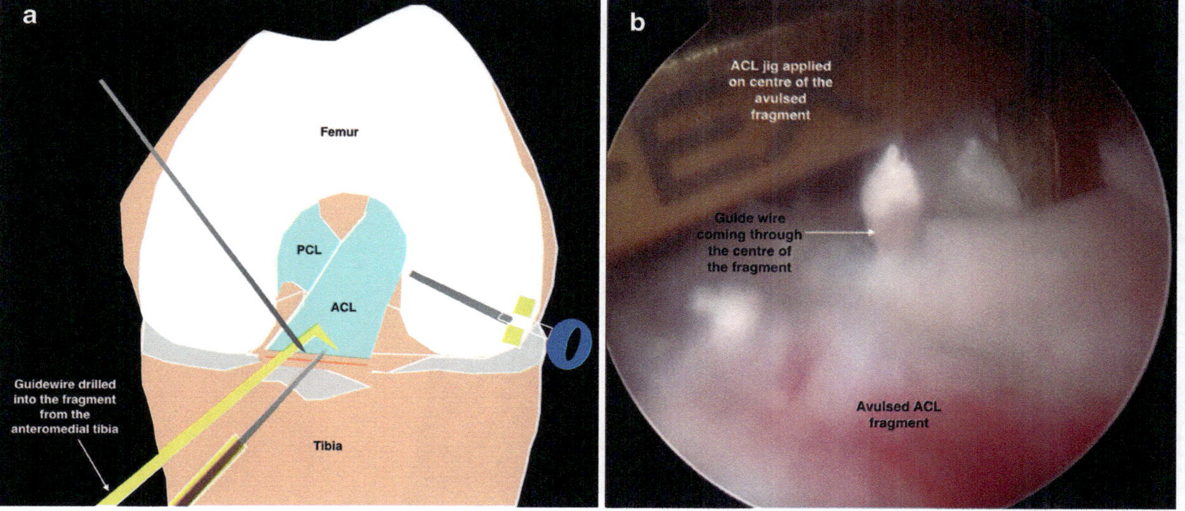


**Fig. 17.8** (**a**) Illustration of the knee while viewing through Portal A showing a guidewire drilled through the jig sleeve from the anteromedial aspect of the knee into the fragment. (**b**) Arthroscopic image of the knee while viewing through Portal A showing the guidewire drilled through the centre of the fragment using a ACL jig through Portal B

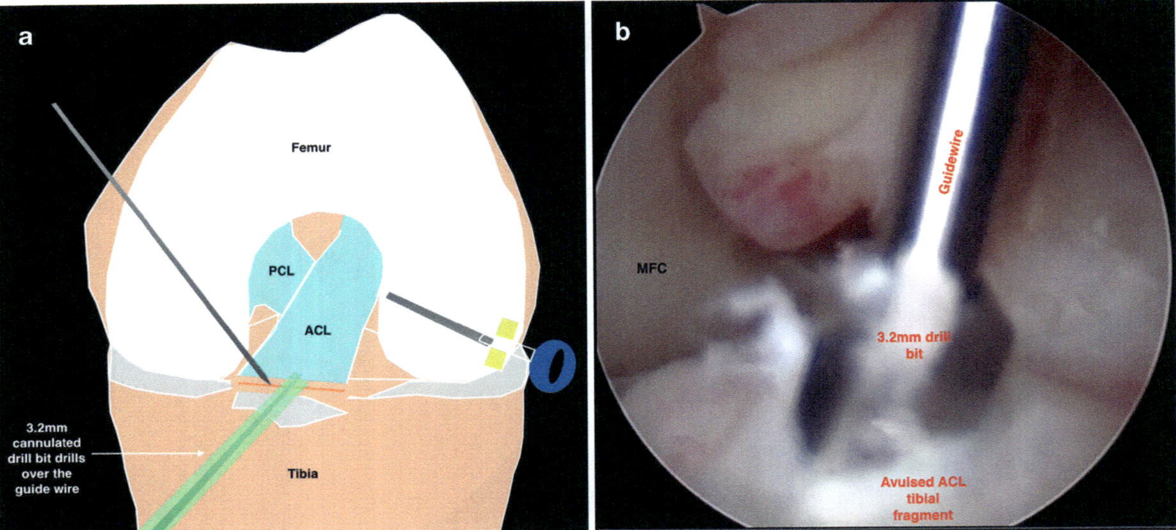


**Fig. 17.9** (**a**) Illustration of the knee while viewing through Portal A showing a 3.2 mm drill bit cannulated over the guidewire and drilling the tibial tunnel from the anteromedial aspect of the tibia into the joint. (**b**) Arthroscopic image of the knee while viewing through Portal A showing a 3.2 mm drill bit coming out over the guidewire while the tibial tunnel is drilled

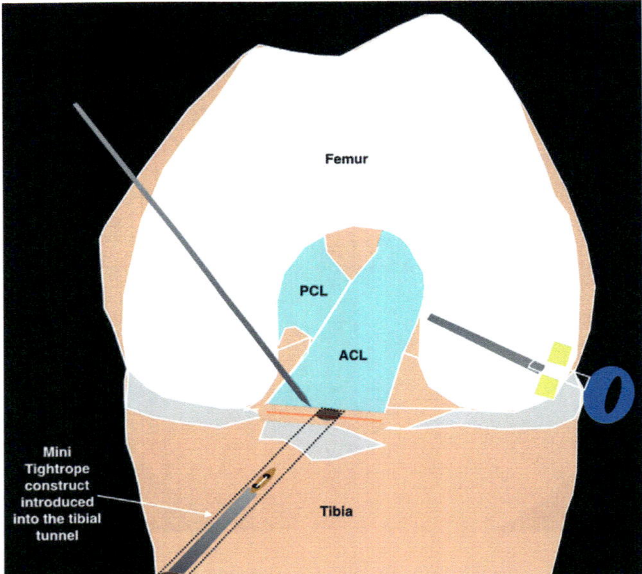


**Fig. 17.10** Illustration of the knee showing the Mini Tightrope construct being introduced through the tibial tunnel into the joint

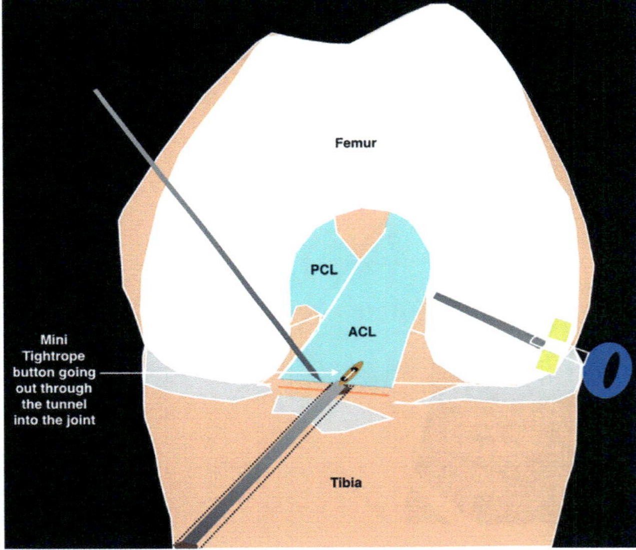


**Fig. 17.11** Illustration of the knee while viewing through Portal A showing the Tightrope button exiting into the knee joint while being introduced through the tibial tunnel

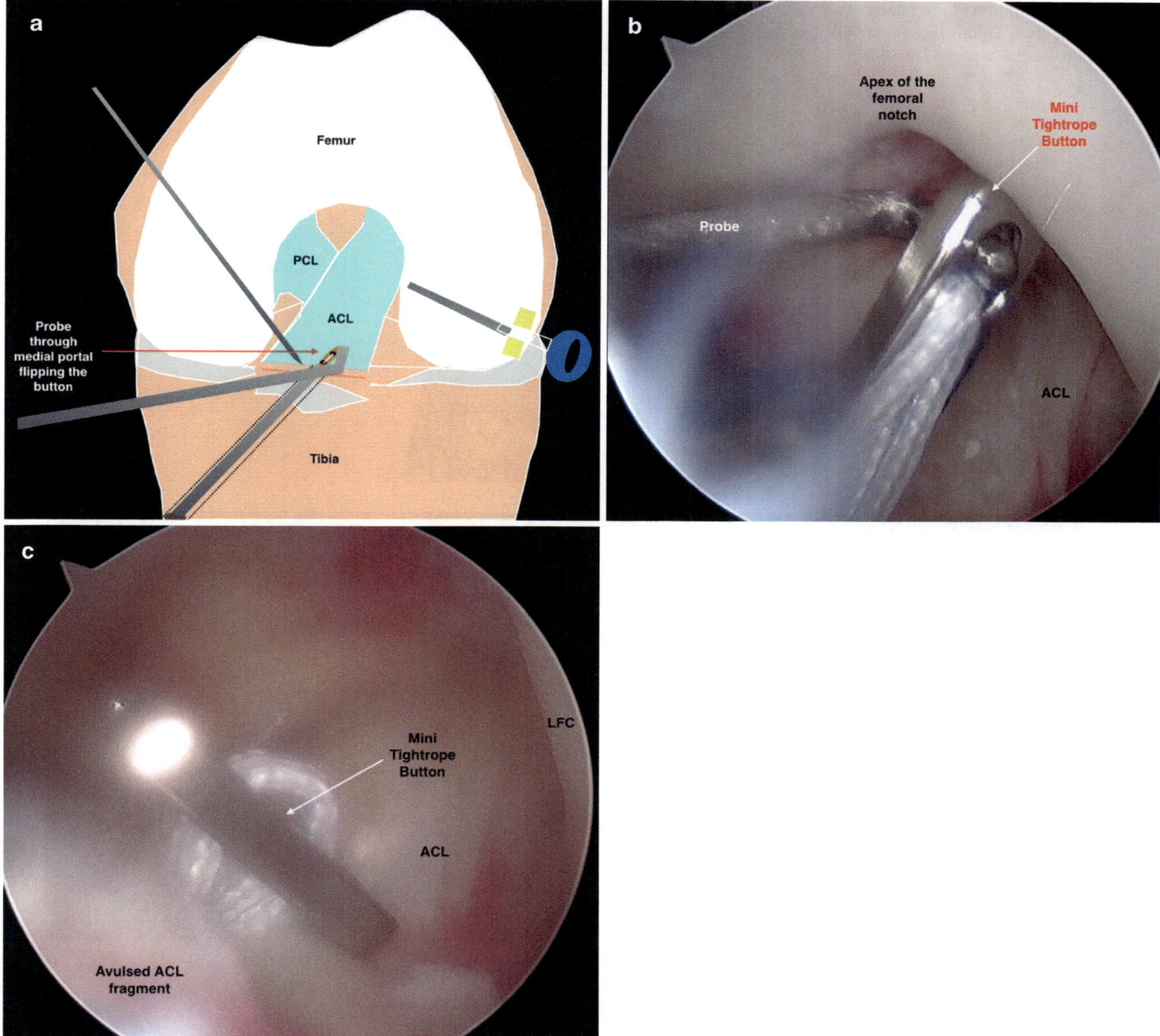


**Fig. 17.12** (**a**) Illustration of the knee while viewing through Portal A showing a probe introduced through Portal B helping flip the Tightrope button in the joint. (**b**) Arthroscopic image of the knee while viewing through Portal A showing a probe introduced through Portal B flipping the Tightrope button that has been introduced through the tibial tunnel into the joint. (**c**) Arthroscopic image of the knee while viewing through Portal A showing the Tightrope button flipped in the joint

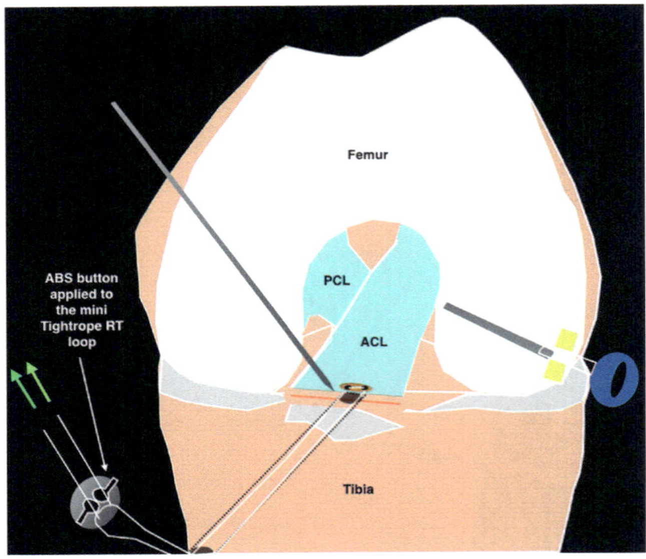


**Fig. 17.13** Illustration of the knee showing the ABS button applied to the mini Tightrope loop outside the tunnel orifice on the anteromedial aspect of the tibia

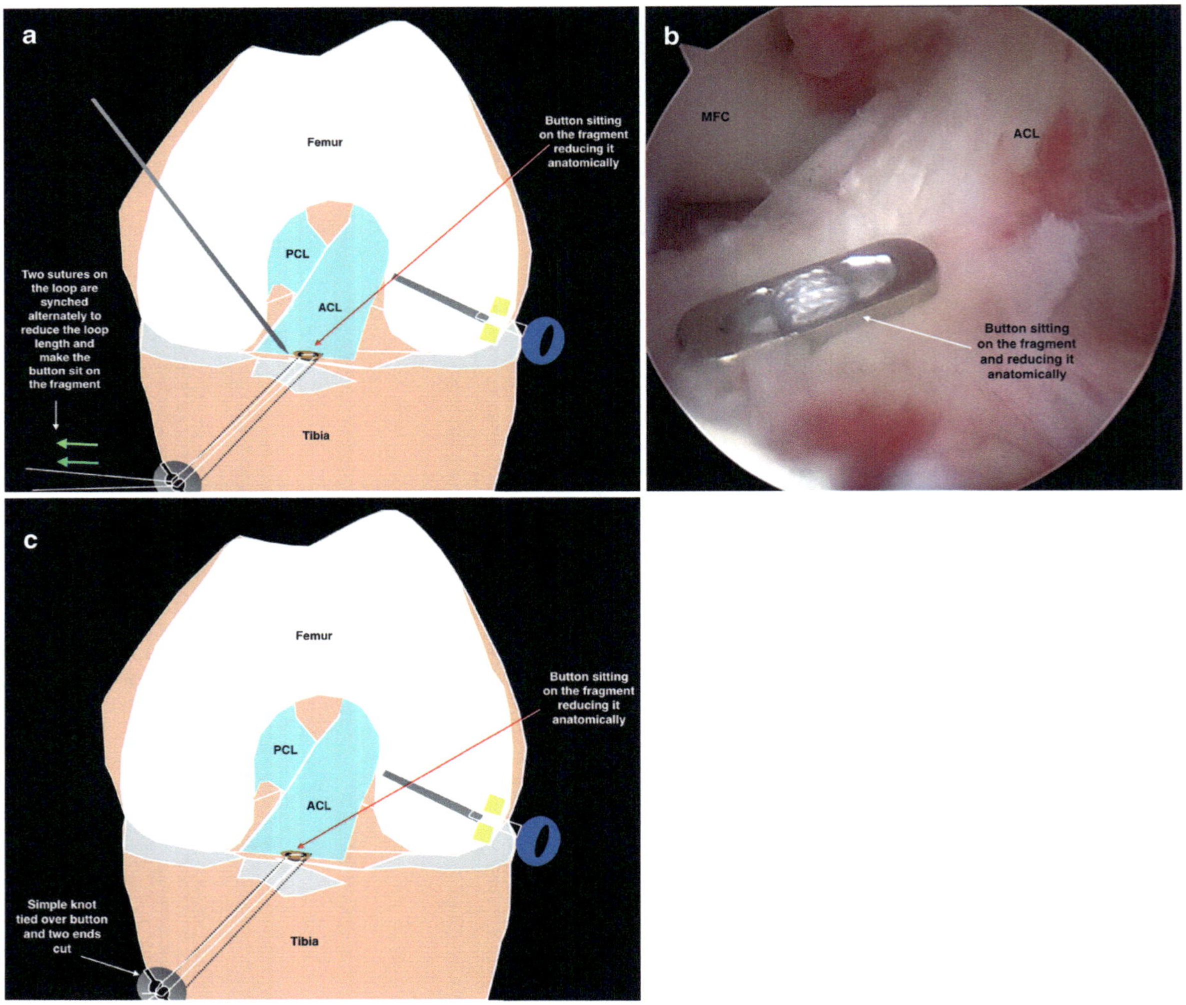

**Fig. 17.14** (**a**) Illustration of the knee showing the two sutures at the end of the loop being pulled alternately to reduce the loop length over the ABS button and make the Tightrope button sit over the avulsed fragment and compress it. (**b**) Arthroscopic image of the knee viewing through Portal A showing the Tightrope button sitting on the fragment and compressing it into its footprint anatomically. (**c**) Illustration of the knee showing the reduced avulsion with the mini Tightrope construct tied over the ABS button with an additional simple knot and two ends of the sutures cut

## 17.6 Tips and Tricks

1. In chronic avulsions clear the footprint of excess granulation tissue that can overgrow. A burr may need to be used if there is bony growth in the footprint.
2. The intermeniscal ligament should be cut if the fragment cannot be reduced as it gets interposed between the fragment and the footprint.
3. The tip of the ACL jig can be used to reduce the fragment before fixing with a 'K' wire.
4. Securely fasten the bullet on the anteromedial tibia and hold it in place while drilling.

## 17.7 Advantages and Disadvantages

### 17.7.1 Advantages

1. No sutures violate the ACL fibres.
2. The button exerts uniform pressure over the fragment preventing comminution.
3. No suture management and a faster technique.

### 17.7.2 Disadvantages

1. Single button may not reduce large fragments anatomically.
2. More expensive and requires specialised equipment.

# Parachute Technique for Fixation of Tibial Spine Avulsion of Anterior Cruciate Ligament

18

Amit Joshi, Bibek Basukala, Nagmani Singh, Rajiv Sharma, Sunil Panta, Sabin Shrestha, Rohit Bista, and Ishor Pradhan

## 18.1 Introduction

Avulsion of the tibial spine is a rare injury with an incidence of 3 per 100,000 per year [1, 2]. Multiple terminologies have been used to describe this injury, such as tibial spine fracture, tibial eminence injury, anterior cruciate ligament (ACL) avulsion, and tibial spine avulsion (TSA) of ACL etc. [3–6]. Among many terminologies, we find that TSA of ACL best explains its nature, mechanism of injury, and future treatment strategies.

Meyer and McKeever's classification is the most commonly used classification system for decision-making in treatment. Type 1 and 2 are usually managed conservatively, while type 3 and 4 are managed surgically [4]. Although some surgeons advocate non-operative treatment for most of these avulsions, citing a high complication rate of stiffness; surgical stabilization and early range of motion has become the gold standard for TSA of ACL. Many fixation methods have been described, like Kirschner wires, screws, stainless steel wire, sutures, anchors, and suture buttons. Since the advancement of arthroscopy techniques, trans-tibial suture pullout technique has become the gold standard for the treatment of TSA of ACL.

Trans-tibial suture pullout fixation options are a very popular technique these days [7]. Multiple modifications of this technique have been described in the literature. All these techniques were modified to simplify the technique and increase stability. However, in none of these techniques, sutures are passed from the posterior aspect of the avulsed fragment to provide fixation from all the directions. In this chapter, we present our technique of TSA of ACL fixation, in which the sutures are passed from anterior to posterior and in mediolateral direction to get a better hold on the fragment. Unlike many other suture-based techniques, this technique gives circumferential compression over the fragment, ensuring the adequate reduction of fragment and optimal tension of ACL.

A. Joshi (✉) · B. Basukala · N. Singh · R. Sharma · S. Panta · S. Shrestha · R. Bista · I. Pradhan
AKB Center for Arthroscopy, Sports Injuries and Regenerative Medicine, B&B Hospital, Lalitpur, Nepal

## 18.2 Steps of the Technique

### 18.2.1 Step 1: Diagnostic Arthroscopy

A thorough diagnostic arthroscopy is always the first step. The patient is positioned on the table with thigh supported on a lateral post and foot kept at foot post. A standard draping and preparation is done. Diagnostic arthroscopy is done with a standard anteromedial and anterolateral portal. A complete diagnostic round of the knee joint is performed during the diagnostic arthroscopy. Any loose bodies in the joint, and cartilage and meniscal injuries are noted and addressed accordingly. Once the diagnostic arthroscopy and treatment of ailment, if any, are completed, the avulsed fragment is addressed.

The extent and comminution of the avulsed fragments are assessed (Fig. 18.1). Anterior root of lateral meniscus is carefully evaluated to define its attachment (Fig. 18.1c); it is often attached with the avulsed fragment.

### 18.2.2 Step 2: Crater Preparation

Crater preparation is an essential step in the surgical management of ACL avulsion. In an acute injury, removing all hematoma from both the crater and the fragment is necessary to evaluate the fragment and surrounding anatomy to achieve adequate reduction. Adequate identification of the crater's anterior, posterior, medial, and lateral margins is essential. Proper crater preparation also helps us plan the tunnel's entry point while doing suture pullout repair.


V. A. Mhaskar, J. Maheshwari (eds.), *Innovative Approaches in Knee Arthroscopy*,
https://doi.org/10.1007/978-981-99-4378-4_18

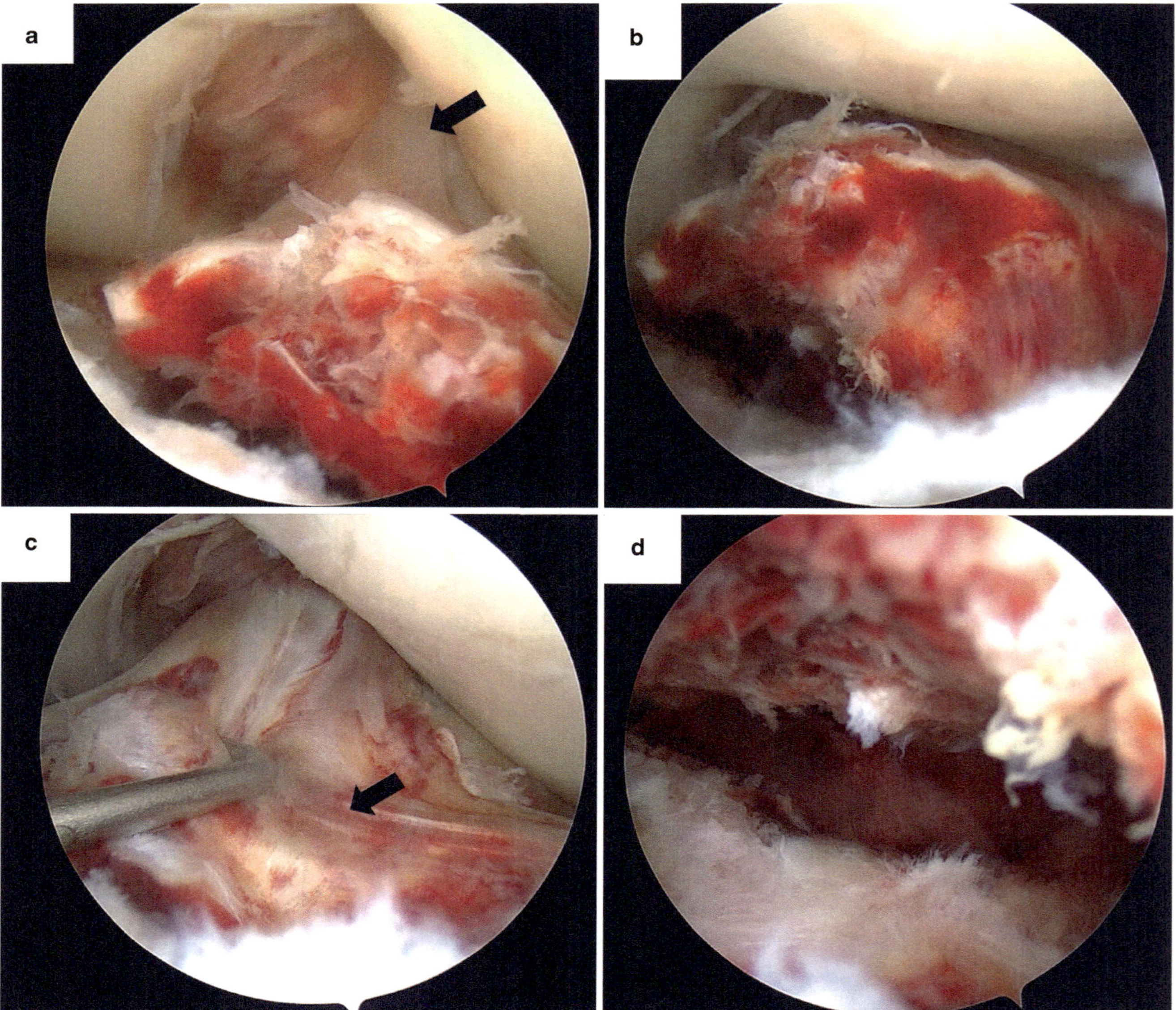


**Fig. 18.1** (**a**) Diagnostic arthroscopy showing avulsed bone fragment with ACL (black arrow) attachment. (**b**) The avulsed fragment is impinging at the notch in full knee extension. (Conservative management will lead to malunion at this position, thus leading to loss of extension). (**c**) Associated injuries have to be noted. It is imperative to see the anterior root of the lateral meniscus, which is often attached to the fragment. The figure shows that (**d**) Diagnostic arthroscopy also includes the crater examination

## 18.2.3 Step 3: Suture Passage

This step is the most important in our technique. We believed that the avulsed fragment should be pulled from all sides (front, back, medial, and lateral) just like a parachute for proper reduction. Many techniques use sutures either anteriorly alone or from a mediolateral direction. If there are reduction sutures from only one direction, the other side tends to lift. If we pass suture mediolaterally, there will be a possibility of anterior or posterior opening.

Similarly, if sutures are pulled anteriorly, the fragment may lift off posteriorly. Therefore, we need a construct in which sutures traverses from both mediolateral and anteroposterior direction to have a circumferential hold on the fragment. This configuration simulates a parachute.

A parachute constitutes the canopy, the canopy skirt, suspensory strings, and the load. We try to mimic this basic construct of the parachute in our technique, as shown in Fig. 18.2.

The most crucial step of this technique is the passage of suture through the ACL and around the bone fragment. This step requires the passage of four strands of sutures, two from anterior to posterior direction and two from medial to lateral direction. For ease of understanding, the step of suture passage is further divided into four stages.

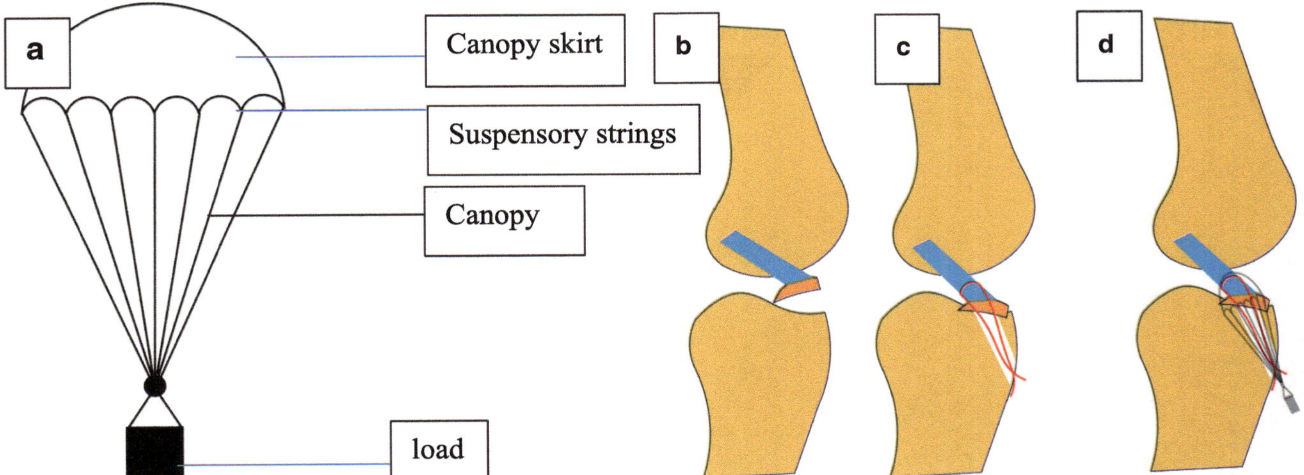


**Fig. 18.2** (**a**) Schematic diagram of parachute showing its parts. (**b**) Diagram showing a lateral view of knee joint with ACL avulsion with displaced tibial spine fragment. (**c**) Same fracture after suture bridge fixation. (**d**) Suture bridge fixation model compared with a parachute by superimposition

1. Posterior, medial to lateral passage
2. Anterior, medial to lateral passage
3. Lateral, anterior to posterior passage
4. Medial, anterior to posterior passage

Here, the first word denotes the thread's location at the base of ACL, second and third word indicates the direction of passage of the thread.

We use two No. 1 orthocord for the procedure, cut into two halves to make four threads. Threads of different colors are preferred for ease of identification and suture management.

(a) **Posterior, medial to lateral passage**

The scope at AL portal and No 1 Prolene loaded at first pass mini is introduced from AM portal. A bite through the substance of ACL was taken at the base as deep (posterior) as possible (Fig. 18.3a, b). The scope was switched to AM portal, and both the limbs of sutures were pulled into AL Portal and held outside with artery forceps.

(b) **Anterior, medial to lateral passage**

The arthroscope is switched back to the AL portal. Again, the first pass mini loaded with second sutures is introduced through the AM portal. This time, the bite is taken from the same medial to lateral direction but more anterior than the previous pass (Fig. 18.3c, d). The two ends are retrieved again at the AL portal.

(c) **Lateral, anterior to posterior passage**

A Touhy epidural needle is used to pass Prolene from the anterior to the posterior direction, which will be used to shuttle an orthocord of different colors. The arthroscope is in the AL portal, and the Touhy epidural needle is introduced inside the joint through the AM portal. From the base of ACL, the needle was introduced from anterior to posterior direction keeping its location on the lateral third of the ACL fibers (Fig. 18.4a). Once the tip of the epidural needle is visible through the posterior border of ACL, the stylet is removed, No. 1 Prolene is pushed through the lumen, and the tail of Prolene is retrieved at AM portal. This Prolene is now used to shuttle the third orthocord through the ACL. These sutures are also retrieved and parked at the AL portal, and ends are secured with artery forceps.

(d) **Medial, anterior to posterior passage**

Keeping the arthroscope in the anterolateral portal, the same epidural needle is now introduced from the anteromedial portal and passed in anterior to posterior direction but this time from the medial one-third fibers of ACL. Once the tip of the needle is visible from the posterior of ACL, the Prolene is passed through its lumen and tip retrieved out through the anteromedial portal. Using the Prolene, the orthocord is shuttled. The suture ends are again retrieved at the AL portal and secured with artery forceps (Fig. 18.5).

At the end of the suture passage, there will be four sutures all together passing through the substance of ACL. Two in medial to the lateral direction and two in anterior to posterior direction. There will be eight suture ends coming out from the AL portal. The respective ends of sutures are held with four artery forceps for identification and future suture management to avoid entanglement.

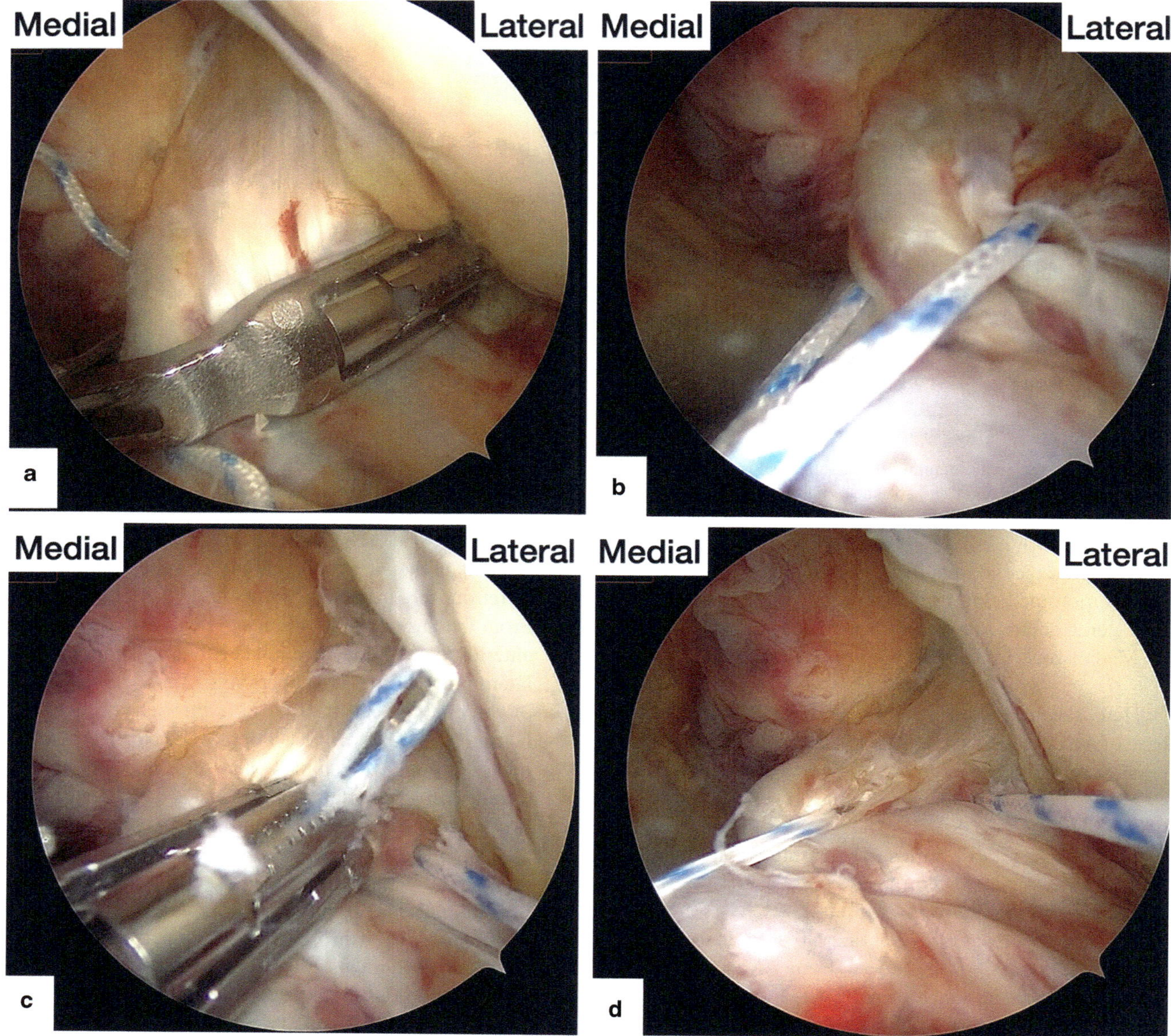


**Fig. 18.3** (**a**, **b**) The first passage of Orthocord from the medial to the lateral direction. Note the passage from the posterior fibers of the ACL. (**c**) Second passage is again from medial to lateral direction. This bite is taken anterior to the previous suture. (**d**) Two fibers of orthocord passed from the medial to the lateral direction. The first fiber wire is passed posteriorly, and the second fiber is passed anteriorly

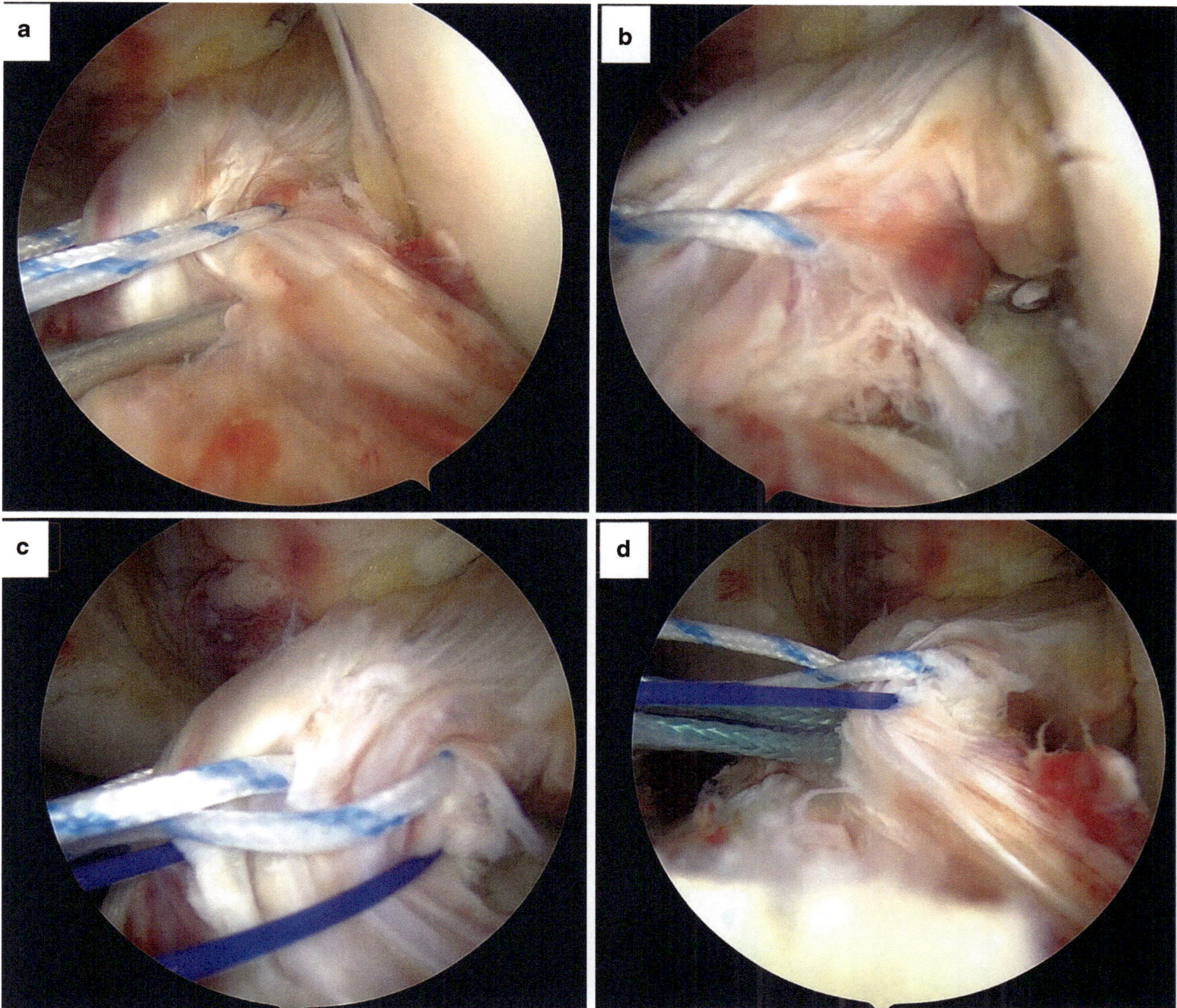


**Fig. 18.4** (**a**, **b**) Third passage will be from the anterior to a posterior direction at the lateral edge of the ACL base. An epidural needle is used as a suture passing device. The first and second sutures are parked at AM portal. (**c**, **d**) No. 1 Prolene is passed through the lumen of the needle, and different coloured thread is shuttled

### 18.2.4 Step 4: Tunnel Preparation

The attention is now focused on the crater for tunnel preparation. Anterior, posterior, medial, and lateral borders of the crater are identified and cleaned. The center of the crater is marked, and an ACL tip aiming zig is used to pass a beath pin from the anteromedial cortex of the tibia into the center of the crater. The beath pin is then reamed with a 4.6 mm endo button reamer (Fig. 18.6).

### 18.2.5 Step 5: Suture Retrieval

This is again a crucial step in our technique. An arthroscopy cannula is placed in the anteromedial portal. Furthermore, this step is divided into four synchronous steps of Prolene loop passage into the crater, retrieval through the cannula at AM portal, pull respective and suture from AL to AM portal, and pull the suture limb through the tunnel out to the anteromedial cortex with the help of Prolene loop. Since there are eight strands of sutures coming out of the AL portal, these steps have to be repeated four times, as two respective limbs are pulled into the tunnel at one time. Sequential shuttling of sutures will prevent sutures entanglement, and suture management becomes easy.

A No. 1 Prolene is passed through the cannulation of the IP needle to form a loop of Prolene at the tip. The needle is introduced from the tunnel to deliver inside the joint at the crater. The Prolene loop is now retrieved through the cannula at AM portal. Next, the medial end of the posterior suture

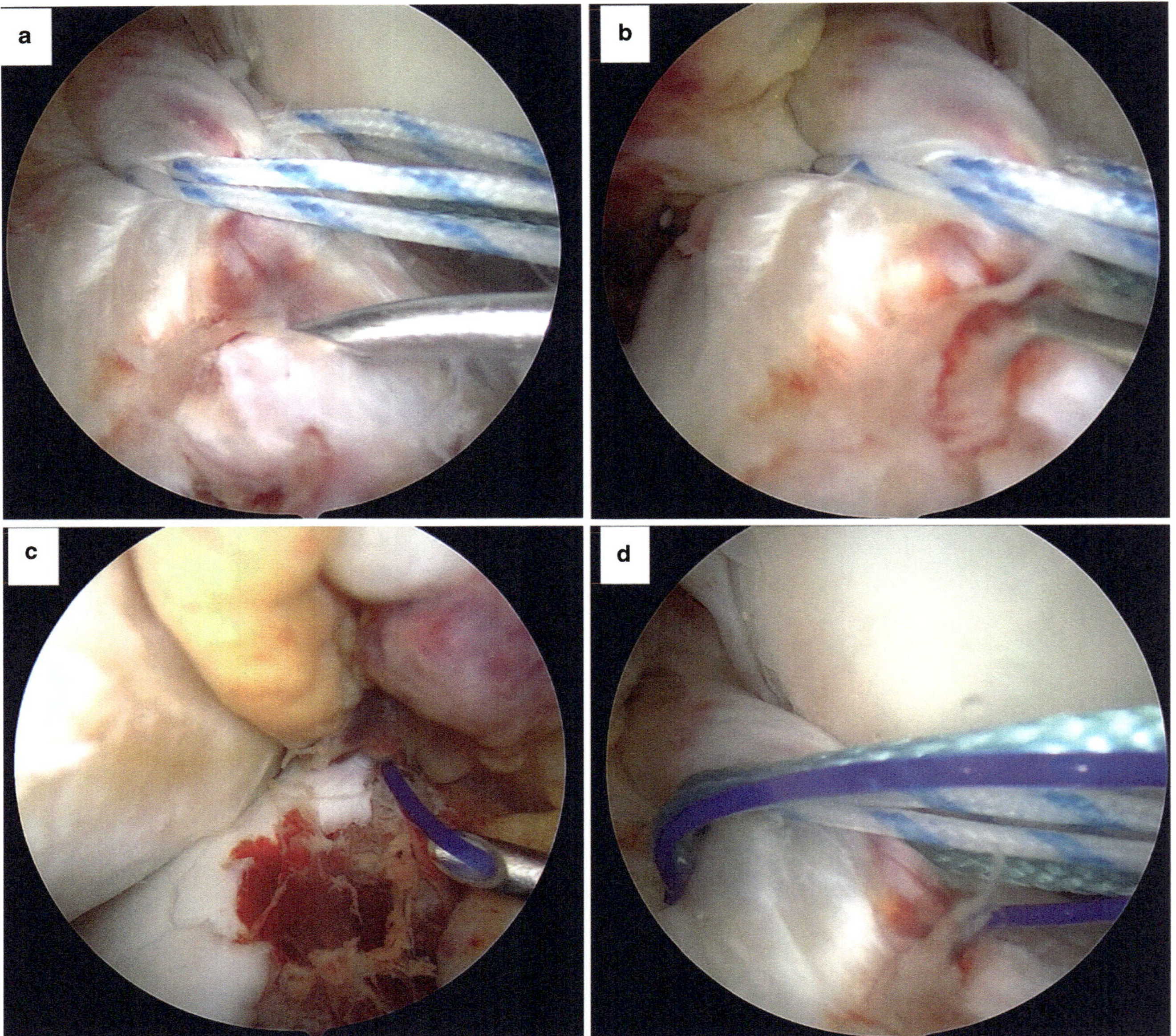


**Fig. 18.5** (**a**, **b**) Fourth passage is done at the medial edge of ACL from anterior to posterior direction. (**c**) Prolene is passed through the lumen. (**d**) Fourth thread is shuttled with the help of prolene

(deep medial to lateral) and posterior end of the 4th suture (medial anterior to posterior) through the cannula at AM portal. Using the Prolene loop, these sutures are now pulled out through the tunnel.

IP needle with the Prolene loop is again introduced, and the loop is pulled out into the AM cannula. Now, the medial end of the 2nd thread (anterior medial to lateral) and the anterior end of the 4th suture (medial anterior to posterior) are retrieved from the AL portal to the AM cannula. Then the limbs of sutures are pulled out through the tunnel and held with artery forceps.

The same process is repeated two more times, first to retrieve the anterior end of the 3rd suture (lateral anterior to posterior) and the lateral end of the second suture (anterior medial to lateral). Then the lateral end of the 1st suture (posterior medial to lateral) and posterior end of the 3rd suture (lateral anterior to posterior) are retrieved out to the tunnel. Each pair will act as the canopy skirt of the parachute and help in achieving and maintaining the proper reduction of the fragment, which will serve as a canopy (Figs. 18.7 and 18.8).

### 18.2.6 Step 6: Reduction of the Fragment

Now with the help of the probe, the threads passed to its respective positions at the fragment. The fragment is reduced with the probe. This may require extension of the knee. Once the fragments are reduced, the respective limbs are pulled

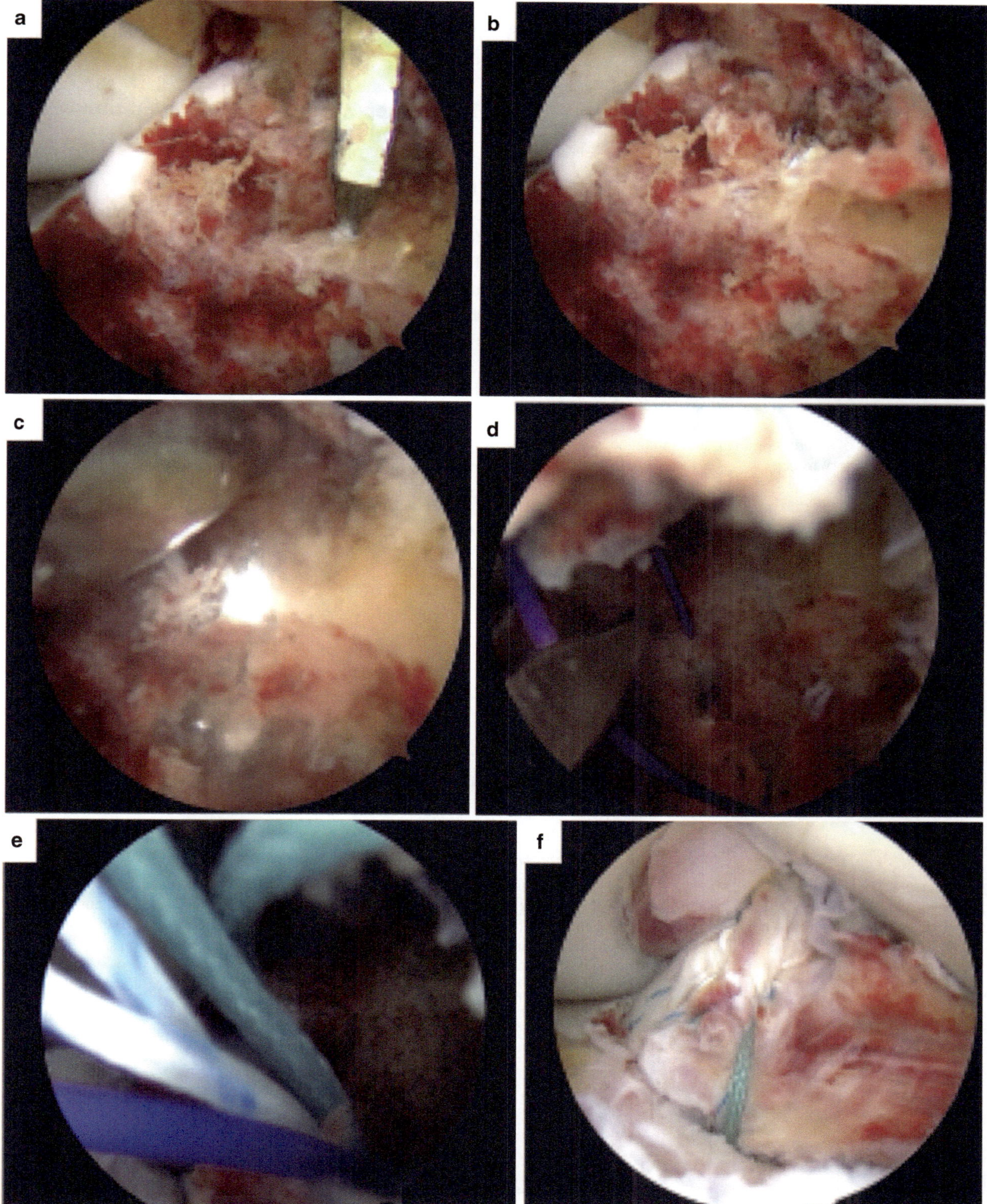


**Fig. 18.6** (**a**) Crater after removal of clot and soft tissues. The center of the crater is marked, and a beath pin is introduced from the anteromedial tibia to the center of crater with the help of tip aiming ACL zig. (**b**) Beath pin entry is confirmed at the desired point of crater. (**c**) Pin is over reamed with 4.6 mm endoscopic reamer. (**d**) Prolene loop in initial puncture (IP) needle is used for suture shuttle. (**e**) Serial shuttle of each pair of threads with the help of prolene loop passed through the IP needle. (**f**) Well, reduced bone fragment showing good anchorage with threads all around mimicking canopy skirt of the parachute

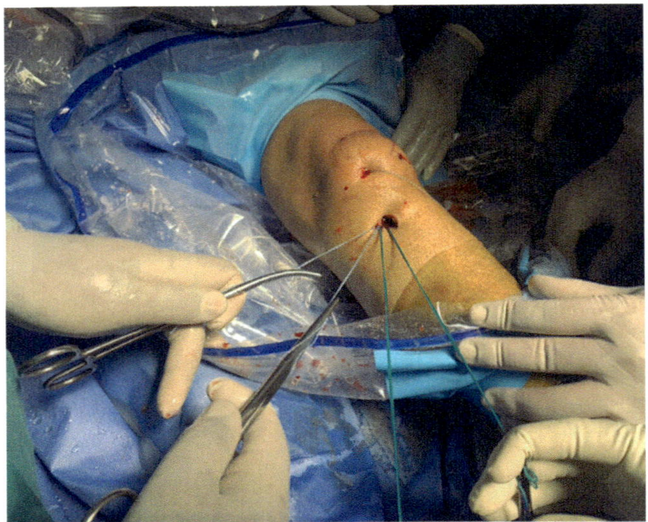

**Fig. 18.7** Four pairs of sutures coming out of the tunnel are held separately with separate artery forceps

and kept on traction to see the reduction. Keeping tension on the sutures, the knee can be flexed to see the reduction.

### 18.2.7 Step 7: Bone Bridge Preparation and Final Knot Tying

The final step is to tie the knots. Our preferred technique of securing the suture is implant less bone bridge fixation [7]. In this technique, an accessory tunnel was created 1 cm away from the aperture of the previous tunnel at the anterior tibia using a beath pin. The tunnel was directed towards the previous tunnel so that both the tunnels are connected with each other inside forming a small triangular bone bridge.

The same IP needle with a loop of No. 1 prolene is inserted from the accessory tunnel towards the primary tunnel. By pushing the Prolene, a loop is created inside the primary tunnel, which is retrieved out through the primary tunnel using an arthroscopy probe. Now one tail each of four pairs is passed through the loop of Prolene and pulled out from the accessory tunnel.

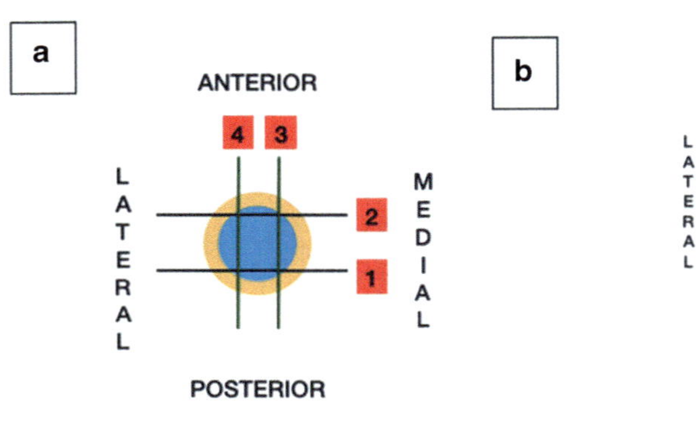


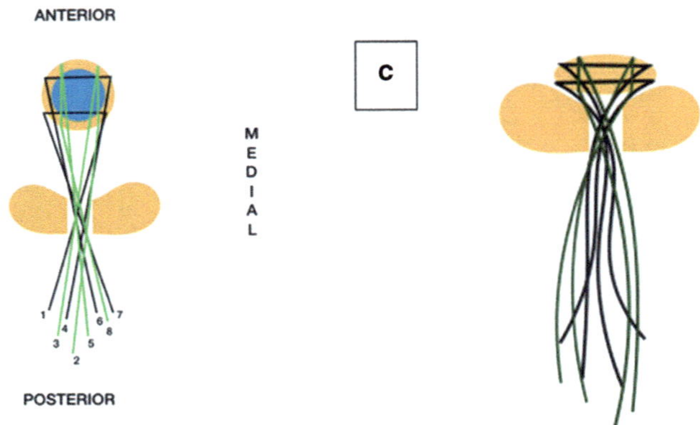


**Fig. 18.8** (**a**) Schematic diagram showing the direction and sequence of suture passage denoted by numbers. Representation: blue circle—ACL substance, yellow circle—bone fragment attached to ACL. (**b**) suture shuttled through the center of the crater with eight suture ends. Lower yellow oval with superior depression represents the crater with the tunnel shown as white at the center. Threads are numbered according to their serial of the shuttle through the tunnel. (**c**) suture configuration, and parachute-like replication after reduction

Arthroscope is inserted into the joint and fragment is visualized. If the fragment has displaced, it is reduced and provisionally stabilized by putting traction on to the sutures. After confirming the reduction, the reciprocal sutures are tied one by one over the bone bridge.

The intra-articular reduction of fragment and final tension of ACL is checked with the help of a probe. Notch impingement with the fragment is evaluated by extending the knee. Wounds closed with non-absorbable simple sutures (Figs. 18.9 and 18.10).

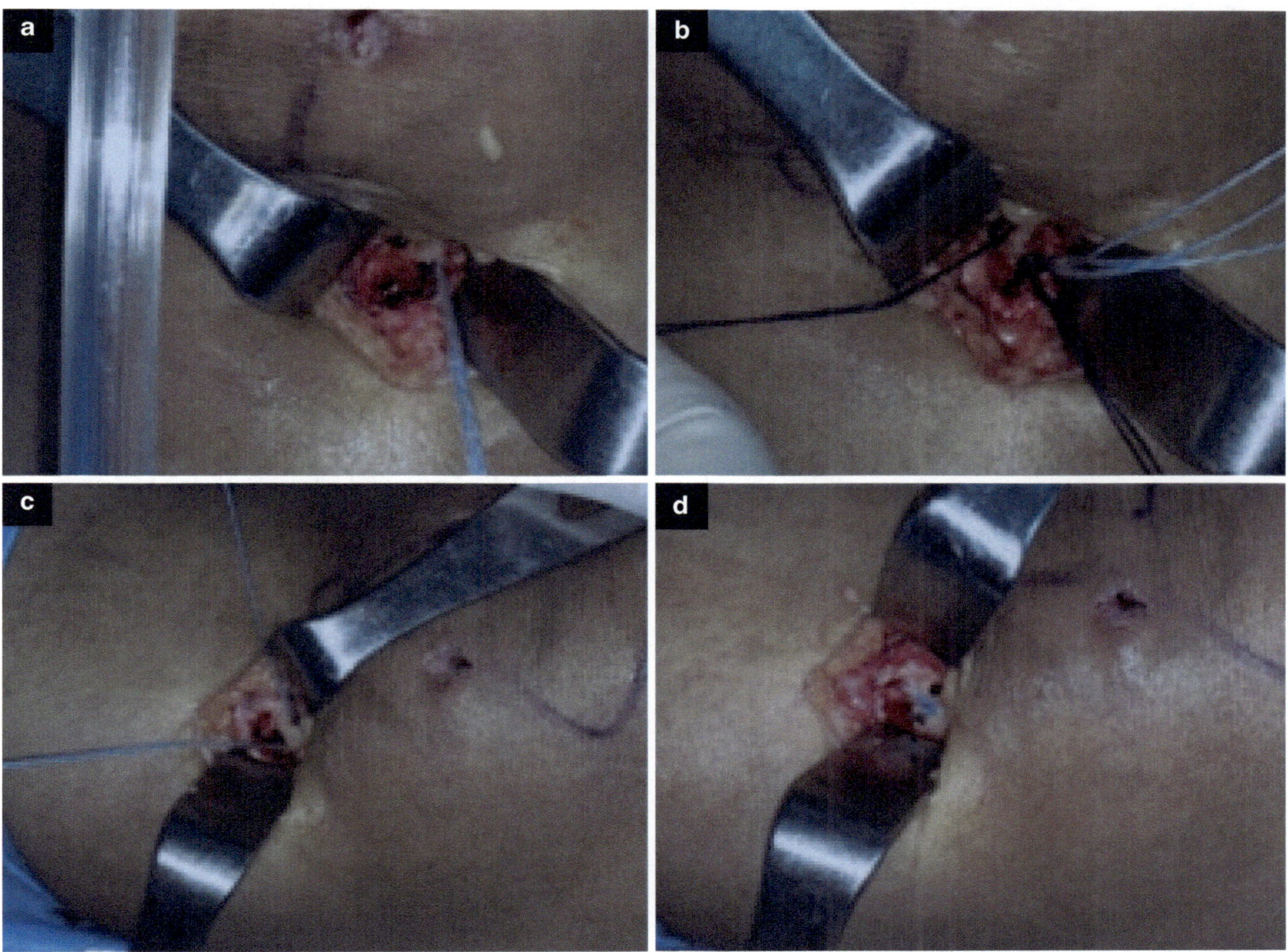


**Fig. 18.9** (**a**–**d**) Steps of creating a bone bridge and final knot tying. (Joshi A, Basukala B, Singh N, Bista R, Tripathi N, Pradhan I. Implant-Free, Trans-tibial, Bone Bridge Fixation for Knee Surgery Including Tibial Spine and Meniscal Root Fixation. Arthroscopy techniques. 2020 Nov 1;9(11):e1837-43)

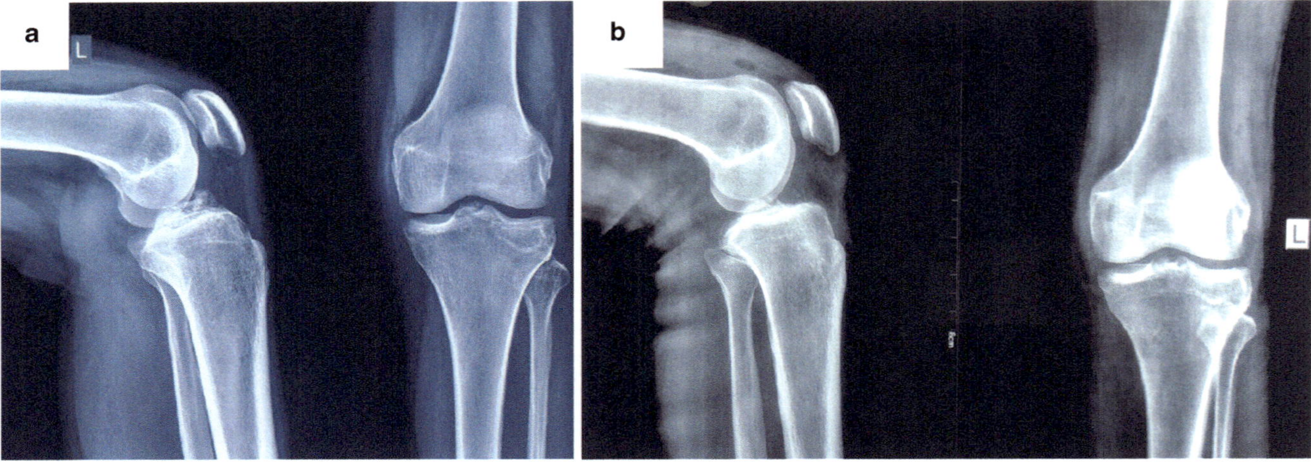


**Fig. 18.10** (**a**) Preoperative Plain X-ray AP and lateral view of the left knee showing displaced Mayer and McKeever type 3 Tibial Spine fracture. (**b**) Postoperative X-ray of the same knee showing very well reduced fracture without any implants

## 18.3 Advantages of the Technique

(a) Achieves good reduction with compression at the fragment from all the direction.
(b) Reproducible and can be done with instruments readily available in an operation theater.
(c) Early full range of motion can be allowed to avoid postoperative stiffness.
(d) Economical beneficial as it avoids any implants, thus avoids implant-related complications too.

## 18.4 Disadvantages of the Technique

(a) Multiple suture ends may lead to confusion and tangling during suture management.
(b) Technically demanding as it requires passage of multiple threads in various directions.

## References

1. Axibal DP, Mitchell JJ, Mayo MH, Chahla J, Dean CS, Palmer CE, et al. Epidemiology of anterior tibial spine fractures in young patients: a retrospective cohort study of 122 cases. J Pediatr Orthop. 2019;39(2):e87–90.
2. Reda A. Tibial spine avulsion fractures: current concepts and technical note on arthroscopic techniques used in manageme. London: IntechOpen; 2013.
3. Kendall NS, Hsu SY, Chan KM. Fracture of the tibial spine in adults and children. A review of 31 cases. J Bone Joint Surg Br. 1992;74(6):848–52.
4. Meyers MH, McKeever FM. Fracture of the intercondylar eminence of the tibia. JBJS. 1959;41(2):209–22.
5. Mclennan JG. The role of arthroscopic surgery in the treatment of fractures of the intercondylar eminence of the tibia. J Bone Joint Surg Br. 1982;64(4):477–80.
6. Van Loon T, Marti RK. A fracture of the intercondylar eminence of the tibia treated by arthroscopic fixation. Arthrosc J Arthrosc Relat Surg. 1991;7(4):385–8.
7. Joshi A, Nagmani S, Basukala B. Tibial spine avulsion of anterior cruciate ligament: current trend and management. London: IntechOpen; 2019.

# Part V

# PCL

# 19 Arthroscopic Trans-septal PCL Reconstruction

Vikram Arun Mhaskar

## 19.1 Introduction

Posterior cruciate ligament tears may require surgical reconstruction in symptomatic patients. Normally the surgery is conducted using two anterior and one posteromedial portal. However, using posterolateral portal in addition helps visualize the PCL tibial footprint well, apart from helping in suture management.

## 19.2 Special Equipment Required (Fig. 19.1)

Vissinger rod-1 (c)
7 mm Cannulae-2 (Arthrex, Naples, FL) (q)
Bone awl (a)
Mallet (b)
PCL jig-1 (Arthrex, Naples, FL) (i)
Beath pin-1 (e, f)
No 5 Ethibond-2 (Ethicon, Rariton, NJ) (e, f)
Passport Cannula-1 (Arthrex, Naples, FL)
Guide wire 1 (Arthrex, Naples, FL) (j)
4.5mm drill bit (Arthrex, Naples, FL) (d)
Flower drill 6–10 mm (Arthrex, Naples, FL) (g)
Standard drill bit 6–10 mm (Arthrex, Naples, FL) (k)
Screw driver (m)
Suture manipulator (l)
Tightrope RT (Arthrex, Naples, FL)
PEEK screw (Arthrex, Naples, FL)

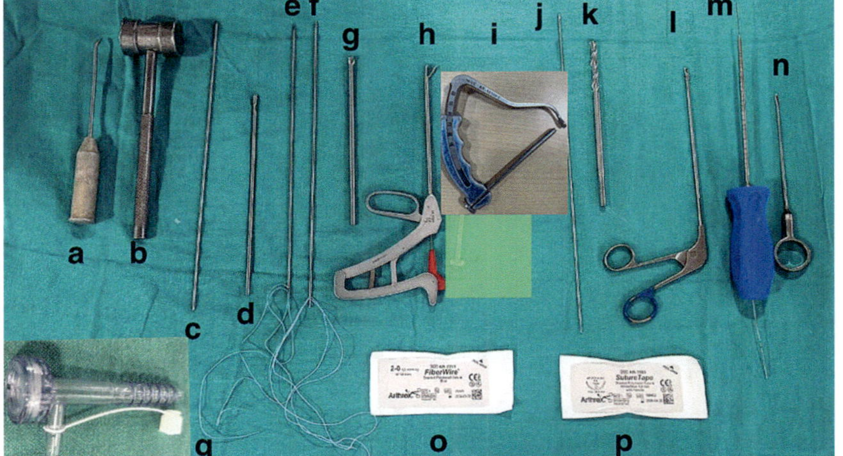


**Fig. 19.1** Instruments required for a PCL reconstruction

V. A. Mhaskar (✉)
F7 East of Kailash, Knee & Shoulder Clinic, New Delhi, India

JMVM Sports Injury Center, Sitaram Bhartia Institute of Science & Research, New Delhi, India


V. A. Mhaskar, J. Maheshwari (eds.), *Innovative Approaches in Knee Arthroscopy*,
https://doi.org/10.1007/978-981-99-4378-4_19

## 19.3 Positioning

The patient is kept supine on the operating table with the knee kept in 70° flexion with a side support on the lateral side and a bolster for the foot. This is such that there is access to the posteromedial and posterolateral aspect of the knee (Fig. 19.2).

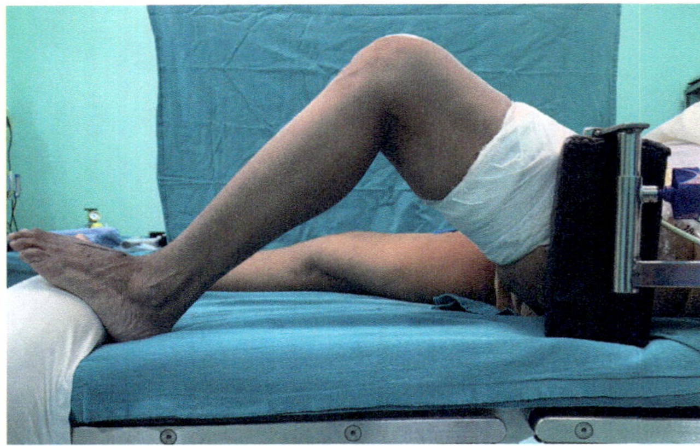

**Fig. 19.2** Image of the knee flexed at 70° flexion with a side support and a bolster at the end of the operation table

## 19.4 Draping

The draping is done in the standard way so as to have the upper 1/3 of the tibia and the distal 1/3 of the thigh exposed.

## 19.5 Portals

1. A standard horizontal anterolateral viewing portal (AL) is made at the soft spot about 5 mm lateral to the lateral border of the patellar tendon (Fig. 19.3a)
2. Another anteromedial (AM) horizontal portal is made at the same level for the Passport cannula for drilling the femoral tunnel (Fig. 19.3a)
3. A high anterolateral (High AL) portal is made at the level of the inferior pole of the patellar tendon just abutting the patellar tendon to view the femoral footprint of the PCL (Fig. 19.3a)
4. A high posteromedial (PM) portal just above the posteromedial fold of synovial tissue is made and acts as a working portal in the back of the knee (Fig. 19.3b)
5. A posterolateral (PL) portal is made by the inside out trans-septal technique such that it is at the level of the PM portal or just lower to it and should be above the biceps femoris tendon (Fig. 19.3b)

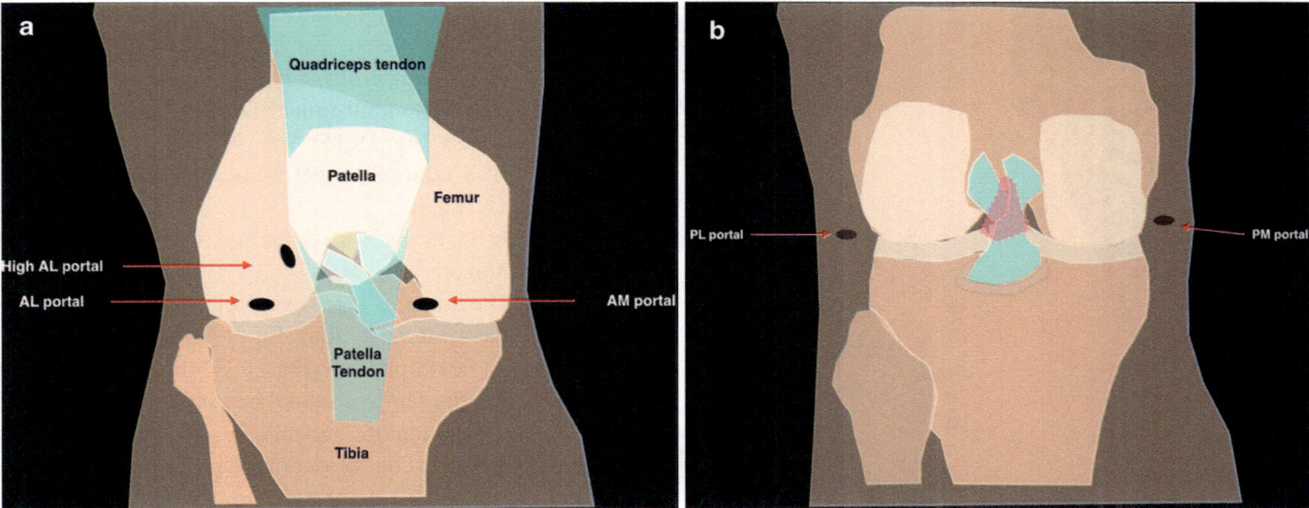


**Fig. 19.3** (**a**) Illustration of the front of the knee showing the position of the AL, High AL and AM portals. (**b**) Illustration of the back of the knee showing the PM and PL portals

## 19.6 Surgical Steps

Step 1: The arthroscope is introduced through the AL portal and PCL tear visualized and pseudolaxity of the ACL is demonstrated. The PCL femoral tunnel is marked at the centre of the PCL insertion on the femoral notch just abutting the cartilage (Fig. 19.4).

Step 2: The arthroscope is introduced between the PCL and Medial Femoral Condyle (MFC) and the PM compartment is visualised and PM portal made under vision (Fig. 19.5).

Step 3: A PL portal is made using the trans-septal technique as described in the PCL avulsion chapter (Fig. 19.6a, b).

Step 4: The arthroscope is then introduced through the PL portal and the tibial footprint of the PCL is visualized end on and cleared using a shaver (Fig. 19.7).

Step 5: A PCL jig set at 70 degree is introduced through the AM portal and between the ACL and PCL and applied to the centre of the PCL tibial footprint and sleeve with ratchet secured over the AM tibial condyle (Fig. 19.8).

Step 6: The jig is drilled with a guide wire that is trapped by a catch on the tip of the jig (Fig. 19.9a–c).

Step 7: Keeping the tip secure over the catch, a 4.5 mm drill bit is cannulated over the guide wire and drilled till the posterior cortex is breached, the penetration of the guide wire into the popliteal vessel is prevented by the catch while drilling (Fig. 19.10a, b).

Step 8: The guide wire is then removed and introduced such that the blunt end comes out posteriorly. This is over drilled with a drill bit the size of the diameter of the graft till the posterior cortex is breached (Fig. 19.11).

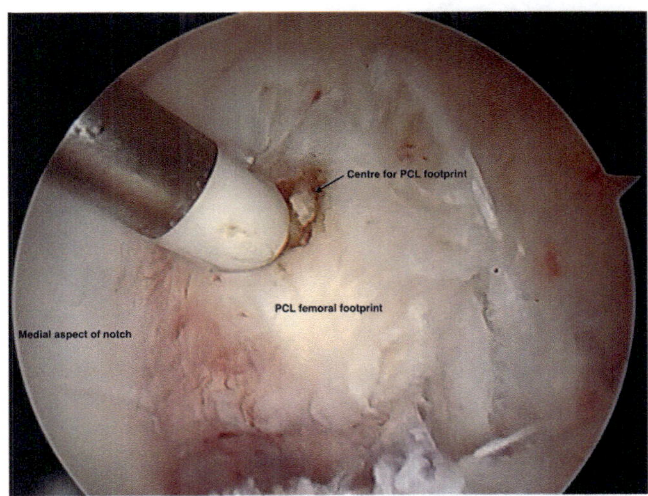


**Fig. 19.4** Viewing through the AL portal a RF through AM portal is used to mark the femoral tunnel at the centre of the PCL footprint

Step 9: A Beath pin carrying a Ethibond loop (Ethicon, Rariton, NJ) is then introduced through this tunnel from the anteromedial tibia to the posterior aspect of the knee (Fig. 19.12a, b).

Step 10: A suture manipulator is introduced through the PM portal to deliver the Ethibond loop through the PM portal (Fig. 19.13).

Step 11: The arthroscope is then introduced through the high AL portal and a Beath pin is applied to the centre of the

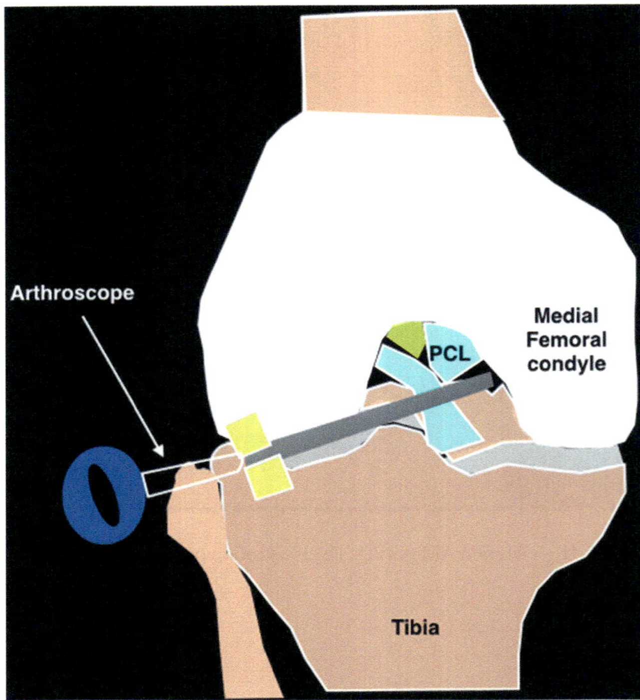


**Fig. 19.5** Illustration of the front of the knee showing the arthroscope in the AL portal being manipulated between the PCL and medial femoral condyle to the posteromedial aspect of the knee

femoral footprint marked initially and tapped in (Fig. 19.14a, b).

Step 12: A 4.5 mm drill bit is then cannulated over the Beath pin and the femoral tunnel is drilled till the medial cortex is breached (Fig. 19.15).

Step 13: The femoral tunnel is measured using a depth gauge (Fig. 19.16a, b).

Step 14: A Beath pin is reversed and then introduced into the femoral tunnel.

Step 15: The tunnel is then over drilled with a drill bit the diameter of the graft for 20 mm (Fig. 19.17a, b).

Step 16: A Beath pin carrying an Ethibond loop is then introduced into the femoral tunnel and the loop is delivered at the orifice of the femoral tunnel (Fig. 19.18a, b).

Step 17: The loop coming out of the posterior tibial cortex and femoral tunnel are delivered through the Passport cannula using a grasper (Fig. 19.19a, b).

Step 18: The loop coming out of the tibial tunnel is pulled such that it becomes a single thread that is tied around the loop coming out of the femoral tunnel through the Passport Cannula (Fig. 19.20).

Step 19: The thread is then pulled out through the tibial tunnel anteriorly to deliver the Ethibond loop from the femoral tunnel through the tibial tunnel (Fig. 19.21).

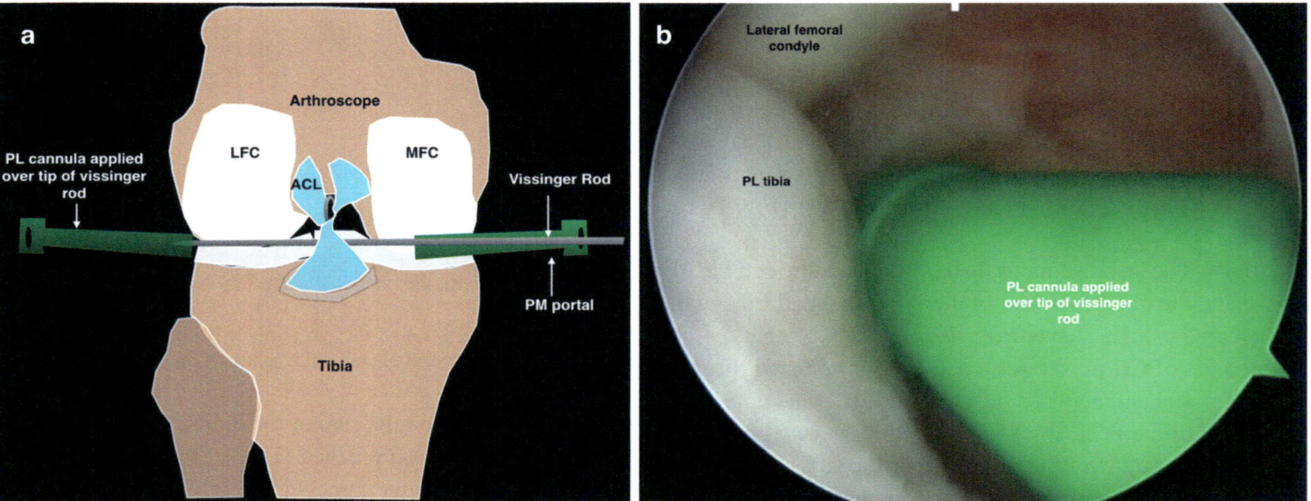


**Fig. 19.6** (**a**) Illustration of the back of the knee showing PL portal being made trans-septal. (**b**) Arthroscopic image of the posterior aspect of the knee showing PL portal with a cannula

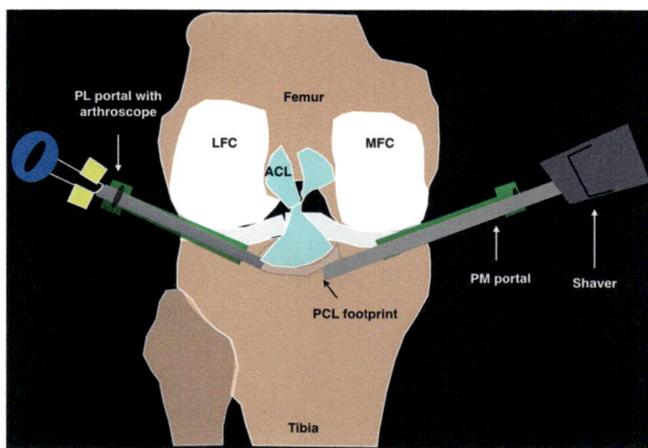


**Fig. 19.7** Illustration of the back of the knee, viewing from the PL portal showing a shaver through the PM portal cleaning the footprint of the PCL on the tibia

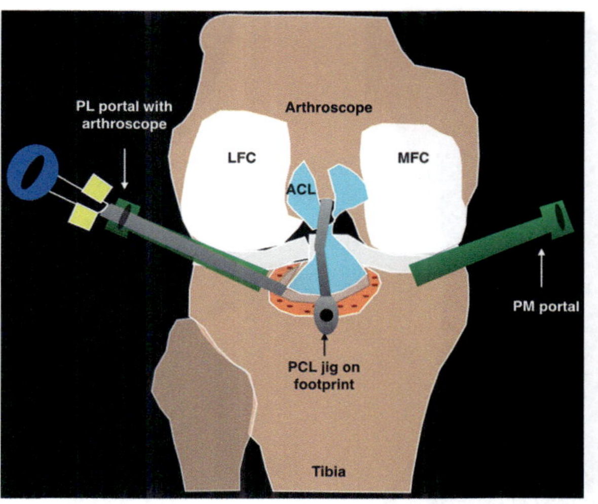


**Fig. 19.8** Illustration of the back of the knee showing the PCL jig set at 70° manipulated between the PCL and ACL placed at the centre of the PCL footprint, while viewing from the PL portal

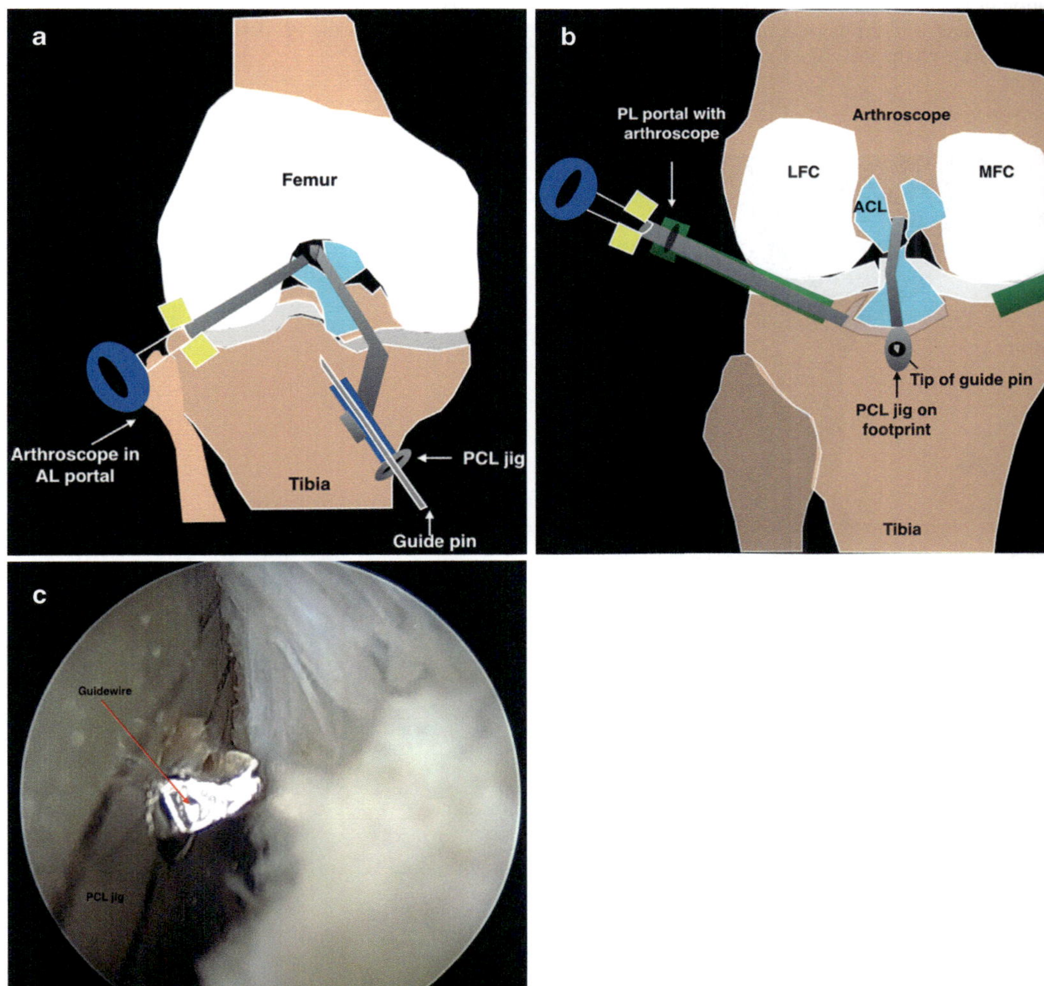


**Fig. 19.9** (**a**) Illustration of the front of the knee showing a guidewire drilled through the PCL jig. (**b**) Illustration of the back of the knee showing the guidewire tip coming out of the centre of the PCL jig trap. (**c**) Arthroscopic image of the back of the knee viewing through the PL portal showing the tip of the guide wire coming out of the centre of the trap of the PCL jig

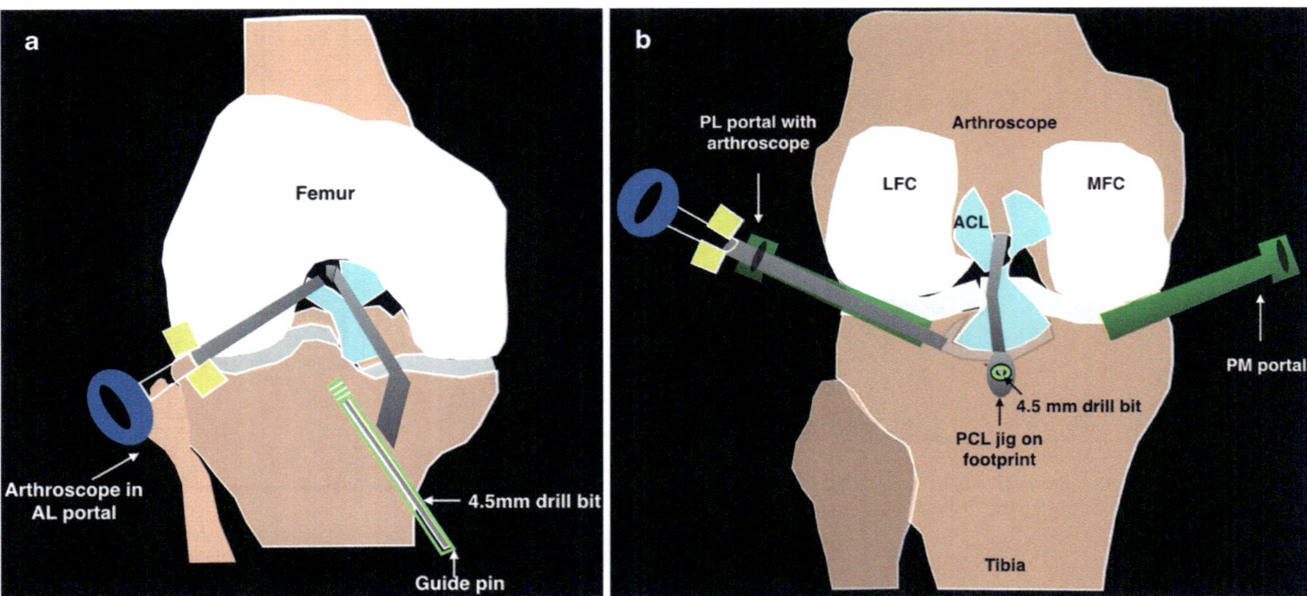


**Fig. 19.10** (**a**) Illustration of the front of the knee showing a 4.5 mm drill bit cannulated over the guide wire drilling the tibial tunnel while holding the tip of the guide wire with the PCL jig. (**b**) Illustration of the back of the knee showing a 4.5 mm drill bit cannulated over the guide wire while viewing from the PL portal and holding the guidewire tip with a PCL jig

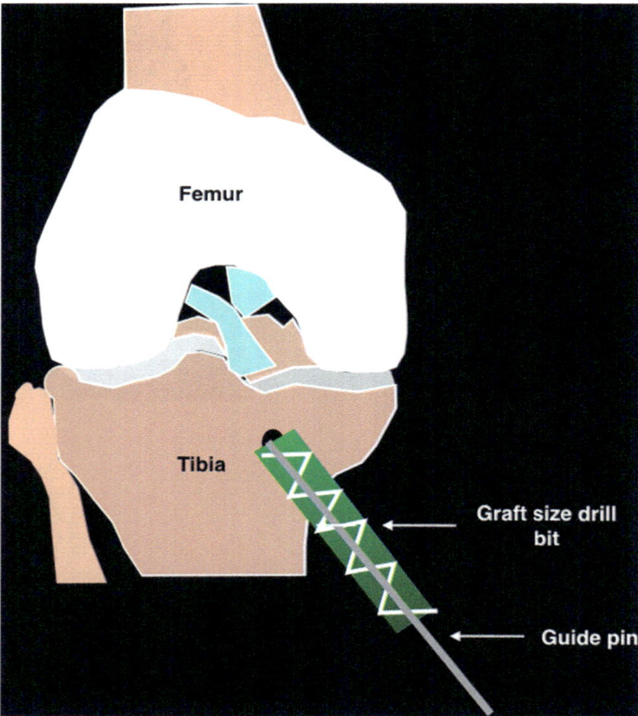


**Fig. 19.11** Illustration of the front of the knee showing a graft sized drill bit drilling the tibial tunnel from anteromedial to the posterior tibia

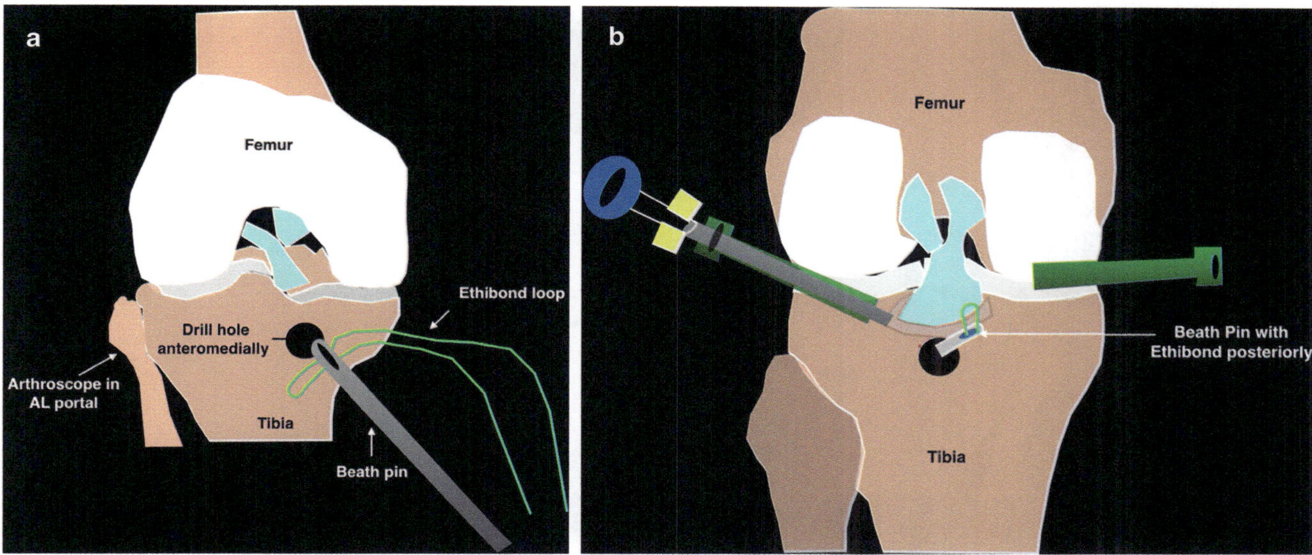


**Fig. 19.12** (**a**) Illustration of the front of the knee showing a Beath pin with a No 5 Ethibond loop introduced through the anteromedial tibial tunnel to the posterior aspect of the knee. (**b**) Illustration of the back of the knee while viewing through the PL portal showing the Ethibond loop on a Beath pin coming out through the tibial tunnel posteriorly

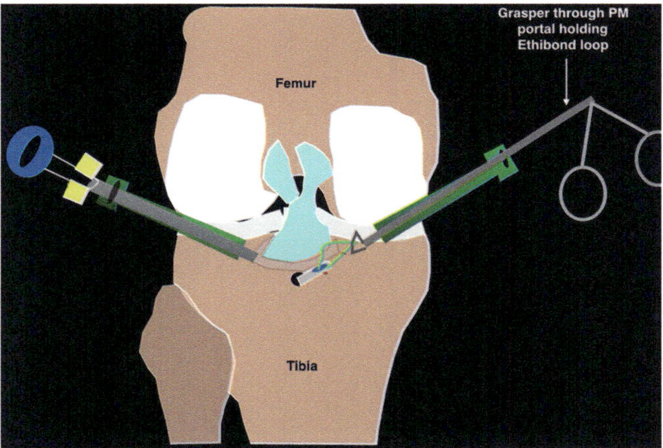


**Fig. 19.13** Illustration of the back of the knee showing a suture manipulator through the PM portal pulling the Ethibond loop while viewing through the PL portal

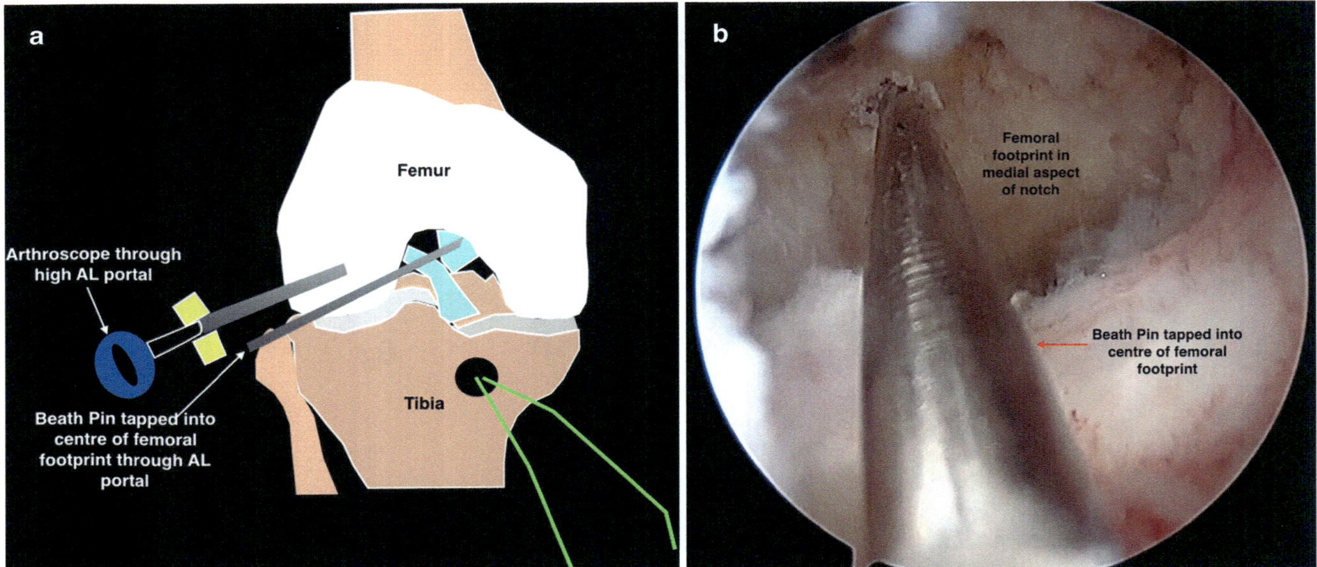


**Fig. 19.14** (**a**) Illustration of the front of the knee showing a Beath pin tapped into the centre of the femoral footprint of the PCL while viewing from the high AL portal. (**b**) Arthroscopic image showing a Beath pin through the AL portal tapped into the centre of the PCL femoral footprint while viewing through the high AL portal

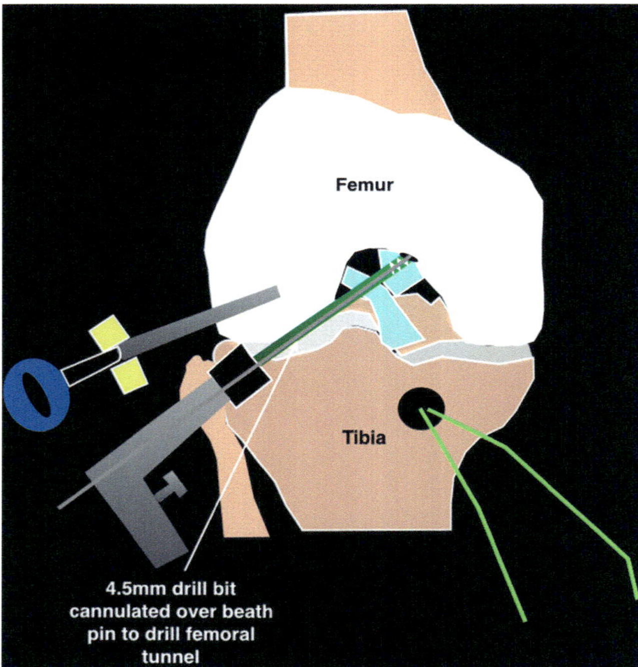


**Fig. 19.15** Illustration of the front of the knee showing a 4.5 mm drill bit through the AL portal cannulated over the Beath pin while viewing through the high AL portal

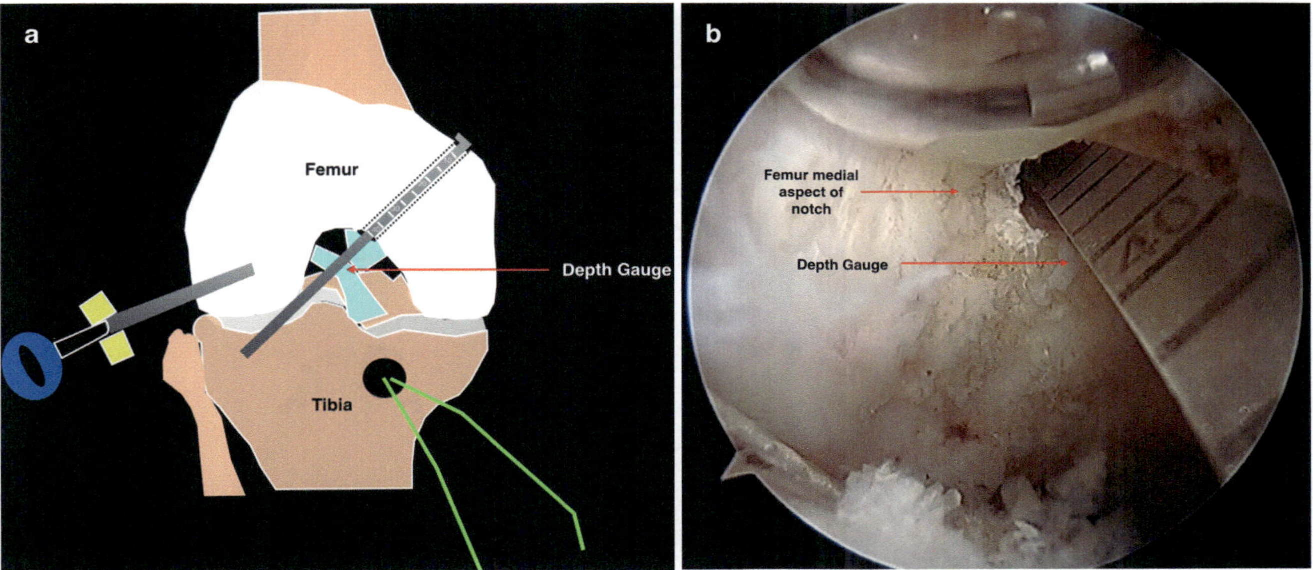


**Fig. 19.16** (**a**) Illustration of the front of the knee showing measuring the femoral tunnel length with a depth gauge. (**b**) Arthroscopic image showing the femoral tunnel being measured with a depth gauge through the AL portal while viewing through the high AL portal

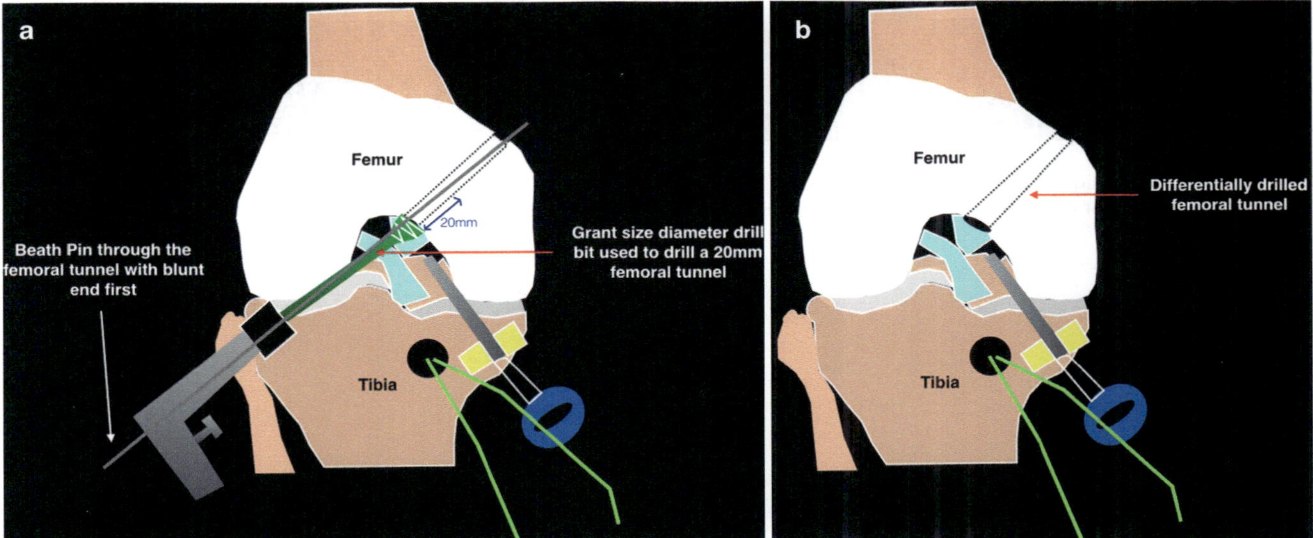


**Fig. 19.17** (**a**) Illustration of the front of the knee showing the femoral tunnel being over drilled to the diameter of the graft till 20 mm while viewing through the AM portal. (**b**) Illustration of the front of the knee showing a differentially drilled femoral tunnel

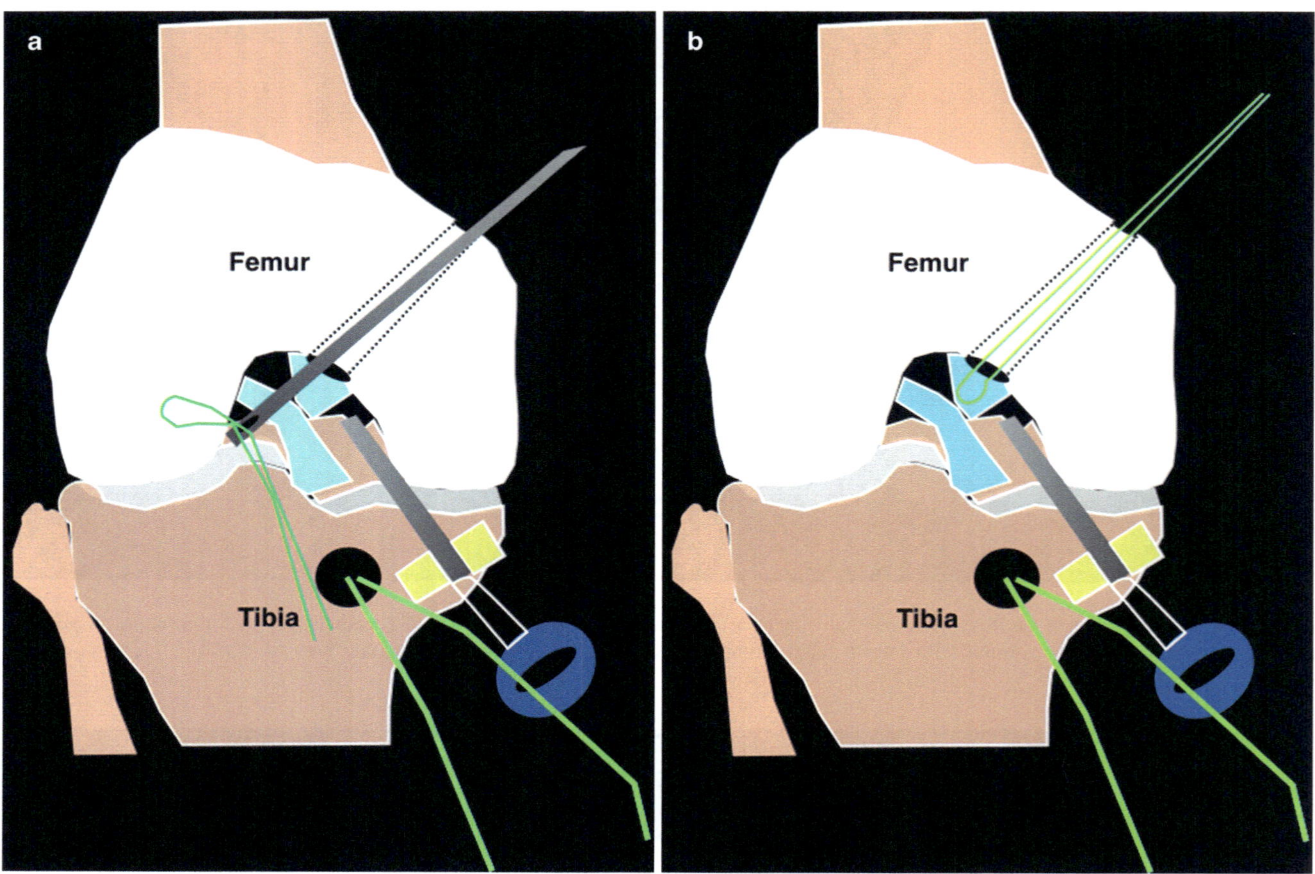


**Fig. 19.18** (**a**) Illustration of the front of the knee showing a Beath pin with an Ethibond loop introduced from the AL portal into the femoral tunnel. (**b**) Illustration of the front of the knee showing the Ethibond loop at the orifice of the femoral tunnel

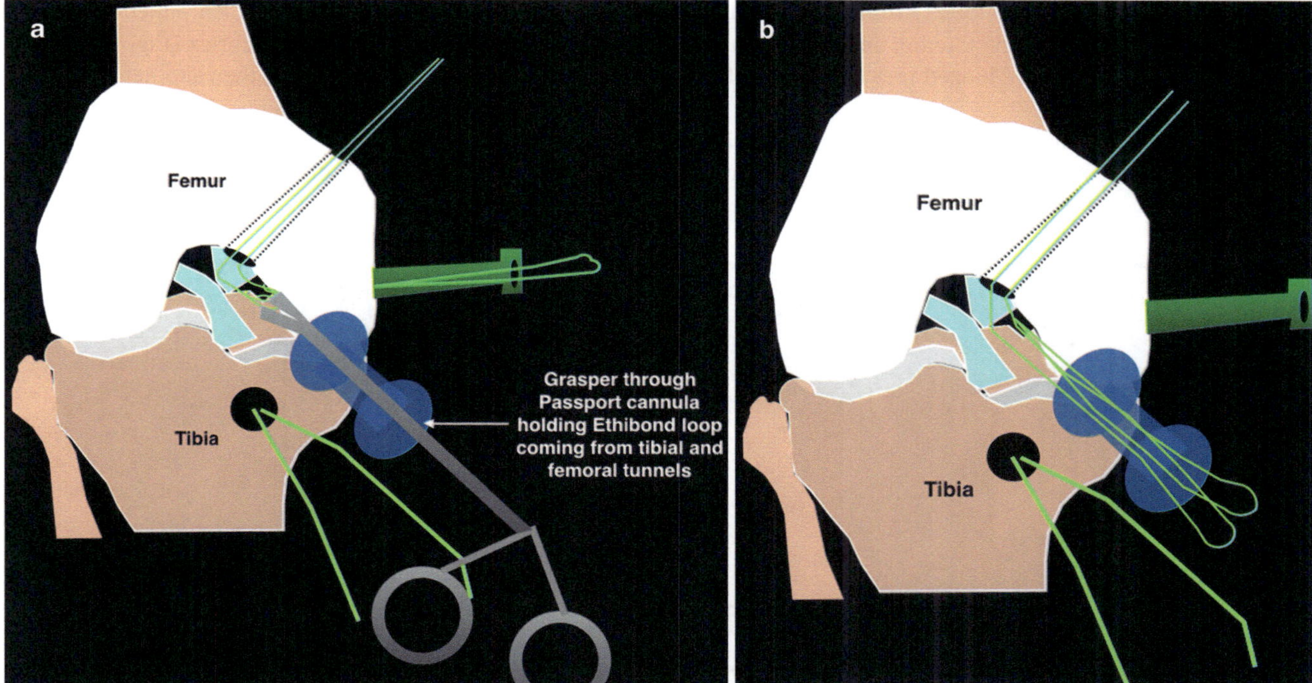


**Fig. 19.19** (**a**) Illustration of the front of the knee showing the Ethibond loop from the tibial and femoral tunnel being held by a grasper through the AM portal. (**b**) Illustration of the front of the knee showing both Ethibond loops from the tibia and femur through the Passport cannula in the AM portal

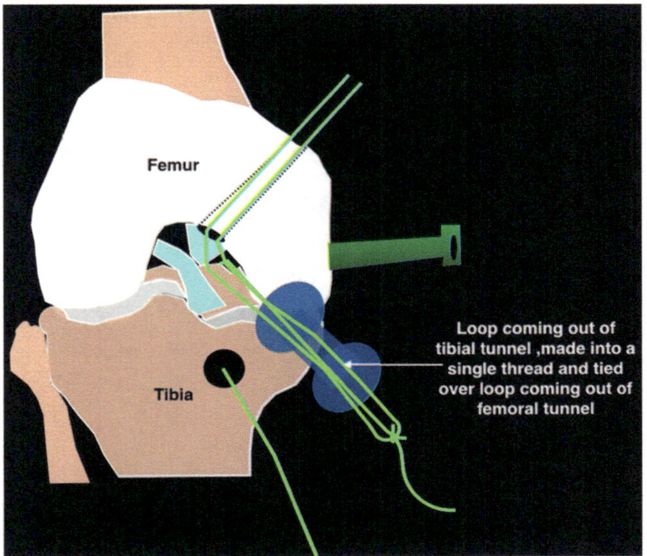


**Fig. 19.20** Illustration of the front of the knee showing the loop from the tibial tunnel being made into a single Ethibond thread and tied over the femoral Ethibond loop to deliver it through the anteromedial tibial tunnel such that the loop is from the femoral tunnel to the tibial tunnel

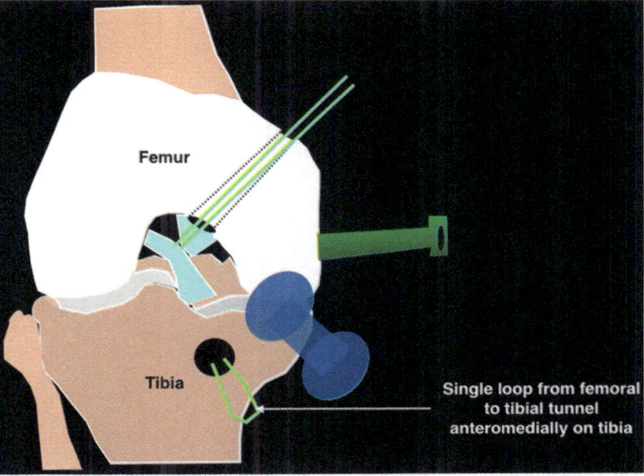


**Fig. 19.21** Illustration of the front of the knee showing an Ethibond loop at the anteromedial aspect of the tibial tunnel, coming from the femoral tunnel

Step 20: The Tightrope RT loop (Arthrex, Naples, FL) is lengthened to 100 mm and the traction and milking sutures coming out of the button are looped into the Ethibond loop (Fig. 19.22).

Step 21: The Ethibond loop is then pulled such that the traction and milking sutures are delivered through the medial cortex of the femur (Fig. 19.23).

Step 22: The traction sutures are then pulled so that the Tightrope button flips on the medial cortex (Fig. 19.24a, b).

Step 23: The milking sutures and then alternatively pulled to pull the graft through the tibial tunnel into the femoral tunnel (Fig. 19.25a–c).

Step 24: A guide wire is then applied through the tibial tunnel posterior to the graft and parallel to it (Fig. 19.26a, b).

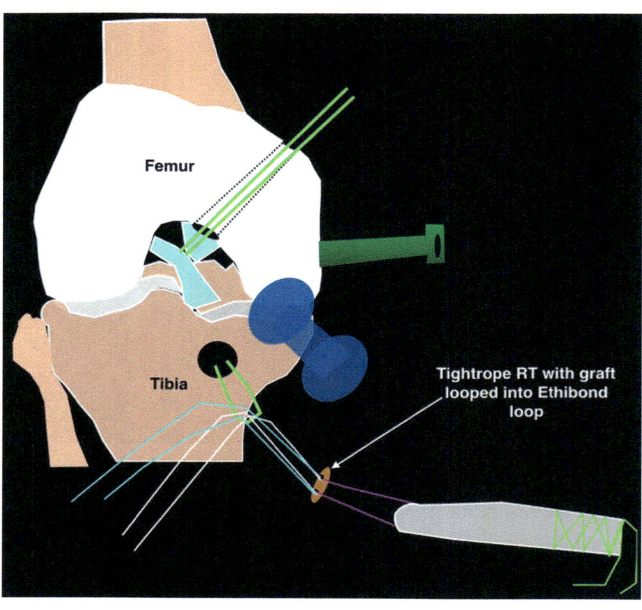


**Fig. 19.22** Illustration of the front of the knee showing the threads attached to the Tightrope button carrying the graft being looped into the Ethibond loop

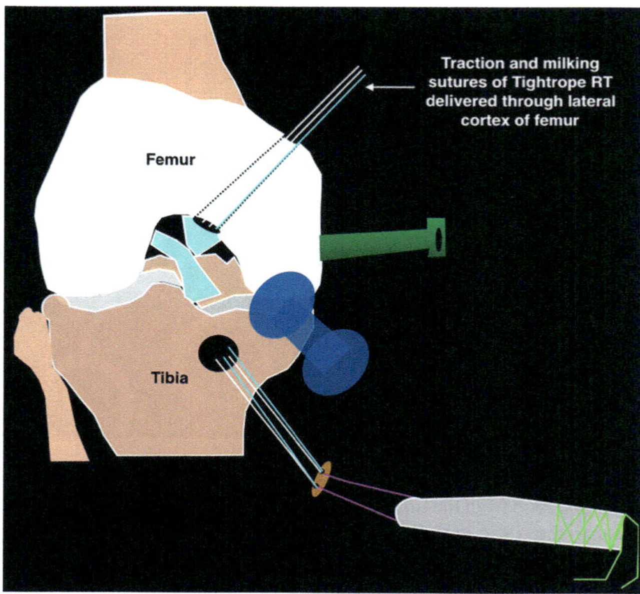


**Fig. 19.23** Illustration of the front of the knee showing the traction and milking sutures of the Tightrope construct delivered through the medial cortex of the femur externally by shuttling them with the Ethibond loop through the tibial and femoral tunnel

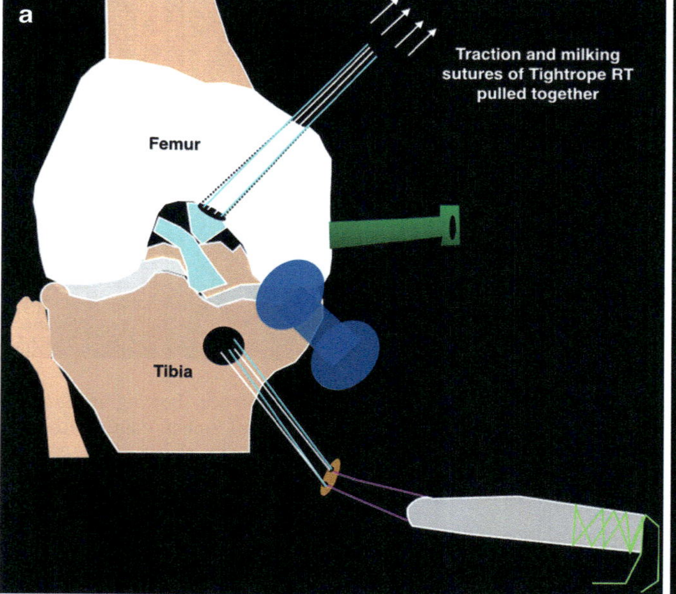


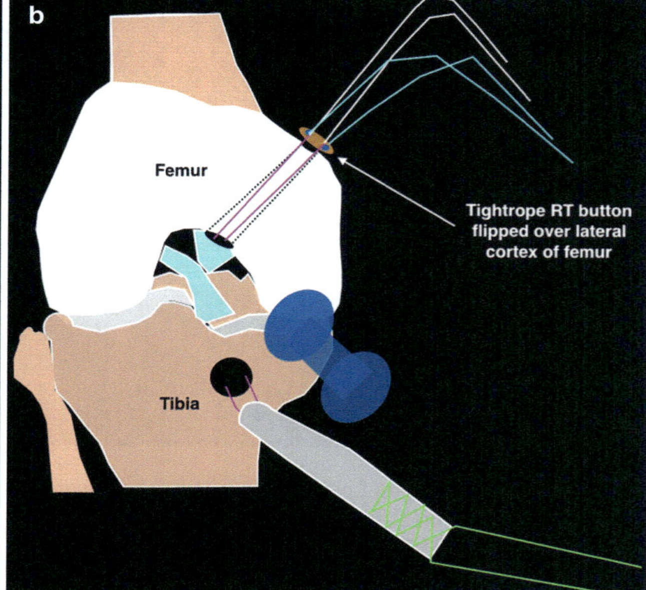


**Fig. 19.24** (**a**) Illustration of the front of the knee showing the traction and milking sutures being pulled simultaneously to pull the Tightrope button up the tunnels. (**b**) Illustration of the front of the knee showing the Tightrope button flipped over the medial cortex of the femur

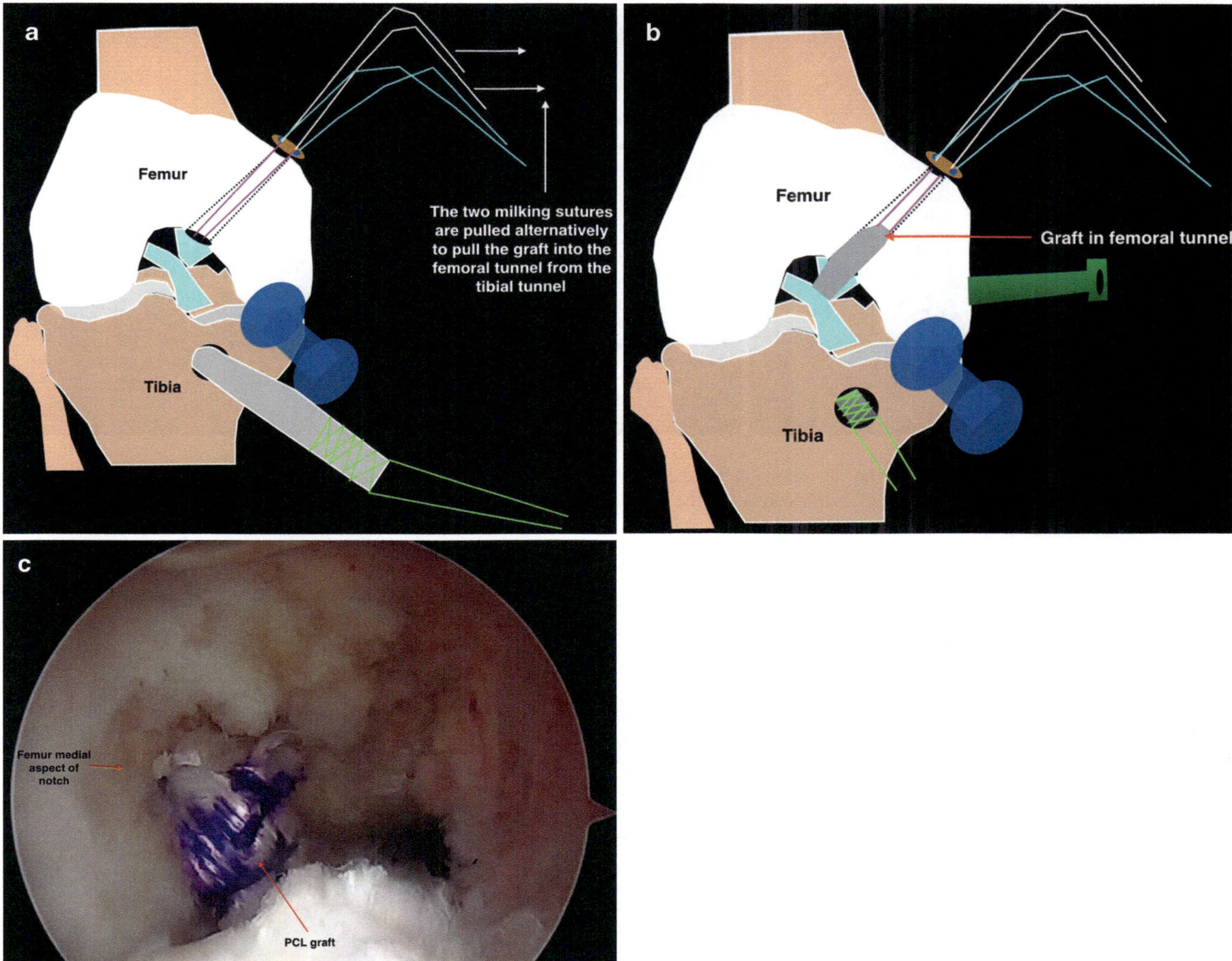


**Fig. 19.25** (**a**) Illustration of the front of the knee showing the milking sutures of the Tightrope device being pulled alternately to pull the graft up the tibial tunnel into the femoral tunnel. (**b**) Illustration of the front of the knee showing the graft pulled up the tibial and femoral tunnels. (**c**) Arthroscopic image of the PCL graft seen in the femoral tunnel in the medial aspect of the notch

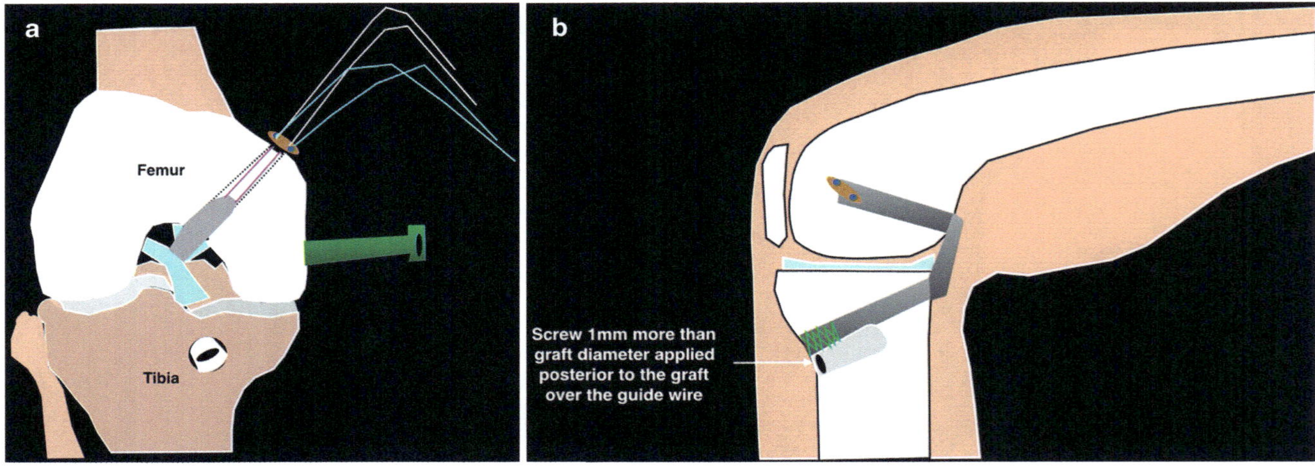


**Fig. 19.27** (**a**) Illustration of the front of the knee showing the interference screw applied to the tibial tunnel parallel and posterior to the graft while giving an anterior drawer force. (**b**) Illustration of the sagittal section of the knee showing the interference screw applied parallel to the graft and posterior to it

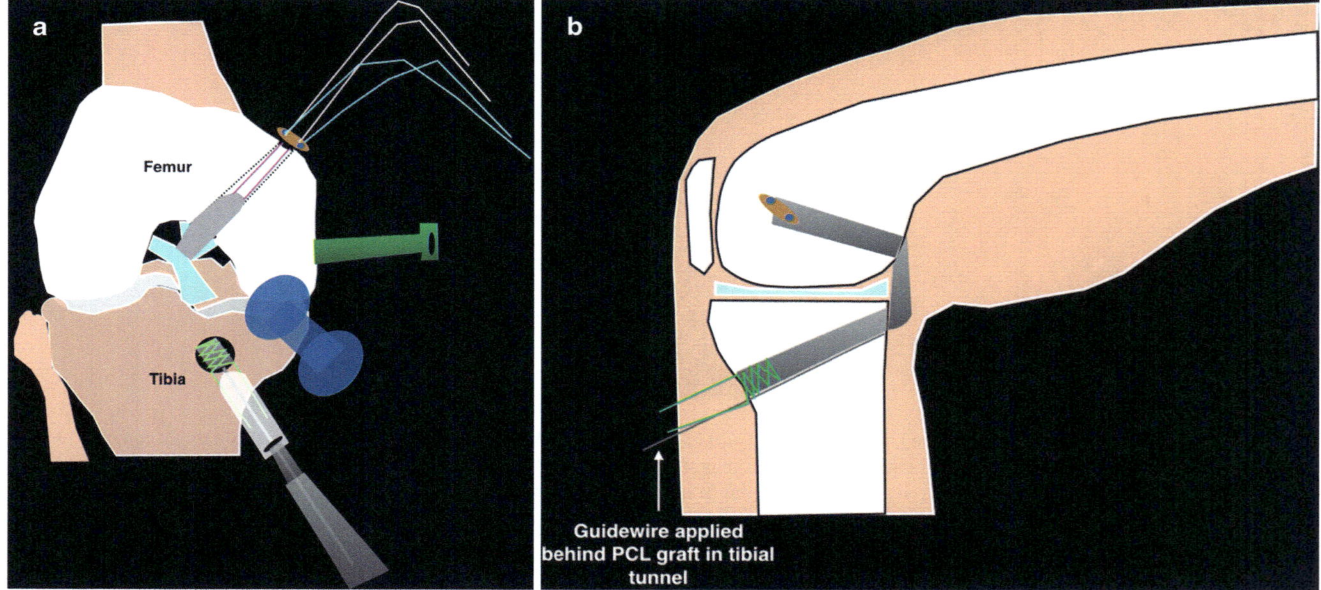


**Fig. 19.26** (**a**) Illustration of the front of the knee showing a guide wire applied posterior to the graft and parallel to it in the tibial tunnel anteromedially with an Interference screw cannulated through it. (**b**) Illustration of the sagittal section of the knee showing a guide wire applied posterior and parallel to the graft in the tibial tunnel anteromedially to apply the interference screw

Step 25: While giving an anterior drawer force on the tibia a crew 1 mm more in diameter to the graft is applied over the guide wire such that it lies posterior to the graft (Fig. 19.27a, b).

## 19.7 Tips and Tricks

1. Hold the tip of the guidewire with the trap in the tibial jig while over drilling with a 4.5 mm drill bit to avoid penetrance into the NV bundle

2. Grasp the loop coming out of the femur and tibia together and deliver through the AM portal if no cannula is used as it can act as a virtual cannula and prevent a soft tissue bridge
3. While passing the graft while sequentially pulling the milking sutures exert an anterior drawer force so that the graft can easily slide from the tibia to the femur

## 19.8 Advantages and Disadvantages

**Advantages**

1. Possibly more anatomical tibial tunnel placement as it is seen end on while drilling it
2. Suture manipulation at the back of the knee is easier as all work on the posterior aspect of the knee is seen and done from posterior portals

**Disadvantages**

1. Learning curve required for making a trans-septal portal
2. Dissection in the posterior compartment can cause fibrosis and possible stiffness later on

# 20 An Innovative Approach to All Inside Posterior Cruciate Ligament Reconstruction

Attique Vasdev, Roshan Wade, Saksham Tripathi, and Ashok Rajgopal

## 20.1 Introduction

Posterior cruciate ligament (PCL) reconstruction is considered one of the challenging arthroscopic procedures in Knee arthroscopic surgery [1, 2]. Non-operative treatment of grade-III posterior cruciate ligament (PCL) injuries leads to a declining knee function and early osteoarthritis [3–7]. The importance of optimizing knee function shown a growing interest in surgical reconstruction of the injured PCL. Double bundle (DB), single bundle (SB), transtibial, and tibial inlay techniques have been described for PCL reconstruction (PCLR) and all are associated with successful clinical outcomes.

LaPrade described qualitatively and quantitatively the locations of the anterolateral and posteromedial bundles of the PCL relative to arthroscopically relevant landmarks to assist with anatomic tunnel placement during both single and double bundle PCL reconstruction surgery. This greatly helped in a better reproduction of antomic placement of tunnels in PCL reconstruction [8].

Newer techniques like all-inside PCL reconstruction (single or double bundle) [9, 10] especially with the development of the GraftLink (Fig. 20.1) (Arthrex, Naples, FL) technique and availability of newer-generation implants and instruments such as the TightRope RT (Arthrex) and FlipCutter (Arthrex) for the all-inside anatomic anterior cruciate ligament (ACL) reconstruction have not only made it possible to perform these surgical procedures by making sockets instead of tunnels but also have less post-operative pain and better cosmesis [9–12]. However, overcoming the killer turn is often a step of discomfort for the surgeon while attempting arthroscopic PCL reconstruction.

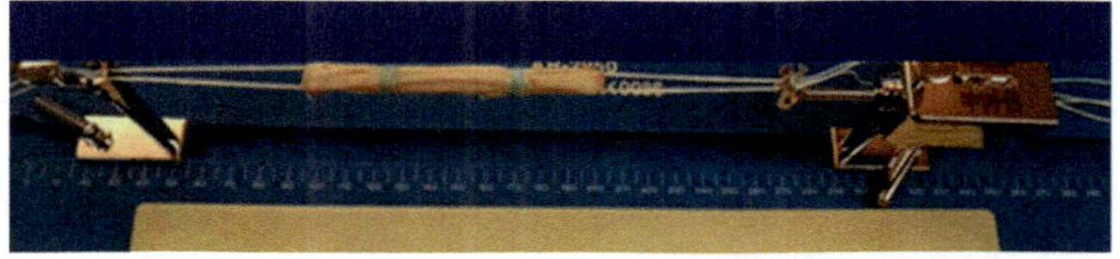

**Fig. 20.1** Graftlink after preparation

In an attempt to overcome the difficulty of the killer turn encountered while performing the arthroscopic PCL reconstruction we described a new way of passing the GraftLink graft construct through the posteromedial (PM) portal while doing the arthroscopic all-inside PCL reconstruction [13].

## 20.2 Patient Positioning and Anesthesia

Supine position, with the affected leg hanging over the side of the operating table in flexion and the foot resting on the surgeon's lap with the surgeon sitting or leg flexed at 90–100° (Fig. 20.2) on the operating table with the surgeon standing.

Anesthesia may be general or Spinal.

**Supplementary Information** The online version contains supplementary material available at https://doi.org/10.1007/978-981-99-4378-4_20.

A. Vasdev (✉) · S. Tripathi · A. Rajgopal
Department of Musculoskeletal Disorders and Orthopaedics, Medanta-The Medicity, Gurugram, Haryana, India

R. Wade
Department of Orthopaedics, Seth GS Medical College and KEM Hospital, Mumbai, India


V. A. Mhaskar, J. Maheshwari (eds.), *Innovative Approaches in Knee Arthroscopy*, https://doi.org/10.1007/978-981-99-4378-4_20

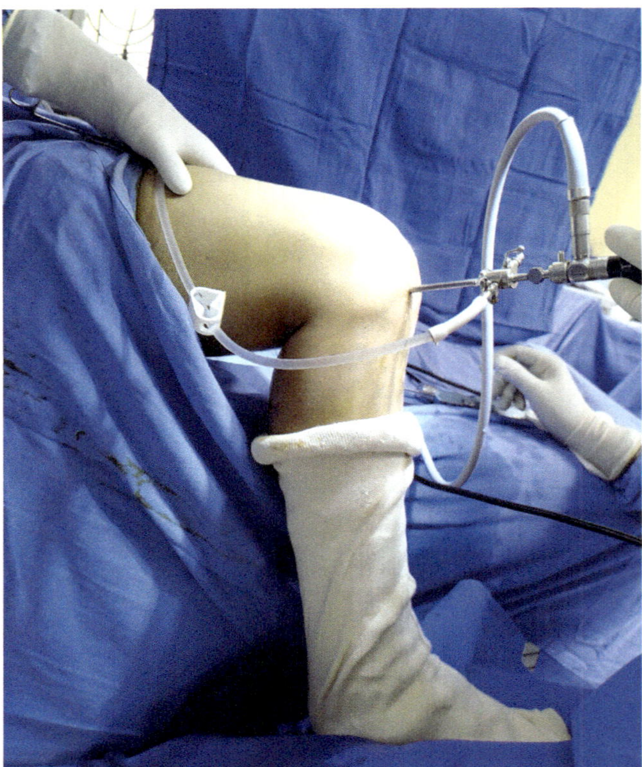

**Fig. 20.2** Position of patient

## 20.3 Surgical Steps

### 20.3.1 Graft Harvesting, Preparation and Length

With the patient under anesthesia sterile draping is done making sure that the posterior aspect of the knee is easily accessed.

Step 1: Under torniquet control, the ipsilateral semitendinosus is harvested (alternately the central quadriceps tendon, (CQT with or without patellar bone block), Peroneus Longus tendon, or various allografts may be used).

Step 2: A GraftLink construct is made using TightRope RT devices with markings at both ends to indicate the desired intraosseous length. Alternately a TightRope RT on one side and an ABS TightRope on the other with an ABS button may be used. The grafts were quadrupled or tripled to achieve a desirable diameter (range, 8–11 mm) and a minimum length of 90 mm (quadrupled or tripled) allowing an intra-articular graft availability of 35–40 mm. The intraosseous socket length should be between 20 and 25 mm in the femur and between 20 and 25 mm in the tibia depending on the length of the available graft. A 5–10 mm larger socket length in the tibia may be taken to use the entire length of the graft which allowing for final re-tensioning and prevents bottoming out.

### 20.3.2 Arthroscopy

Step 3: Initial arthroscopic examination is performed using a 30° arthroscope with the knee in 90° of flexion via standard anterolateral (AL) and anteromedial (AM) portals. To improve intra articular vision the torn PCL may be debrided with a motorised shaver from the anterior standard portals.

Step 4: A posteromedial (PM) portal is then created (Fig. 20.3). The 30° arthroscope is switched with a 70° arthroscope for better visualization and debridement of the tibial PCL footprint which is done by passing a shaver through the PM portal.

### 20.3.3 Socket Drilling and Shuttle Passage

Step 5: With the knee in 90° of flexion an TibialPCL guide (Arthrex) is passed through the AM portal 16 mm below the posterior edge of the tibia in the center of the PCL footprint (Fig. 20.4) with the guide fixed at 65°. The all-inside pin sleeve (Arthrex) is tapped into the tibia anteriorly to achieve a 7-mm bone bridge (alternately this may be tapped in after the flip cutter has been drilled).

Step 6: A flip cutter 0.5 mm larger than the size of the graft is drilled into the tibia until it hits the tibial PCL guide and could not be advanced any further (this step is done always keeping the tibial PCL guide in the posterior aspect of the knee under vision via PM or AL portal to prevent any injury to the posterior neurovascular bundle). The tibial PCL guide is then removed.

Step 7: The flip cutter is then slowly advanced, just enough to allow for the flipping to occur (under direct vision of the 70° arthroscope).

Step 8: A curette can be passed through the PM portal once the jig is removed to prevent any injury to the neurovascular bundles by the flip cutter tip (Fig. 20.5).

Step 9: Depending on the length of the graft, a socket 5–10 mm larger in length is created. The Flip Cutter is then removed, keeping all inside pin sleeve in position, and a fiber stick (Fig. 20.6) is passed through the and suture pulled out through the PM portal with the help of a suture retriever (Fig. 20.7).

Step 10: The 70° arthroscope is then switched back for a 30° arthroscope and then transferred from the AL portal to the AM portal. A drill pin for the TightRope with a spade tip is passed through the AL portal in the center of the PCL stump on the medial femoral condyle (Fig. 20.8) and a socket of the desired length made, drilling from inside the joint through the AL portal with the arthroscope in the AM portal (alternately an Arthrex outside in guide can be used for this step especially in multiligament injury situations).

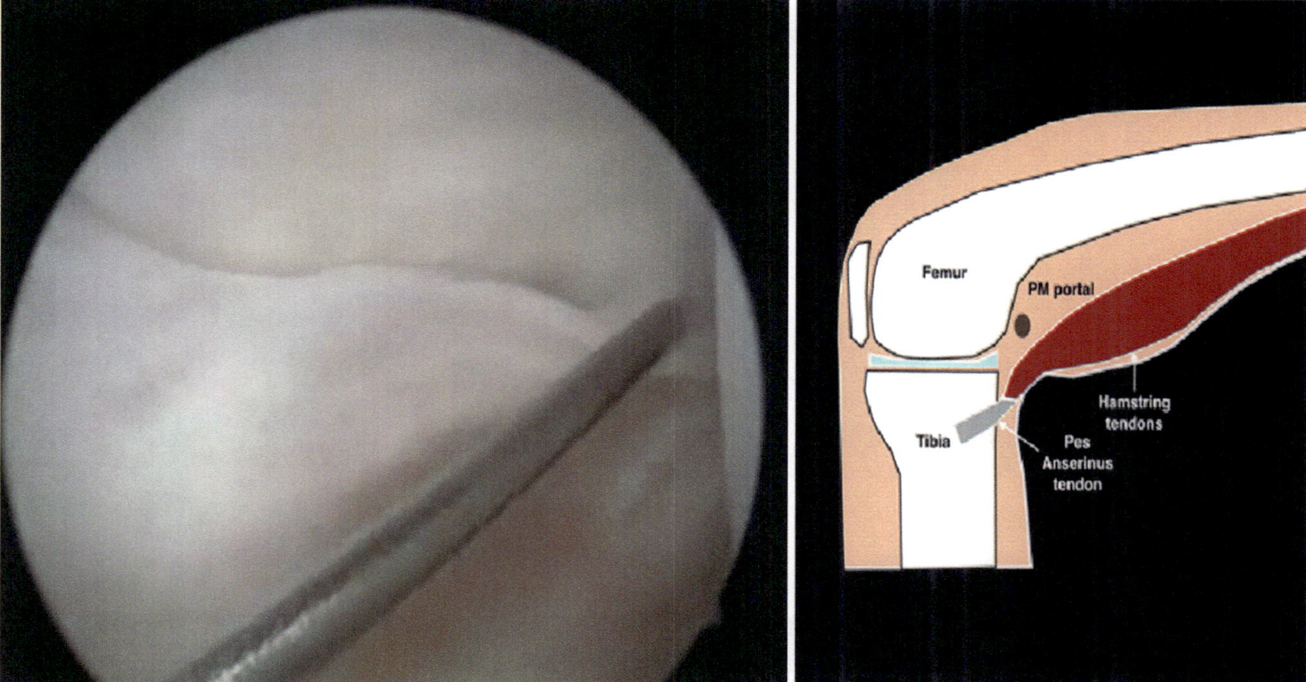


**Fig. 20.3** PM portal

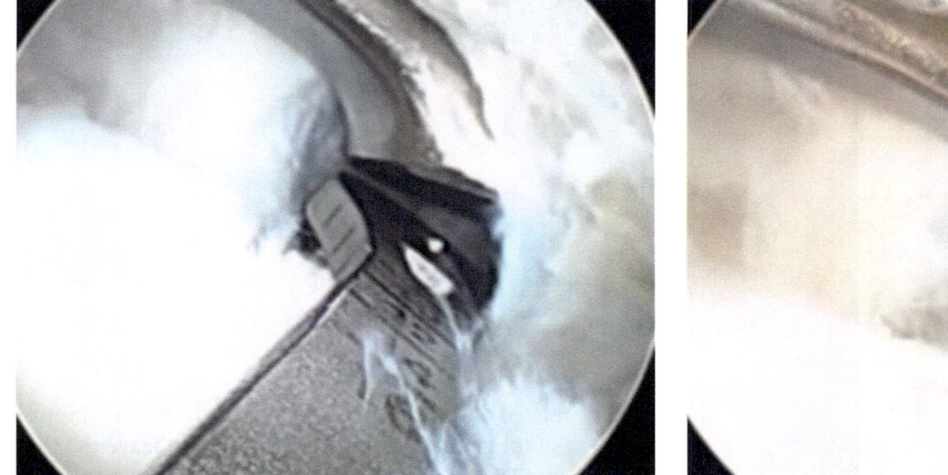

**Fig. 20.4** PCL tibial jig

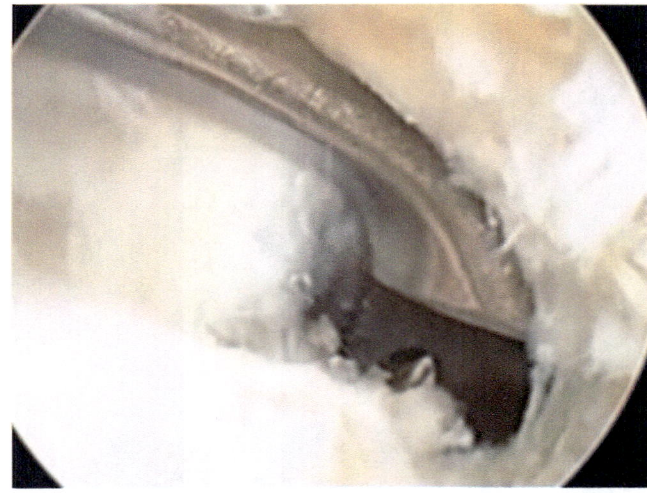

**Fig. 20.5** Flippcutter for tibia tunnel

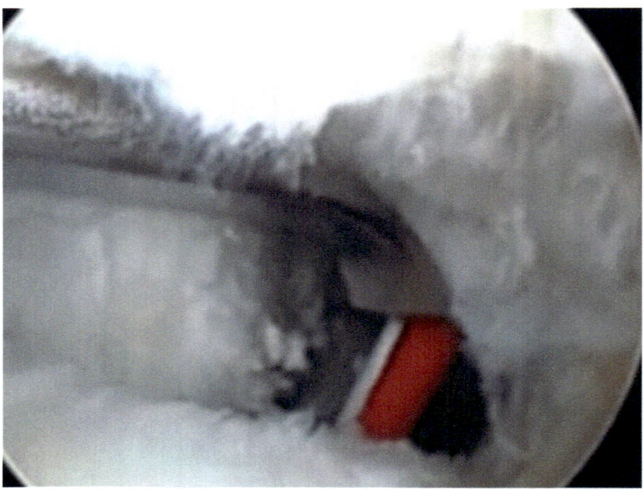

Fig. 20.6 Fibrestick through tibial tunnel

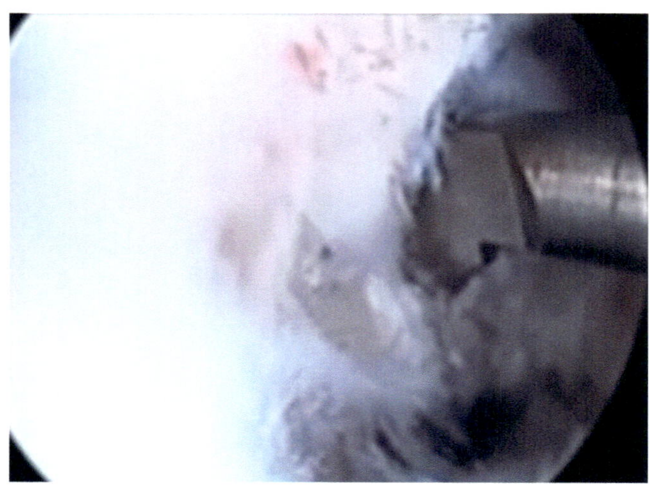

Fig. 20.8 Femoral guide pin

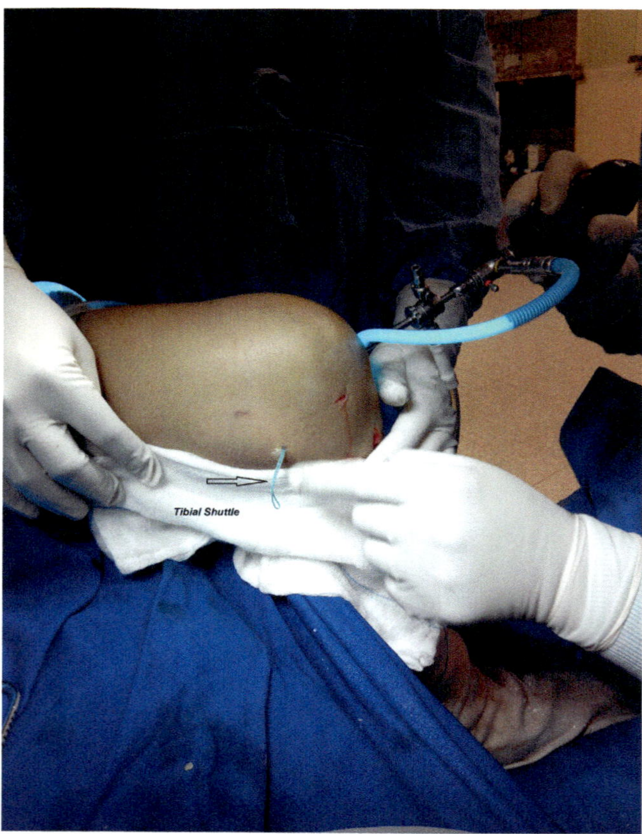


Fig. 20.7 Tibial shuttle

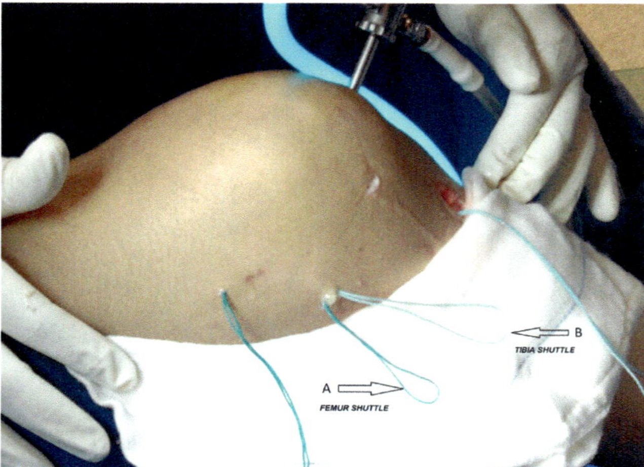


Fig. 20.9 Suture shuttles from tibia and femur

Step 11: A suture shuttle is then passed into the joint by pulling out the spade drill pin, making sure to leave the loop in the joint. The arthroscope was transferred back to the AL portal, and with the help of the suture retriever, the loop was delivered into the posterior compartment of the joint and pulled out of the PM portal. The PM portal now has two shuttles, 1 from the tibial socket and 1 from the femoral socket (Fig. 20.9).

### 20.3.4 Graft Passage and Tensioning

Step 12: Both the Tibial and Femoral end TightRopes are lengthened and suture tails are individually pulled via tibial and femoral shuttles out of their respective tibia and femoral sockets leaving the graft in the vicinity of the PM portal. The femoral TightRope Button is not flipped at this stage (Fig. 20.10).

Step 13: The femoral TightRope was then pulled under direct vision of the femoral socket in the medial femoral condyle (via the arthroscope in the AL portal) until the button of the TightRope RT flips over the outer cortex of the medial femoral condyle.

Step 14: The graft is then pulled into the femoral socket (Fig. 20.11). A similar procedure is performed on the tibial side with the TightRope RT pulled until the TightRope button is visualized outside the anterior tibia (Fig. 20.12).

Step 15: The graft was then pulled into the socket by tightening the TightRope RT, keeping the knee in 70–90° of flexion with a strong anterior drawer pull for single bundle reconstructions (In case of double bundle PCL reconstruction Anterolateral bundle tensioned first at 90° of flexion and then Posteromedial bundle is tensioned at 30° of flexion).

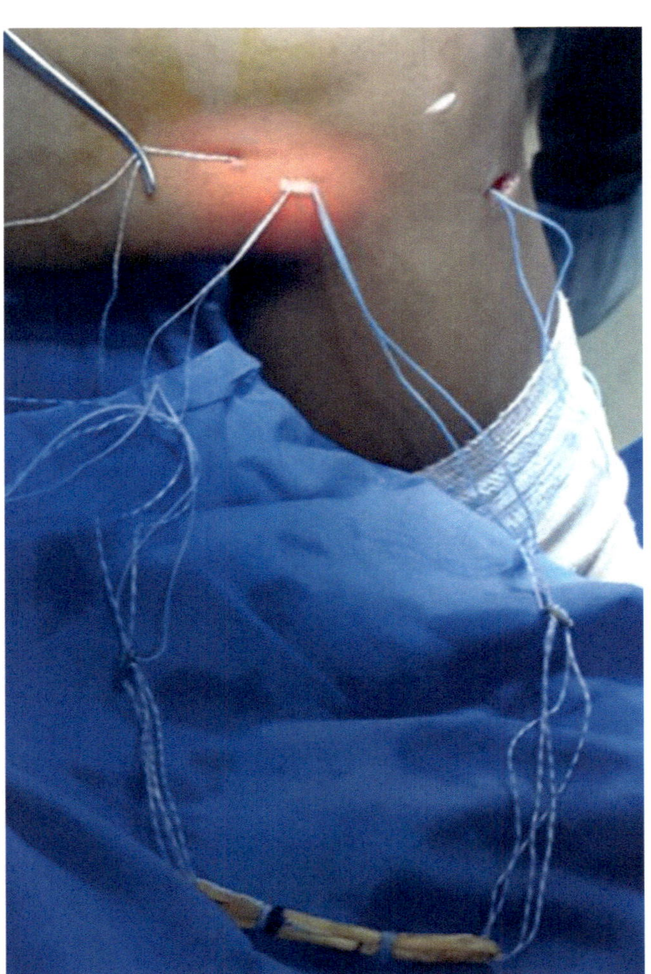

**Fig. 20.10** Graftlink ready for passage

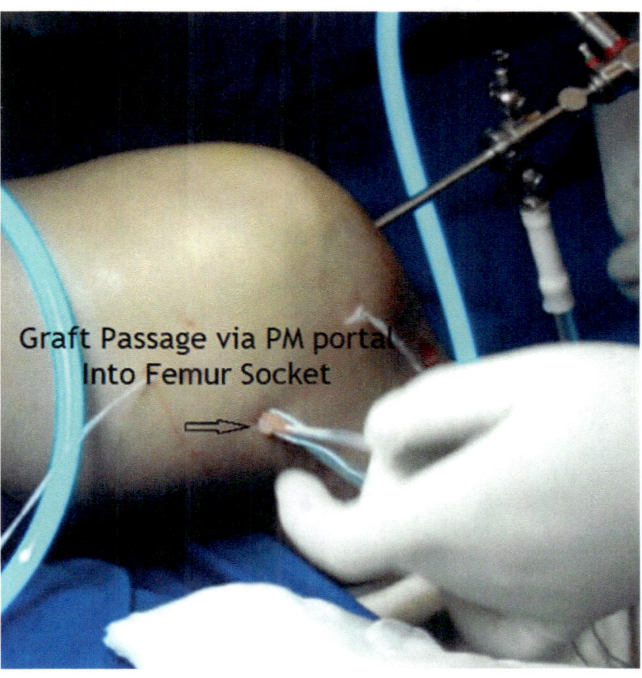


**Fig. 20.11** Graft passage via the PM portal into the femoral socket

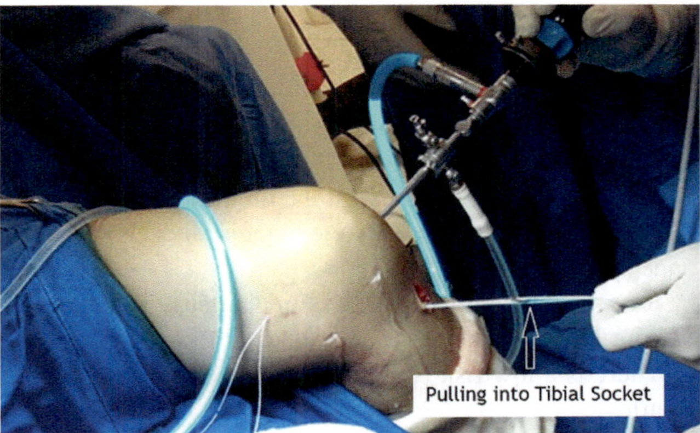


**Fig. 20.12** Graft passage via the PM portal into the tibial socket

Step 16: The knee is then moved through a cyclic range of motion multiple times, and the tensioning of the TightRope RT is performed again at both ends, keeping the knee in 90 degrees of flexion with the proximal end of the tibia thrust anteriorly.

Step 17: A final arthroscopy is then performed and probed for the position of the PCL (Fig. 20.13). Knots are tied over the buttons to prevent any slippage of the TightRope [14].

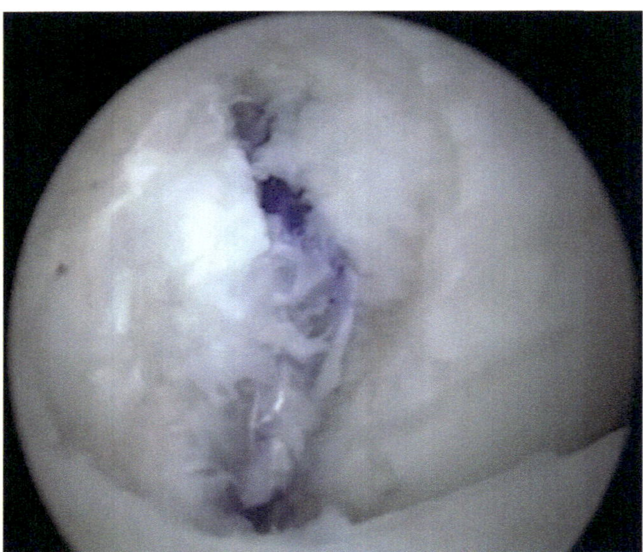

**Fig. 20.13** Reconstructed PCL

## 20.4 Advantage and Disadvantages of All-Inside PCL Reconstruction

### 20.4.1 Advantages

The technique overcomes the killer turn by passing the graft directly into the sockets from the Posteromedial Portal.

Anterolateral viewing with a 70° arthroscope allows visualization of both PCL stumps at the tibia and the femur.

Bony bridges with incomplete tunnels (sockets) allow for bone sparing.

Retrograde reaming with the Flip Cutter reduces the risk of injury to the neurovascular bundle.

There is a low risk of a tissue bridge or crossing over of shuttles.

Overcrowding of the joint space is prevented because graft is passed through the posteromedial portal.

Graft may be passed into either the femoral or tibial socket first, as per the surgeon's choice.

Suspensory fixation in sockets may reduce tunnel widening.

Simultaneous tensioning of both femoral and tibial suspensory systems is possible.

The technique can be used for graft passage in conventional PCL reconstructions.

Technique can be used for both single and double bundle reconstructions.

Useful in the pediatric population.

## 20.5 Limitations

Graft length is critical to prevent bottoming out of graft in sockets.

The posteromedial portal cannot be used for visualization of graft passage into sockets because graft is passed from this portal.

The inside-out technique for the femoral socket through the anterolateral portal leads to oblique tunnels, giving the appearance of the femoral socket being distal and posterior on radiographs (This can be overcome by the outside-in technique using the Flip Cutter).

Smaller semitendinosus graft may allow only a tripled graft instead of a quadrupled graft, leading to graft of smaller diameter (this can be overcome by attaching the gracilis (Fig. 20.14) to the semitendinosus is to increase the length to make a quadruple graft).

Injury to the saphenous vein and sartorial branch of the saphenous nerve may occur while making the posteromedial portal.

A postoperative X-ray is included for reference (Fig. 20.15)

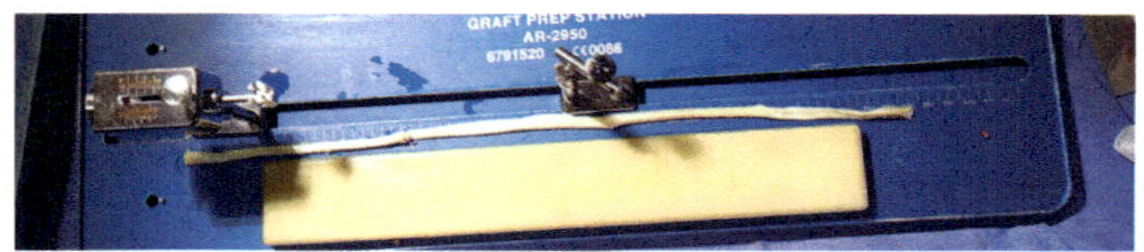

**Fig. 20.14** Gracillis attached to Semitendinosus to increase length

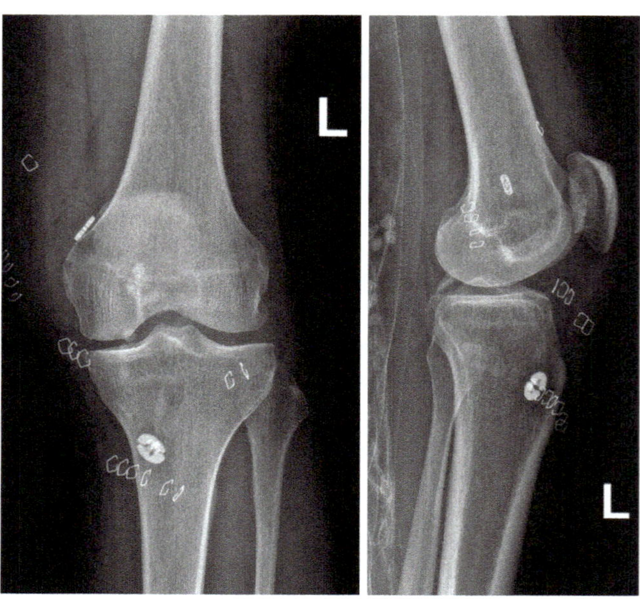


**Fig. 20.15** Immediate post operative X-rays

## References

1. Campbell RB, Jordan SS, Sekiya JK. Arthroscopic tibial inlay for posterior cruciate ligament reconstruction. Arthroscopy. 2007;23:1356.
2. Kim SJ, Kim TE, Jo SB, Kung YP. Comparison of the clinical results of three posterior cruciate ligament reconstruction techniques. J Bone Joint Surg Am. 2009;91:2543–9.
3. Fanelli GC, Beck JD, Edson CJ. Current concepts review: the posterior cruciate ligament. J Knee Surg. 2010;23(2):61–72.
4. Boynton MD, Tietjens BR. Long-term follow-up of the untreated isolated posterior cruciate ligament-deficient knee. Am J Sports Med. 1996;24(3):306–10.
5. Covey CD, Sapega AA. Injuries of the posterior cruciate ligament. J Bone Joint Surg Am. 1993;75(9):1376–86.
6. Dejour H, Walch G, Peyrot J, Eberhard P. The natural history of rupture of the posterior cruciate ligament. Rev Chir Orthop Réparatrice Appar Mot. 1988;74(1):35–43.
7. Keller PM, Shelbourne KD, McCarroll JR, Rettig AC. Nonoperatively treated isolated posterior cruciate ligament injuries. Am J Sports Med. 1993;21(1):132–6.
8. Anderson CJ, Ziegler CG, Wijdicks CA, et al. Arthroscopically pertinent anatomy of the anterolateral and posteromedial bundles of the posterior cruciate ligament. J Bone Joint Surg Am. 2012;94:1936–45.
9. Adler GG. All-inside posterior cruciate ligament reconstruction with a GraftLink. Arthrosc Tech. 2013;2:e111–5.
10. Slullitel D, Galan H, Ojeda V, Seri M. Double-bundle "all inside" posterior cruciate ligament reconstruction. Arthrosc Tech. 2012;1:e141–8.
11. Lubowitz JH, Amhad CH, Anderson K. All-inside anterior cruciate ligament graft-link technique: Second generation, no-incision anterior cruciate ligament reconstruction. Arthroscopy. 2011;27:717–27.
12. Benea H, d'Astorg H, Klouche S, Bauer T, Tomoaia G, Hardy P. Pain evaluation after all-inside anterior cruciate ligament reconstruction and short term functional results of a prospective randomised study. Knee. 2014;21:102–6.
13. Noonan BC, Dines JS, Allen AA, et al. Biomechanical evaluation of an adjustable loop suspensory anterior cruciate ligament reconstruction fixation device: the value of retensioning and knot tying. Arthroscopy. 2016;32(10):2050–9.
14. Vasdev A, Rajgopal A, Gupta H, et al. Arthroscopic all-inside posterior cruciate ligament reconstruction: overcoming the "killer turn". Arthrosc Tech. 2016;5:e501–6.

# 21 Arthroscopic Trapdoor Technique of Fixing a PCL Avulsion

Vikram Arun Mhaskar

## 21.1 Introduction

This technique involves fixing the posterior cruciate ligament (PCL) when it avulses off the tibia with a piece of bone. It can be used for both large and small fragment avulsions. Fixing the PCL avulsion back anatomically requires proper visualization of the footprint that cannot be provided adequately with just viewing it from the anterior aspect of the knee. Another important aspect of the technique is to manipulate the instruments and jigs to their correct location that is difficult to do when just a single portal is made posteriorly. This technique also uses few cost effective implants to fix the fragment back in place. A variation in the technique has also been described that uses just suture tapes and no metallic implants.

## 21.2 Special Equipment Required (Fig. 21.1)

1. 7 mm arthroscopic cannulae-2 (Arthrex, Naples, FL) (q)
2. Flexible cannula (Passport Cannula)-1 (Arthrex, Naples, FL)
3. Vissinger rod-1 (c)
4. Knee scorpion/suture passers-1 (Arthrex, Naples, FL) (h)
5. PDS suture/Fiberwire 2-0 (Arthrex, Naples, FL) (o)
6. Suture tape (Arthrex, Naples, FL) (p)
7. No 5 ethibond-2 (Ethicon, Rariton, NJ)
8. Knot pusher-1 (Arthrex, Naples, FL) (n)
9. PCL jig (Arthrex, Naples, FL) (i)
10. Guide wires (Arthrex, Naples, FL) (l)
11. 4.5 mm drill bit (Arthrex, Naples, FL) (d)

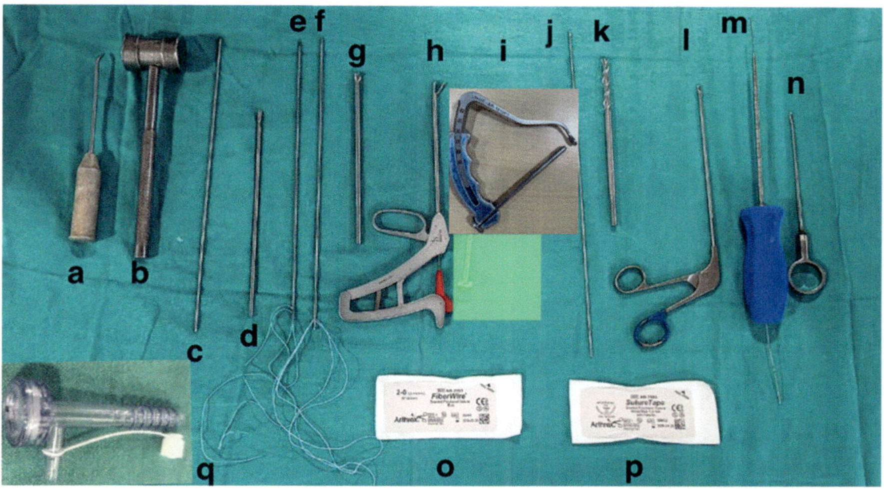


**Fig. 21.1** Instruments used (c) Vissinger rod (d) 4.5mm drill bit (e) Beath pin with No5 Ethibond loop (h) Knee Scorpion (i) PCL jig set at 70 degrees (j) Guidewire (l) Suture manipulator (n) Knot Pusher (o) 2-0 Fiberwire (p) Suture tape (q) 7 mm cannula

V. A. Mhaskar (✉)
F7 East of Kailash, Knee & Shoulder Clinic, New Delhi, India

JMVM Sports Injury Center, Sitaram Bhartia Institute of Science & Research, New Delhi, India


V. A. Mhaskar, J. Maheshwari (eds.), *Innovative Approaches in Knee Arthroscopy*,
https://doi.org/10.1007/978-981-99-4378-4_21

## 21.3 Positioning

The patient is positioned supine on an operating table with a bolster at the foot end and a side support, so as to position the knee at 70° flexion.

The key to this step is to have adequate access to the back of the knee both on the posteromedial and posterolateral aspect (Fig. 21.2).

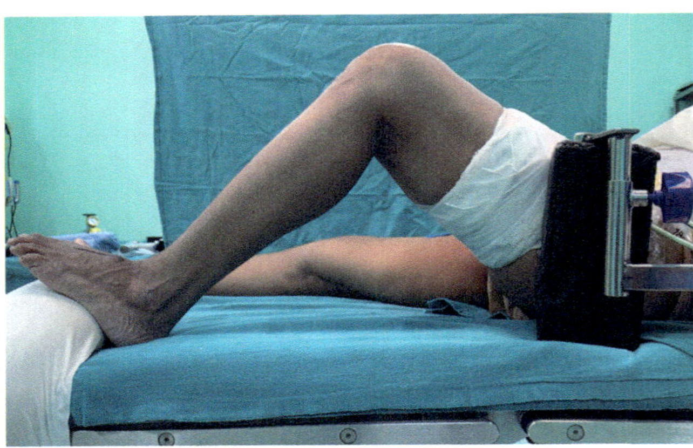

**Fig. 21.2** The knee in 70 degrees flexion with a side support and bolster at the foot

## 21.4 Draping

The draping is done in the standard way so as to have the upper 1/3 of the tibia and the distal 1/3 of the thigh exposed (Fig. 21.3)

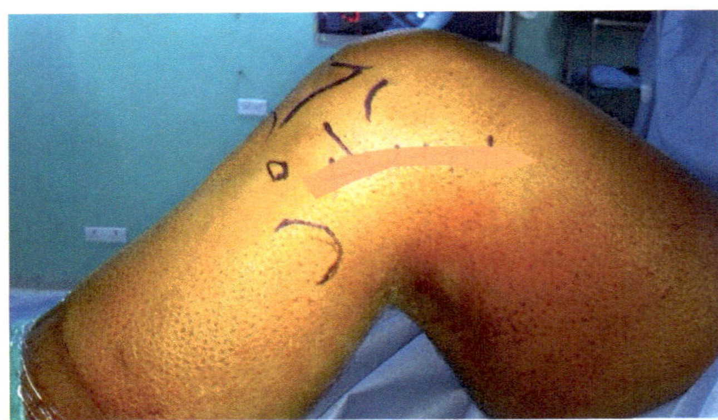

**Fig. 21.3** The knee draped such that distal 1/3 of the thigh and proximal 1/3 of the leg exposed and adequate access to posterior aspect of the knee

## 21.5 Portals

1. A standard horizontal anterolateral viewing portal (AL) is made at the soft spot about 5 mm lateral to the lateral border of the patellar tendon (Fig. 21.4a)
2. Another antero medial (AM) horizontal portal is made at the same level for manipulation of the knee scorpion and suture management anteriorly (Fig. 21.4a).
3. A high posteromedial (PM) portal just above the posteromedial fold of synovial tissue is made and acts as a working portal in the back of the knee, helping in suture management and tying knots posteriorly (Fig. 21.4b).
4. A posterolateral (PL) portal made by the inside out transseptal technique such that it is at the level of the PM portal or just lower to it and should be above the biceps femoris tendon (Fig. 21.4c).

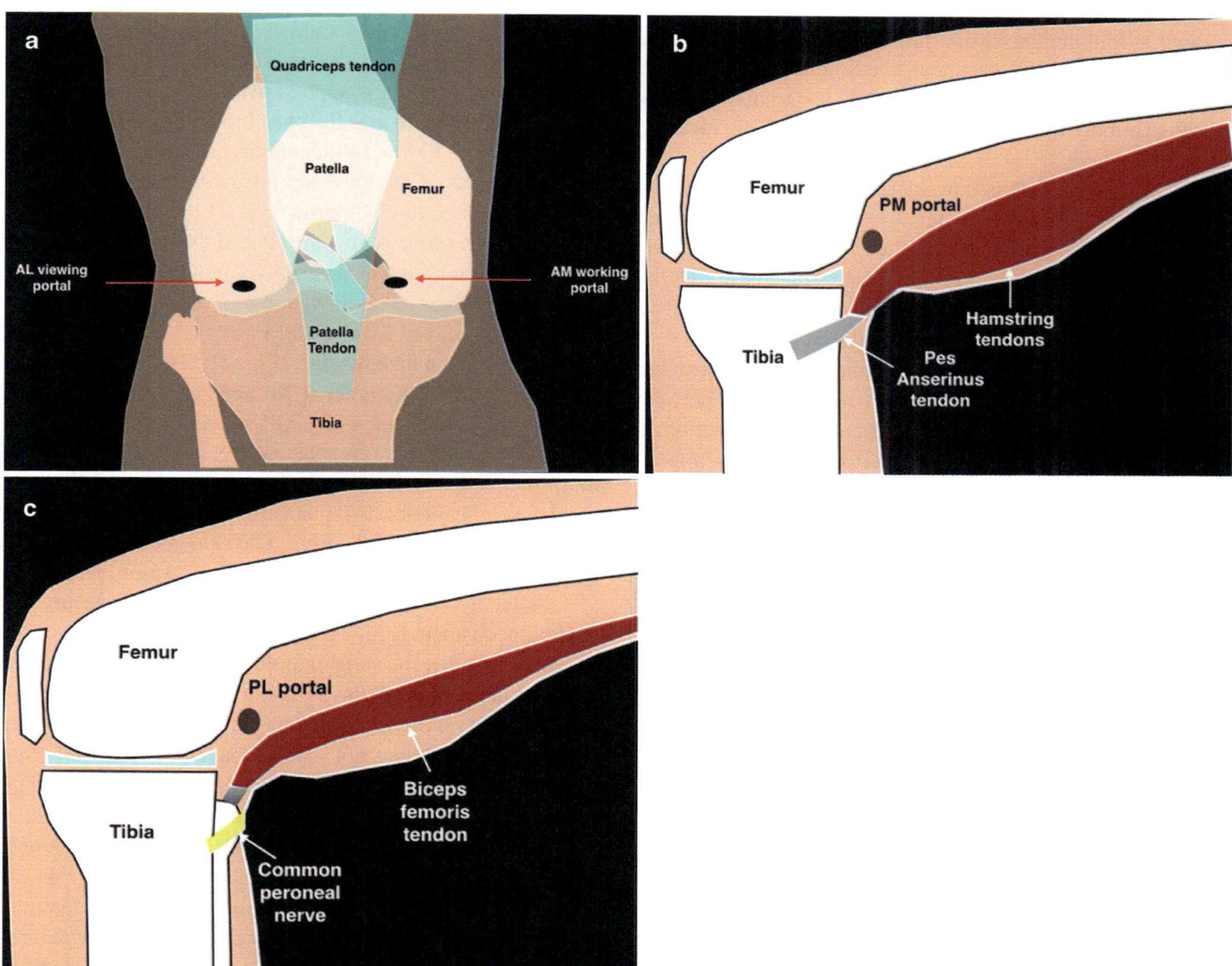


**Fig. 21.4** (**a**) Illustration of the knee from front showing the AL viewing and AM working portals made at the soft spot. (**b**) Illustration of the knee from the medial side showing the PM portal position. (**c**) Illustration of the knee from the lateral side showing PL portal made above the biceps femoris tendon and common peroneal nerve

## 21.6 Surgical Steps

Step 1: A standard anterolateral portal (AL) is made at the soft spot lateral to the patellar tendon which is used as a viewing portal for the anterior compartment. An anteromedial portal is made in the soft spot medial to the patellar tendon and is used as a working portal in the anterior compartment (Fig. 21.4a).

Step 2: The arthroscope is introduced into the posteromedial compartment by manipulating the scope through the PCL and medial femoral condyle (Fig. 21.5).

Step 3: Making the PM portal: Once the arthroscope is in the posteromedial compartment it is important to visualize the synovial fold that acts as the lighthouse to make the PM portal. Turning the camera cable to view more medially helps in doing this.

An 18 G LP needle is introduced such that it is above the synovial fold as it is easier to introduce the cannula (Fig. 21.6a). A 1 cm incision is then made vertically at this level (Fig. 21.6b). A Vissinger rod is introduced through this and a 6.5 mm cannula applied over it such that two threads of the cannula at least are protruding inside (Fig. 21.6c).

Step 5: Viewing through the anterolateral portal, a shaver is introduced through the AM portal and the space between the ACL and PCL is cleared from the anterior aspect of the notch till the end of the notch posteriorly and the septum is removed. The scope is then re-introduced between the ACL and medial femoral condyle (MFC) to the PM compartment and a shaver introduced through the PM portal to remove the rest of the septum (Fig. 21.7a–e).

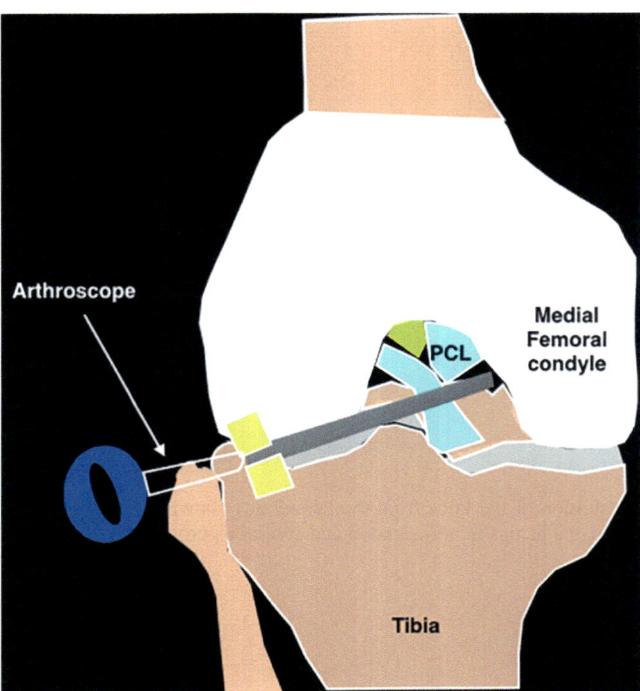


**Fig. 21.5** Arthroscope introduced through the AL portal and manipulated to the posterior compartment of the knee between the PCL and medial femoral condyle

Step 6: Making a trans-septal portal: The arthroscope is then introduced to the posterior aspect of the knee in between the ACL and PCL using the AL portal. A Vissinger rod is introduced through the PM portal (Fig. 21.8a, b). The rod is visualized and the knee is placed in 110° flexion, then under vision it is advanced to the posterolateral compartment of the knee, just along and touching the lateral femoral condyle. This is further advanced till the tip of the rod is seen projecting from the skin above the biceps femoris tendon on the posterolateral aspect of the knee (Fig. 21.8c). A 1 cm incision is made over it and a 6.5 mm cannula is applied over it (Fig. 21.8d) and the rod removed. Only then is the knee brought into 70° flexion.

Step 7: Both PM and PL cannulas can then be seen in the posterior aspect of the knee when viewing between the ACL and PCL through the AL portal (Fig. 21.9a, b).

Step 8: The scope is now introduced through the PL portal and the avulsed fragment is visualized end on (Fig. 21.10a, b).

Step 9: A shaver followed by a radiofrequency (RF) device is introduced from the PM portal is used to clear the footprint and visualize it better (Fig. 21.11a–c).

Step 10: A PCL jig is set at 70° and is introduced through the anteromedial portal while still viewing from the PL portal and advanced between the ACL and PCL to the tibial footprint of the PCL. The jig is positioned just below the tibial footprint of the PCL and the bullet is applied to the anteromedial aspect of the tibia. The skin is incised from the point where the bullet touched the skin, 3 cm proximally. The bullet is advanced to touch the bone and secure the ratchet mechanism (Fig. 21.12a–c).

Step 11: While the surgeon holds the PCL jig in place, the assistant drills through the jig using a guide wire. The tip of the jig sitting on the footprint has a trap mechanism to make sure the guide pin does not advance beyond it. It is, however, important to hold the jig steadily while the drilling is happening. The tip of the jig is constantly visualized while the drilling process is happening and the tip of the guidewire is seen (Fig. 21.13a–c).

Step 12: The trap mechanism is secured over the tip of the guide wire and held in place while the bullet on the anteromedial aspect of the tibia is disengaged. This is done to accommodate the 4.5 mm drill bit over the drill bit and prevent the guidewire from advancing. The 4.5 mm drill bit is then cannulated over the guidewire and the tibia is drilled while keeping the tip of the guidewire secure with the PCL jig (Fig. 21.14a–d).

Step 13: A Beath pin with an Ethibond loop is passed through the tunnel from the anteromedial aspect of the tibia to the tibia footprint. A suture manipulator is introduced from the PM portal and the loop is delivered into the PM cannula (Fig. 21.15a, b).

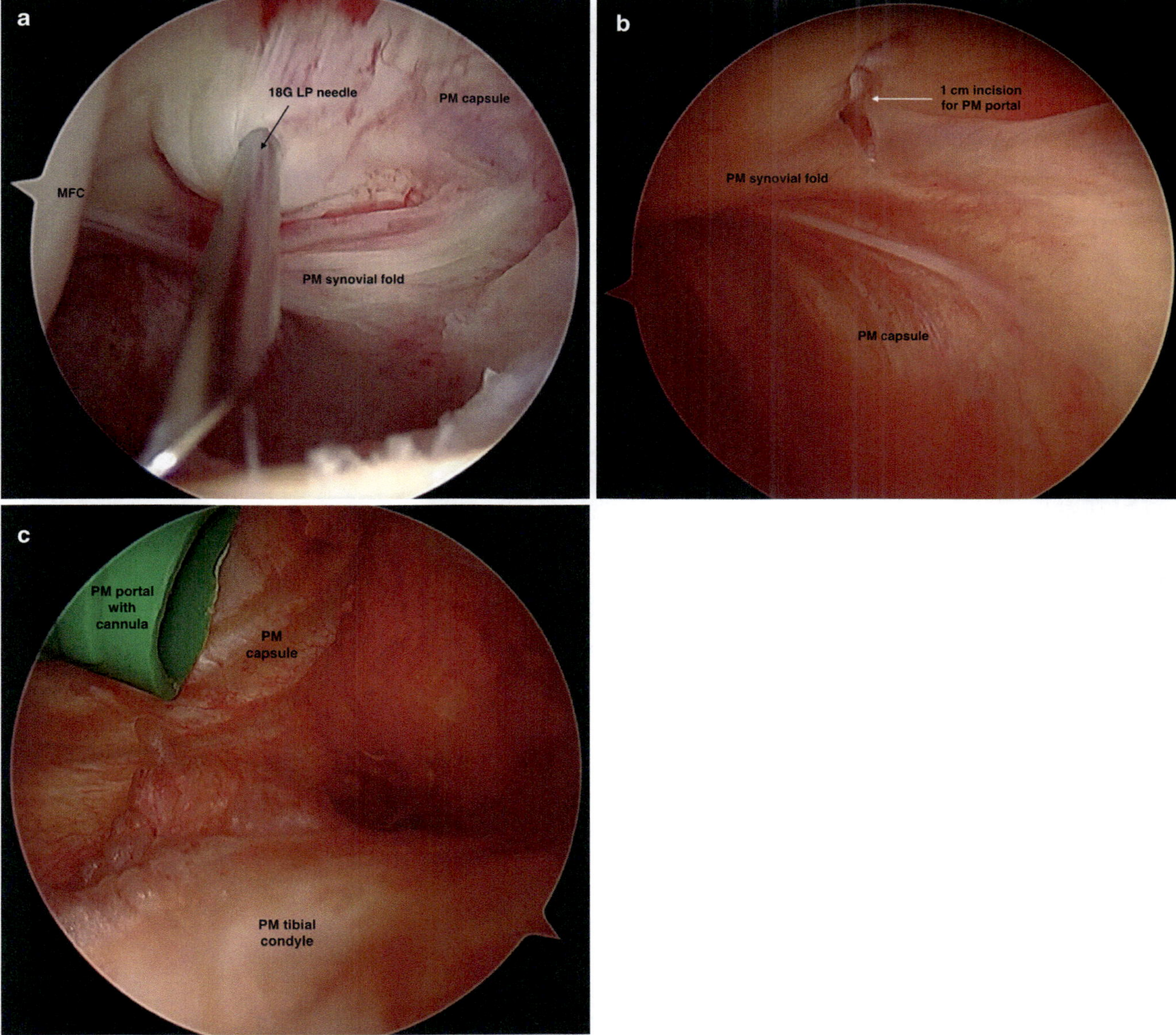


**Fig. 21.6** (**a**) View of PM aspect of the knee viewing through AL portal showing an 18 G LP needle is introduced just above the synovial fold to localize the portal position. (**b**) View of PM aspect of the knee with scope through AL portal showing a 1 cm portal incision made at the level of the LP needle introduced above the synovial fold. (**c**) View of PM aspect of the knee with scope in AL portal showing a 6.5 mm cannula introduced through the incision for the PM portal

Step 14: The arthroscope is now introduced through the AL portal. A flexible passport cannula is introduced into the AM portal (Fig. 21.16).

Step 15: A Knee Scorpion (Antegrade suture passer) is loaded with a 2-0 Fiber wire and a bite is taken through the mid substance of the PCL. This Fiberwire is used to shuttle a Suture Tape through it. Another bite is taken just distal to the previous bite with the 2-0 Fiberwire and one end of the Fiberwire is used to shuttle one end of the suture tape. This forms a knot like configuration of the suture tape around the PCL (Fig. 21.17a–d).

Bites can also be taken through the PCL using a suture passer with PDS to shuttle a suture tape.

Step 16: One end of the Suture Tape is held with a grasper and taken to the PM part of the knee between the PCL and MFC while visualizing through the AL portal. Once posterior, the grasper is shifted to the PM portal and the end delivered through it (Fig. 21.18a, b)

Step 17: The same is repeated for the other end of the suture that is passed between the ACL and PCL, with this end also delivered through the PM portal (Fig. 21.19a, b).

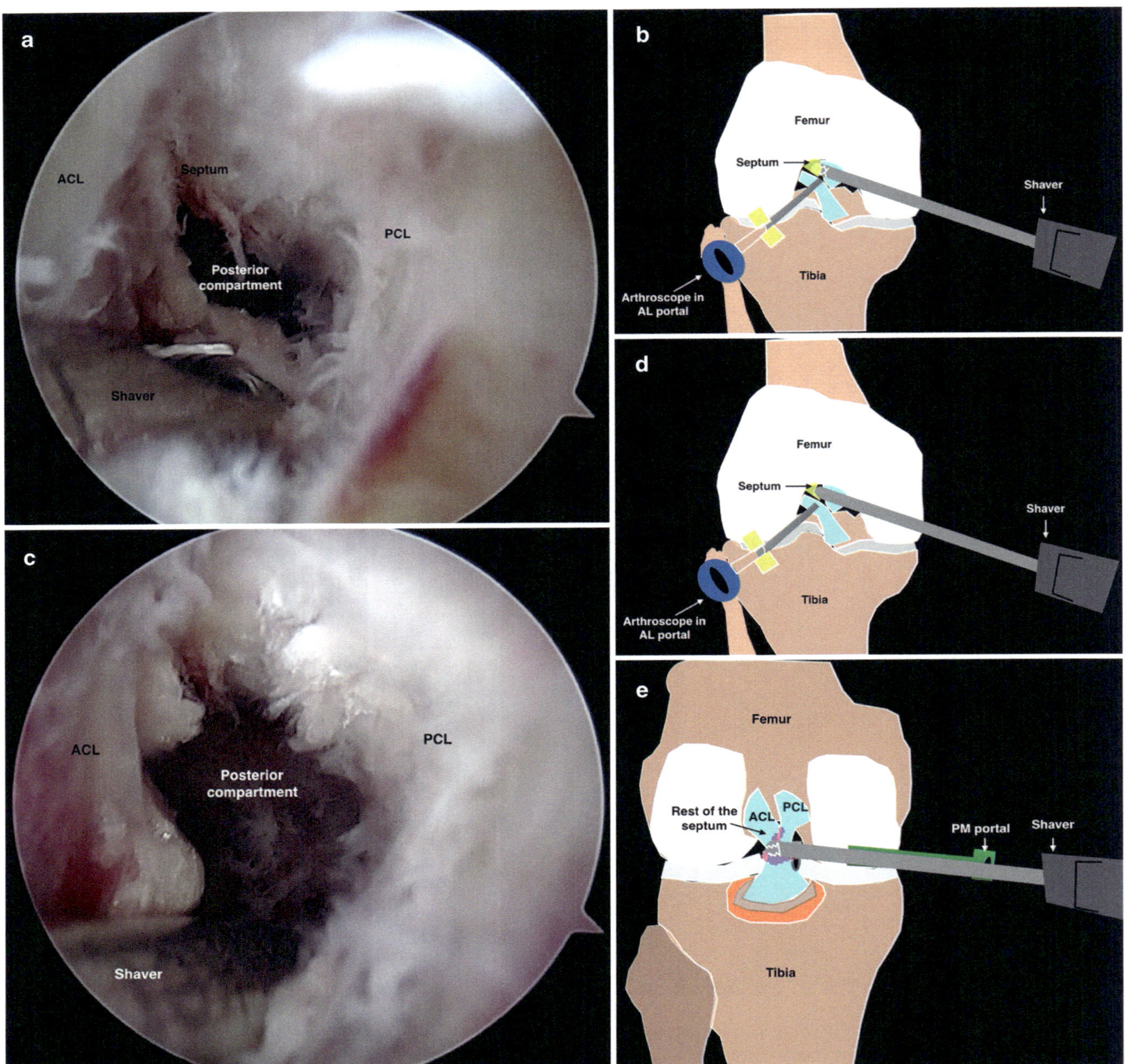


**Fig. 21.7** (**a**) View of the space between ACL and PCL with scope through AL portal and a shaver through AM portal removing the septum and fat between ACL and PCL. (**b**) Illustration of the front of the knee with scope through AL portal and shaver through AM portal shaving the septum and fat pad between ACL and PCL. (**c**) View of the posterior compartment between the ACL and PCL after removing the septum with the scope in the AL portal. (**d**) Illustration of the knee showing removal of the septum between the ACL and PCL while viewing from the AL portal and shaver from the AM portal. (**e**) Illustration of the posterior aspect of the knee with the scope through the AL portal between the PCL and MFC and the shaver through the PM portal removing the rest of the septum posteriorly

Step 18. The scope is now shifted to the PL portal. The PM portal now contains the Ethibond loop and the two ends of the Suture Tape. The two ends are applied to an arthroscopic knot pusher and multiple simple knots are tied around the PCL such that they are tight but do not strangle the PCL. At least 4–5 knots should be tied (Fig. 21.20a, b).

Step 19: The two ends of the suture tape in the PM portal are then looped through the Ethibond loop. The Ethibond is then pulled from the anteromedial tunnel and the loop with the two suture tapes are delivered anteromedially (Fig. 21.21a, b).

Step 20: While viewing from the PL portal a grasper is used to manipulate the two ends of suture over the frag-

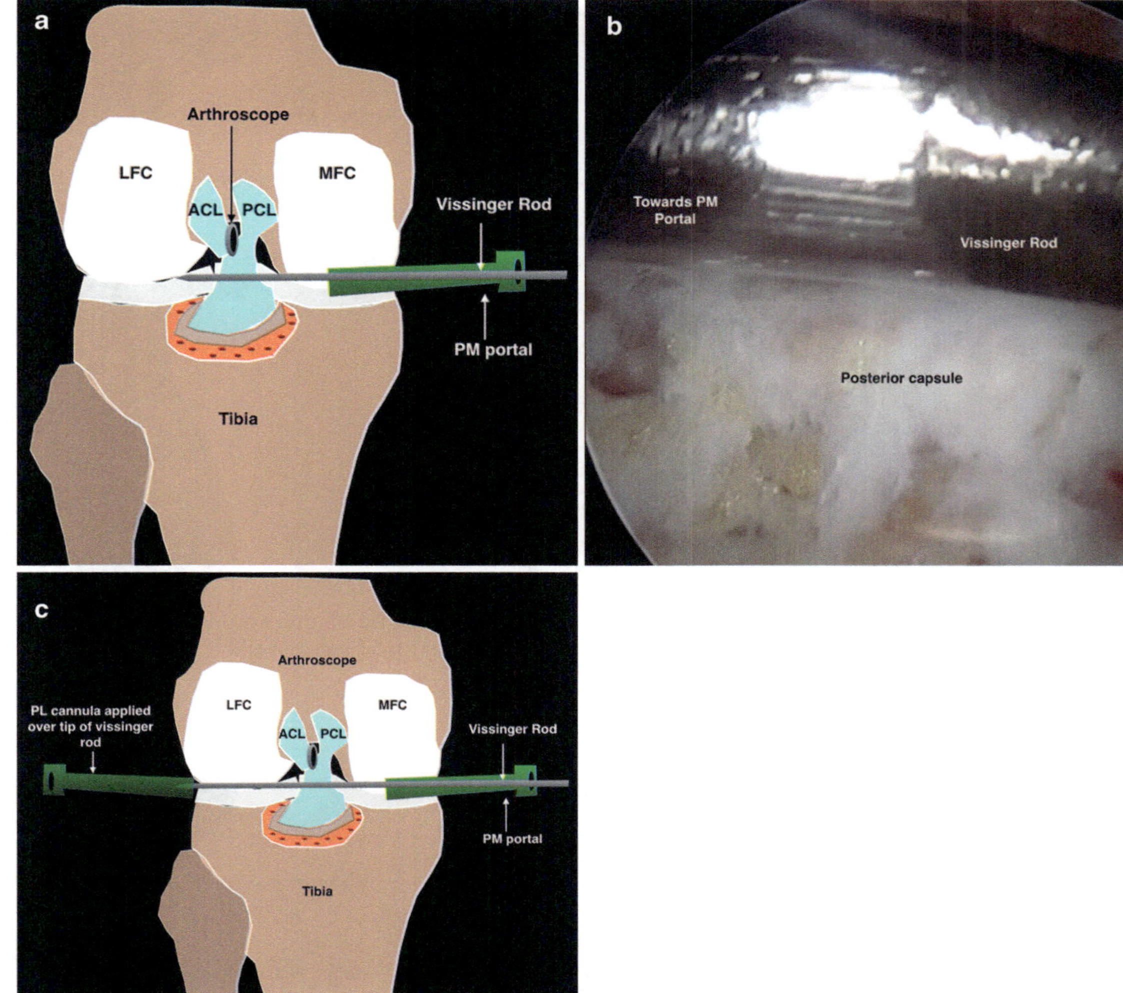


**Fig. 21.8** (**a**) Illustration of the posterior aspect of the knee with the scope between the ACL and PCL and a Vissinger rod introduced through the PM portal along the MFC towards the PL aspect. (**b**) View of the posterior aspect of the knee with scope through the AL portal between the ACL and PCL showing the Vissinger rod going from the PM and PL aspect of the knee along the MFC and LFC. (**c**) Illustration of the posterior aspect of the knee with the scope through the AL portal between the ACL and PCL showing the Vissinger rod coming out through the PL aspect of the knee and a 6.5 mm cannula applied over it and the knee in 110° flexion

ment such that they produce a uniform compression to make the avulsed fragment sit anatomically when traction is applied over the two ends anteromedially (Fig. 21.22a, b).

Step 21: The two ends are then tied over an ABS button with multiple simple knots (at least 4) anteromedially while viewing the fragment from the PL portal to make sure it does not shatter or displace (Fig. 21.23a, b).

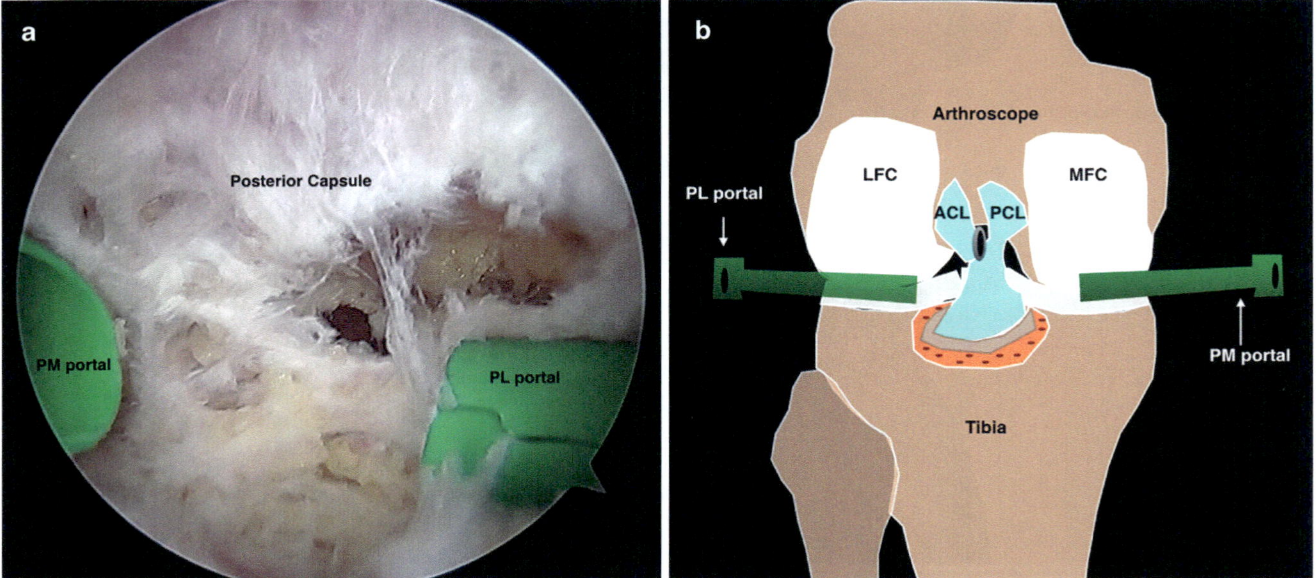


**Fig. 21.9** (**a**) View of the posterior aspect of the knee with the scope through the AL portal and between the ACL and PCL showing the PM and PL 6.5 mm cannulas. (**b**) Illustration of the posterior aspect of the knee with the scope through the AL portal and between the ACL and PCL showing the PM and PL 6.5 mm cannulas

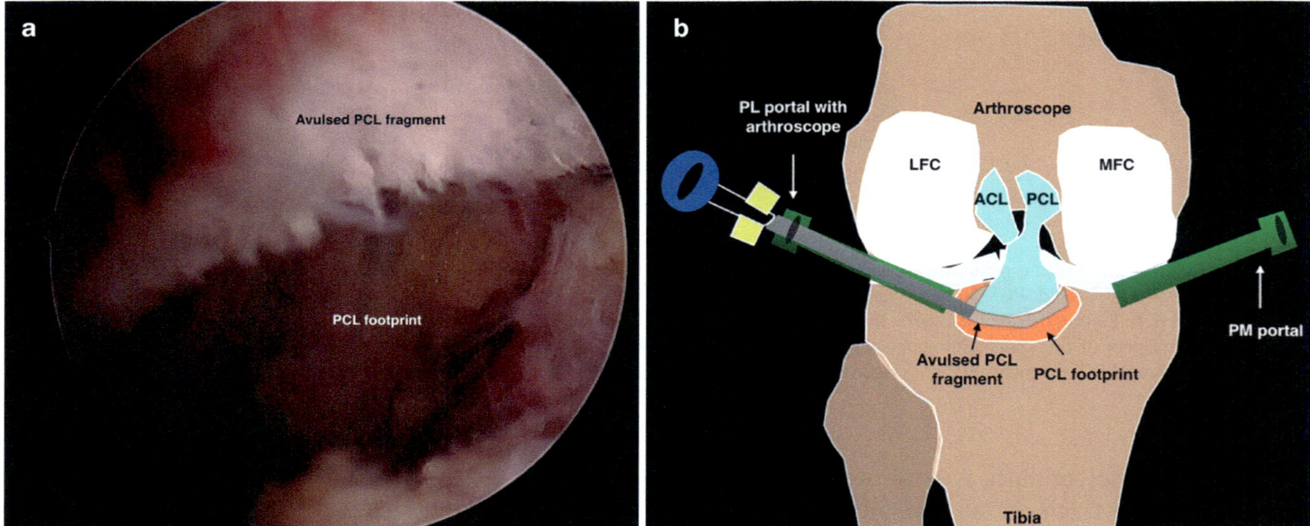


**Fig. 21.10** (**a**) View of the PCL avulsion from the tibia with the scope in the PL portal. (**b**) Illustration of the posterior aspect of the knee with the scope through PL portal viewing the tibial PCL avulsion

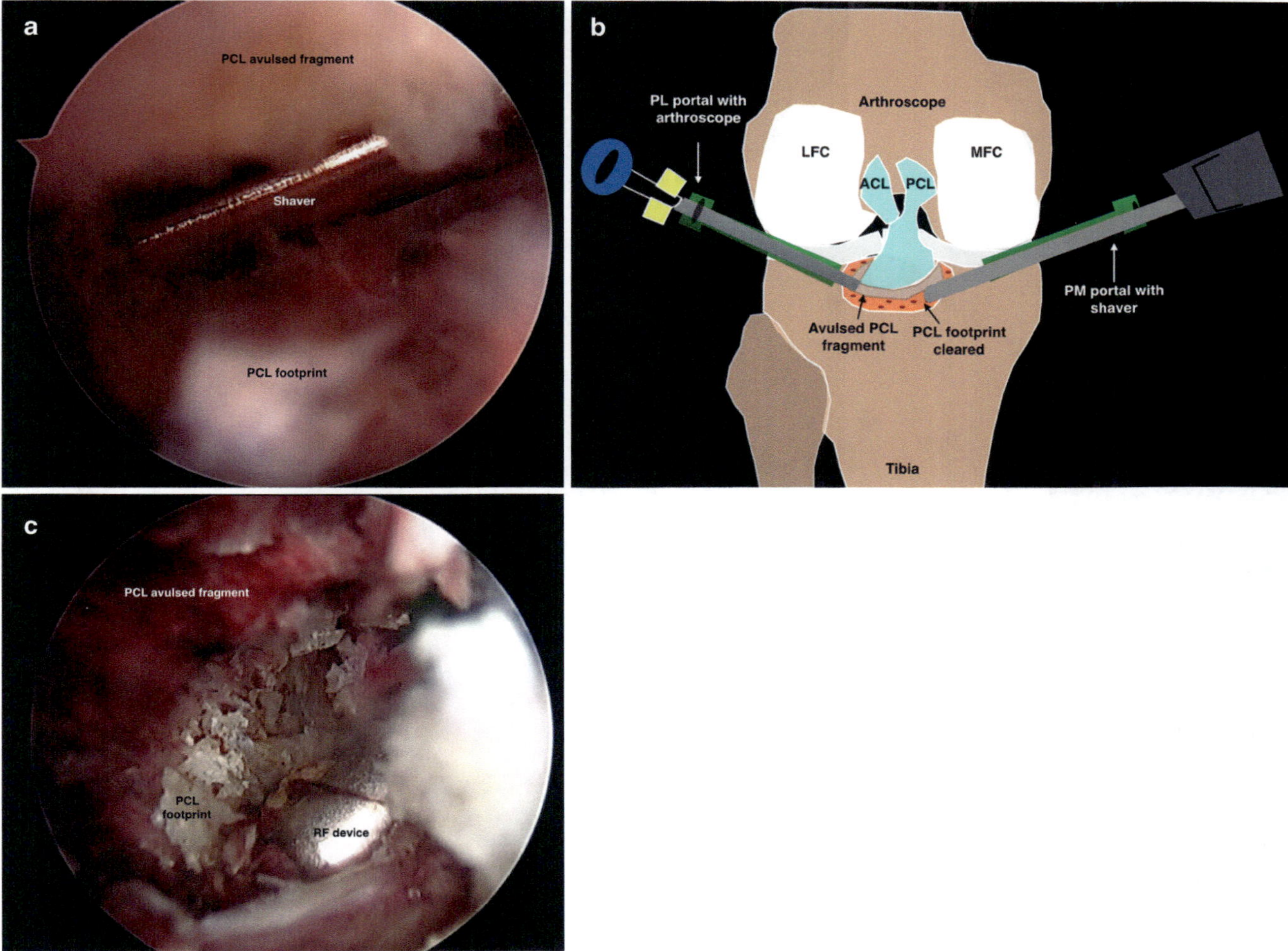


**Fig. 21.11** (**a**) View of the PCL footprint on the tibia with the scope through the PL portal and a shaver introduced through the PM portal to clear the footprint. (**b**) Illustration of the posterior aspect of the knee with the scope through the PL portal and shaver through the PM portal clearing the PCL footprint on the tibia. (**c**) View of the PCL footprint on the tibia with the scope through the PL portal and a RF introduced through the PM portal to clear the footprint

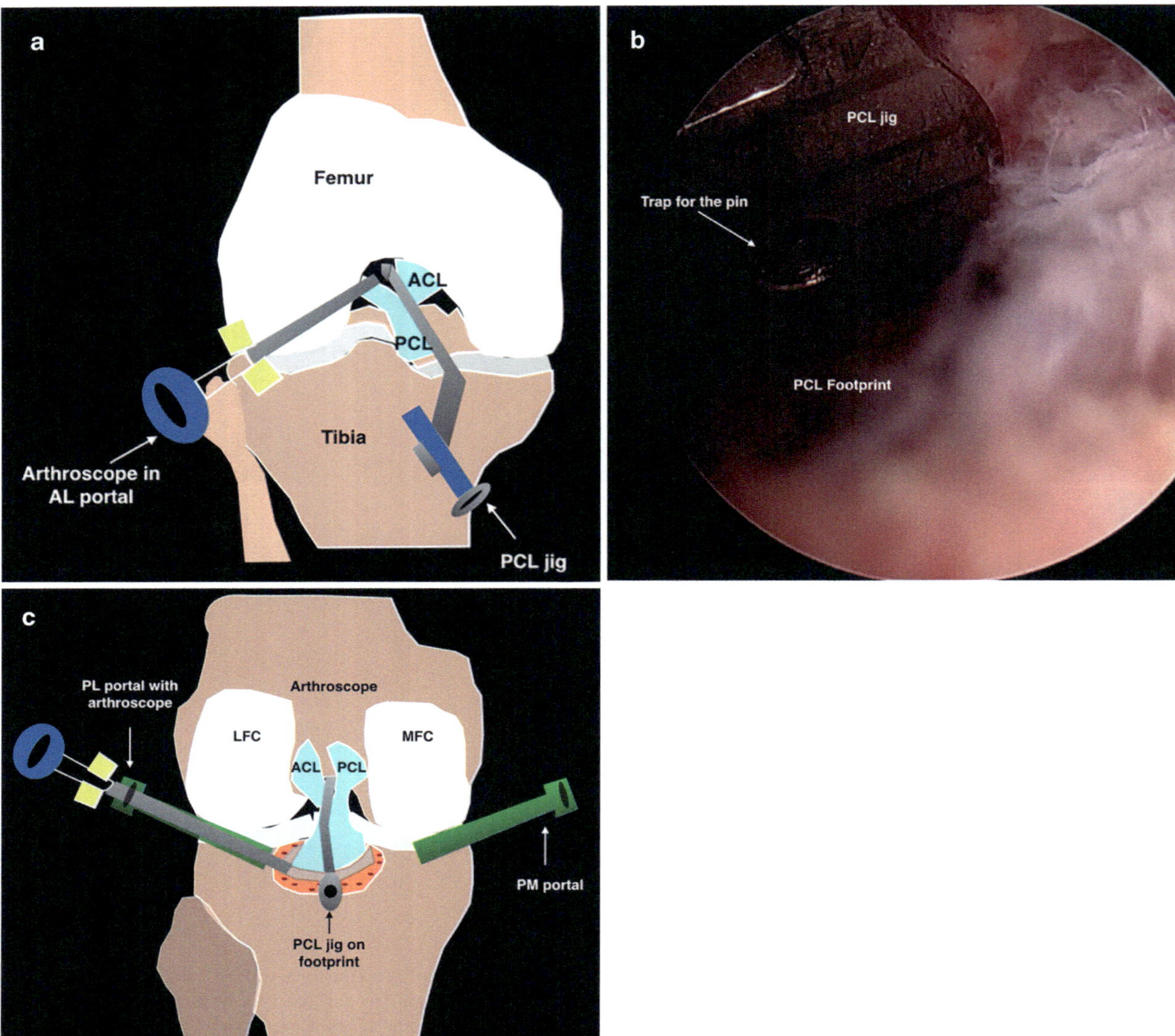


**Fig. 21.12** (**a**) Illustration of the anterior aspect of the knee with the scope through the AL portal and PCL jig introduced through the AM portal and applied to the PCL footprint by manipulating it between the ACL and PCL. (**b**) View of the PCL jig on the tibial footprint with scope in the PL portal. (**c**) Illustration of the posterior aspect of the knee showing the PCL jig on the tibial footprint of the PCL and scope through the PL portal

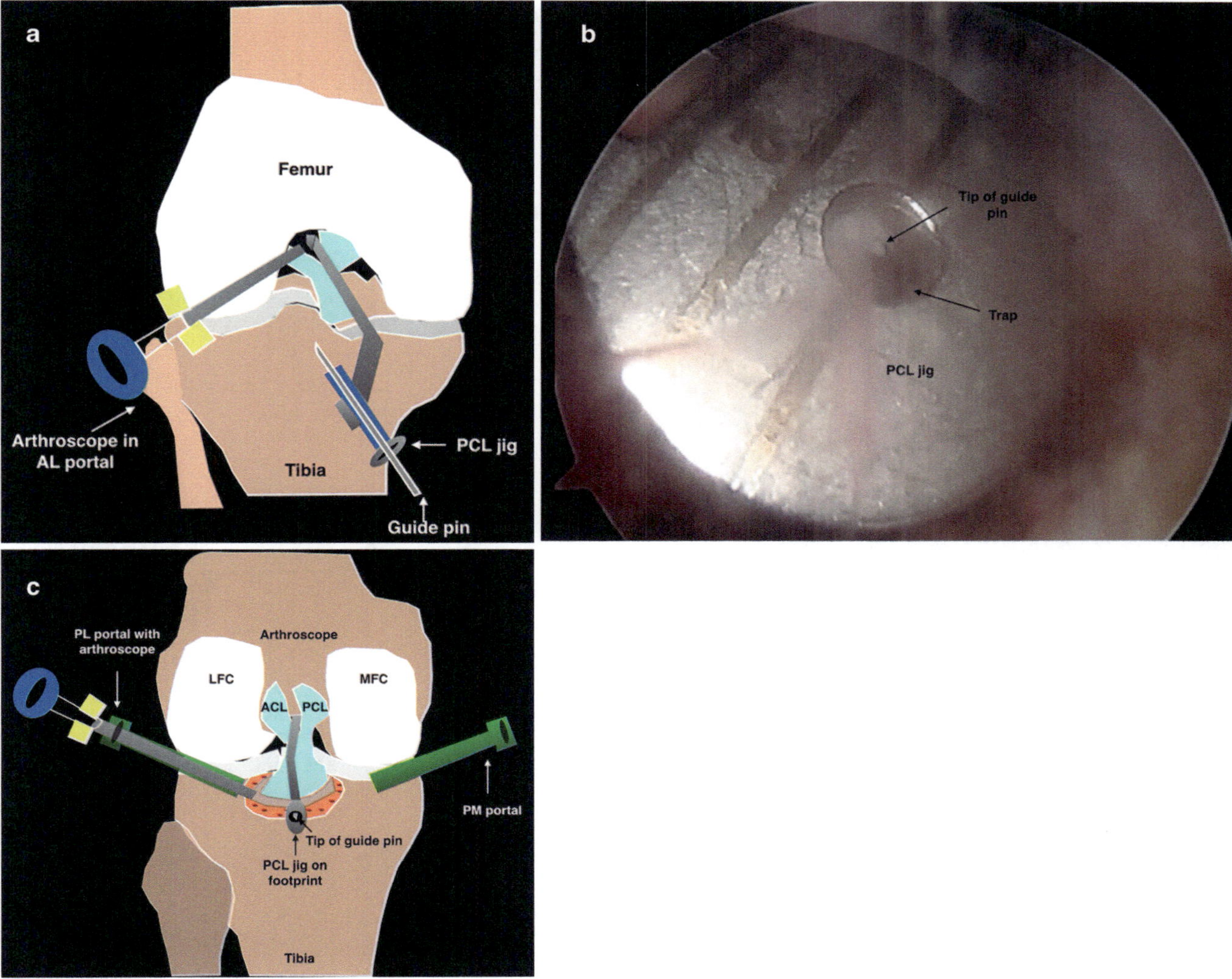


**Fig. 21.13** (**a**) Illustration of the anterior aspect of the knee with PCL jig bullet applied to the AM aspect of the knee and a guidewire drilled from AM to posterior aspect of the knee. (**b**) View of the guidewire coming out of the center of the trap on the PCL jig posteriorly with the scope in the PL portal. (**c**) Illustration of the posterior aspect of the knee showing the guide wire coming out of the center of the trap on the PCL jig with scope in the PL portal

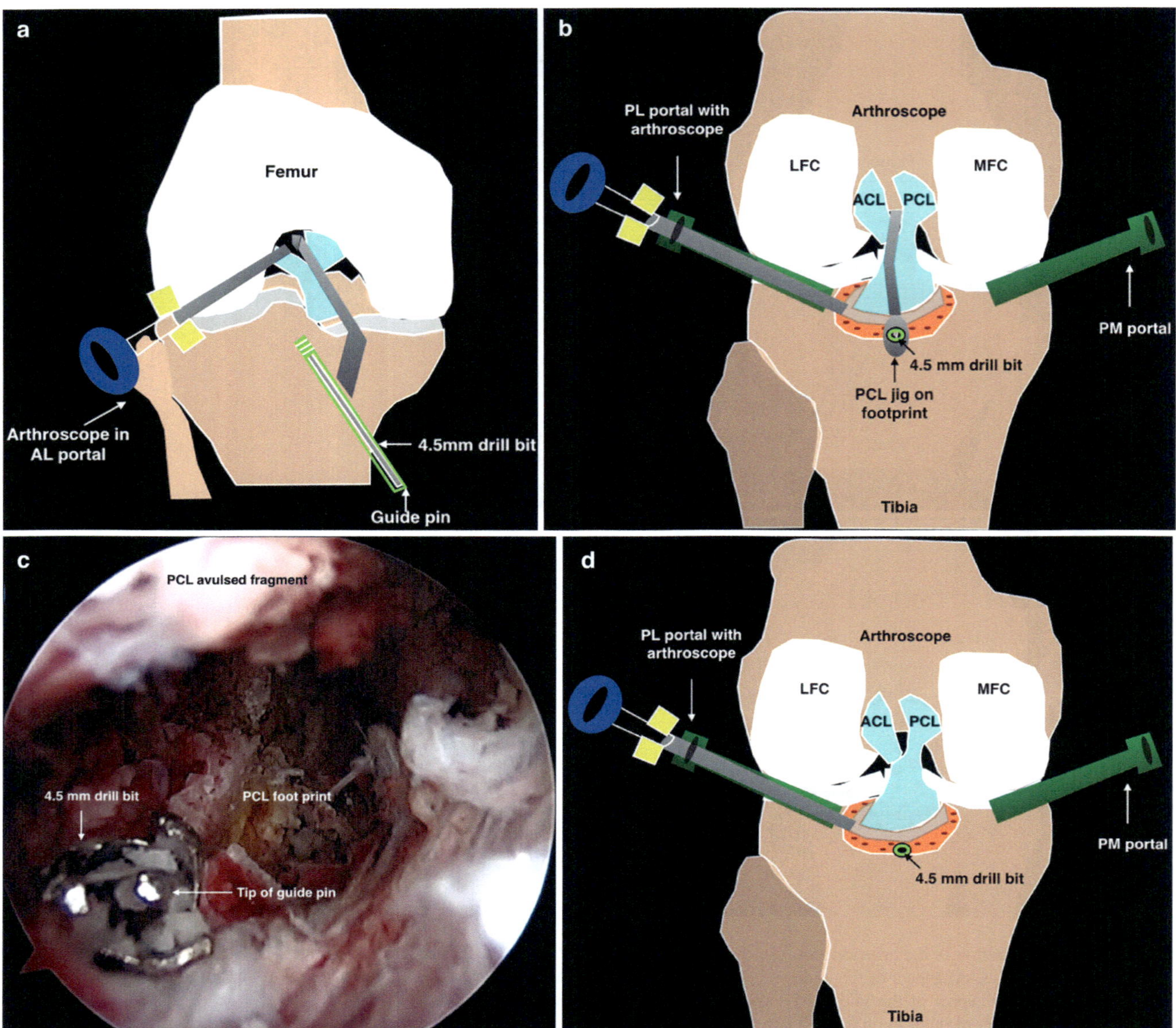


**Fig. 21.14** (a) Illustration of the tibial tunnel drilled with a 4.5 mm drill bit from the AM aspect of tibia to the center of the tibial footprint of the PCL, scope through the AL portal between the ACL and PCL. (**b**) Tibial foot print drilled with 4.5 mm drill bit with scope in PL portal and trap of the PCL jig over tip of guide wire to prevent migration of the wire. (**c**) View of the PCL tibial footprint showing the tip of the guidewire and 4.5 mm drill bit at the center of the footprint with scope through the PL portal. (**d**) Illustration of the back of the knee showing PCL footprint and 4.5 mm drill bit at the center of it and scope in the PL portal

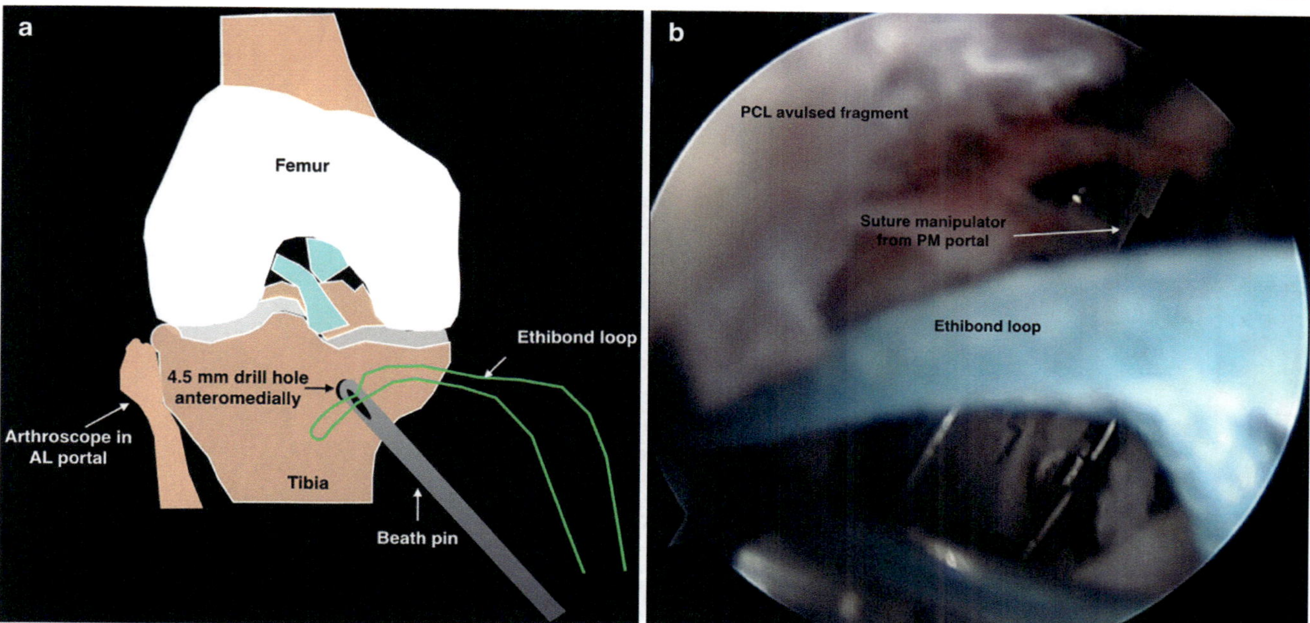


**Fig. 21.15** (**a**) Illustration of anterior aspect of the knee with Beath pin carrying an Ethibond loop being introduced through the tibial tunnel orifice on the AM aspect of the tibia. (**b**) Ethibond loop delivered through the PCL tibial footprint 4.5 mm tunnel and being held by a suture manipulator, scope through the PL portal

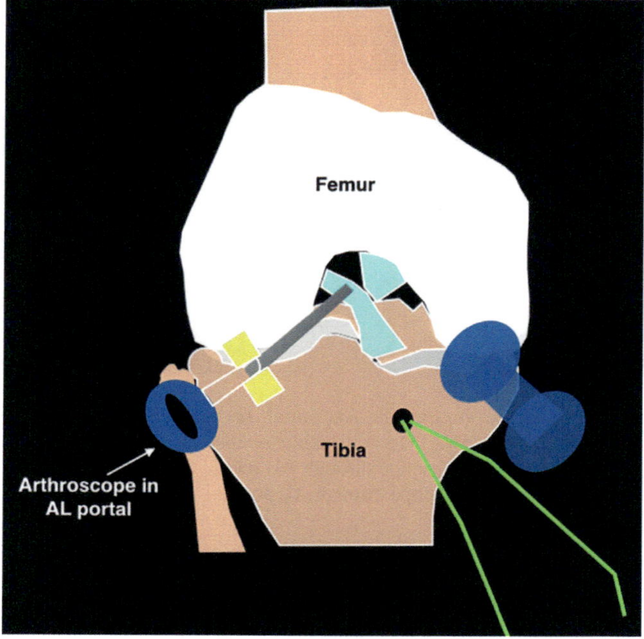


**Fig. 21.16** Illustration of anterior aspect of the knee showing Passport Cannula through the AM portal, scope through the AL portal and Ethibond suture ends through the tibial tunnel on the AM aspect of the tibia

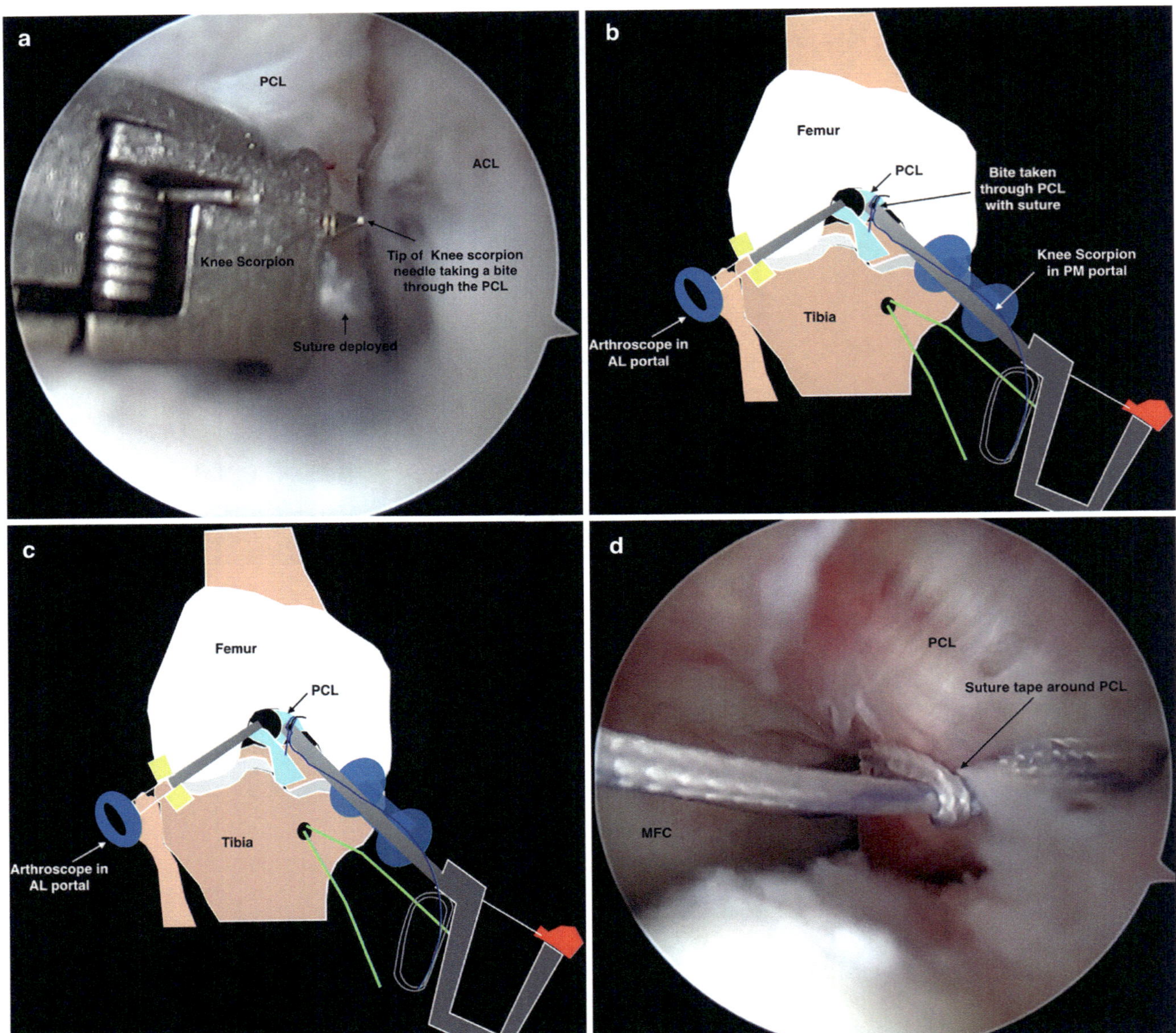


**Fig. 21.17** (**a**) Arthroscopic image showing the Knee Scorpion taking a bite through the PCL showing the tip of the needle that is carrying a 2-0 Fiberwire. Knee scorpion through the Passport Cannula, scope through the AL portal. (**b**) Illustration of the anterior aspect of the knee showing a Knee Scorpion taking a bite through the PCL with a 2-0 Fiberwire, scope through the AL portal. (**c**) Knee Scorpion through Passport Cannula in AM portal taking second bite through the PCL using a 2-0 Fiberwire, scope through AL portal. (**d**) Knot around PCL with Suture Tape and scope through AL portal

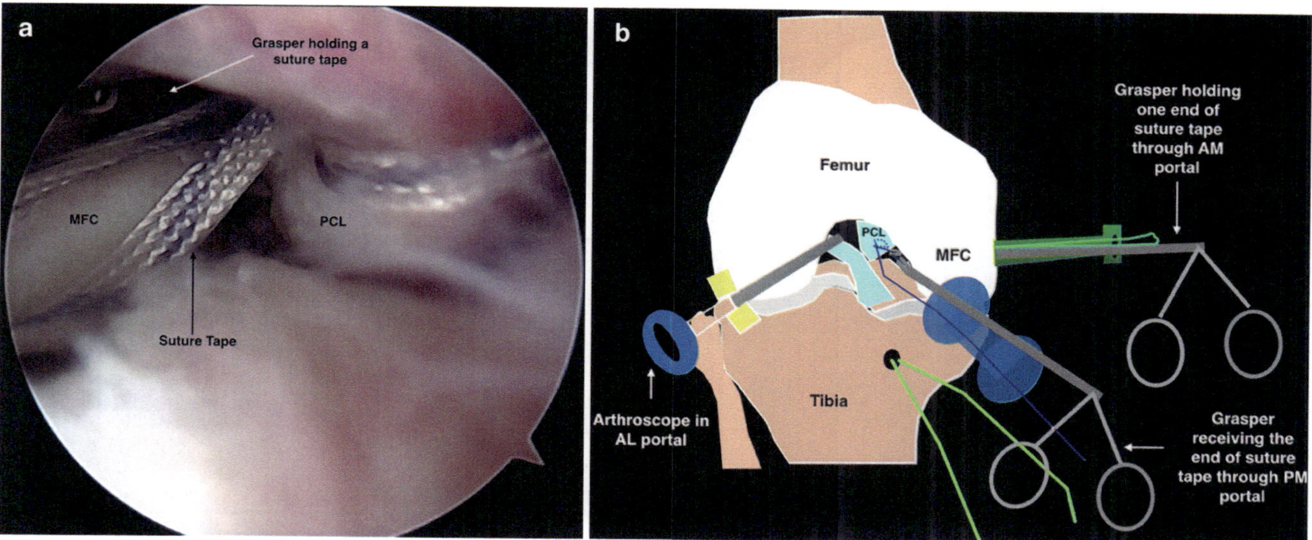


**Fig. 21.18** (**a**) One end of the Suture Tape being taken to the posterior aspect of the knee between the MFC and PCL using a grasper introduced through the AM portal and scope through the AL portal. (**b**) Illustration of the anterior aspect of the knee showing one end of the Suture Tape being taken to the posterior aspect of the knee between the PCL and MFC using a grasper through the AM portal and a grasper introduced through the PM portal posteriorly retrieving it through the PM portal, scope through the AL portal

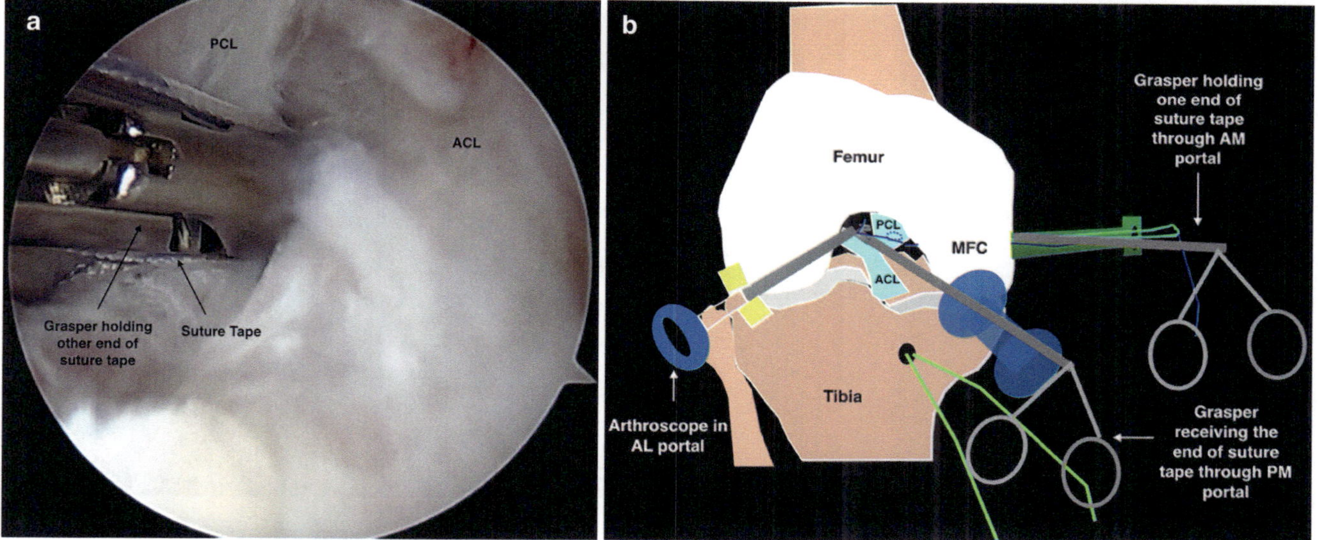


**Fig. 21.19** (**a**) The other end of the Suture Tape held by a grasper in the AM portal and delivered to the posterior aspect of the knee between the ACL and PCL, scope through the AL portal. (**b**) Illustration of the anterior aspect of the knee and a grasper from the AM portal holding the other end of the Suture Tape and passing it to the posterior aspect of the knee between the ACL and PCL and retrieved by a grasper introduced through the PM portal

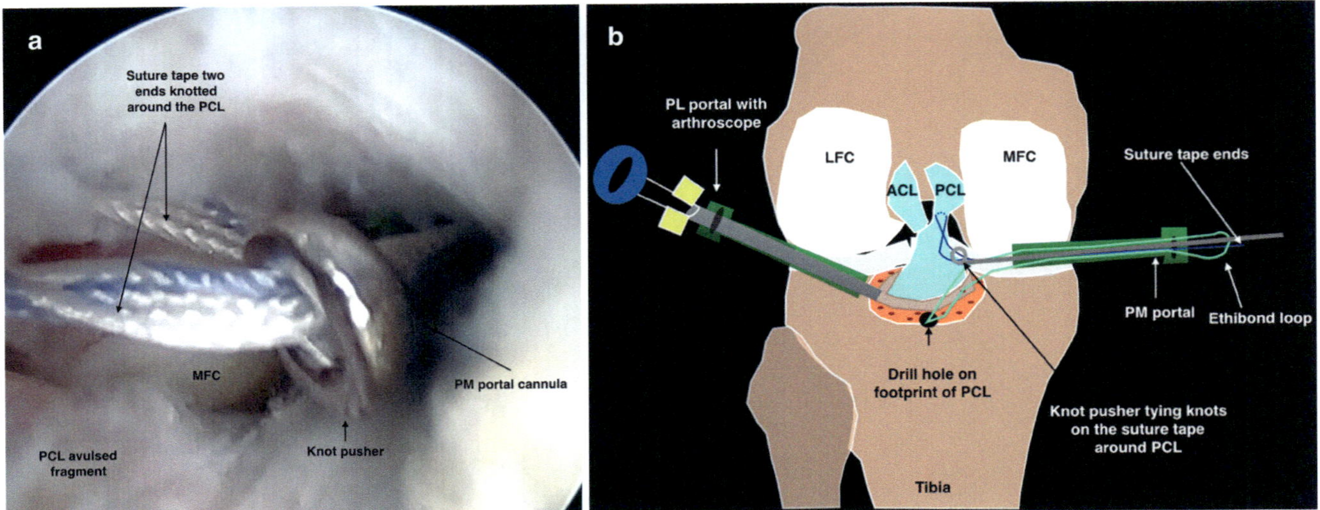


**Fig. 21.20** (**a**) A knot pusher introduced through the PM portal tying multiple simple knots to the two ends of the Suture Tape around the PCL posteriorly, scope through the PL portal. (**b**) Illustration of a knot pusher in the PM portal tying multiple simple knots with two ends of the Suture Tape around the PCL posteriorly, scope through the PL portal

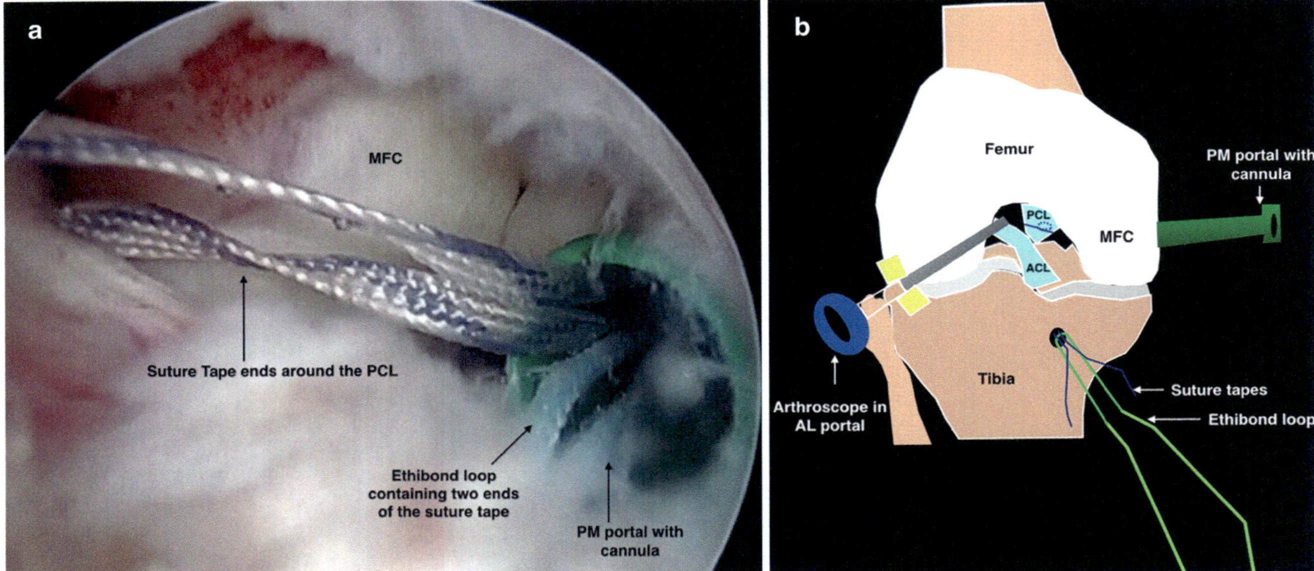


**Fig. 21.21** (**a**) The two ends of the Suture Tape looped through the No 5 Ethibond loop through the PM portal, scope through the PL portal. (b) Illustration of the Ethibond loop pulling with it the two ends of the suture tape looped through it through the AM aspect of the tibial tunnel

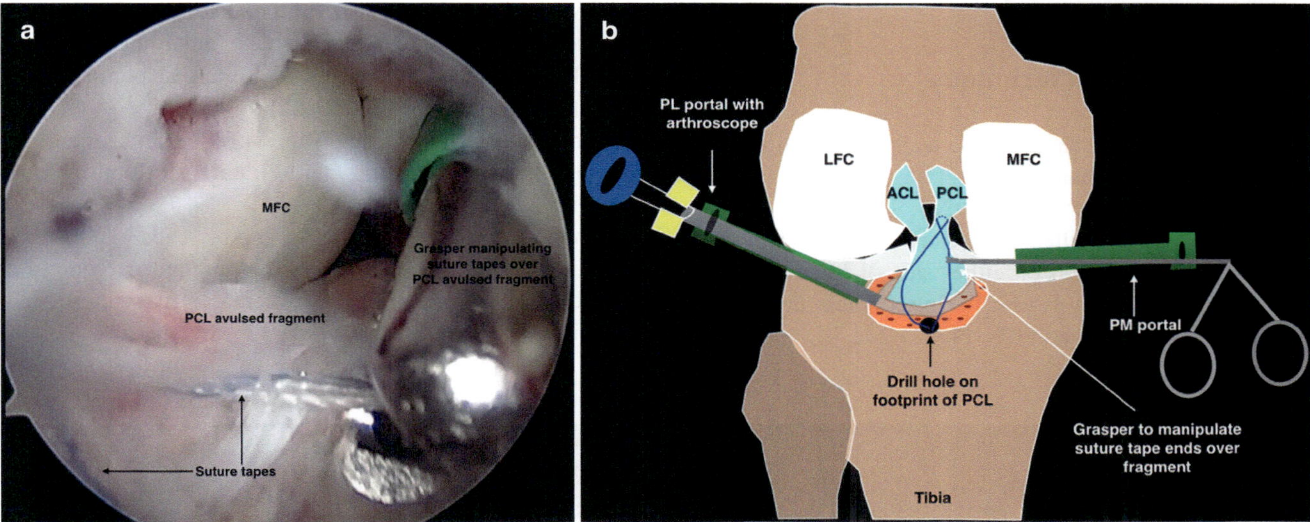


**Fig. 21.22** (**a**) Grasper through PM portal manipulating the ends of the Suture Tape over the avulsed PCL fragment so as to exert uniform compression over it, scope through the PM portal. (**b**) Illustration of grasper manipulating the two ends of the Suture Tape over the avulsed PCL fragment so as to exert uniform pressure over it, scope through PL portal

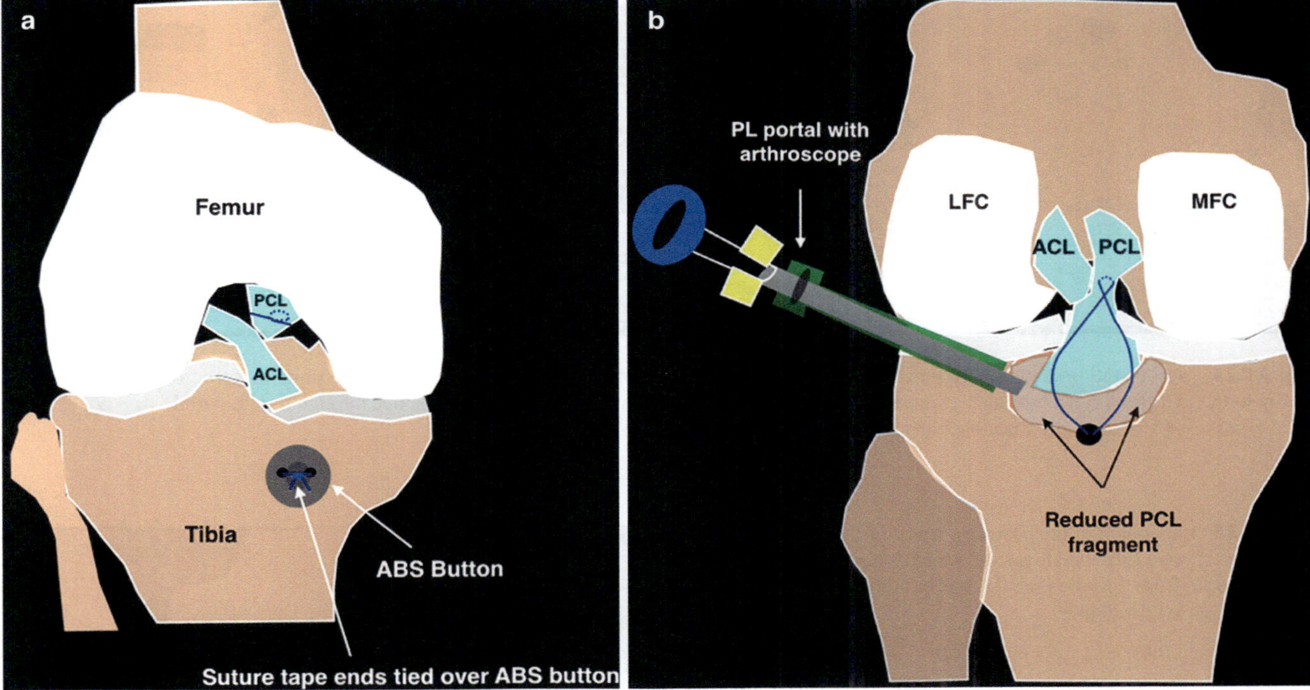


**Fig. 21.23** (**a**) Illustration of the anterior aspect of the knee showing two ends of the Suture Tape being tied over an ABS button with multiple simple knots (at least 4) anteromedially over the tibia. (**b**) Illustration of the posterior aspect of the knee showing the reduced PCL avulsion and two ends of the Suture Tape exerting uniform compression over the fragment after the two ends are tied over an ABS button, scope through the PL portal

## 21.7 Variation

### 21.7.1 Two Tunnel Technique

The portals used are same in this technique. It differs from the single tunnel technique in

1. Two tunnels are drilled in the same way with a guidewire and 4.5 mm drill bit on either side of the avulsed PCL footprint and just below it, introducing the PCL jig between the ACL and PCL (Fig. 21.24a, b).
2. Two Beath pins with an Ethibond loop each are introduced from individual tunnels anteromedially and Ethibond loop delivered through the PM portal using a suture manipulator (Fig. 21.25).
3. One end of each Suture Tape shuttled anteromedially on the tibia using individual Ethibond loops (Fig. 21.26a, b).
4. The individual Suture Tape ends are tied anteromedially over the tibia. No implant is required as there is a bone bridge between the two suture ends (Fig. 21.27).

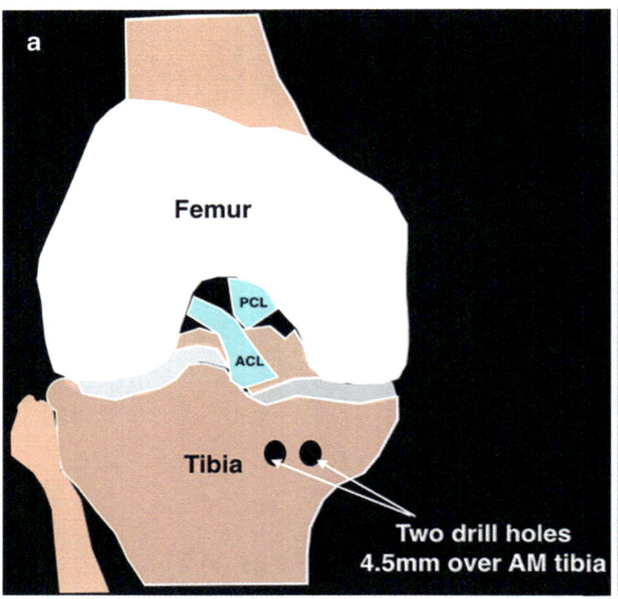


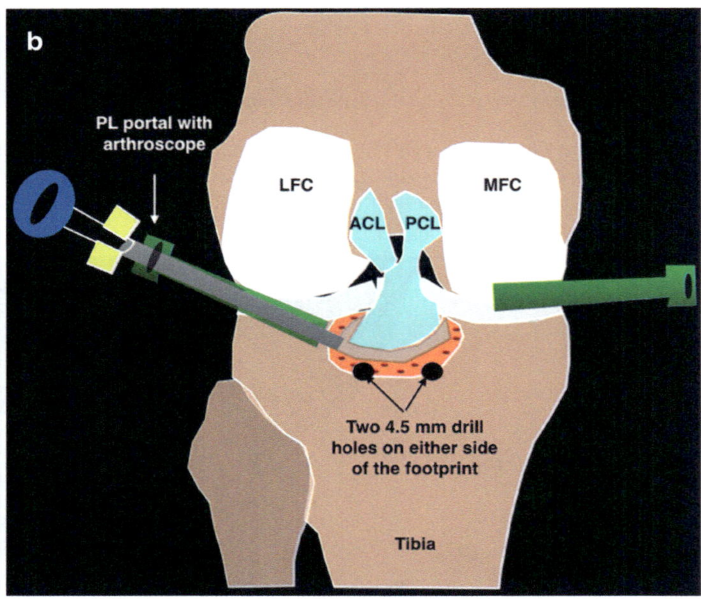


**Fig. 21.24** (**a**) Illustration showing two tunnels drilled from anteromedially to the PCL footprint posteriorly using a PCL jig. (**b**) Illustration of the posterior aspect of the knee showing two tunnels drilled from anteromedially on the tibia to the tibial footprint on either side of the avulsed PCL fragment, scope through the PL portal

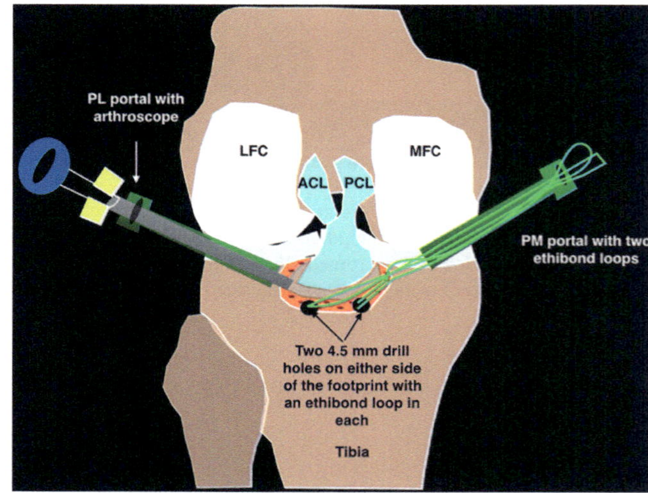


**Fig. 21.25** Illustration of the posterior aspect of the knee showing two Ethibond loops delivered through the PM portal from the anteromedial aspect of the tunnel using two Beath pins

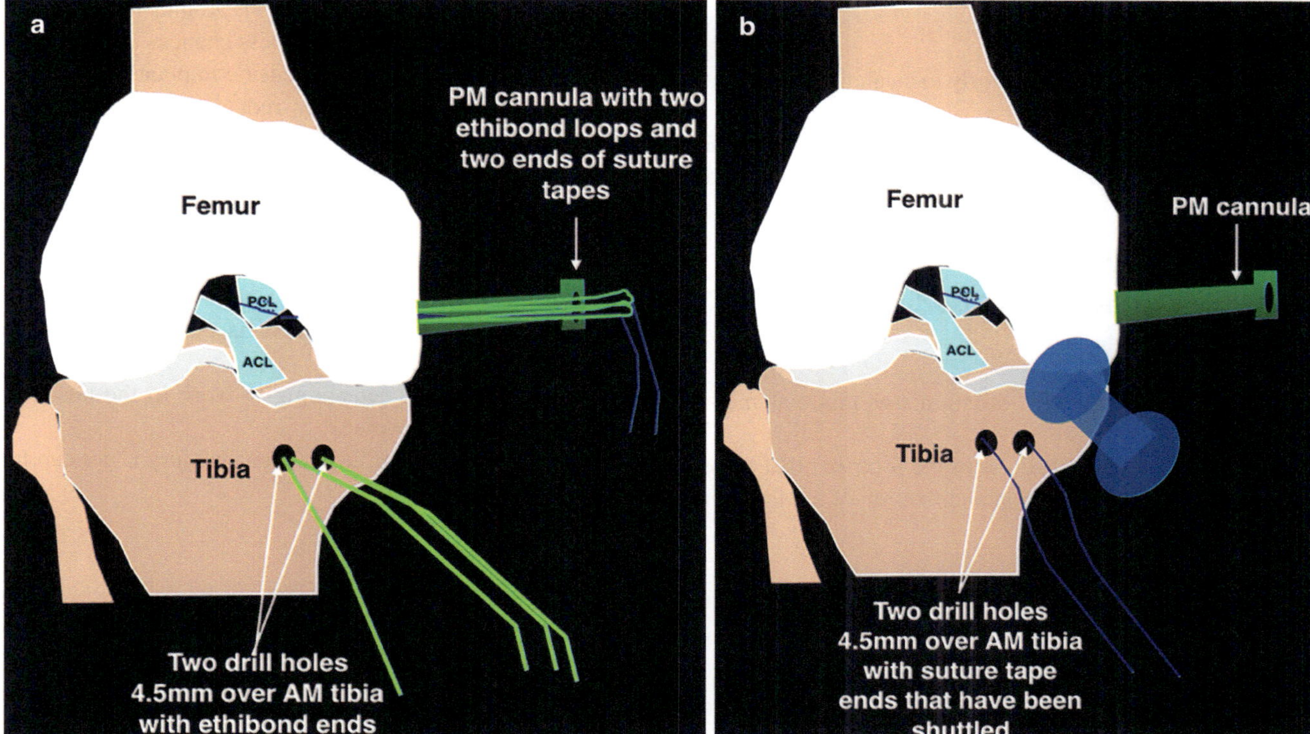


**Fig. 21.26** (**a**) Illustration of the anterior aspect of the knee showing two ends of each Ethibond loop at the end of each tunnel on the anteromedial aspect of the tibia and PM portal containing the two Ethibond loops and suture tape ends with each end looped through one Ethibond loop. (**b**) Illustration of each of the Suture Tapes delivered through one tunnel each on the anteromedial aspect of the tibia using the Ethibond loops

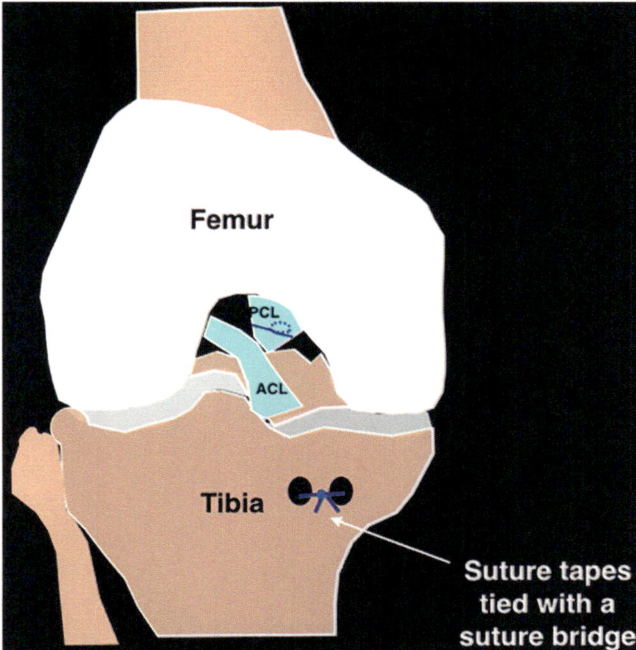


**Fig. 21.27** Illustration of the anterior aspect of the knee showing two ends of the Suture Tape tied to each other over a bone bridge between them using four simple knots

## 21.8 Tips and Tricks

1. RF can also be used posteriorly to clean the footprint as it controls bleeding
2. Drilling the tibial tunnel just below the footprint helps in making sure the avulsed fragment sits anatomically over the footprint
3. Bites through the PCL and knots around it posteriorly make the construct stable with less chances of a cut out
4. The two -tunnel technique needs no implant anteromedially to tie the sutures over reducing the cost of the surgery
5. Manipulation of the two ends of the suture tape over the PCL avulsed fragment is not required in the two tunnel technique

## 21.9 Advantages and Disadvantages

**Advantages**

1. This technique and its variation use minimal metallic implants.
2. There is direct visualization of the footprint that helps in more anatomical reduction and fixation of the fragment.

**Disadvantages**

1. Possibility of stiffness as there is posterior dissection arthroscopically
2. Can be technically demanding to work in the posterior compartment of the knee
3. The is a possibility of neurovascular injury if not careful while drilling

# Part VI
# Miscellaneous

# 22 Arthroscopic Stiff Knee Release

Vikram Arun Mhaskar and J. Maheshwari

## 22.1 Introduction

Stiff knee can be a consequence of trauma, surgery or infection. There could be an inability to flex the knee completely, with or without a flexion deformity. Stiffness can be intra- or extraarticular. Arthroscopic release has the advantage of being minimally invasive and allowing access to all aspects of the knee. Flexion deformity can be due to a posterior capsular contracture, retro patellar fibrosis or synovitis in the notch. Inability to flex can be due to adhesions in the supra patellar pouch, lateral and medial gutters or adhesion of the quadriceps tendon to the femur. We describe a technique to arthroscopically release the knee.

## 22.2 Specialised Equipment

1. Radiofrequency device (Stryker,Kalamazoo,MI).
2. 4.5 mm shaver (Stryker,Kalamazoo,MI)
3. Narrow osteotome (Arthrex,Naples,Fl).
4. 6 mm cannulas (Arthrex,Naples,Fl)
5. Arthroscopic punches (Smith & Nephew, Watford,UK).

## 22.3 Positioning (Fig. 22.1)

Supine on an operating table with a side support and a bolster at the end of the table in whatever degree of flexion the knee can be kept.

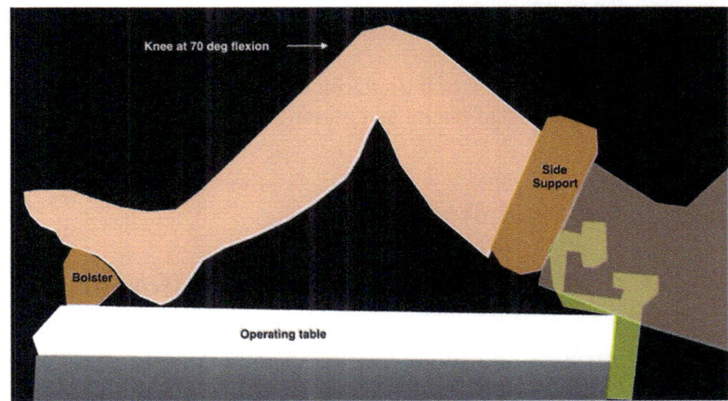


**Fig. 22.1** Knee in 70° flexion on an operating table with a side support and bolster at the end of the bed

## 22.4 Portals (Fig. 22.2a, b)

Portal A: Lateral portal made in the soft spot just lateral to the inferior pole of the lateral aspect of the patella just lateral to the patellar tendon.

Portal B: Medial portal made in the soft spot just medial to the medial border of the patellar tendon.

Portal C: Superolateral portal made under guidance of a LP needle.

Portal D: Superomedial portal made under guidance of a LP needle.

Portal E: Posteromedial portal (PM) made just above the synovial fold under LP needle guidance in the posteromedial aspect of the knee and has a 7 mm cannula.

Portal F: Posterolateral portal (PL) made trans septally inside out with a switching stick and has a 7 mm cannula.

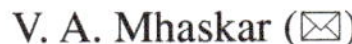

V. A. Mhaskar (✉)
F7 East of Kailash, Knee & Shoulder Clinic, New Delhi, India

JMVM Sports Injury Center, Sitaram Bhartia Institute of Science & Research, New Delhi, India

J. Maheshwari
F7 East of Kailash, Knee & Shoulder Clinic, New Delhi, India
e-mail: drjmaheshwari@jmvmsportsinjury.com


V. A. Mhaskar, J. Maheshwari (eds.), *Innovative Approaches in Knee Arthroscopy*,
https://doi.org/10.1007/978-981-99-4378-4_22

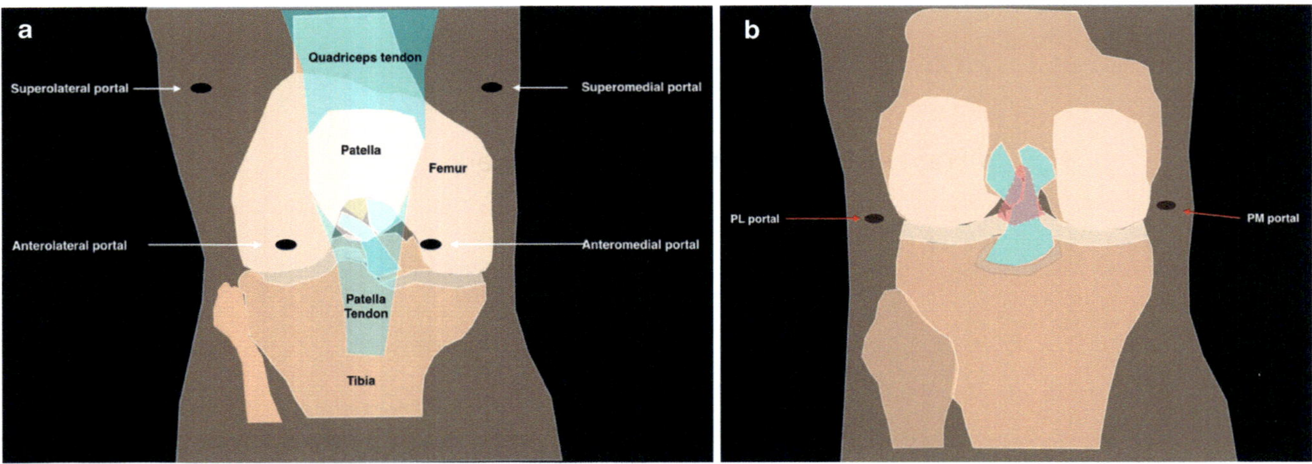


**Fig. 22.2** (**a**) Illustration of the anterior knee showing anterolateral, anteromedial, superomedial and superolateral. (**b**) Illustration of the back of the knee showing posterolateral and posteromedial portals

## 22.5 Surgical Steps

### 22.5.1 Stiff Knee Without a Flexion Deformity

Step 1: Introduce the scope through Portal A and try to visualise the notch.

Step 2: If not visualised introduce the shaver through Portal B and clear the tissue obstructing it.

Step 3: Remove the synovitis in the notch and clear it of excessive tissue (Fig. 22.3a, b).

Step 4: Through the AL portal manipulate the scope into the suprapatellar pouch.

Step 5: Introduce the shaver and clear the supra patellar space of fibrosis and synovitis, superiorly and inferiorly. Sometimes the quadriceps tendon is adherent to the femur and using an osteotome through the AM portal into the suprapatellar pouch to detach the scar tissue from the femur (Fig. 22.4a–e).

Step 6: Make the superolateral portal introduce the shaver and through it and while viewing the lateral gutter, it is cleared of synovitis and adhesions are released (Fig. 22.5a, b).

Step 7: The superomedial portal is then made, the scope through the AL portal is manipulated into the medial gutter and the shaver through the superomedial portal to clear the synovitis and adhesions in the medial gutter.(Fig. 22.6a, b).

The RF device is used along with the shaver intermittently to release tissues.

Step 8: With the scope in the superolateral portal a RF device is introduced through the superomedial portal and tissues behind the patellar tendon are released all the way down to its insertion of the tibia (Fig. 22.7a, b).

Step 9: Gently manipulate the knee by flexing it after lowering the table and keeping the two thumbs on the patellar tendon insertion on the tibia.

### 22.5.2 In Case of Posterior Capsular Contracture Causing a Flexion Deformity

Step 1: Introduce the scope into the posteromedial compartment by manipulating it between the PCL and the medial femoral condyle with a little valgus force at the knee.

Step 2: A posteromedial portal is made and a shaver introduced through a 7 mm cannula in the PM portal that is used to release the menisco capsular junction. An RF can also be used with the shaver alternately to release the menisco capsular tissue and septum(Fig. 22.8).

Step 3: The PL portal is made trans septally and while viewing through the PL portal tissue the menisco capsular tissue is released in the posteromedial aspect of the knee, the scope is then interchanged into the PM portal and the PL meniscocapsular scar tissue released (Fig. 22.9a–d).

Step 4: Keep a folded drape under the heel and extension is the facilitated so that the back of the knee touches the bed.

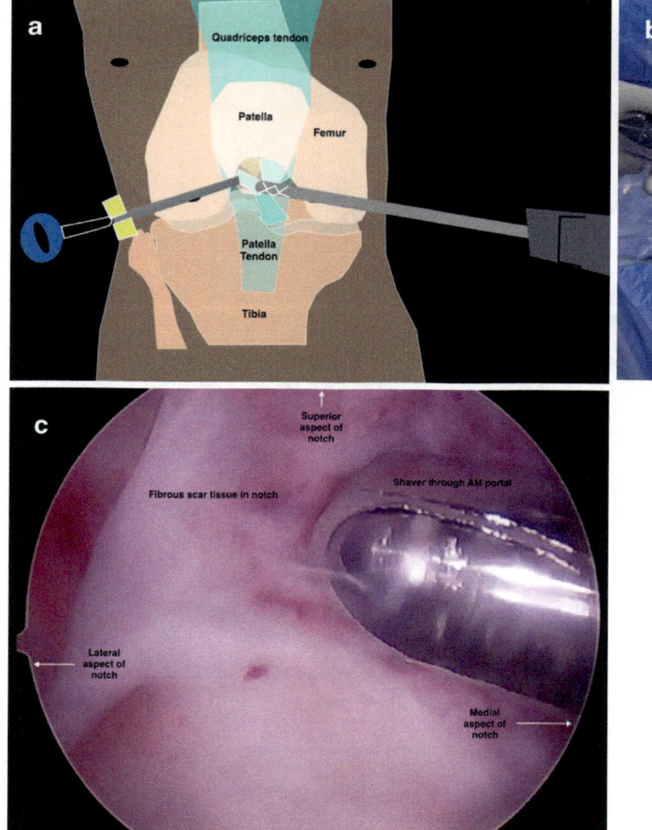


**Fig. 22.3** (**a**) Illustration of the front of the knee showing the arthroscope through the anterolateral portal looking into the notch and a shaver through the anteromedial portal clearing the notch of scar tissue. (**b**) External image showing the arthroscope from the anterolateral portal and shaver from the anteromedial portal. (**c**) Arthroscopic image of the notch while viewing through the anterolateral portal showing scar tissue and a shaver through the anteromedial portal

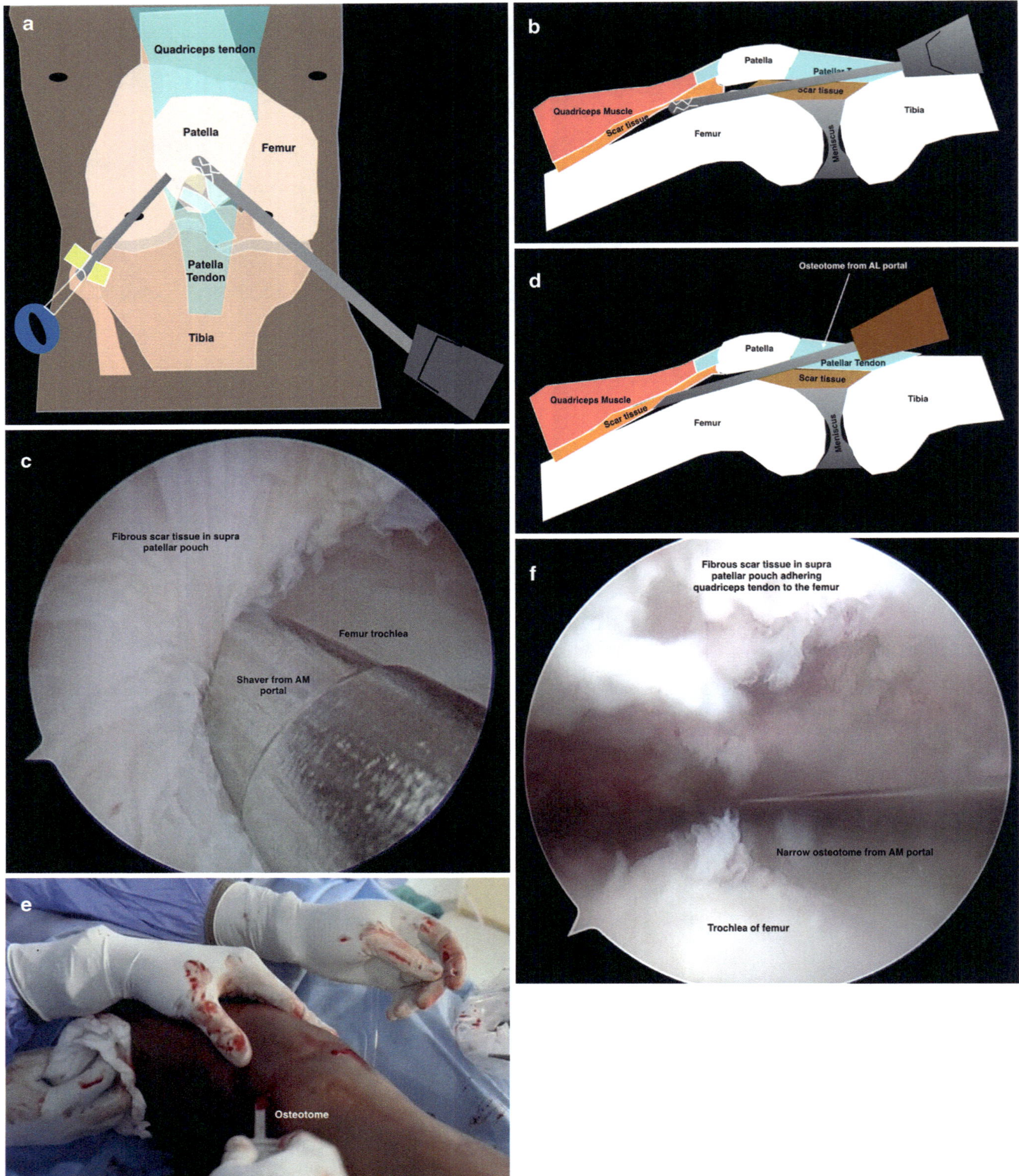


**Fig. 22.4** (**a**) Illustration of the knee showing scope from the AL portal introduced into the suprapatellar pouch and shaver through the AM portal to the suprapatellar pouch clearing the scar tissue. (**b**) Illustration of the knee seen laterally showing the shaver through the AM portal clearing scar tissue in the supra patellar space. (**c**) Arthroscopic image of the supra patellar pouch showing scar tissue being removed with a shaver introduced through the AM portal while viewing through the AL portal. (**d**) Illustration of the knee viewed laterally showing an osteotome introduced through the AM portal releasing the adhered quadriceps tendon from the femur. (**e**) External image showing the osteotome through AL portal releasing the suprapatellar pouch and quadriceps tendon from the femur. (f) Arthroscopic image of the suprapatellar pouch while viewing through the AL portal showing an osteotome releasing the quadriceps adhesions to the femur

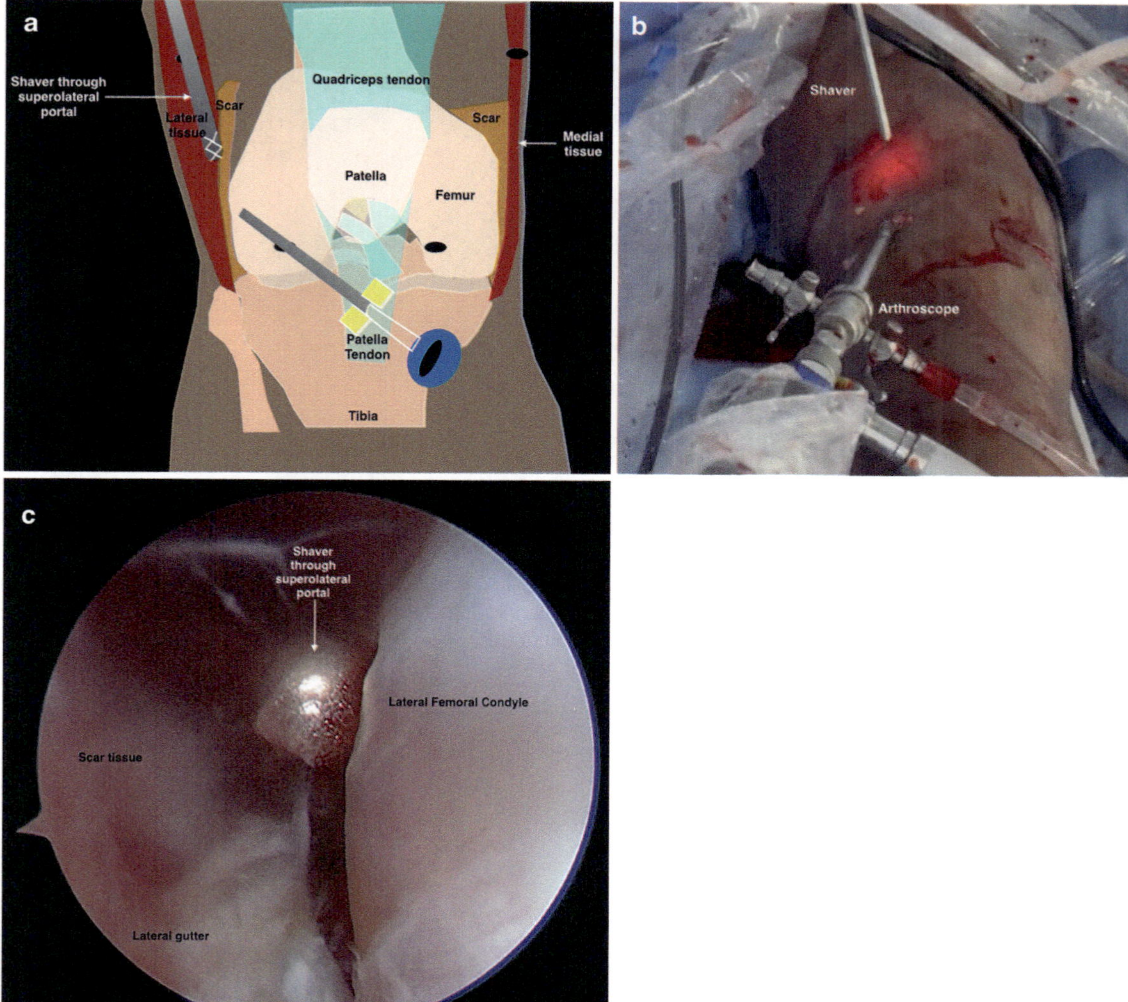


**Fig. 22.5** (**a**) Illustration of the knee showing the scope through the AL portal and shaver through the superolateral portal removing the adhesions between the femur and tissues of the lateral gutter. (**b**) External image showing the arthroscope through the anterolateral portal and shaver through superolateral portal to clear the lateral gutter. (**c**) Arthroscopic image of the lateral gutter showing a shaver removing adhesions between the lateral tissue and the lateral femoral condyle

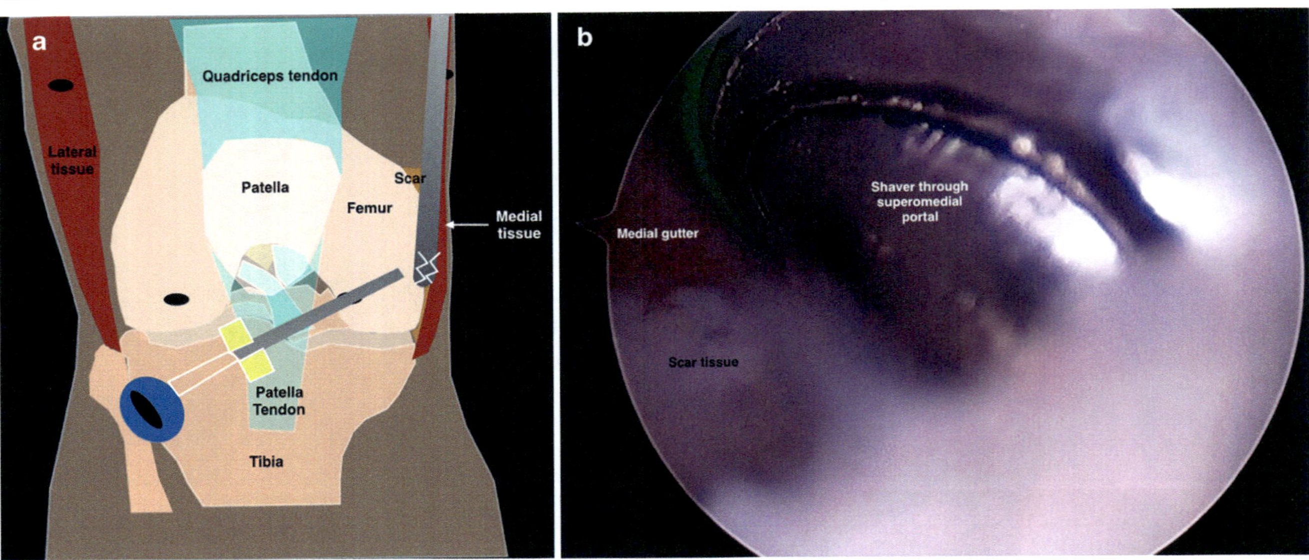


**Fig. 22.6** (a) Illustration of the knee showing the scope through the AL portal viewing the medial gutter and a shaver from the superomedial portal removing scar tissue in the medial gutter. (b) Arthroscopic image of the medial gutter showing the shaver from the superomedial portal while viewing from the AL portal removing scar tissue in the medial gutter

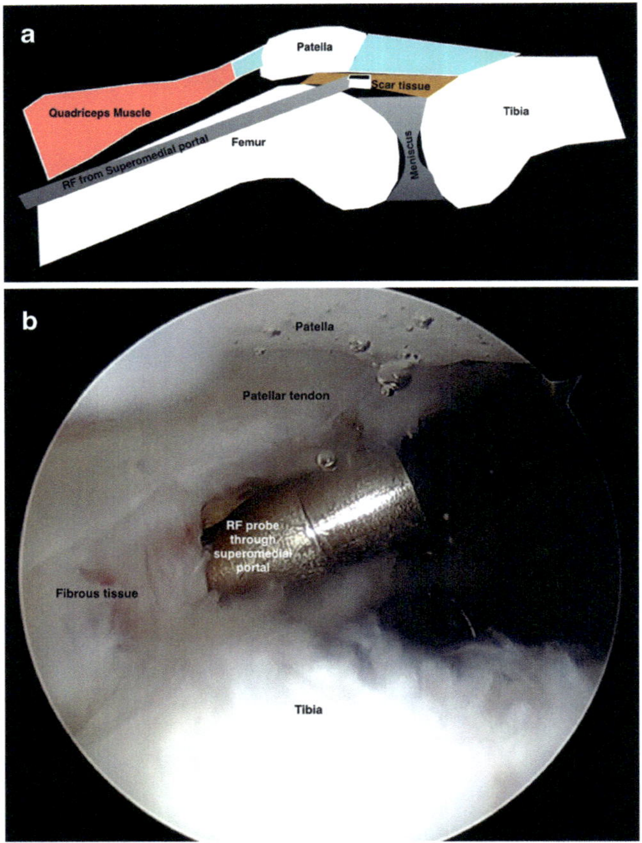


**Fig. 22.7** (**a**) Illustration of the lateral aspect of the knee showing a RF from the superomedial portal removing scar tissue behind the patellar tendon while viewing from the superolateral portal. (**b**) Arthroscopic image of the area behind the patellar tendon while viewing from the superolateral portal with the RF from the superomedial portal removing scar tissue behind the patellar tendon

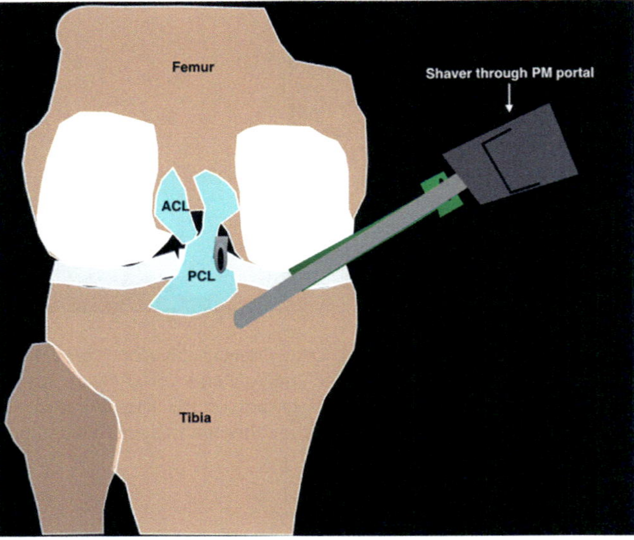


**Fig. 22.8** Illustration of the back of the knee showing the scope from the AL portal introduced between the PCL and medial femoral condyle to the posterior aspect of the knee and a shaver through the PM portal releasing the menisco capsular tissue

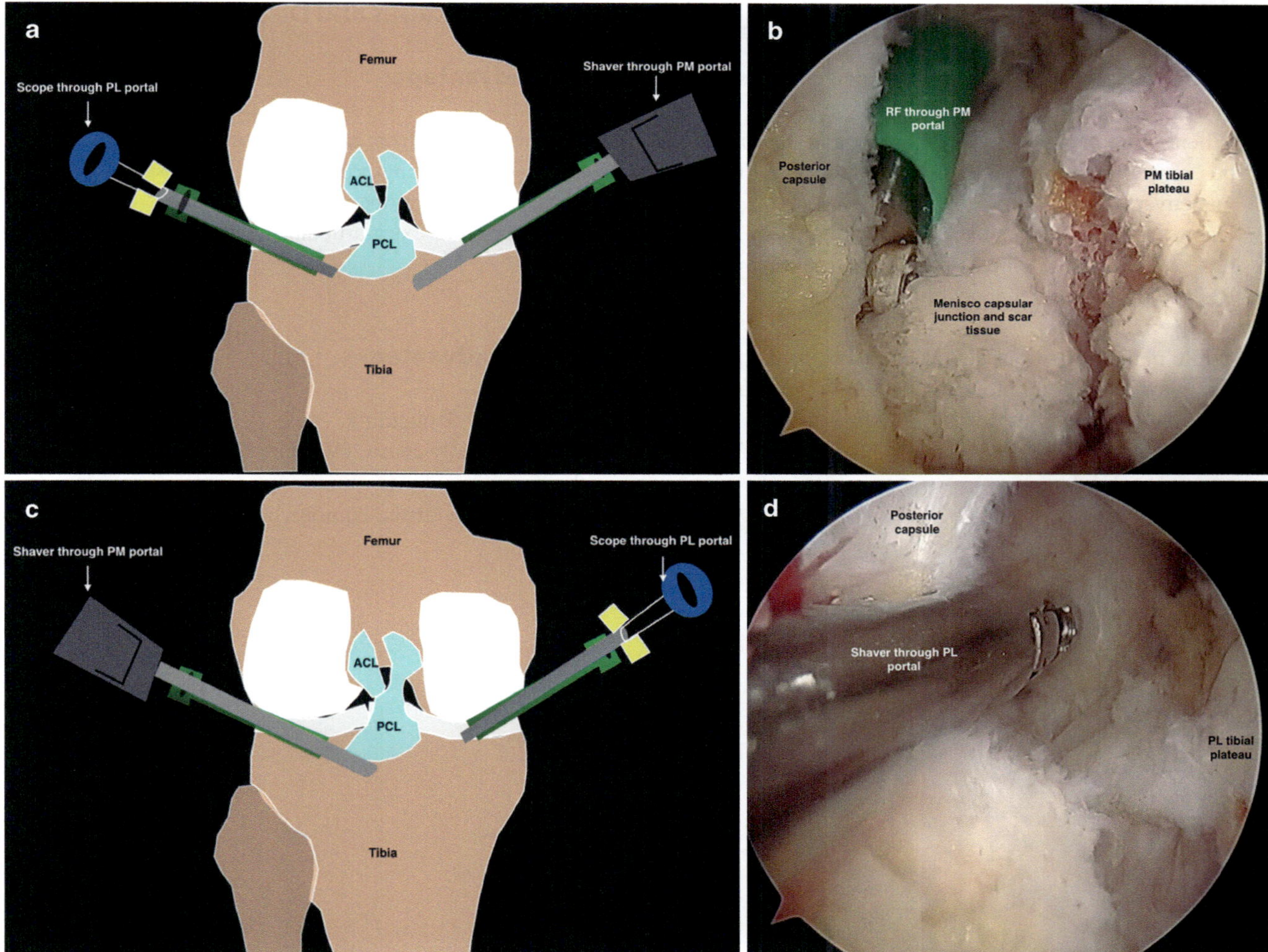


**Fig. 22.9** (**a**) Illustration of the back of the knee showing the scope through the PL portal and a shaver through the PM portal trans portally releasing the menisco capsular junction on the medial side. (**b**) Arthroscopic image of the back of the knee showing an RF through the PM portal releasing the scar tissue in the PM aspect of the knee along the menisco capsular junction. (**c**) Illustration of the back of the knee showing the scope through the PM portal and shaver through the PL portal releasing the scar tissue along the menisco capsular junction in the PL part of the knee. (**d**) Arthroscopic image of the posterior aspect of the knee showing a shaver through the PL portal clearing scar tissue along the menisco capsular junction in the PL part of the knee

## 22.6 Tips and Tricks

1. Touch the scope technique helps if you cannot see much in the knee due to fibrosis.
2. When you enter the supra patellar pouch, the trocar can be moved medial/lateral to create space for easy maneuverability.
3. Using cannulas at the back of the knee help maintain pressure within the joint as there are multiple portals.
4. RF should be interchangeably used with the shaver to remove scar tissue.
5. While making the trans septal portal, point the tip of the vissinger rod upwards towards the femoral end and introduce the cannula after dilating it with a dilator.
6. Pointing the RF towards the bone (tibia/femur) prevent neurovascular damage.

## 22.7 Advantages and Disadvantages

### 22.7.1 Advantages

1. The whole knee front and back can be accessed well.
2. Less wound healing problems than open surgery.
3. Earlier rehab than open surgery.
4. Both intra and extra-articular causes of stiffness can be treated.

### 22.7.2 Disadvantages

1. Technically demanding.
2. Can potentially cause NV injury in the posterior aspect of the knee.
3. Requires specialised equipment.

# 23 Ultrasound Guided Arthroscopic Popliteal Cyst Excision

Vikram Arun Mhaskar

## 23.1 Introduction

Popliteal cysts may present with pain or an inability to flex the knee completely. They may be just incidental findings on an MRI or ultrasound and in these cases can be left alone. However, those that cause symptoms need to be removed. Arthroscopic removal has the advantage of being minimally invasive but is technically demanding. Using intra-operative ultrasound helps in confirming the location of the lesion and whether it has been removed completely [1]. We describe our technique of decompressing a popliteal cyst arthroscopically using ultrasound guidance.

## 23.2 Specialised Equipment

1. Arthroscopic punch (Acufex,Smith &Nephew,Watford,UK).
2. 18G LP needle (Becton, Dickinson & Company, Franklin Lakes,NJ)
3. Ultrasound machine (Sonosite, Bothell, Washington,USA).
4. Sterilised arthroscope cover and tape (Karl Storz,Tuttlingen,Germany).
5. Betadine solution (Avrio Health,NY,USA).
6. Arthroscopicpunch(Acufex,Smith&Nephew,Watford,UK).
7. Shaver with tip (Stryker,Kalamazoo,MI).
8. Radiofrequency device (Stryker,Kalamazoo,MI).

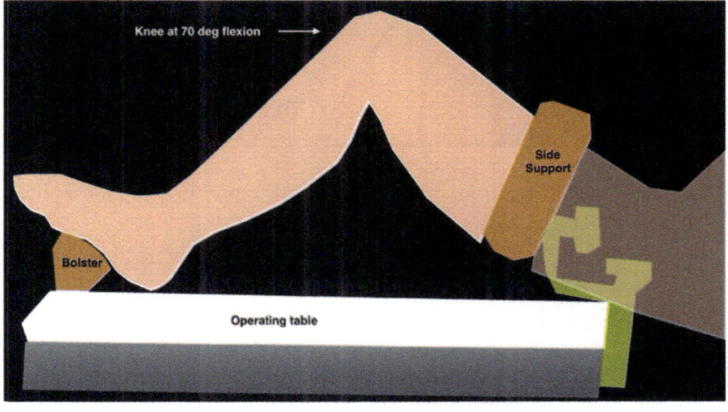


**Fig. 23.1** Positioning of the limb at 70 degrees flexion on an operating table with a side support and bolster at the end of the table

## 23.3 Positioning (Fig. 23.1)

Knee flexed at 70 degrees on the operating table with a bolster at the end of the table and a side support on the lateral aspect of the thigh.

The ultrasound machine is on the same side as the surgeon stands and the arthroscopic trolley on the opposite side.

## 23.4 Portals (Fig. 23.2a, b)

Portal A: Standard anterolateral (AL) viewing portal made just lateral to the patellar tendon just below the inferior pole of the patella in the soft spot.

Portal B: Made under vision by introducing an 18G LP needle just above the posteromedial (PM) soft tissue fold in the PM compartment.

Portal C: High posteromedial (High PM) portal made above the PM portal about 5 cm proximal to it under vision using an 18 G LP needle.

V. A. Mhaskar (✉)
F7 East of Kailash, Knee & Shoulder Clinic, New Delhi, India

JMVM Sports Injury Center, Sitaram Bhartia Institute of Science & Research, New Delhi, India


V. A. Mhaskar, J. Maheshwari (eds.), *Innovative Approaches in Knee Arthroscopy*,
https://doi.org/10.1007/978-981-99-4378-4_23

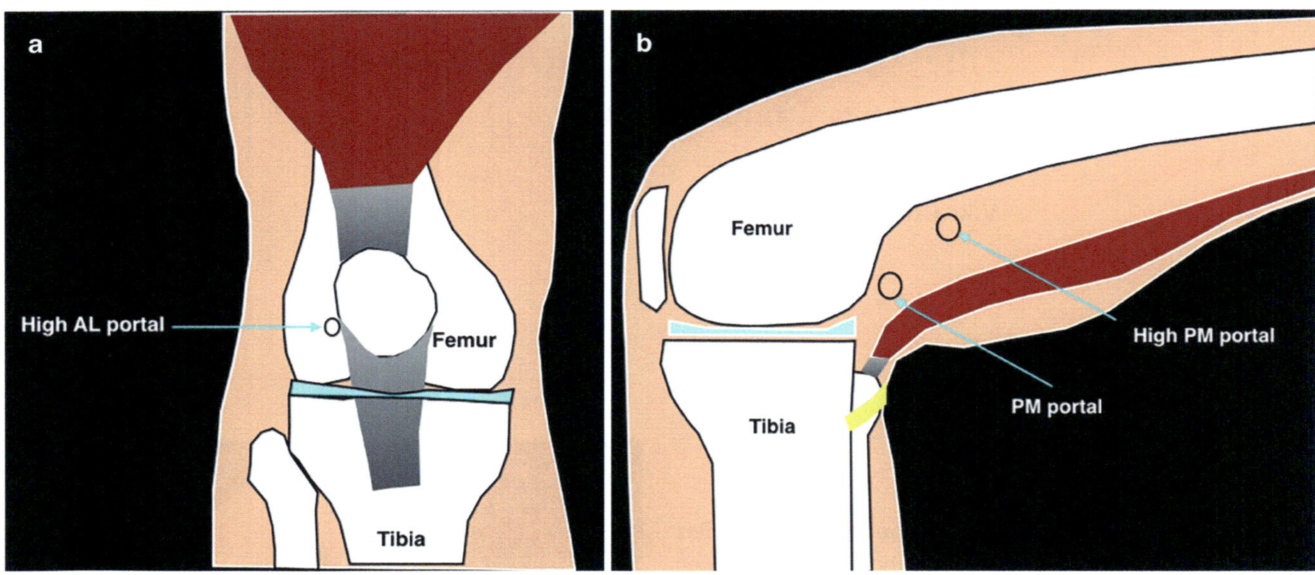


**Fig. 23.2** (**a**) Illustration showing Portal A made just lateral to the patellar tendon at the inferior pole of the patella. (**b**) Illustration showing postero-medial and high postero-medial portal

## 23.5 Surgical Steps

Step 1: The ultrasound probe is introduced into the arthroscope cover and the secured with a sterile sticky tape at the base of the probe. The whole probe and wire connecting it to the monitor are covered with the arthroscope cover (Fig. 23.3).

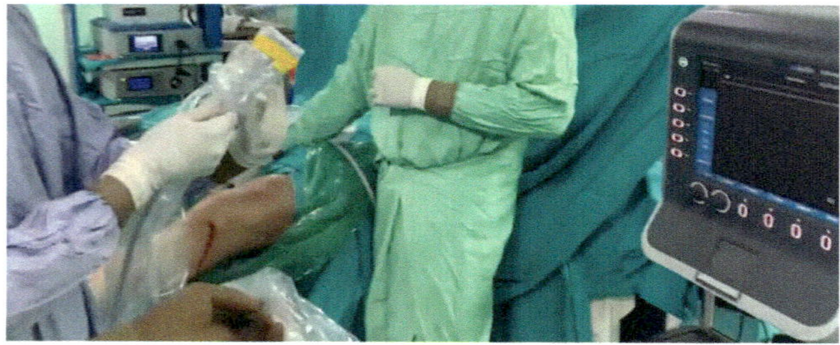

**Fig. 23.3** Picture showing the ultrasound probe covered in a sterile cover with a sticky tape applied to the bottom of the probe

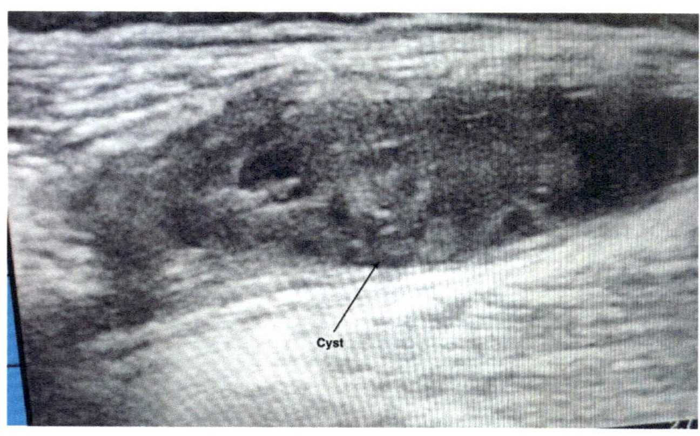


Step 2: The probe is applied to the PM aspect of the knee after dipping it in the Betadine solution to visualise the cyst and the point is marked with a marking pen (Fig. 23.4).

Step 3: The arthroscope is introduced through Portal A between the medial femoral condyle (MFC) and PCL to the PM compartment of the knee (Fig. 23.5).

Step 4: An 18G LP needle is introduced from the skin in the PM aspect of the thigh just above the PM capsular fold by trans illuminence and Portal B is made (Fig. 23.6).

Step 5: An arthroscopic punch is then introduced through this portal and the PM capsular fold is cut using the punch, which communicates the popliteal cyst with the knee joint, and the cyst fluid can be seen which the shaver sucks (Fig. 23.7).

Step 6: The shaver is then introduced through Portal A and the fluid sucked out (Fig. 23.8).

Step 7: A higher PM portal is made about 5 cm proximal to Portal B by transilluminence and the shaver is introduced through it (Fig. 23.9).

Step 8: The arthroscope is then introduced through Portal B and the shaver through Portal C (Fig. 23.10).

Step 9: Now the cyst is visualised from within and the rest of the septae can be shaved off (Fig. 23.11).

Step 10: The ultrasound is used to confirm if the cyst has been decompressed adequately (Fig. 23.12).

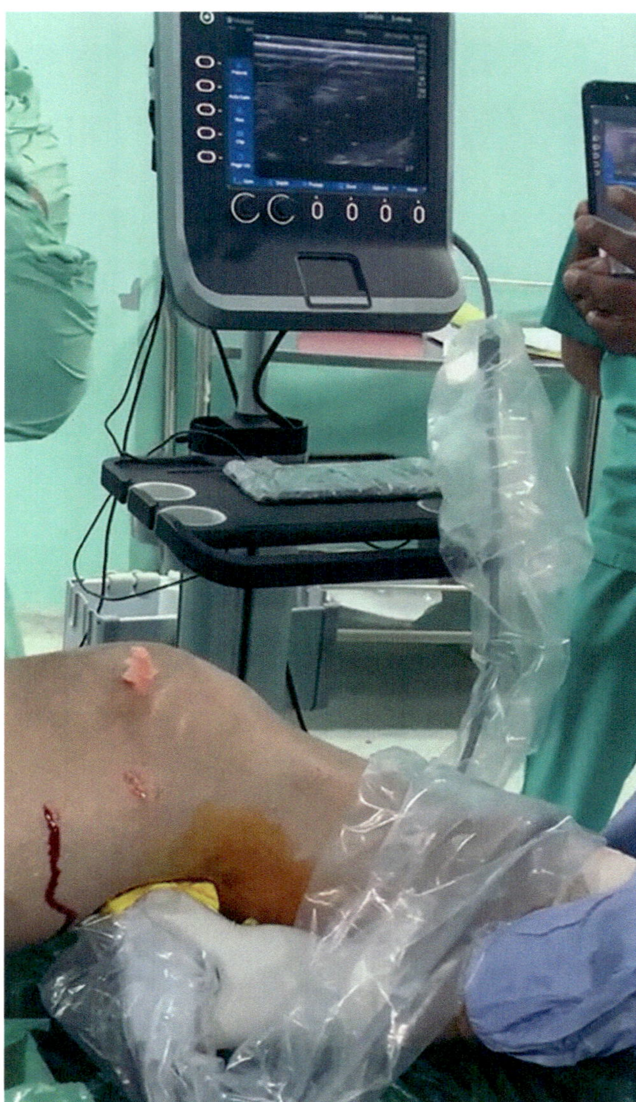

**Fig. 23.4** Picture showing the ultrasound probe covered in a sterile arthroscopic sheath applied to the posteromedial aspect of the knee to visualise the cyst on the monitor

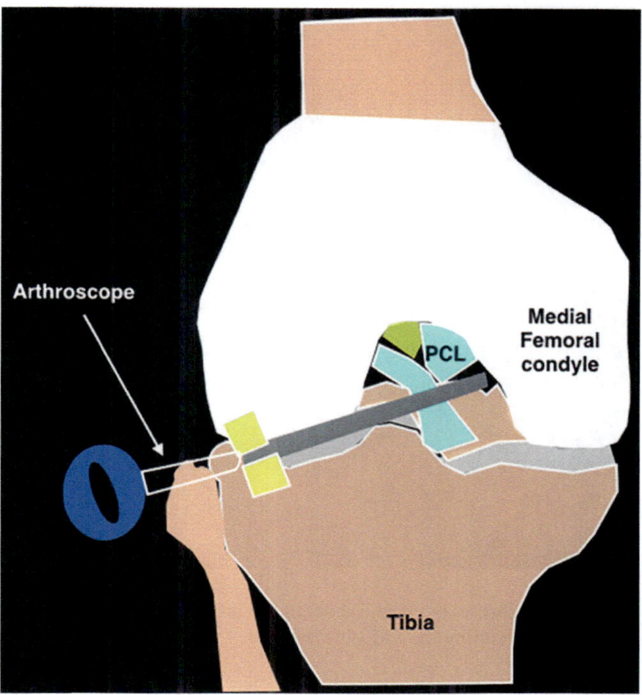


**Fig. 23.5** Illustration showing the arthroscope introduced between the PCL and medial femoral condyle into the posteromedial aspect of the knee

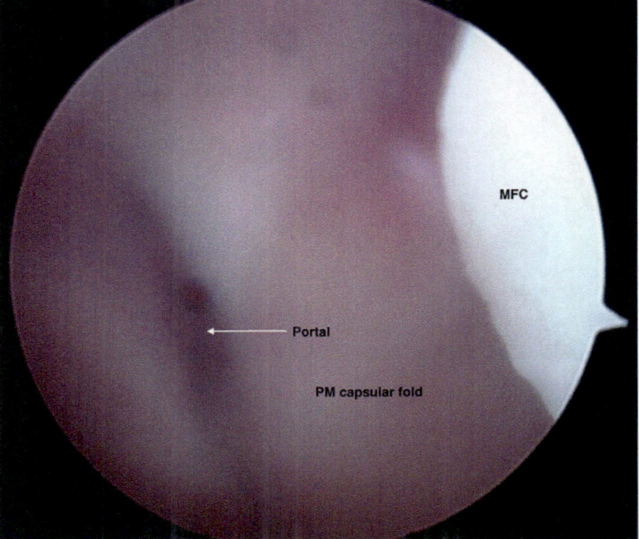


**Fig. 23.6** Arthroscopic image showing the high PM portal made above the PM capsular fold

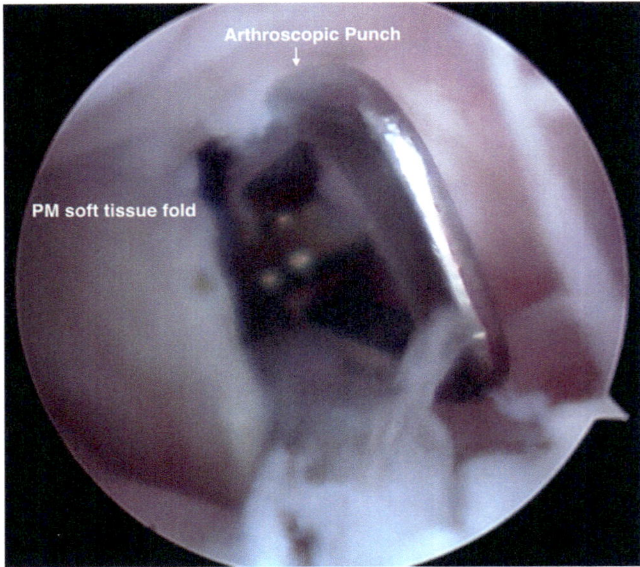


**Fig. 23.7** Arthroscopic image showing the arthroscopic punch through the PM portal cutting the PM synovial fold

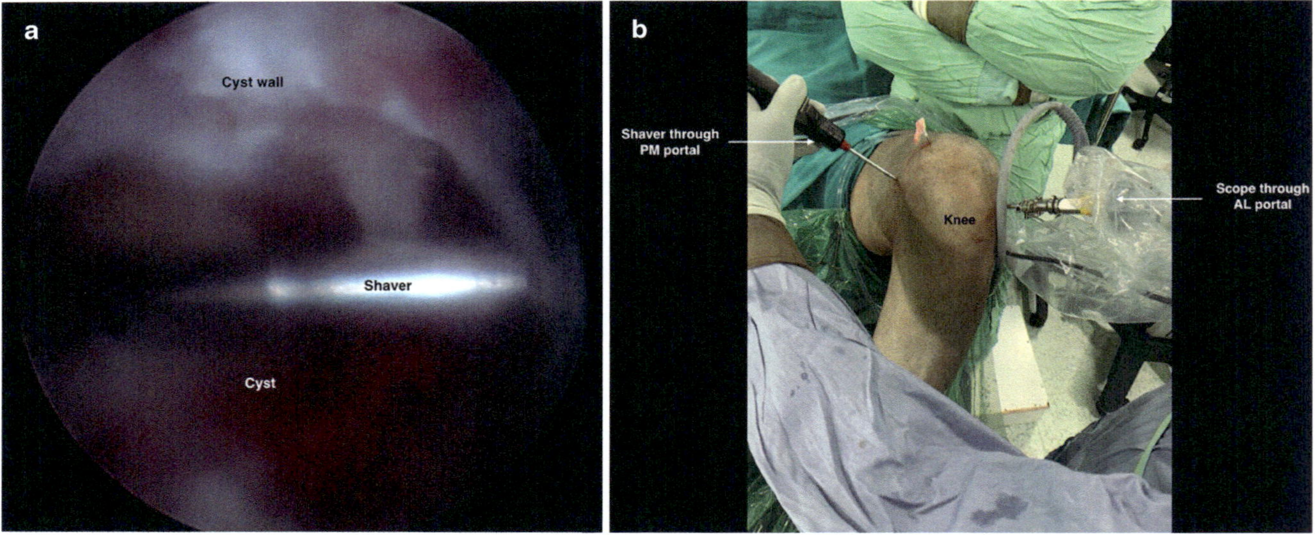


**Fig. 23.8** (**a**) Arthroscopic image showing the shaver introduced through the PM portal and sucking the cyst fluid debriding it while viewing through the AL portal. (**b**) External Image showing the shaver through Portal B (PM portal) while viewing through Portal A (AL portal) with the knee in 70 degrees flexion on the operating table

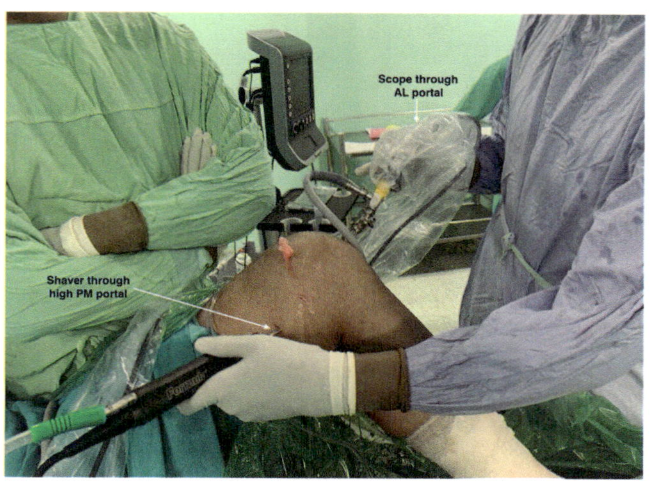


**Fig. 23.9** Shaver through Portal C the high PM portal sucking the cystic fluid while viewing through Portal A (AL portal)

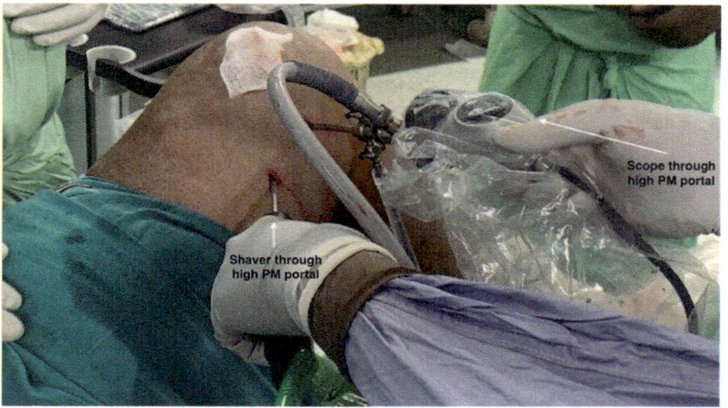


**Fig. 23.10** External image showing the scope through Portal B (PM portal) while the shaver is in Portal A (High PM portal)

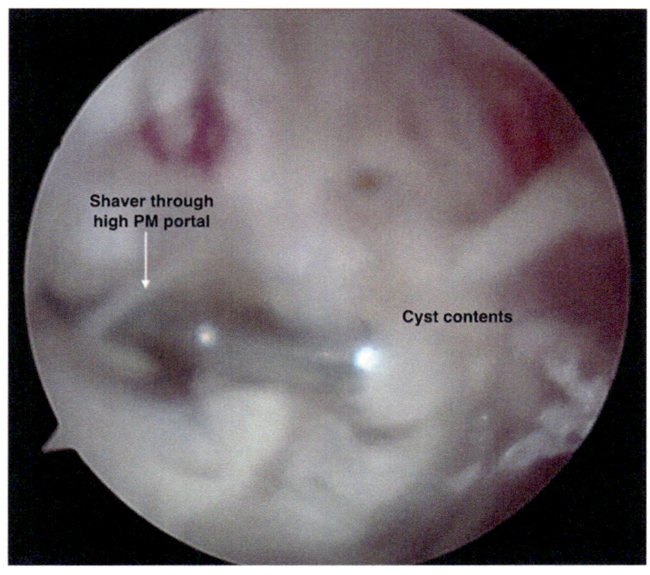


**Fig. 23.11** Arthroscopic image showing the Shaver through Portal C (High PM portal) while viewing through Portal B (PM portal)

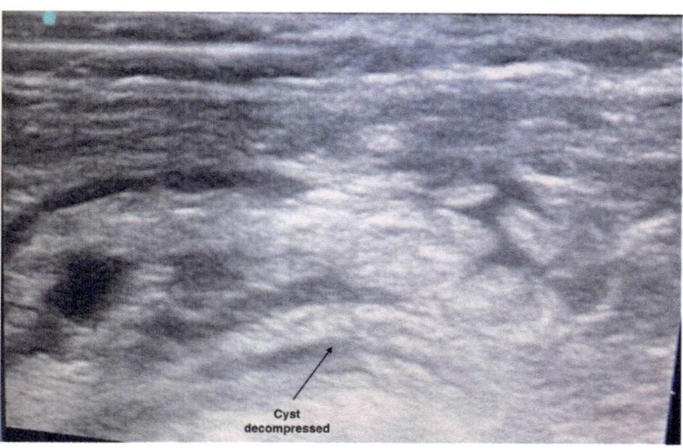


**Fig. 23.12** Ultrasound showing the decompressed cyst intra-operatively

## 23.6 Tips and Tricks

1. The arthroscope cover should be tightly wound around the probe and fixed with a sticky tape at its base but the surface of the probe applied to the skin should have no folds of plastic over it for better visualisation.
2. The high PM Portal C should be made such that the instrumentation does not collide with the arthroscope.

## 23.7 Advantages and Disadvantages

### 23.7.1 Advantages

1. Purely arthroscopic technique with advantages of arthroscopic surgery.
2. Ultrasound helps localise the cyst and confirm its evacuation.

### 23.7.2 Disadvantages

1. Technically demanding.
2. Potential injury to neurovascular structures.
3. Knowledge of interpreting the ultrasound and holding the probe appropriately as at times if not held properly could lead to anisotropy.

## Reference

1. Mhaskar VA, Agrahari H, Maheshwari J. Ultrasound guided arthroscopic meniscus surgery. J Ultrasound. 2022;26:1–5.

# 24 Arthroscopic Popliteus Tendon Reconstruction

Sheetal Gupta and Anmol Sharma

## 24.1 Introduction

Popliteus tendon is the part of posterolateral corner of the knee. The popliteus muscle originates from the posteromedial surface of the proximal tibia, courses superiorly and laterally to form the popliteus tendon which enters the popliteus hiatus. The popliteus tendon then passes under the lateral collateral ligament and inserts into the lateral femoral condyle. Popliteus tendon is regarded as static fifth ligament of the knee. Cadaveric studies have shown that sectioning of the tendon results in significant increase in external rotation, and some increase in internal rotation, Varus angulation and anterior translation.

Popliteus tendon tear is a rare injury. Popliteus tendon tear is seen in athletes suffering rotational injury with foot on the ground or after sudden hyperextension of the knee.

Patient with popliteus tendon tear presents with knee effusion, pain on lateral aspect of knee, sharp pain on palpating the popliteus tendon at popliteus groove, sign of instability may be or may not be present. Injury to posterolateral corner generally present as increase in external rotation with minimal Varus laxity.

Popliteus tear is suspected clinically and on MRI and confirmed on arthroscopic examination.

Arthroscopic assessment of the posterior compartment of the knee and the posterior aspect of the proximal tibia is challenging due to the relative proximity of the neurovascular bundle. Care must be taken when drilling tibial and femoral tunnel for popliteus tendon reconstruction.

## 24.2 Special Instruments Required (Fig. 24.1)

1. Arthroscopic Cannula.
2. Knee Scorpion/ suture passer.
3. Knot pusher.
4. Flexible cannula (passport cannula).
5. Spinal needle.
6. No. 2 fiberwire (multi strand, long chain ultra-high molecular weight polyethylene core braided with polyester).
7. Switching Rod.
8. PCL tibial zig.

S. Gupta (✉) · A. Sharma
Galaxy Knee & Shoulder Hospital, Bhopal, Madhya Pradesh, India


V. A. Mhaskar, J. Maheshwari (eds.), *Innovative Approaches in Knee Arthroscopy*,
https://doi.org/10.1007/978-981-99-4378-4_24

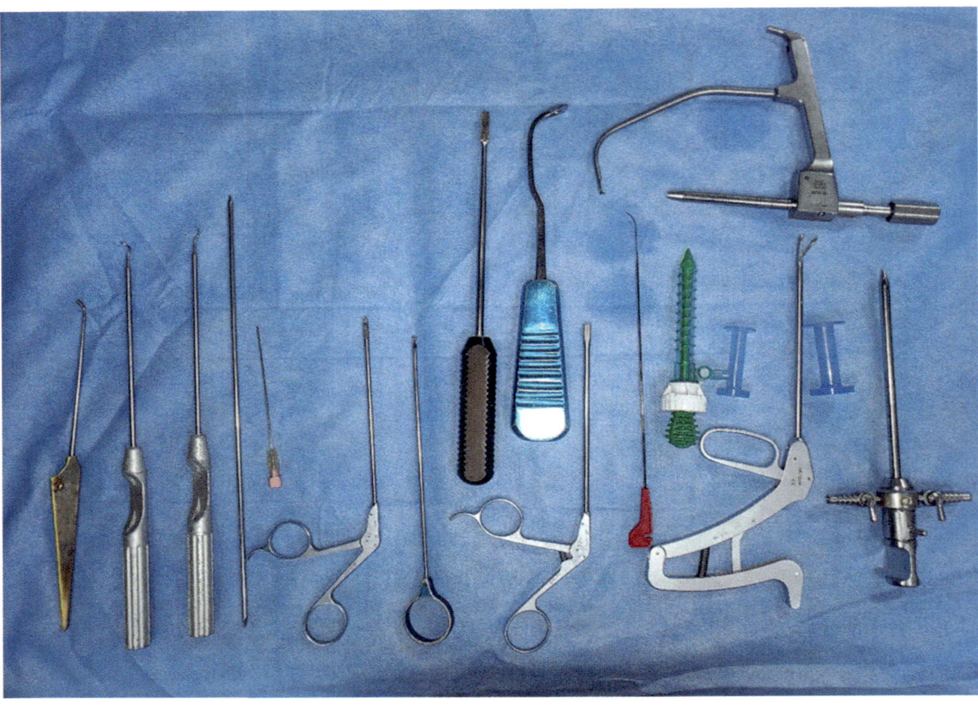

**Fig. 24.1** Special instruments used in arthroscopic popliteus tendon reconstruction

## 24.3 Positioning (Fig. 24.2)

Under spinal anesthesia, patient is in supine position with the knee at $90^0$ degrees of flexion at the edge of the table on the affected side to allow full range of motion and exposure to the back of the knee. Tourniquet is placed high on the thigh with the thigh supported by a post.

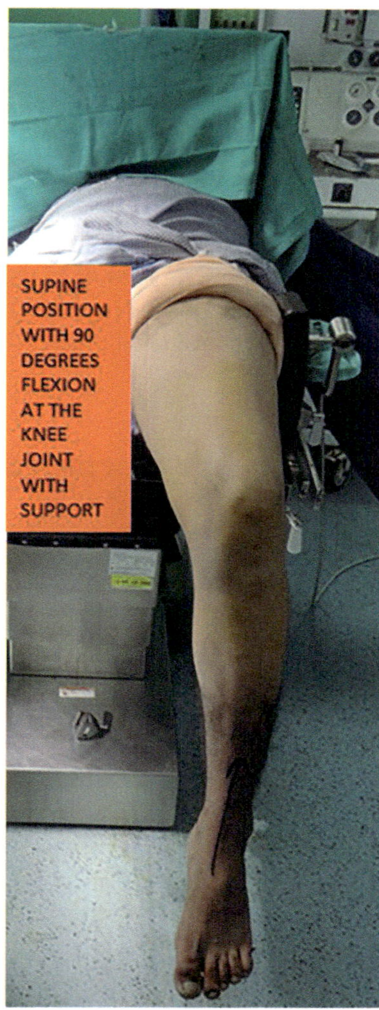


**Fig. 24.2** Positioning of the patient

### 24.3.1 Draping (Fig. 24.3)

Standard draping is done with all sterile technique to expose distal 1/third of thigh and proximal 1/third of leg followed by exsanguination and inflation of tourniquet.

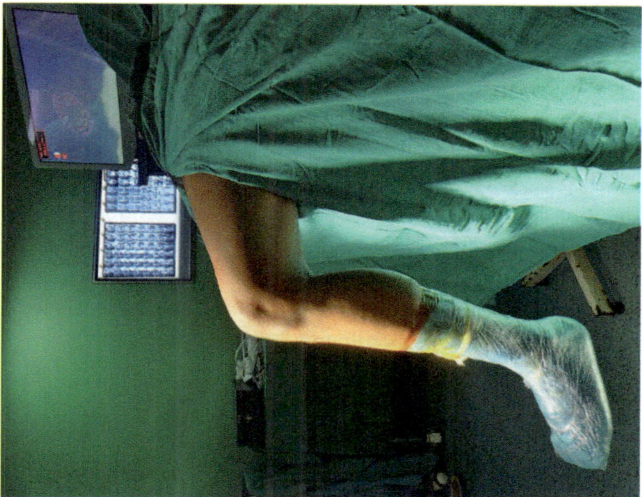

**Fig. 24.3** Draping

## 24.4 Portals

- Standard anterolateral portal—A standard anterolateral portal is made 1 cm above the joint line and just next to the patellar tendon in a palpable soft spot. It is used as a viewing portal for arthroscopic evaluation.
- Standard anteromedial portal—placed 1 cm above the joint line and 1 cm medial to the patellar tendon in a palpable soft spot.
- Low posteromedial portal—just above the joint line.
- High posteromedial portal—4 cm above the joint line.
- Posterolateral portal—posterior to the fibular collateral ligament and popliteus tendon at the level of the joint line for adequate access to the popliteus tendon.

## 24.5 Surgical Steps

### 24.5.1 Graft Preparation

Usually, a semitendinosus hamstring tendon autograft is harvested and prepared for popliteus tendon reconstruction. The diameter of the graft is between 5 and 6 mm. For whip stitching each end of the graft, no. 2 Fiberwire suture is used.

### 24.5.2 Operative Technique

Step 1: A standard anterolateral portal is made 1 cm above the joint line and just next to the patellar tendon in a palpable soft spot. It is used as a viewing portal for arthroscopic evaluation.

Step 2: A second anteromedial portal is made 1 cm above the joint line and 1 cm medial to the patellar tendon in a palpable soft spot. The placement of anteromedial portal can be confirmed with a spinal needle using the arthroscope. This portal is used as a working portal in the anterior compartment through which instruments are passed.

Step 3: A diagnostic arthroscopy is performed first. The popliteus is visualised through the lateral compartment and lateral gutter with the help of 30-degree arthroscope and popliteus tendon tear is confirmed.

Step 4: Two posteromedial portals are made. A low posteromedial portal is made just above the joint line by transillumination technique. An 18 G spinal needle is passed followed by portal creation with a no. 11 blade scalpel and a haemostat under direct vision (Fig. 24.4a and Fig. 24.5). An 8 mm arthroscopic cannula/ passport is then placed for ease of instrumentation through this portal (Fig. 24.4b).

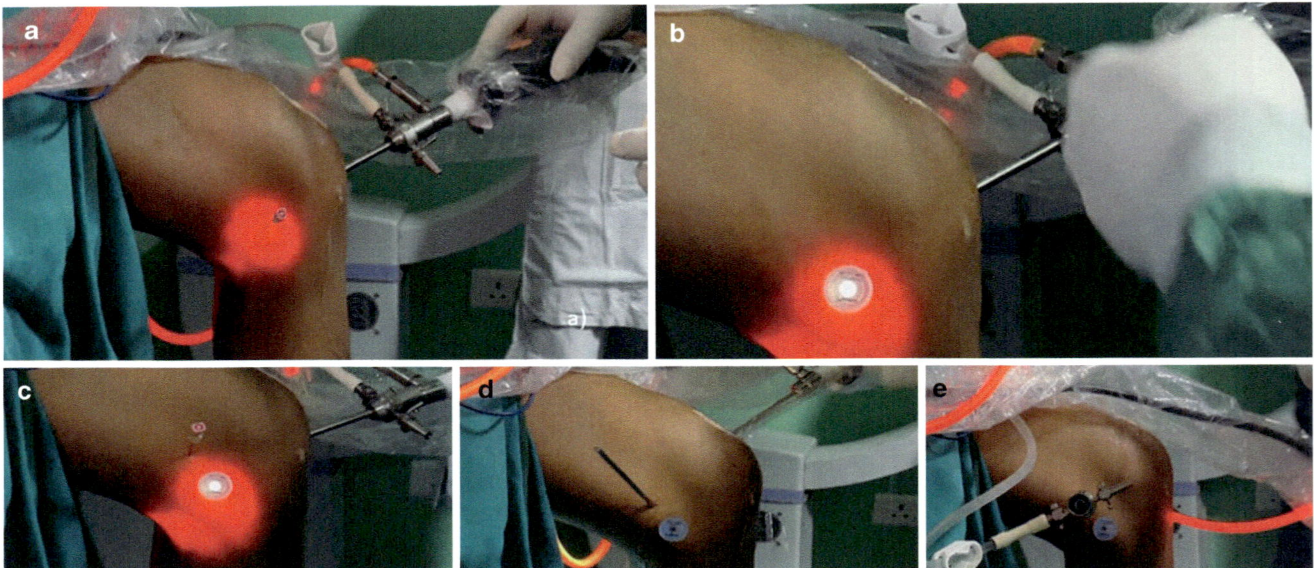

**Fig. 24.4** (**a**) Spinal needle for low posteromedial portal using Transillumination technique and doing needle test at the same time. (**b**); Passport cannula through low PM Portal. (**c**); Spinal needle for high PM Portal. (**d**); switching stick through high PM portal for shifting scope for visualisation port. (**e**); Arthroscopic sheath through high PM portal

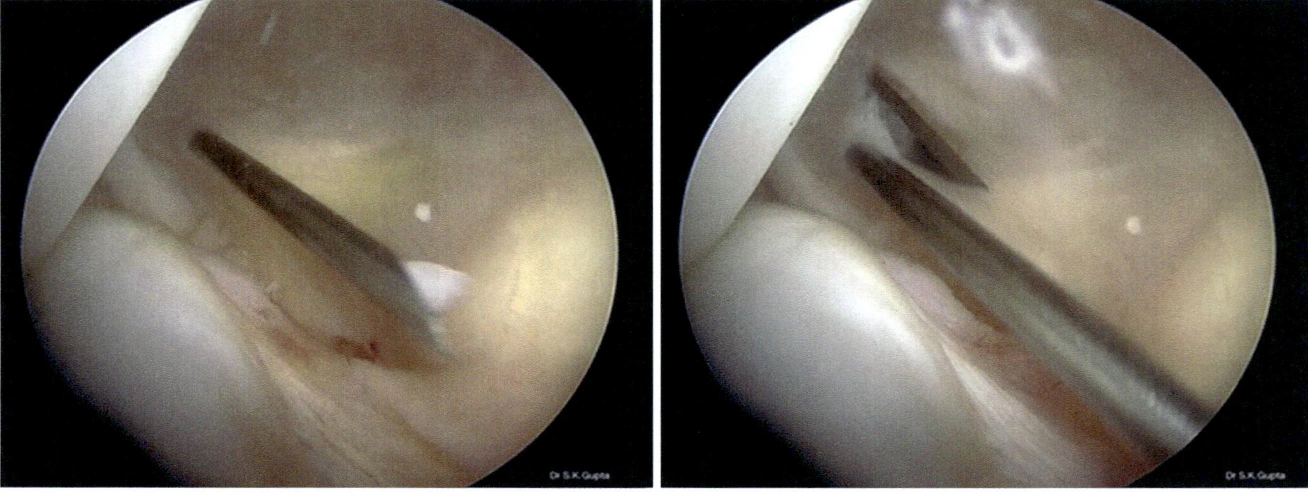

**Fig. 24.5** Low posteromedial portal creation with the help of 18 G spinal needle and 11 no. blade scalpel under direct vision by Transillumination technique

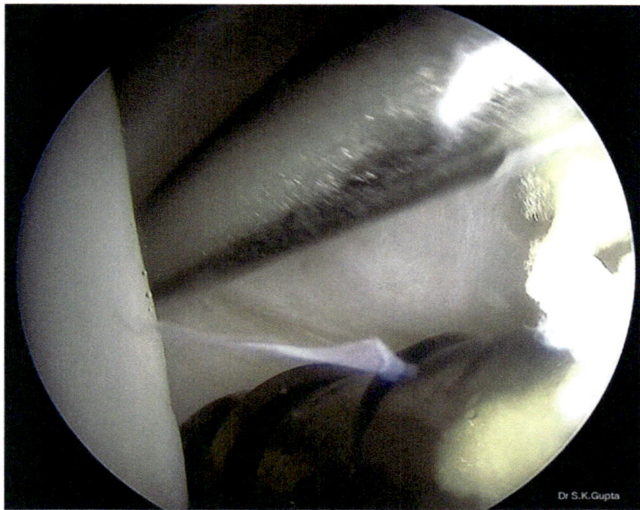


**Fig. 24.6** High posteromedial portal creation with low posteromedial portal showing an 8 mm cannula for ease of instrumentation

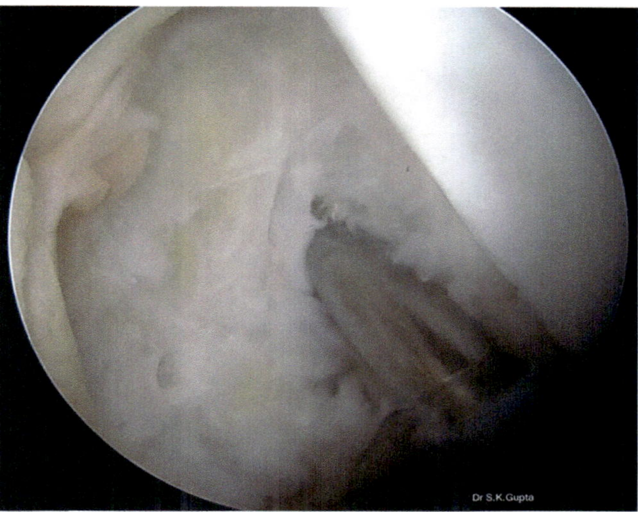


**Fig. 24.7** making way through central inferior septum with the help of shaver

A high posteromedial portal is made in the same manner 4 cm above the joint line (Fig. 24.4c). A switching rod is then passed and the arthroscope is switched to high posteromedial portal (Fig. 24.4d, e and Fig. 24.6).

Step 5: The arthroscope is placed through the high posteromedial portal to access the posteromedial compartment. The shaver is then introduced through the low posteromedial portal to gently remove the central inferior septum to avoid iatrogenic injury to the middle genicular vessels (Fig. 24.7). The shaver is faced towards the joint and away from the posterior neurovascular bundle. The septum is carefully released from medial to lateral. The shaver is kept in this position posterior to the PCL.

Step 6: The posterolateral portal is established under direct arthroscopic visualisation with the help of transillumination technique to avoid neurovascular injury. The spinal needle is positioned at the soft spot between the posterior border of the iliotibial band and the anterior border of biceps femoris (Fig. 24.8). An 11-no. blade is inserted in line with the spinal needle to make entry into the joint which is further widened with the help of haemostat. The portal should be placed posterior to the fibular collateral ligament and popliteus tendon at the level of joint line for adequate access to the popliteus tendon.

Insert the shaver into the posterolateral portal and resect the septum all the way to the level of the PCL.

The lateral meniscus, popliteus and posterior capsule are identified (Fig. 24.9). The posterior capsule and gastrocnemius muscle fibres are seen distally and the space between popliteus and gastrocnemius is opened.

To expose the popliteus musculotendinous junction, the synovium is debrided with the help of shaver. Posterolateral capsule is separated from the posterior horn of lateral meniscus for more than 10 mm downward from the articular surface. Posterolateral tibia is exposed and the popliteus musculotendinous junction is completely identified. The cutting surface of shaver is kept in anteroinferior direction to prevent damage to lateral inferior genicular artery.

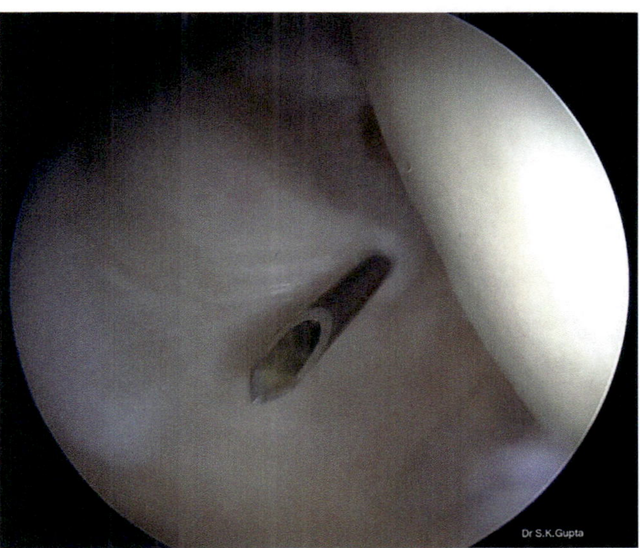


**Fig. 24.8** Posterolateral portal creation under direct vision using trans-illumination technique

Step 7: A PCL tibial guide is passed through the Anterolateral portal, advanced towards the popliteus musculotendinous junction area on the posterior tibia (Fig. 24.10). A small incision is given just lateral to the patellar tendon and directly over the Gerdy's tubercle.

A guide wire is passed from the anterior tibial cortex to posterior aspect of the lateral tibial plateau. This guide wire should exit at the point of the popliteus musculotendinous

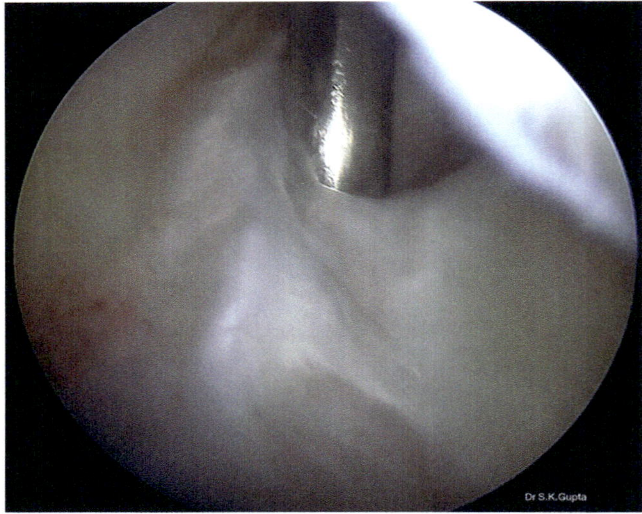


**Fig. 24.9** Identification of posterolateral capsule and gap creation to reach the popliteus musculotendinous junction

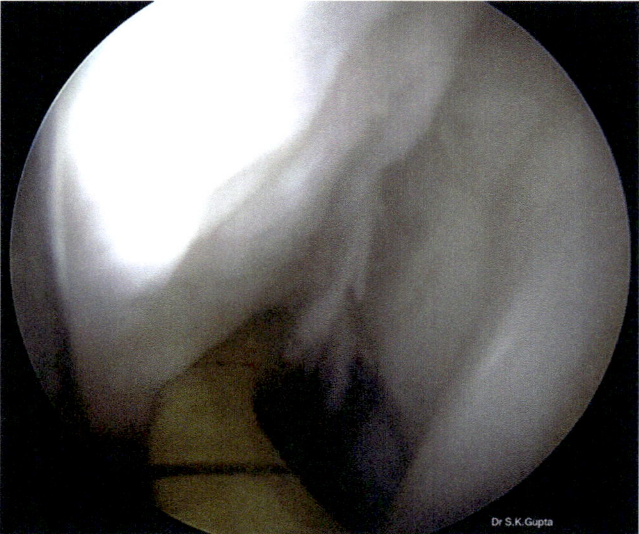


**Fig. 24.10** The PCL tibial guide is positioned over the posterior tibia such that the guide pin exits at the popliteus musculotendinous junction in the popliteus groove

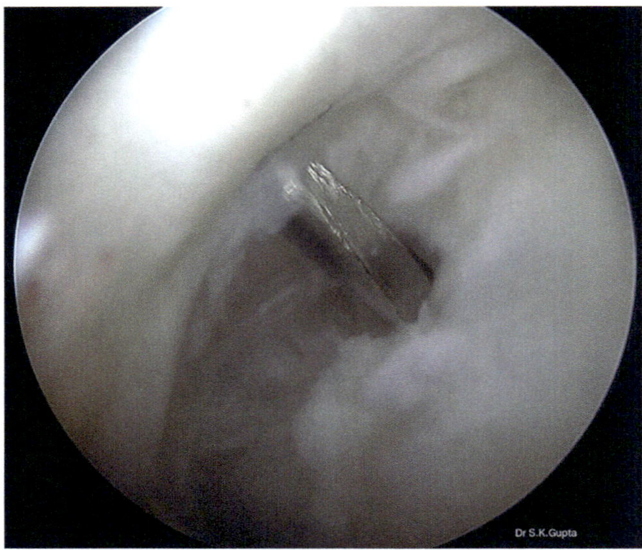


**Fig. 24.11** The drill exiting at the popliteus musculotendinous junction in the shallow popliteus groove

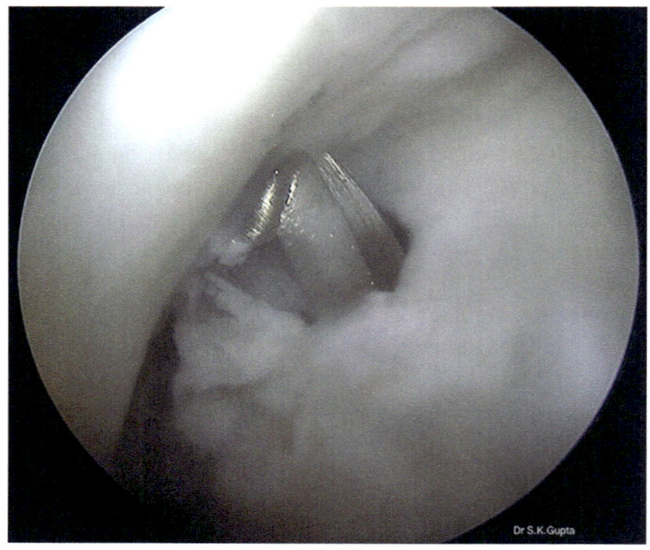


**Fig. 24.12** Creation of tibial tunnel by using cannulated drill

junction. The optimal point for the guide pin to penetrate is taken in the middle of the posterior tibia about 1 cm below the joint line, exactly in the shallow groove of the popliteus tendon (Fig. 24.11).

After positioning of the guide pin, a tibial tunnel is made with a cannulated reamer depending on the diameter of the graft taken (Fig. 24.12). During this procedure, care is taken to protect the lateral inferior genicular artery.

Step 8: Passing suture is used to pass the harvested graft, with the help of a suture manipulator or grasper suture is taken out through posterolateral portal (Fig. 24.13). Suture at the tibial end is tied to graft at the anterior tibial tunnel and suture from posterolateral portal is pulled to relay the graft. The suture with graft tied to it is pulled through the posterolateral portal and parked there (Fig. 24.14).

Step 9: A radiofrequency device is introduced through the posterolateral portal to separate the posterolateral capsule from the posterior horn of lateral meniscus for 2 cm to visualise the popliteus sulcus.

Electrocautery is used to mark the central point of femoral footprint. An eyelet guide pin is drilled into the centre of the footprint and a femoral tunnel of about 6–7 mm diameter and approximately 25 mm depth is created over the guide pin (Fig. 24.15).

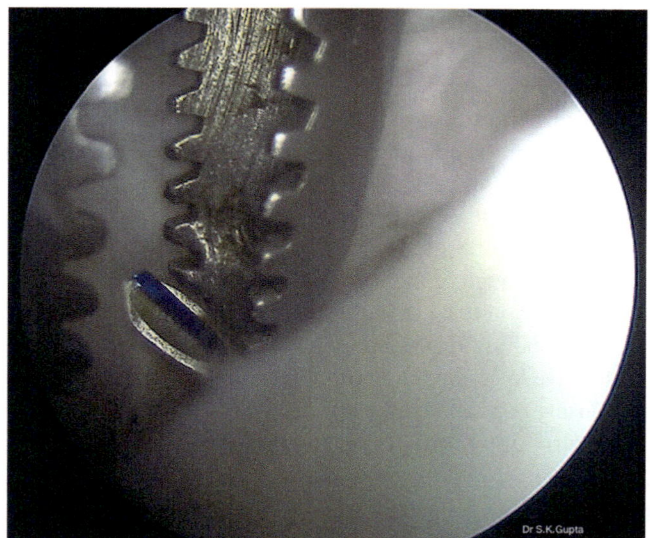


**Fig. 24.13** Passing suture is grasped and carried out through posterolateral portal

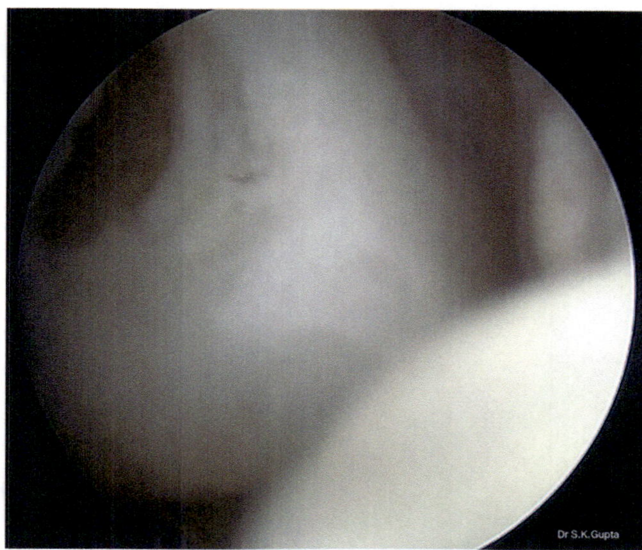


**Fig. 24.15** Femoral tunnel created at the popliteus femoral foot print

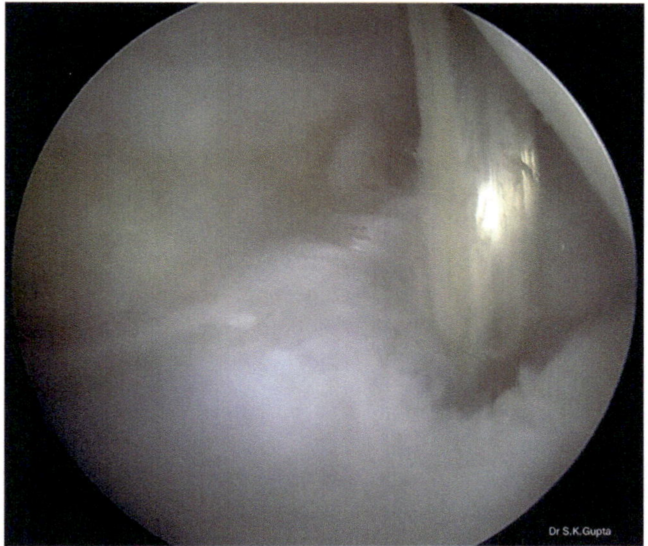


**Fig. 24.14** Graft passed with the help of passing suture and taken out of posterolateral portal

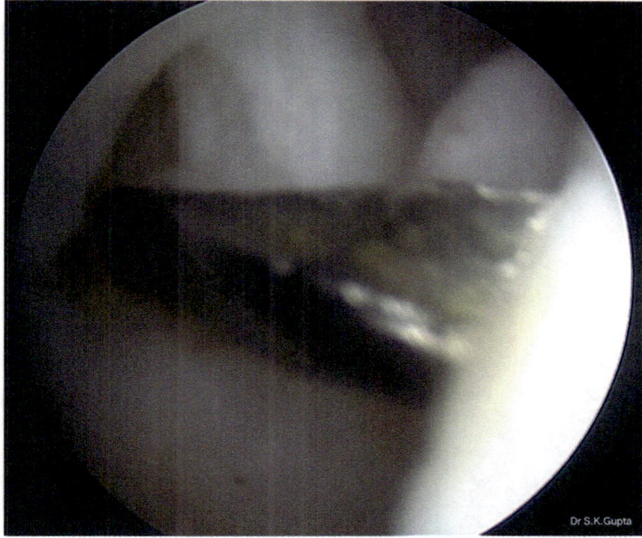


**Fig. 24.16** An eyelet guide pin passed into femoral tunnel to pass the passing suture followed by the harvested graft

Step 10: Now, the passing suture is introduced into the femoral tunnel by using guide pin (Fig. 24.16) and pulled through the medial side of the knee. The graft is then pulled through the femoral tunnel (Fig. 24.17).

Step 11: The popliteus reconstruction is completed by pulling the passing suture and tensioning the graft from the medial side of the knee. When the graft sits well in the femoral tunnel (Fig. 24.18), it is fixed with a bioabsorbable screw usually 1 size larger than the tunnel diameter. Similarly, after tensioning the graft is fixed in tibial tunnel with a bio-interference screw which is advanced to the posterior aspect of the tunnel. In osteoporotic cases, the tibial fixation can be further secured by tying the attached suture over a post on the anterolateral aspect of tibia.

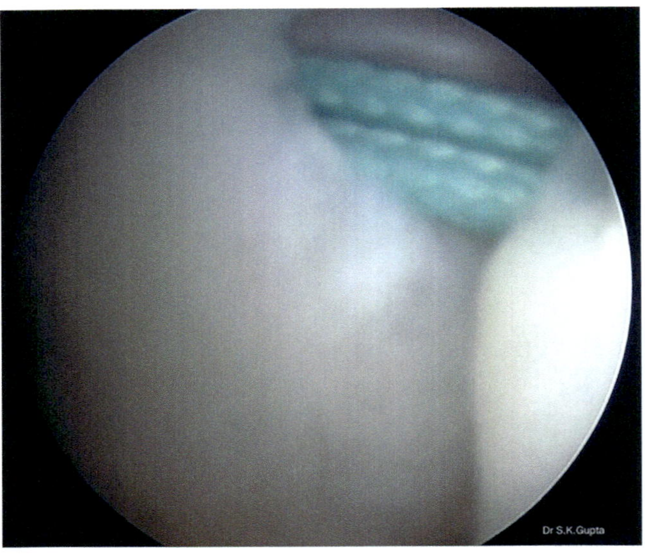


**Fig. 24.17** The whipstitched end of harvested graft being passed through femoral tunnel

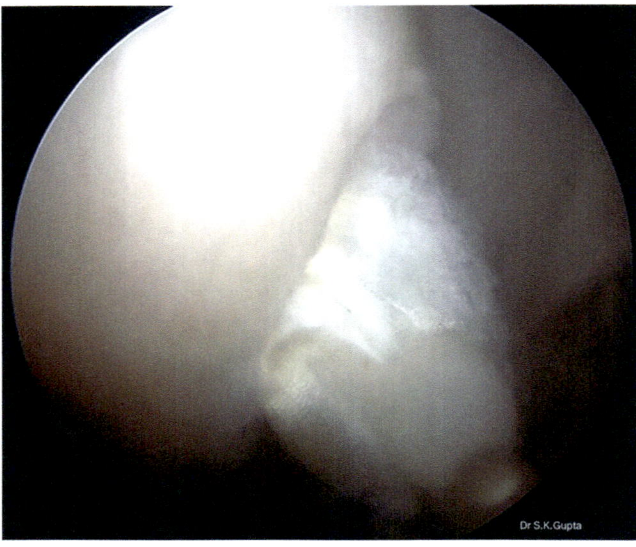


**Fig. 24.18** The harvested graft is passed through femoral tunnel

## 24.6 Postoperative Rehabilitation

- Postoperatively, immobilisation and protected weight bearing is encouraged till 6 weeks.
- Long leg brace is preferred as these control leg external rotation for 3 weeks.
- Passive range of motion exercises are begun at 2 weeks to avoid arthrofibrosis.
- Limited range of motion 0—20 for 2 weeks.
  - 0—45 in third to fourth week
  - 0—60 in fiffth—sixth week.
- Passive knee flexion in prone position against quadriceps muscle resistance up to $60^0$ allowed.
- Return to sports after nine months only.

## 24.7 Advantages and Disadvantages

### 24.7.1 Advantages

- Precise positioning of the musculotendinous junction of the popliteus.
- Avoid the morbidity of the open technique.
- Decrease the potential iatrogenic injury to the genicular arteries.
- Allows for simultaneous arthroscopic transtibial reconstruction of the posterior cruciate ligament.
- Can also be used in combination with LCL reconstruction in PLC injuries.

### 24.7.2 Disadvantages

- Arthroscopic exploration of musculotendinous junction is difficult.
- Positioning of popliteus femoral insertion is difficult due to lack of visualisation and less space in lateral gutter.
- Risk of injury to lateral inferior genicular artery.
- Iatrogenic compartment syndrome risk due to extravasation of irrigating fluid.
- Subcutaneous effusion or interstitial oedema.

# 25 All Arthroscopic: Anatomic Posterolateral Reconstruction of Knee

Sameer Salim Shaikh, Amol Umakant Gowaikar, and Santosh Dattatray Takale

## 25.1 Introduction

All landmarks of PLC can be arthroscopically visualised in detail allowing safe and effective treatment of PLC injuries. The PLC consists primarily of the lateral collateral ligament (LCL) and popliteus complex (PTC), which includes the popliteus muscle tendon (PLT) unit and the arcuate complex. The arcuate complex contains the popliteofibular ligament (PFL), fabellofibular ligament and popliteomeniscal fibres. Functionally, the arcuate complex acts as a static stabiliser of the tibia against external rotation and in synergy with PLT against posterior translation [1–3].

Arciero introduced a fibula-based technique with an anatomic transfibular tunnel placement, from anterolateral to posteromedial, in accordance with the native functional anatomy of the LCL and PTC injury with subsequent posterolateral rotational instability [4]. Here we introduce an all arthroscopic technique for posterolateral stabilisation in accordance with the procedure devised by Arciero & Larsons, using the semitendinosis graft.

This technique is indicated for posterolateral instabilities, Fanelli grades B and C. With the technique described in this technical note, lateral (varus) instability and the external rotational instability can be addressed. In most patients, an additional posterior instability is present which is treated by additional remnant preserving PCL reconstruction [5].

This technical note describes a reproducible arthroscopic surgical approach to identify and expose the PT, posterior fibular head, LCL, PFL and Biceps femurs tendon without exposing the popliteal nerve. The arthroscopic approach may be used in any case of posterolateral reconstruction. It has the advantage of a smaller skin incision, lower infection rates, more precise localisation of anatomic landmarks for graft positioning and nerve injury can be avoided.

## 25.2 Special Instruments Required

1. 5.5/6 mm arthroscopic cannula –2
2. Wissinger rod - 1.
3. No 5 and 2.0 Ethibond / fibrewire.
4. PDS Suture - 2.0 and no. 1.
5. Knot pusher.
6. PCL Jig with long arm.
7. Guide Wires - 2.4 mm.
8. Drill bits of various sizes ranging from 4.5 to 10 mm.

## 25.3 Positioning

Patient is placed in the supine position, with lateral post just proximal to the knee, at the level of the padded tourniquet, hanging knee position with knee in 90 degrees flexion. This allows the knee to be moved freely through its range of movement while preventing the hip from externally rotating (Fig. 25.1).

## 25.4 Diagnostic Arthroscopy

A diagnostic arthroscopy of the knee is done to assess the intraarticular status of PLC and PCL (Fig. 25.2).

**Supplementary Information** The online version contains supplementary material available at https://doi.org/10.1007/978-981-99-4378-4_25.

S. S. Shaikh (✉) · A. U. Gowaikar · S. D. Takale
Department of Arthroscopy, Sports Injuries & Joint Replacement, Shaikh Institute of Orthopaedics & Trauma, Miraj, Maharashtra, India


V. A. Mhaskar, J. Maheshwari (eds.), *Innovative Approaches in Knee Arthroscopy*, https://doi.org/10.1007/978-981-99-4378-4_25

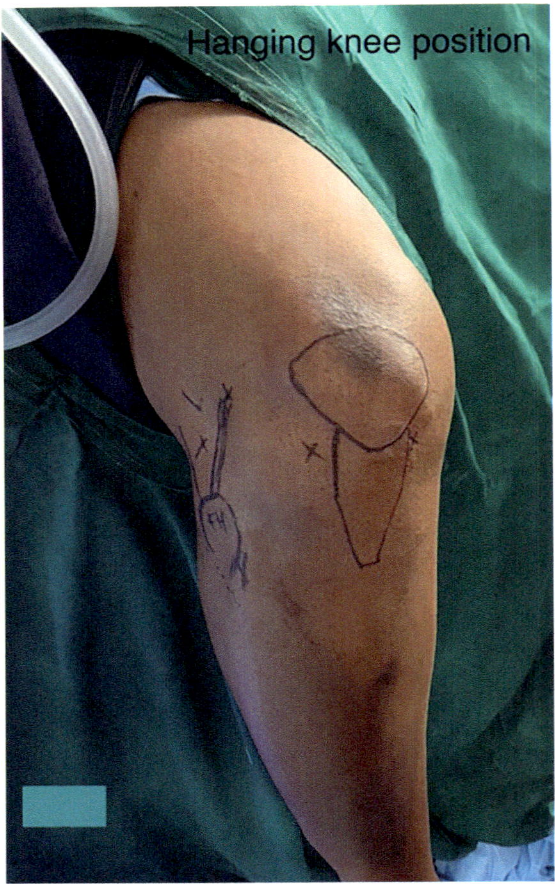


**Fig. 25.1** Hanging leg on table in supine position

Amount of lateral compartment opening: Usually >10 mm of lateral compartment opening when there is grade 3 posterolateral corner injury.

1. During arthroscopy it is important to determine whether this is a meniscofemoral or a meniscotibial injury. When the meniscus stays with the femur - it usually indicates a significant lateral capsular or second variant soft tissue or bony avulsion pattern. If meniscus stays with tibia - it usually indicates femoral based avulsions or intrasubstance stretch injury of the popliteus tendon and probably also FCL Injury.
2. Up to 75% of the patients - anteroinferior popliteomeniscal fascicle to the lateral meniscus tear is seen - Lateral meniscal hyper mobility.
3. Lateral gutter examination shows popliteus tendon injury at femoral attachment site.

## 25.5 Surgical Technique (Video 25.1)

Step 1: Portal creation (Fig. 25.3a–e).

Arthroscopic posterolateral stabilisation requires five portals: high anterolateral, high anteromedial, high posteromedial, low posteromedial and superolateral.

Anterolateral (AL) portal.

Place the standard anterolateral portal far enough lateral to work in lateral gutter and avoid impingement with lateral femoral condyle.

Anteromedial (AM) portal.

Anteromedial portal is added by introducing the needle medial to patellar tendon margin above the medial meniscus to allow easy passage through the intercondylar notch into posterior compartment.

Superolateral (SL)portal.

Insert a spinal needle at the midpoint of the lateral border of the patella with the knee flexed at 90 degrees to confirm access to both the lateral epicondyle and popliteus tendon.

Posteromedial (PM)portal.

After AL and AM portals were created, the arthroscope from AL portal is passed into posteromedial recess by removing the septum and approaching between the ACL and PCL. To develop a high and low posteromedial portal, the needle should be used to localise the correct placement under arthroscopic vision before the stab incision is made.

Posterolateral (PL) portal.

A shaver is introduced through the low PM portal and view through high PM portal, dorsal septum is carefully resected (transeptal approach). Keep the opening of the shaver blade anteriorly to avoid popliteal nerves and vessels (**e**) Needle from outside in method for PL portal viewing from PM portal.

The arthroscope from the high PM portal is advanced into the posterolateral compartment. Palpate the soft spot between the posterior border of iliotibial band and anterior border of biceps femoris. Using an outside in technique an LP needle used to create posterolateral portal posterior to the popliteus for adequate access to the fibular head.

Step 2: Posterolateral capsulotomy, fibular head, identification and preparation of plc (Fig. 25.4).

The 30 degree arthroscope is introduced through in the high PM portal and passed transseptally into the PL compartment. A radio frequency device is then introduced through the PL portal to separate the posterolateral capsular fibres from the lateral meniscus posterior horn dorsal to the popliteus tendon.

Identification of the fibular head is of paramount importance to identify the remaining PLC structures. Directly lateral and distal to the popliteus tendon, the fibular head can be palpated and subsequently exposed by gentle preparation of the surrounding tissue.

During preparation of fibular head, risk of injuring the peroneal nerve is minimised by continuous visualisation, avoidance of preparation past its posterior edge and nerve identification.

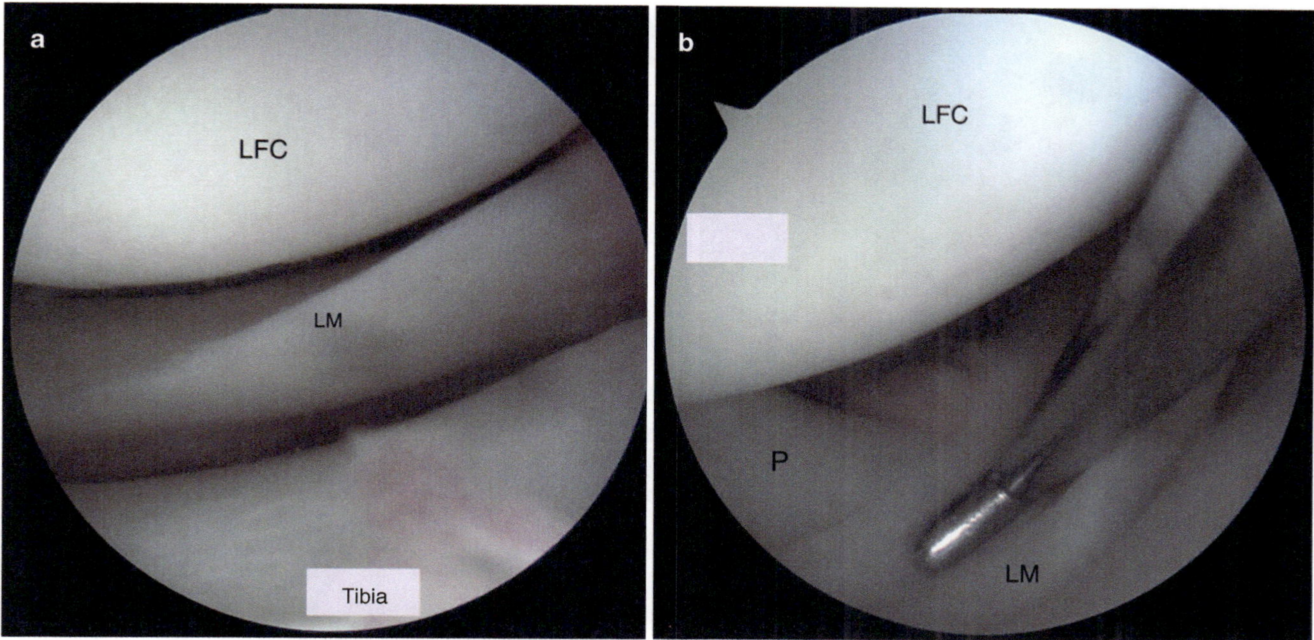


**Fig 25.2** (**a**, **b**) (lateral opening >10 mm which indicates grade III PLC Corner injury.) *LFC* lateral femoral condyle, *LM* lateral meniscus, *P* popliteus

Step 3: Graft preparation (Fig. 25.5).

Semitendinosis tendon is used for the posterolateral stabilisation. At least 20 cm graft is needed to achieve perfect graft fixation.

Step 4: Fibular tunnel placement.

Incision made for the fibular tunnel entry point starting just above the tip of fibula for 1.5cms, while palpating it. With the arthroscope placed in the PM portal, a PCL tibial drill guide is inserted through the posterolateral portal and placed on the posteromedial surface of the fibular head. A small stab incision is made on the anterolateral portion of fibular head and the guide wire is inserted in the anterolateral to posteromedial direction under arthroscopic visualisation. It is then over drilled with a cannulated drill that is the same diameter of the graft which is usually 6–7 mm and care must be taken to avoid blow out of the fibular head. We have seen smaller fibular heads in Indian patients and have not used a screw for fixation in osteoporotic patients (Fig. 25.6).

Step 5: Suture passage.

The passing suture is inserted through the fibular tunnel, viewing through PM portal. An arthroscopic grasper is inserted into the PL compartment and the passing suture retrieved through the PL portal which is retrieved from a lateral incision via the popliteus hiatus.

Step 6: Femoral footprint Preparation and tunnel placement.

Viewing from AL portal and working from SL portal, femoral attachment of popliteus and FCL are exposed. Addition of a stay suture can be helpful to retract the iliotibial band, providing better visualisation. Eyelet beath pins are

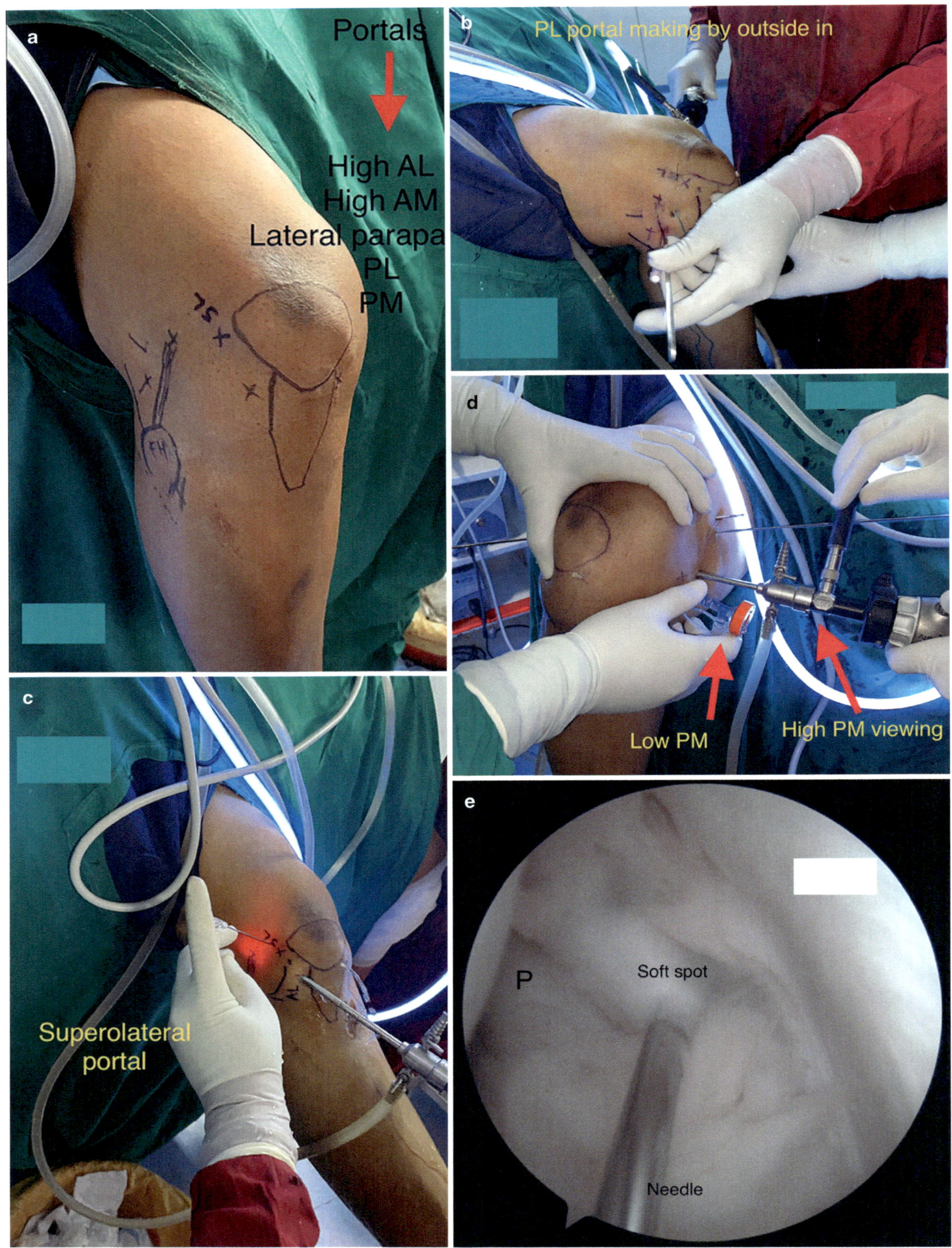


**Fig. 25.3** (**a**) Portals for PLC stabilisation. (**b**) Posterolateral portal making viewing from PM portal. (**c**) superolateral portal. (**d**) Shows high and low PM portals

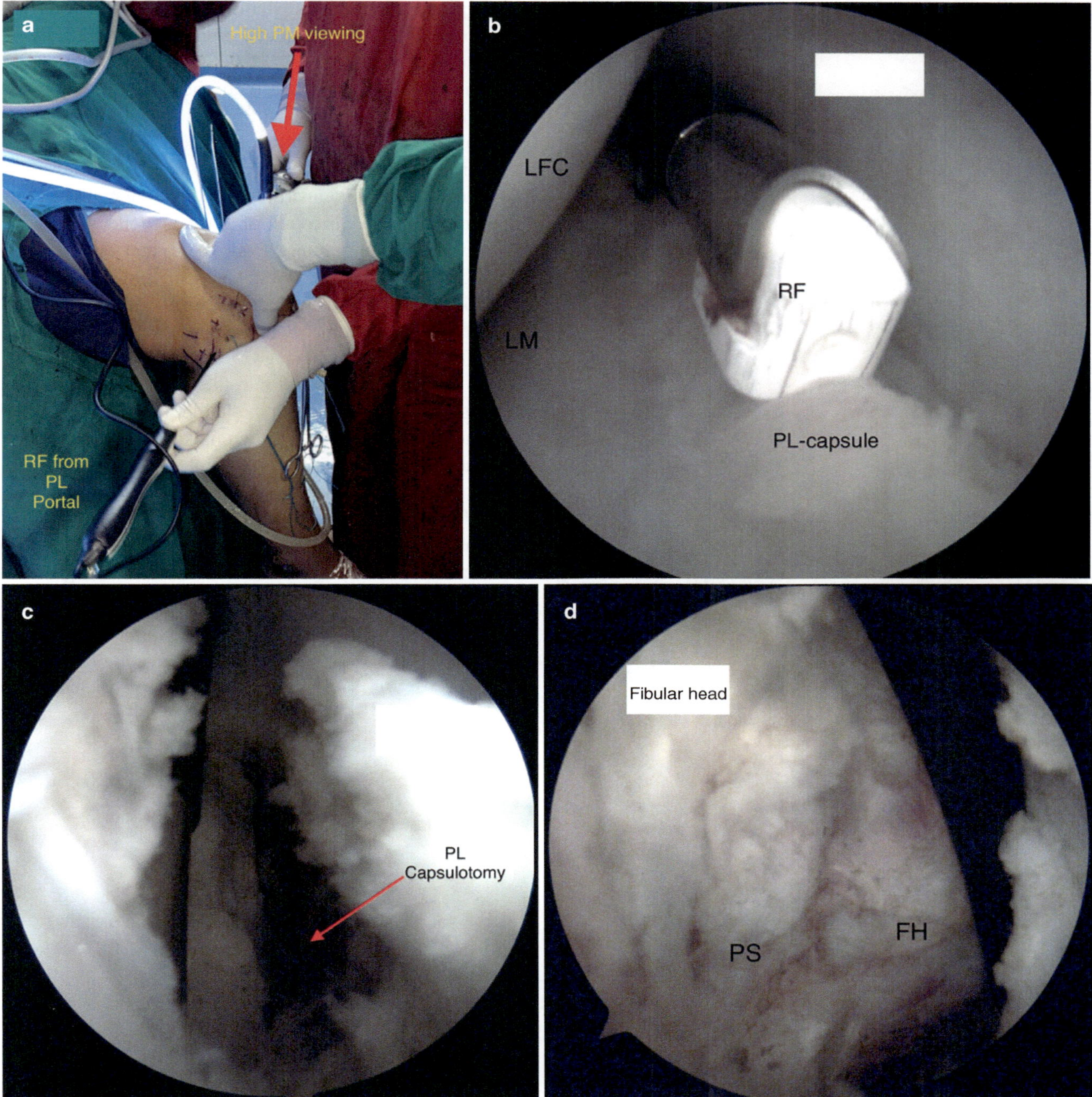


**Fig. 25.4** (**a**) PM viewing and radiofrequency probe from PL portal for posterolateral capsulotomy. (**b**) RF in PL portal, posterior to popliteus and viewing from PM portal. (**c**) Posterolateral capsulotomy posterior to lateral meniscus posterior horn. (**d**) Posterior aspect of fibular head palpated with RF.) *PS* popliteal sulcus, *FH* fibular head, *LFC* lateral femoral condyle, *LM* lateral meniscus, *RF* radio frequency probe

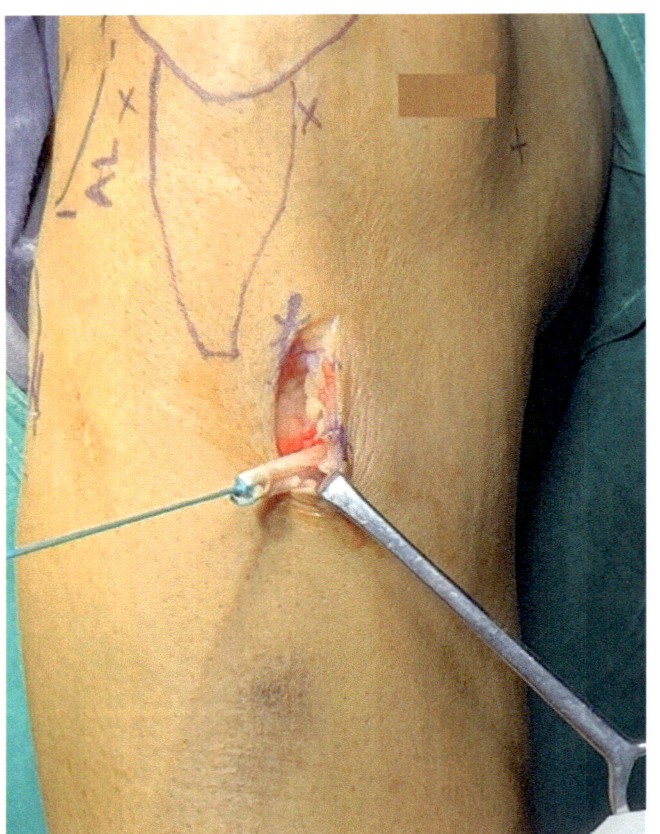

**Fig. 25.5** Ipsilateral harvesting of semitendinosis graft for PLC stabilisation

then drilled through lateral stab incision into femoral footprints of the LCL (proximal and posterior to lateral epicondyle) and PLT. Distance between two guide wires is approximately 18.5 mm, which are then over drilled with a cannulated drill (Fig.25.7).

Step 7: Graft passage and fixation.

Insert the curved artery forceps into lateral stab incision to reach posterolateral compartment through the popliteus hiatus along the native direction of popliteus tendon. Retrieve the previous passing suture from the lateral stab incision viewing from PM portal. First, the semitendinosis graft is pulled into femoral PLT tunnel and fixed with a bioabsorbable/titanium interference screw under arthroscopic visualisation from the AL portal (Fig. 25.8).

The graft is then shuttled into the knee, along the native popliteus tendon and through the fibular tunnel in the posterior to anterior direction. It is then fixed in the fibular tunnel with another bioscrew with the knee at 90 degrees. In osteoporotic Indian patients and small fibulas, where screw insertion will lead to a blowout the screw is not placed.

Finally, the graft is pulled into LCL tunnel and fixed with a bioscrew/titanium interference screw, at 30 degrees of flexion.

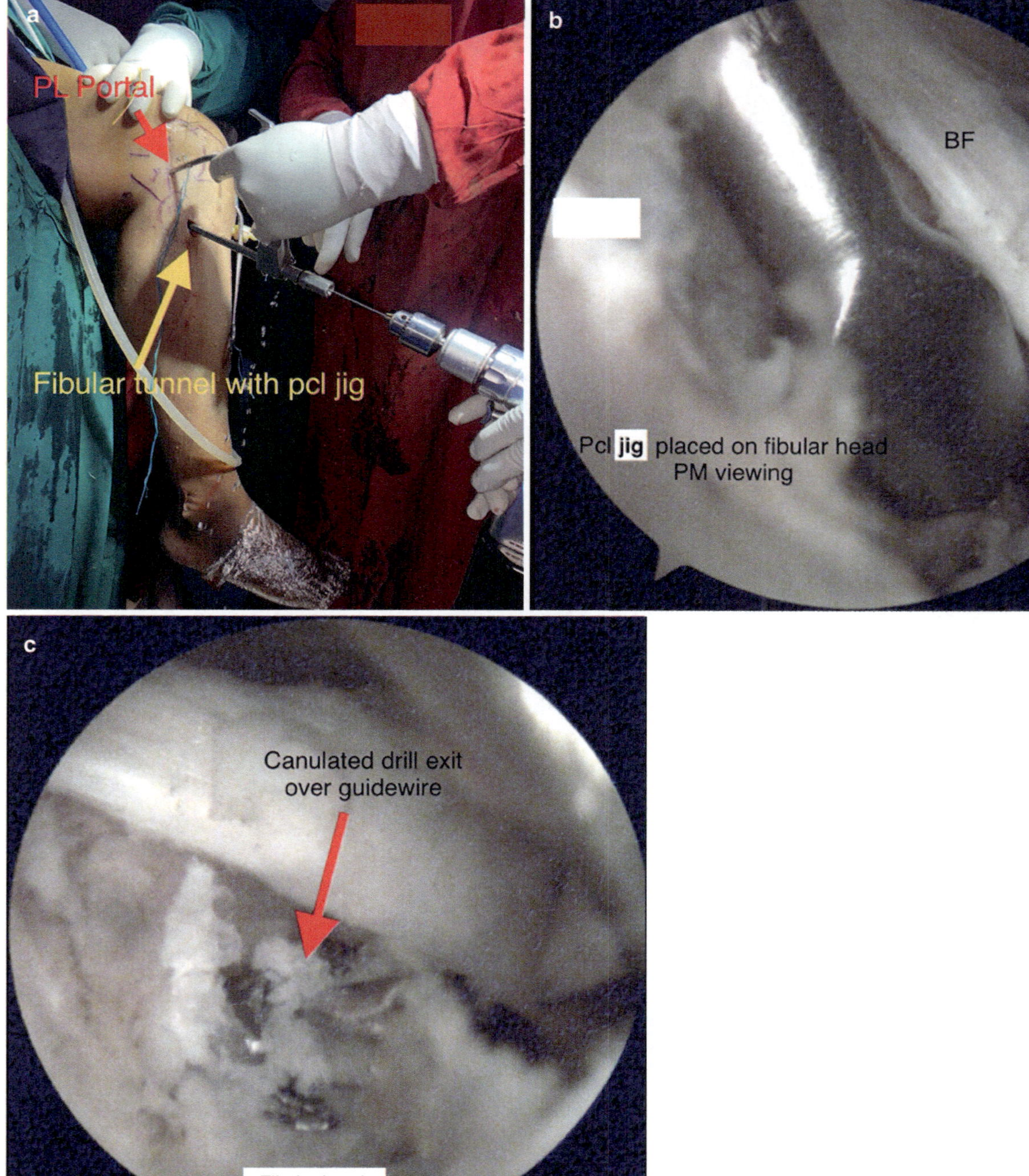


**Fig. 25.6** (**a**) PCL tibial Jig used for fibular tunnel making and guide wire passed from anterolateral to posteromedial direction viewing from PM portal. 6 (**b**) Arthroscopic view from PM portal - jig placed over the posteromedial part of fibular head posteriorly. (**c**) Guide wire exiting posteromedially from anterolateral aspect of fibula with cannulated drill. *BF* biceps femoris

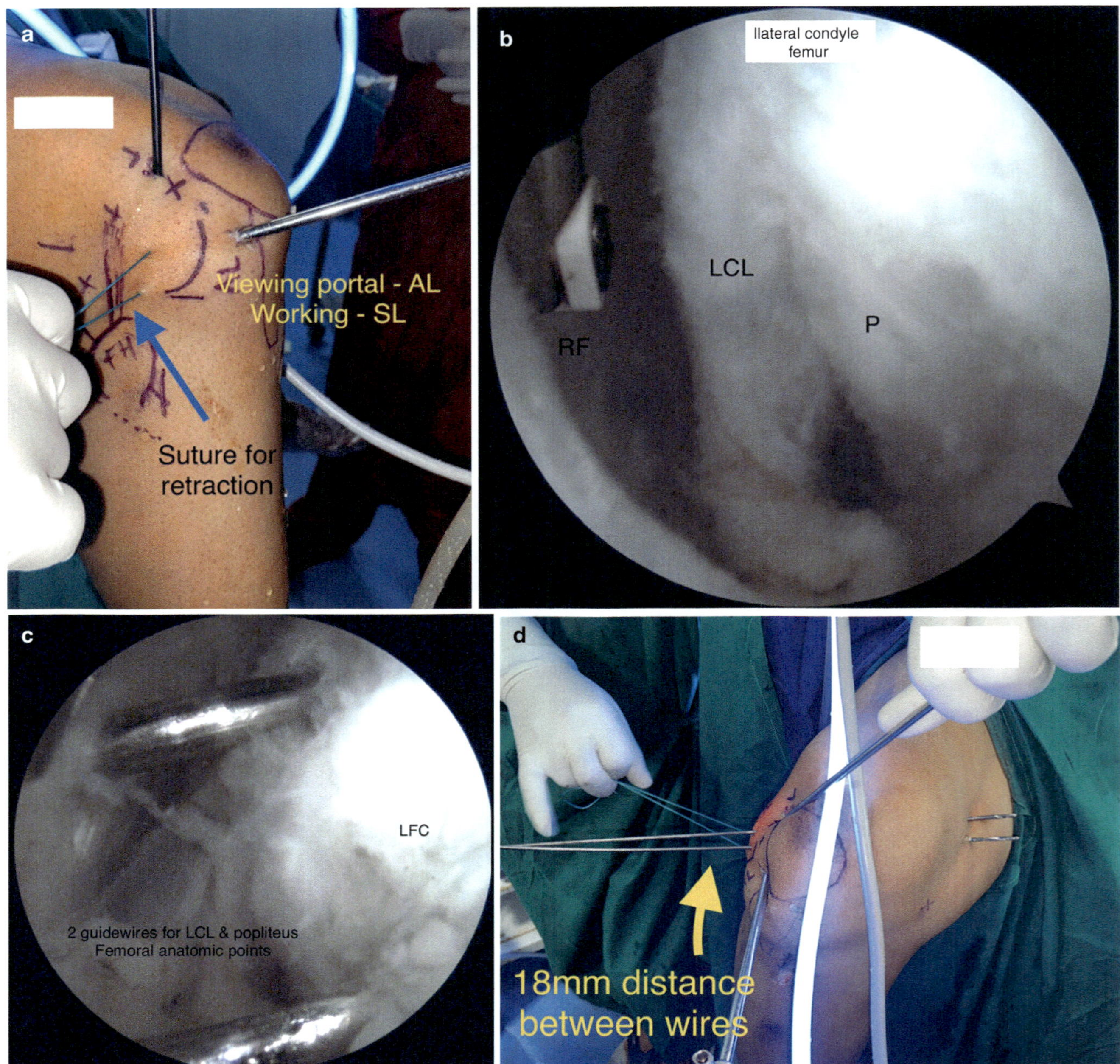


**Fig. 25.7** (**a**) Stay suture used for retraction of iliotibial band during femoral footprint preparation for good viewing from high AL portal and working from SL portal (**b**) LCL and popliteus anatomic marking with RF (**c**) Guidewires at anatomic femoral insertion of LCL and popliteus. (**d**) Popliteus and LCL guide wires in situ with distance between two wires 18.5 mm approx

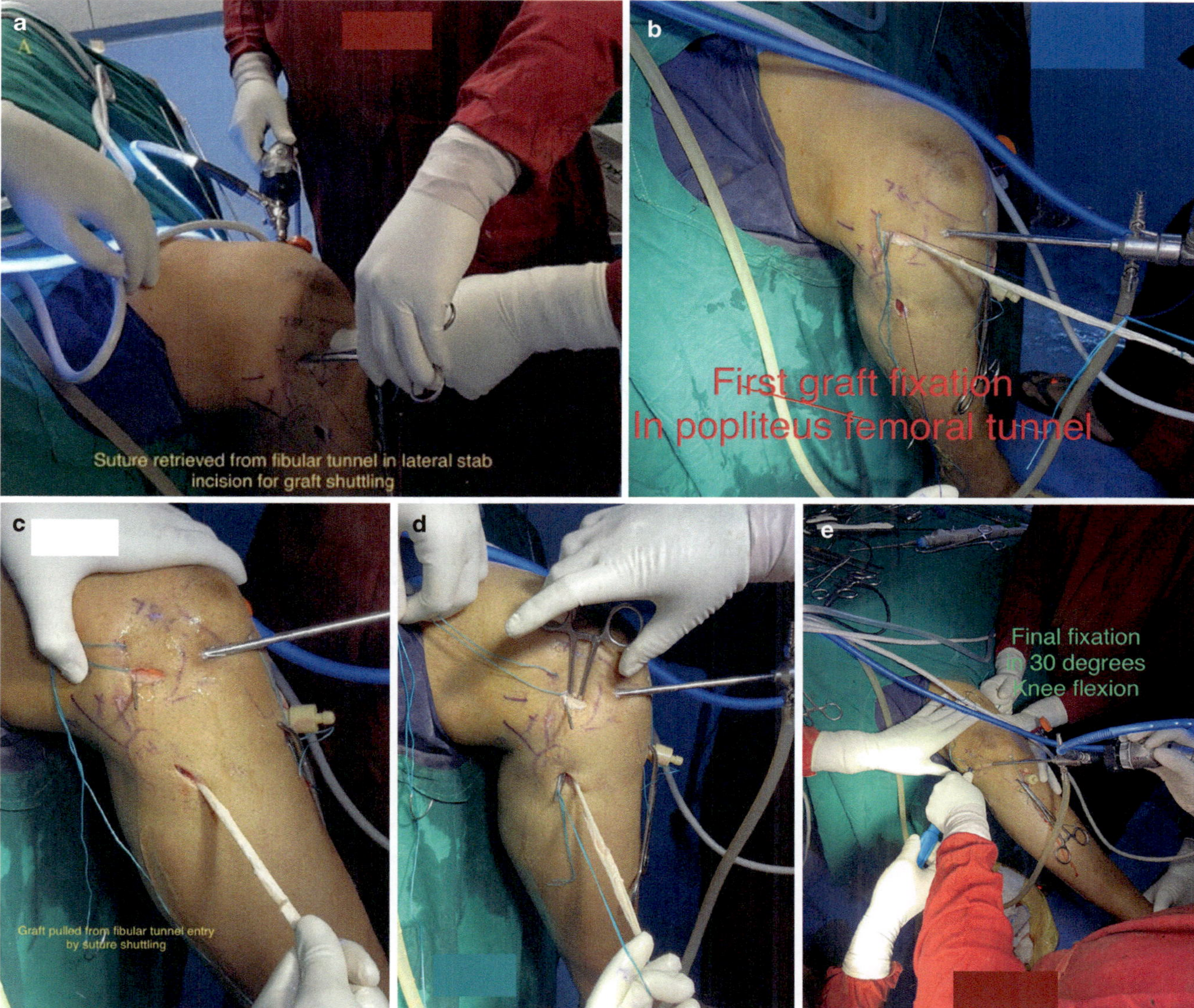


**Fig. 25.8** (**a**) Suture retrieval from lateral stab incision while pulling from the fibular tunnel (**b**): Popliteus graft fixation at popliteus femoral tunnel with Titanium interference screw/bioscrew. (**c**) Shuttling of the graft, along the native popliteus tendon, and through fibular tunnel in the posterior to anterior direction. (**d**) Graft pulled from anterior fibular tunnel into LCL femoral tunnel beneath the iliotibial band. (**e**) Final fixation of the graft into LCL femoral tunnel at 30 degrees of knee flexion

## 25.6 Rehabilitation

Isolated injuries of PLC are rare. Combined PLC + PCL, PLC + ACL, PLC + PCL + ACL injuries are seen. There is no standardised rehabilitation protocol after PLC reconstruction.

Long knee brace with posterior tibial support is recommended to protect the knee from varus stress. Mobilisation should be restricted to partial weight bearing for 6 weeks, and joint mobilisation should be limited to passive motion with limited flexion as per pain tolerance for about 6 weeks depending on injury pattern. Full weight bearing is allowed after 6 weeks.

## 25.7 Advantages and Disadvantages

### 25.7.1 Advantages

1. Minimally invasive technique with good results.
2. Exact location of anatomic landmarks is possible.
3. Precise tunnel placement and anatomic graft positioning.

### 25.7.2 Disadvantages

1. Requires profound knowledge of the complex posterolateral anatomy.
2. Technically demanding as advanced arthroscopic skills required.
3. Peroneal nerve injury and tunnel mismatch can occur.

## 25.8 Technical Tips and Tricks for all Arthroscopic Anatomic Plc Reconstruction of Knee

1. Posterolateral portal is placed close to the femoral condyle to gain full access to the fibular head.
2. Fibular head preparation: First landmark to be spotted and is the best point to start dissection for better visualisation. The fibular head is palpated from outside using the push–pull method to visualise through the posteromedial portal and working through posterolateral portal.
3. Peroneal nerve: is located 2–3 cm distal to popliteus tendon. Sudden muscle contraction may indicate proximity to the nerve. Common peroneal nerve safety is preserved when the work area is at the level of the tip of the fibular head.
4. Femoral tunnel preparation: A stay suture is used to retract Iliotibial band to provide more space and better visualisation.

## References


1. Thaunat M, Pioger C, Chatellard R, Conteduca J, Khaleel A, Sonnery-Cottet B. The arcuate ligament revisited: role of the posterolateral structures in providing static stability in the knee joint. Knee Surg Sports Traumatol Arthrosc. 2014;22:2121–7.
2. Shon O-J, Park J-W, Kim B-J. Current concepts of posterolateral corner injuries of the knee. Knee Surg Relat Res. 2017;29:25.
3. Domnick C, Frosch KH, Raschke MJ. Kinematics of different components of the posterolateral corner of the knee in the lateral collateral ligament-intact state: a human cadaveric study. Arthroscopy. 2017;33:1821–30.
4. Arciero RA. Anatomic posterolateral corner knee reconstruction. Arthroscopy. 2005;21:1147.
5. Khanduja V, Somayaji H, Harnett P, Utukuri M, Dowd G. Combined reconstruction of chronic posterior cruciate ligament and posterolateral corner deficiency: a two-to nine-year follow-up study. Bone Joint J. 2006;88:1169–72.

# Implant-Less Bone Bridge Fixation

# 26

Amit Joshi, Nagmani Singh, Bibek Basukala,
Rajiv Sharma, Sunil Panta, Sabin Shrestha, Rohit Bista,
and Ishor Pradhan

## 26.1 Introduction

Over the last couple of decades, knee arthroscopy has grown by leaps and bounds. Several conditions involving the knee, which were managed by open surgical techniques, are now being treated efficiently by arthroscopy. Recent advancement in knee arthroscopy has also been paralleled by advances in fixation techniques and implants. Ligamentous and meniscal injuries are commonly treated with implant fixations [1].

Implants used in knee arthroscopy can be broadly classified into metallic and non-metallic implants, and these are used in a variety of conditions. These implants, however, have their own advantages and disadvantages. Metallic implants can cause tissue irritation and allergic reactions, increased chances of infection, problems with migrations and loosening, and the need for complicated removal surgeries for implants in cases that require revisions. Also, these metallic implants may produce altered signal disturbances during Magnetic resonance imaging (MRI) if MRI is needed to evaluate the lesion around the knee. To counter these adverse effects of metallic implants, non-metallic implants were devised. But these implants also have shown to cause several side effects, especially premature absorption, non-absorption, and foreign body reactions like pretibial synovial cyst formation [2].

Due to the disadvantages mentioned above, several researchers worldwide have started trying to find ways to avoid these implants and achieve implant-less fixation [3]. Several authors have described their modifications of press-fit with successful outcomes [4, 5]. Most of them reported that it has strength and stiffness similar to those with implants and have added advantage of decreasing cost and resulting in the direct bone to bone healing [6].

The complications related to implants are more prominent on the tibial side than on the femoral side. The tibia is a subcutaneous bone; hence, even the smallest of the implant becomes prominent and palpable, which may cause irritation and discomfort. It has been noted in our practice that several of these metallic implants used as a fixation post have to be removed subsequently due to prominence and discomfort. Pandey et al., in a paper on tibial spine fracture fixation, mentioned that even a tiny endo button has to be removed because of prominence and irritation [7]. Apart from these complications, these implants are expensive and may not be affordable to many, especially in low- and middle-income countries with less developed health systems.

In contrast to femoral implant-less fixation techniques, tibial implant-less fixation techniques are becoming popular as the complications related to implants are more common on the tibial side. The tibial implant-less fixation can be extremely useful for a variety of ailments of the knee which require tibial fixation [8]. To avoid the complications related to the implants, we described a "suture bridge technique," which is cost-effective, easy to perform, and can be used for various conditions and has become the workhorse for many surgeries. The indications of implant-less fixations on the tibia are ever-expanding and can be used for multiple conditions (Table 26.1). This chapter describes our transtibial pull-out root repair technique of medial meniscus and implant-less

A. Joshi (✉) · N. Singh · B. Basukala · R. Sharma · S. Panta
S. Shrestha · R. Bista · I. Pradhan
AKB Center for Arthroscopy, Sports Injuries and Regenerative Medicine, B&B Hospital, Lalitpur, Nepal


V. A. Mhaskar, J. Maheshwari (eds.), *Innovative Approaches in Knee Arthroscopy*,
https://doi.org/10.1007/978-981-99-4378-4_26

**Table 26.1** Indications for suture bridge fixation on the tibial side

| | Indications |
|---|---|
| 1 | Ligamentous surgeries- ACL reconstruction and PCL reconstructions. |
| 2 | Meniscal surgeries- root repairs, trans osseous repair of radial tear of the meniscus. |
| 3 | Avulsion injuries- ACL and PCL bony avulsion injuries. |

fixation over a bone bridge. The same implant-less fixation technique can be used in various other conditions. This implant-less technique is our first choice in root repairs; hence, this technique is described in detail.

## 26.2 Special Equipment Required (Fig. 26.1)

The significant advantages of this technique are low cost, and it can be performed with equipment readily available in the arthroscopy armamentarium of an operation theater. The minimum equipment required for this technique are listed below and demonstrated in Fig. 26.1.

(a) Beath pin.
(b) Arthroscopic probe.
(c) Initial Puncture (IP) Needle.
(d) No. 1 Prolene.

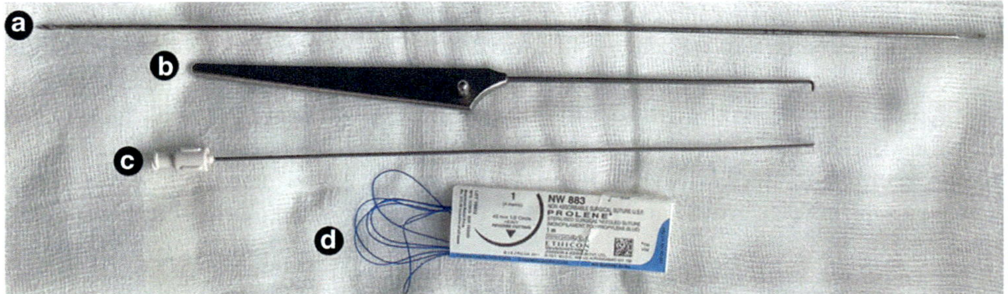


**Fig. 26.1** Materials required for implant-less bone bridge fixation for meniscal root repair. (**a**) Beath pin with eyelet. (**b**) Arthroscopic probe. (**c**) Initial puncture (IP) needle. (**d**) No. 1 Prolene

## 26.3 Positioning

The position of the patient depends on the type of index surgery. For implant-less bone bridge fixation, the leg has to be free so that it can be flexed and extended as and when required.

## 26.4 Surgical Steps

This technique can be implemented in any suture pullout technique in which sutures are delivered in the anterior tibia through a tunnel. This implant less bone bridge fixation technique is completed in the following five steps.

1. Exposing the primary tunnel.
2. Creating an accessory tunnel;
3. Passage of shuttle suture (Prolene) from the accessory tunnel to the primary tunnel;
4. Shuttling of pull-out sutures through the accessory tunnel using shuttle suture (Prolene) loop; and.
5. Knot tying over the bone bridge.

Each step is further elaborated in detail below.

### 26.4.1 Exposure of Primary Tunnel

The tibial tunnel through which the meniscal sutures were pulled out is now named as the primary tunnel, and the sutures are labeled as pull-out sutures. The aperture of the primary tunnel is cleaned, and a 1-cm area lateral to the aperture is exposed (Fig. 26.2a, b).

### 26.4.2 Creating an Accessory Tunnel

A beath pin is inserted through the primary tunnel for the reference of the direction of the tunnel (Fig. 26.3b). A point 1 cm away from the aperture of the primary tunnel is marked using electro-cautery (Fig. 26.3c). Using another beath pin in a drill, an accessory tunnel was created from the marked point directing towards the interior of the primary tunnel (Fig. 26.3d). While creating this tunnel, the direction has to be guided by the beath pin inserted into the primary tunnel. When the accessory tunnel connects to the primary tunnel, the beath pins are removed, and the aperture of both primary and accessory tunnels are cleaned (Fig. 26.3e).

### 26.4.3 Passage of Shuttle Suture (Prolene) from the Accessory Tunnel to the Primary Tunnel

The stylet is withdrawn from an initial puncture (IP) needle. A no. 1 Prolene suture is pushed through the needle's lumen, and the limb emerging from the tip is drawn back to make a loop at the needle's tip (Fig. 26.4a). The IP needle and looped Prolene are then introduced via the accessory tunnel's aperture into the primary tunnel (Fig. 26.4b, c). A loop of Prolene is formed inside the primary tunnel by carefully inserting the Prolene suture to the interior of the primary tunnel while simultaneously withdrawing the IP needle by a few millimeters. After that, an arthroscopy probe is advanced into the primary tunnel until it reaches the needle tip, which can be confirmed by the probe hitting the needle tip (Fig. 26.4d, e). The probe's hook is then used to catch the Prolene loop (achieved by back and forth move-

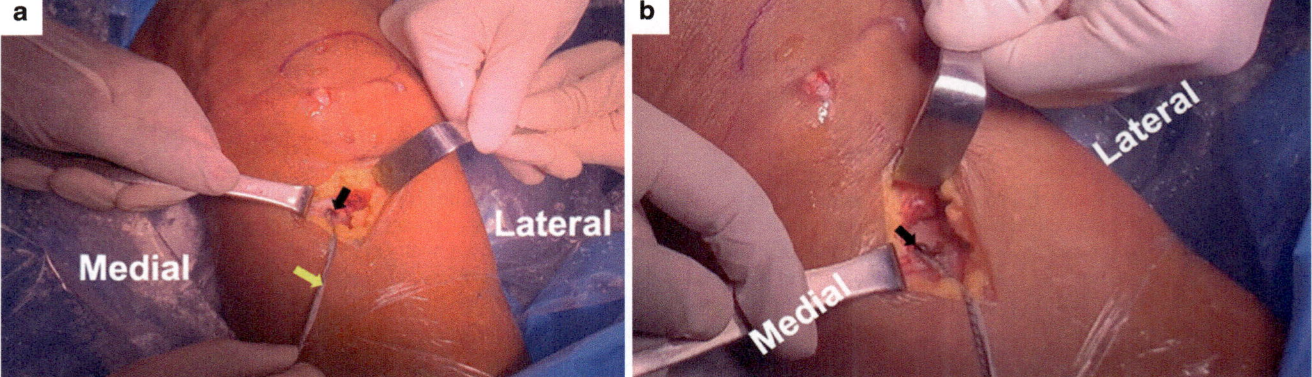


**Fig. 26.2** Superior view of left knee depicting primary tunnel and exposure of bone 1 cm lateral to the primary tunnel. (**a**) Primary tunnel (black arrow) through which sutures (yellow arrow) have come out. (**b**) Bone exposed one cm lateral to the primary tunnel (black arrow)

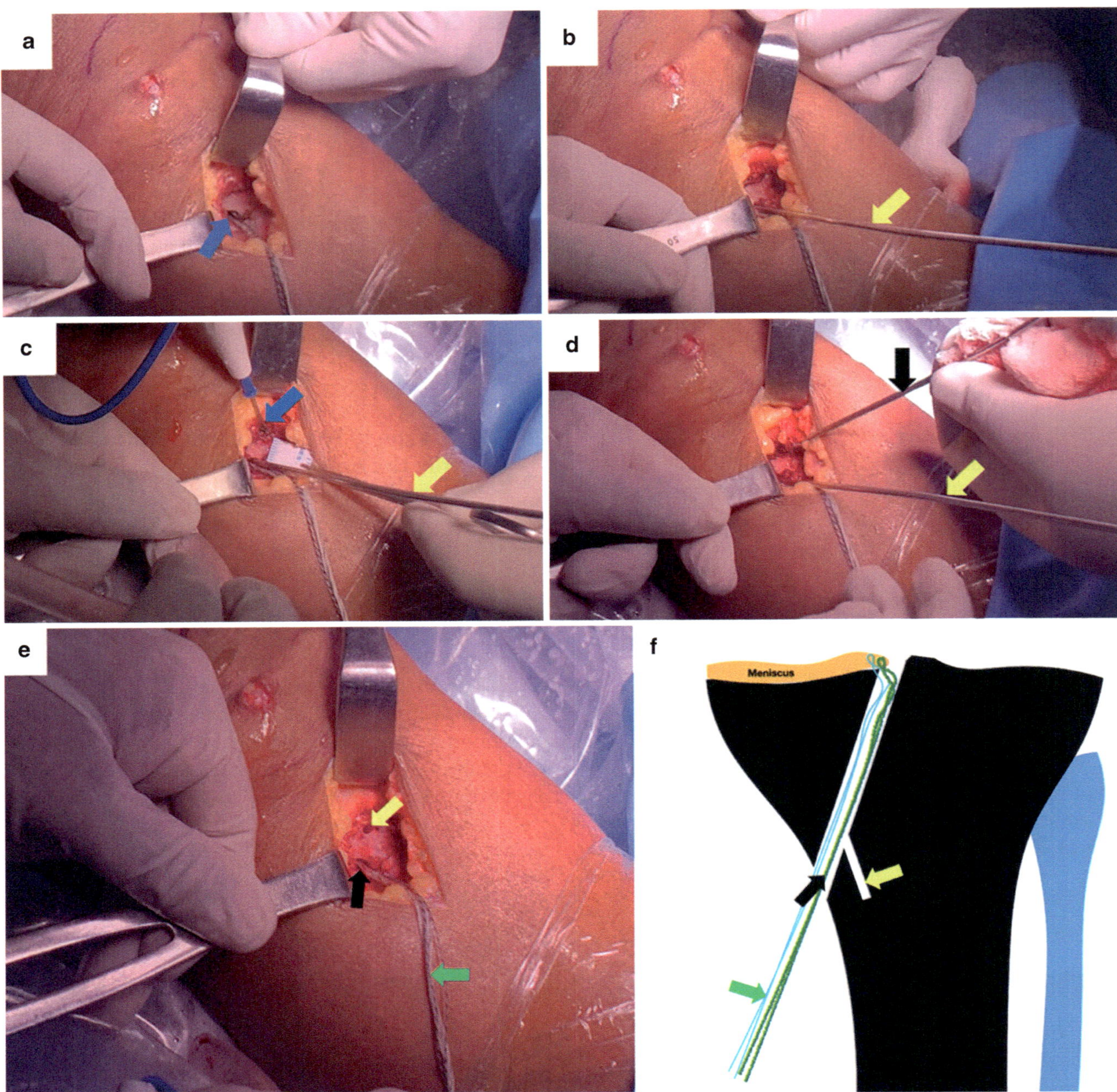


**Fig. 26.3** Medial aspect of a left proximal tibia depicting the steps of making an accessory tunnel. (**a**) Area 1 cm lateral to the tibial tunnel aperture (blue arrow) was cleared. (**b**) A beath pin (yellow arrow) is inserted through the primary tunnel as a guide for the direction of the secondary tunnel. (**c**) A point 1 cm lateral to the aperture of the primary tunnel is marked with electro-cautery (blue arrow). (**d**) using another beath pin in a drill, an accessory tunnel was created from the previously marked point. The beath pin (black arrow) is drilled such that it converges at the primary tunnel inside; the direction is guided by the beath pin in the primary tunnel. (**e**) figure depicting the aperture of the primary tunnel (black arrow) and accessory tunnel (yellow arrow). (**f**) Diagrammatic representation of primary and secondary tunnel

ment and rotational movement of the probe). The loop is collected by the probe and retrieved to the outside through the primary tunnel's opening (Fig. 26.4f, g). If the probe hook does not capture the Prolene loop, this maneuver may need to be repeated multiple times. In our original technique, we used an epidural needle to pass the Prolene, but because of its curvature and sharp tip, we found difficulty in the passage of the needle from the accessory tunnel to the primary tunnel. Of late, we started using the IP needle, this needle is straight, and the tip is blunt, making it easier to negotiate into the primary tunnel.

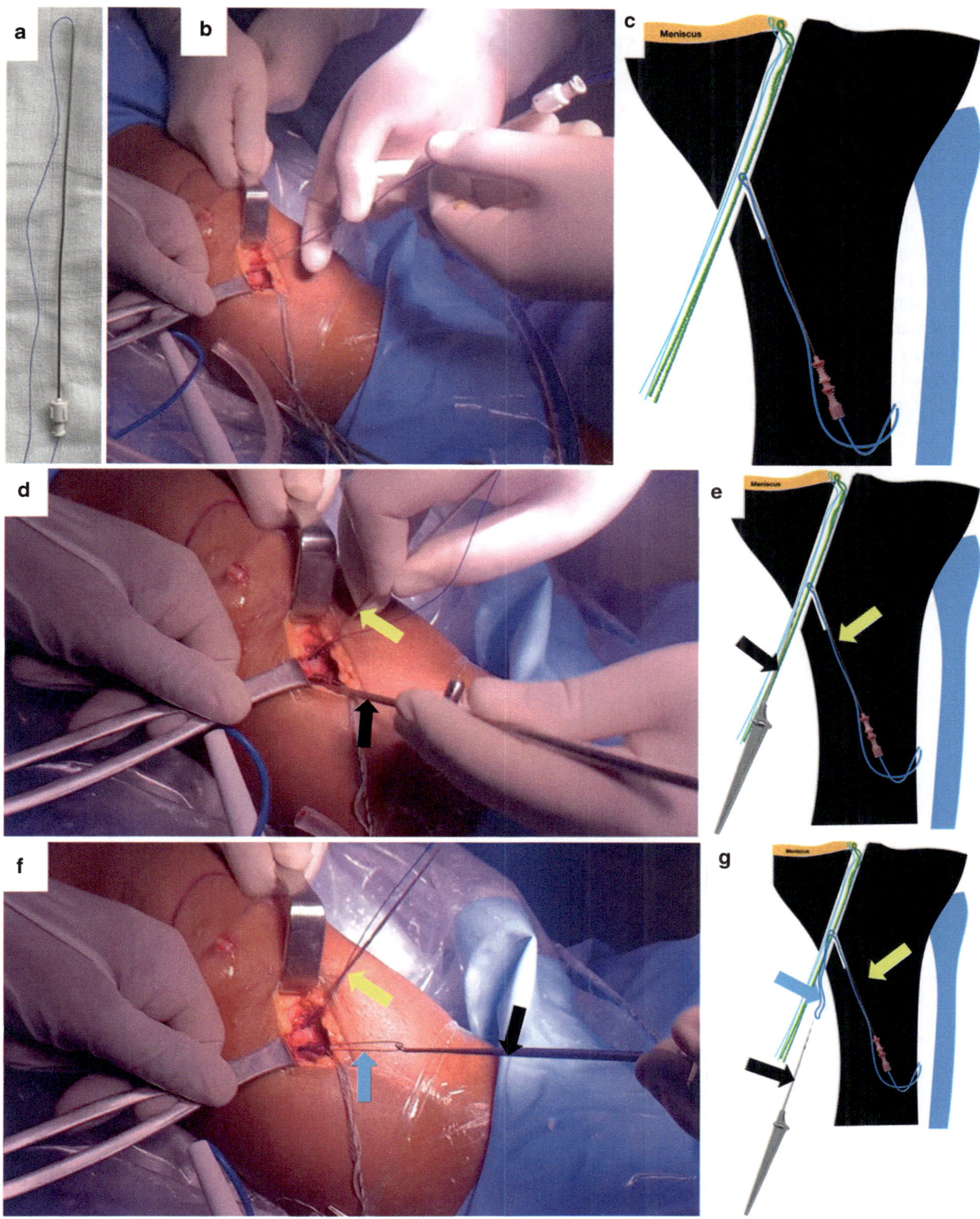


**Fig. 26.4** Steps of passing the Prolene loop from the accessory tunnel to the primary tunnel. (**a**) A number one Prolene suture is passed through the lumen and looped at the tip. (**b**) the IP needle with Prolene passed through the accessory tunnel to the primary tunnel. (**c**) Diagrammatic representation of IP needle passage from the accessory tunnel to the primary tunnel. (**d**) An arthroscopy probe (black arrow) is inserted through the primary tunnel to meet the IP needle (yellow arrow) coming from the accessory tunnel. (**e**) Diagrammatic representation of probe (black arrow) passed through the primary tunnel to meet IP needle (yellow arrow). (**f**) The Prolene loop (blue arrow) is hooked by the probe (black arrow) and delivered out through the aperture of the primary tunnel. (**g**) Diagrammatic representation of Prolene loop (blue arrow) being pulled out through the primary tunnel using arthroscopy probe (black arrow)

### 26.4.4 Shuttling of Pull-out Sutures through the Accessory Tunnel Using a Shuttle Suture (Prolene) Loop

The IP needle is withdrawn once the Prolene loop is out of the primary tunnel aperture, taking care not to pull out the Prolene suture loop (Fig. 26.5a, b). The pull-out sutures are then threaded through the loop of Prolene (Fig. 26.5c, d) and drawn out through the accessory tunnel (Fig. 26.5e, f). If there are many pairs of pullout sutures, complimentary limbs from each pair are shuttled through the accessory tunnel. While pulling the pull-out sutures, one should confirm that complimentary suture strands are looped into the Prolene loop. If many sutures are utilized, different-colored or differently marked sutures are recommended for easier identification. The steps of suture shuttling are depicted in Fig. 26.5 (a–f).

### 26.4.5 Knot Tying over the Bone Bridge

After the complementary strands of sutures have been pulled out through the two tunnels, a knot is placed over the bone bridge using two complementary limbs of pull-out sutures exiting from each tunnel. If there are several sutures, each marked/same colored suture exiting from two tunnels is identified and tied one by one over the bone bridge. The steps of knot tying over the bone bridge are depicted in Fig. 26.6a–d).

After the knots were secured over the bone bridge, the wounds were closed in two layers, and the standard dressing was applied.

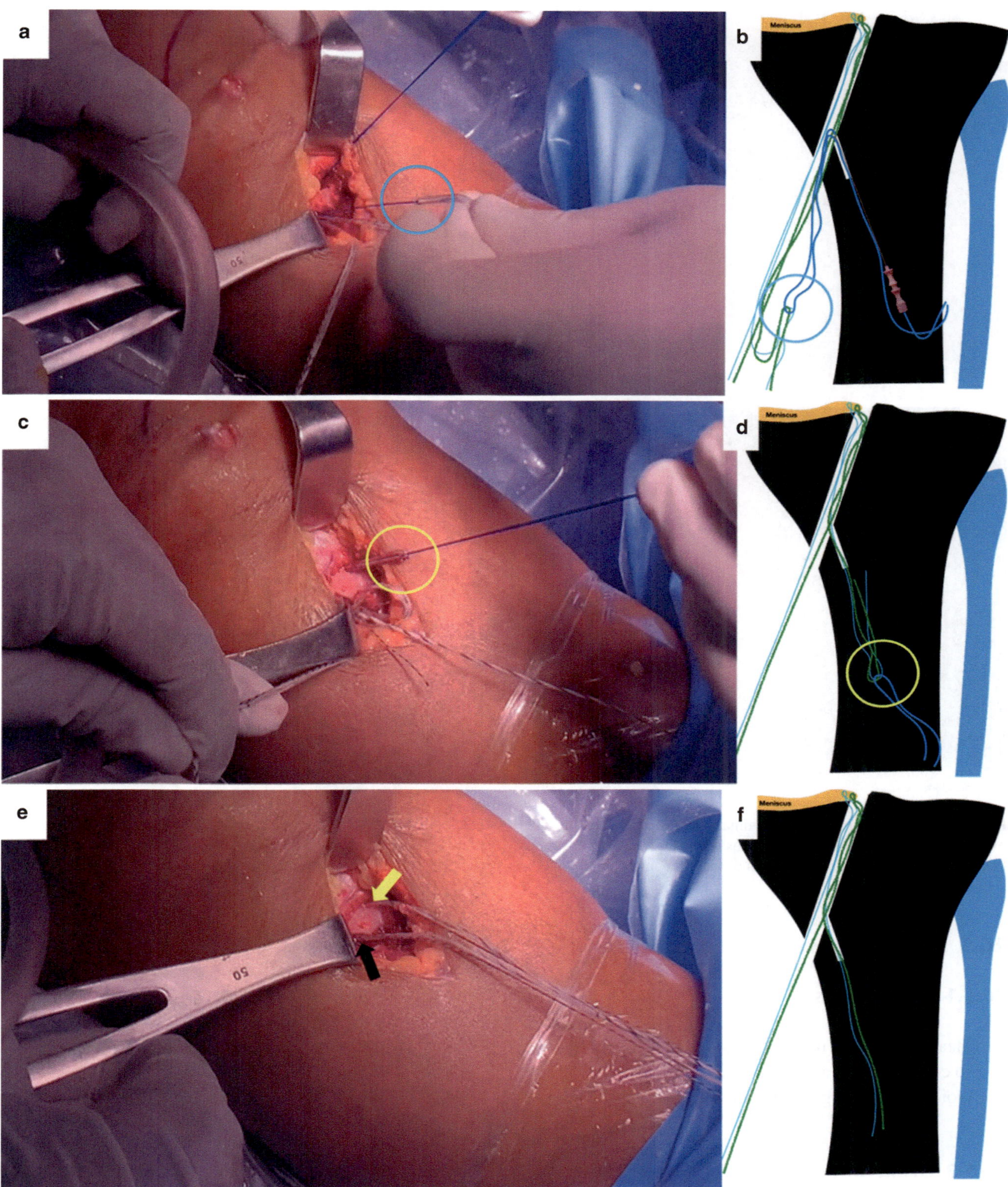


**Fig. 26.5** Intraoperative and diagrammatic pictures of pulling each limb of meniscal suture through the accessory tunnel. (**a**) Intraoperative picture of one limb each from tape and orthocord is looped in the loop of Prolene shown by the blue circle. (**b**) Diagrammatic representation of one limb of tape and orthocord looped in the loop of Prolene depicted in the blue circle. (**c**) The alternating limb of meniscal sutures is pulled out from the accessory tunnel, and the Prolene loop is depicted inside the yellow circle. (**d**) Diagrammatic representation of half of the meniscal suture being pulled out through the accessory tunnel using the Prolene loop (yellow circle). (**e**) External view of the proximal tibia, showing alternate sutures coming from the primary tunnel (black arrow) and accessory tunnel (yellow arrow). (**f**) Diagrammatic representation of the alternate sutures exiting from the primary and secondary tunnel

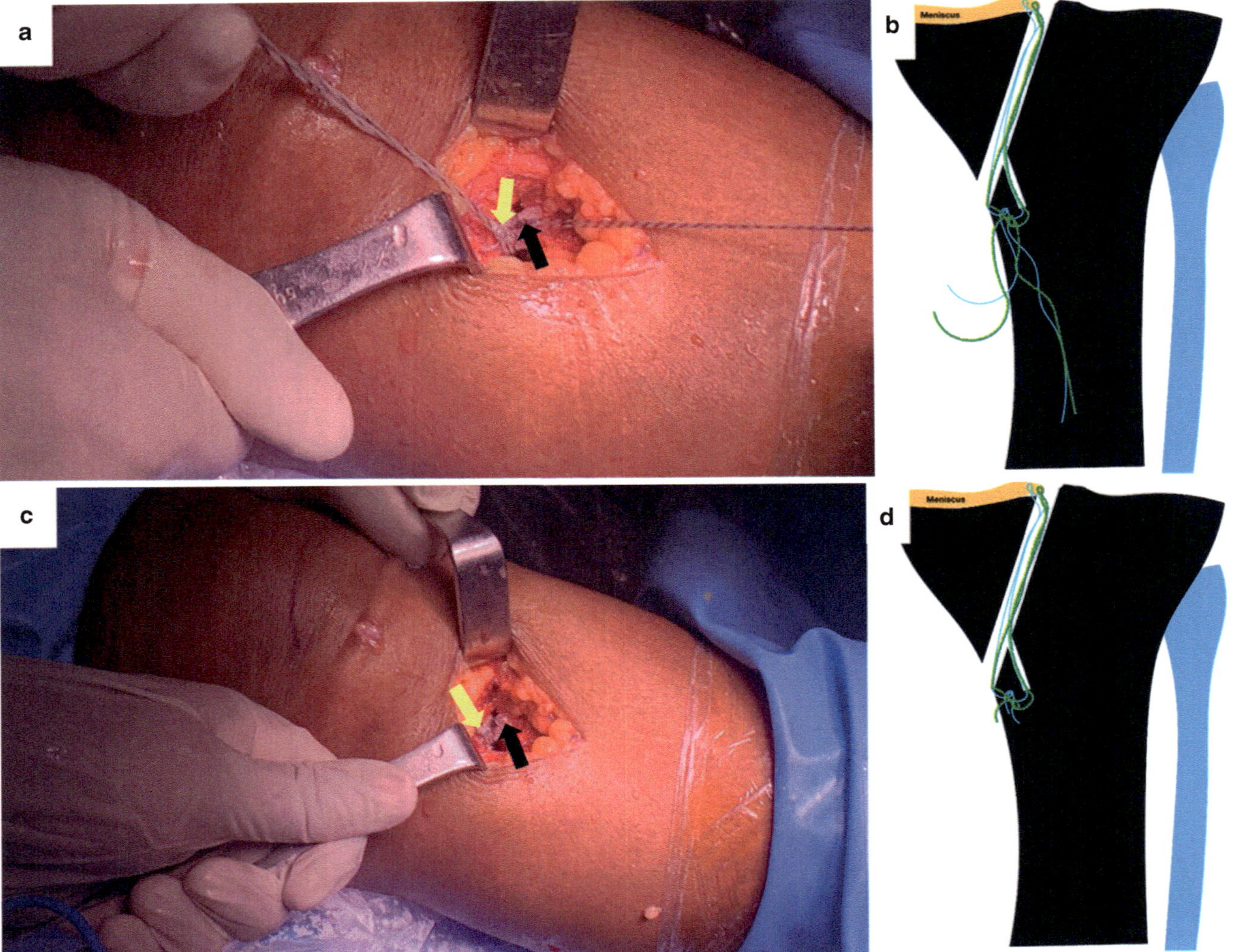


**Fig. 26.6** Intraoperative and diagrammatic representation of knots tied over the bone bridge. (**a**) Both the limbs of the tape (yellow arrow) are tied together. Subsequently, the limbs of the orthocord are tied together (black arrow). (**b**) Diagrammatic representation of respective limbs of sutures are tied over the bone bridge. (**c**) Sutures are cut (yellow and black arrow). (**d**) diagrammatic representation after cutting the sutures

## 26.5 Advantages and Disadvantages

### 26.5.1 Advantages

1. Cheap as it avoids the cost of an implant.
2. No complications associated with implants.
3. Avoids second surgery to remove the implant.

### 26.5.2 Disadvantages

1. Time-consuming.
2. Suture abrasion and wrapping around the beath pin while making the accessory tunnel.
3. A small bone bridge may lead to a bone bridge collapse and tunnel coalition.
4. Bone bridge cut out in osteoporotic bones.
5. Suture cut out with a sharp cortical edge.

In summary, implant-less fixations are gaining popularity amongst many arthroscopy surgeons due to their cost-effectiveness and ease of performing the procedure. These techniques avoid implant-related complications and are found to have fixation strengths comparable to those with implants. These techniques can be very useful and reproducible for fixation in a variety of conditions, especially for the tibial side fixation.

## References


1. Biazzo A, Manzotti A, Motavalli K, Confalonieri N. Femoral press-fit fixation versus interference screw fixation in anterior cruciate ligament reconstruction with bone-patellar tendon-bone autograft: 20-year follow-up. J Clin Orthop Trauma. 2018;9(2):116–20. https://doi.org/10.1016/j.jcot.2018.02.010. Epub 2018 Feb 23. Erratum in: J Clin Orthop Trauma. 2020 Nov-Dec;11(6):1175. PMID: 29896012; PMCID: PMC5995157.
2. Paessler HH, Mastrokalos DS. Anterior cruciate ligament reconstruction using semitendinosus and gracilis tendons, bone patellar tendon, or quadriceps tendon-graft with press-fit fixation without hardware. A new and innovative procedure. Orthop Clin North Am. 2003;34(1):49–64. https://doi.org/10.1016/s0030-5898(02)00070-6. PMID: 12735201.
3. Joshi A, et al. Implant-free, transtibial, bone bridge fixation for knee surgery including tibial spine and meniscal root fixation. Arthrosc Tech. 2020;9(11):e1837–43.
4. Barber FA. Complications of biodegradable materials: anchors and interference screws. Sports Med Arthrosc Rev. 2015;23(3):149–55. https://doi.org/10.1097/JSA.0000000000000076. PMID: 26225575.
5. Carr AJ, Price AJ, Glyn-Jones S, Rees JL. Advances in arthroscopy-indications and therapeutic applications. Nat Rev Rheumatol. 2015;11(2):77–85. https://doi.org/10.1038/nrrheum.2014.174. Epub 2014 Oct 28. PMID: 25348038.
6. Hertel P, Behrend H, Cierpinski T, Musahl V, Widjaja G. ACL reconstruction using bone-patellar tendon-bone press-fit fixation: 10-year clinical results. Knee Surg Sports Traumatol Arthrosc. 2005;13(4):248–55. https://doi.org/10.1007/s00167-004-0606-5. Epub 2005 Feb 3. PMID: 15690197.
7. Pandey V, Cps S, Acharya K, Rao SK. Arthroscopic suture pull-out fixation of displaced Tibial spine avulsion fracture. J Knee Surg. 2017;30(1):28–35. https://doi.org/10.1055/s-0036-1579682.
8. Pache S, Aman ZS, Kennedy M, Nakama GY, Moatshe G, Ziegler C, Laprade RF. Meniscal root tears: current concepts review. Arch of Bone Joint Surg. 2018;6(4):250–9. https://pubmed.ncbi.nlm.nih.gov/30175171/.

# Innovative Techniques of Analgesia for Knee Surgeries

# 27

Nitin Bahl, Puja Bahl, and Vikram Arun Mhaskar

## 27.1 Introduction

*"Pain" is an unpleasant sensory and emotional experience associated with actual or potential tissue damage or described in terms of such damage.*

Knee joint is the most commonly affected joint by trauma and degenerative changes. Hence knee surgeries are the most frequently performed surgeries. The range of operative procedures ranges from diagnostic arthroscopies to total knee replacement. Presently regional analgesia like Neuraxial blocks (Subarachnoid block, Epidural analgesia, combined spinal epidural analgesia) are being given for such procedures. But these leads to unwanted side effects like urinary retention, delayed mobility and chances of epidural hematomas. The advent of ultrasound into the regional analgesia practice opened avenue for area specific and procedure-specific, motor-sparing, opioid-sparing techniques of regional analgesia.

## 27.2 Regional Analgesia for Knee Surgeries

The regional analgesia techniques for knee surgeries have been evolving over the years. A conceptual revolution came in with the introduction of ultrasound into the regional analgesia practice.

Various regional analgesia techniques are as follows:

1. Subarachnoid block:
   (a) Epidural Analgesia,
   (b) Combined Spinal Epidural Analgesia.
2. Plexus block:
   (a) Lumbar plexus block.
   (b) Sacral plexus block.
3. Non-motor-sparing peripheral nerve blocks:
   (a) Femoral.
   (b) Sciatic.
   (c) Obturator nerves block.
4. Motor-sparing blocks:
   (a) Subsartorial blocks/ Adductor canal block.
5. Infiltrations techniques:
   (a) Infiltration between Popliteal Artery and Capsule of Knee (IPACK) block.
   (b) Local Infiltration Analgesia (LIA).

## 27.3 Motor-Sparing Blocks for the Knee

### 27.3.1 Subsartorial (Adductor Canal Block)

The adductor canal block (ACB) is an interfascial plane which blocks the saphenous nerve in the thigh at the level of the adductor canal.

The saphenous nerve is a terminal sensory branch of the femoral nerve supplying superficial structures of the knee, medial aspect of the leg up to the level of ankle and/or mid-foot. Hence block at the level of adductor canal provides anaesthesia to knee, the medial aspect of the lower leg and ankle without motor blockade.

## 27.4 Indications

- Total and uni-compartmental knee replacement surgery.
- Knee arthroscopy.
- Anterior Cruciate Ligament Reconstruction.
- Surgery involving lower leg, foot and ankle involving areas of skin supplied by the saphenous nerve.

The original version of the chapter has been revised. A correction to this chapter can be found at https://doi.org/10.1007/978-981-99-4378-4_28

N. Bahl
JMVM Sports Injury Center, Sitaram Bhartia Institute Of Science & Research, Qutub Institutional Area, New Delhi, India

P. Bahl
Sitaram Bhartia Institute of Science & Research, New Delhi, India

V. A. Mhaskar (✉)
F7 East of Kailash, Knee & Shoulder Clinic, New Delhi, India


V. A. Mhaskar, J. Maheshwari (eds.), *Innovative Approaches in Knee Arthroscopy*,
https://doi.org/10.1007/978-981-99-4378-4_27

## 27.5 Applied Anatomy

The sartorius muscle forms the roof of the adductor canal in the lower half of the thigh as it descends medially from lateral aspect of upper anterior thigh. Here it appears trapezoid in shape below the subcutaneous tissue. The lateral walls of the triangular adductor canal are formed by the vastus medialis laterally and the adductor longus /magnus medially. The femoral vein, femoral artery and saphenous nerve are seen within the triangle at a depth of 2–3 cm. The artery and nerve show colour filling whereas the saphenous nerve is seen as a small, round, hyperechoic structure anterior to the artery.

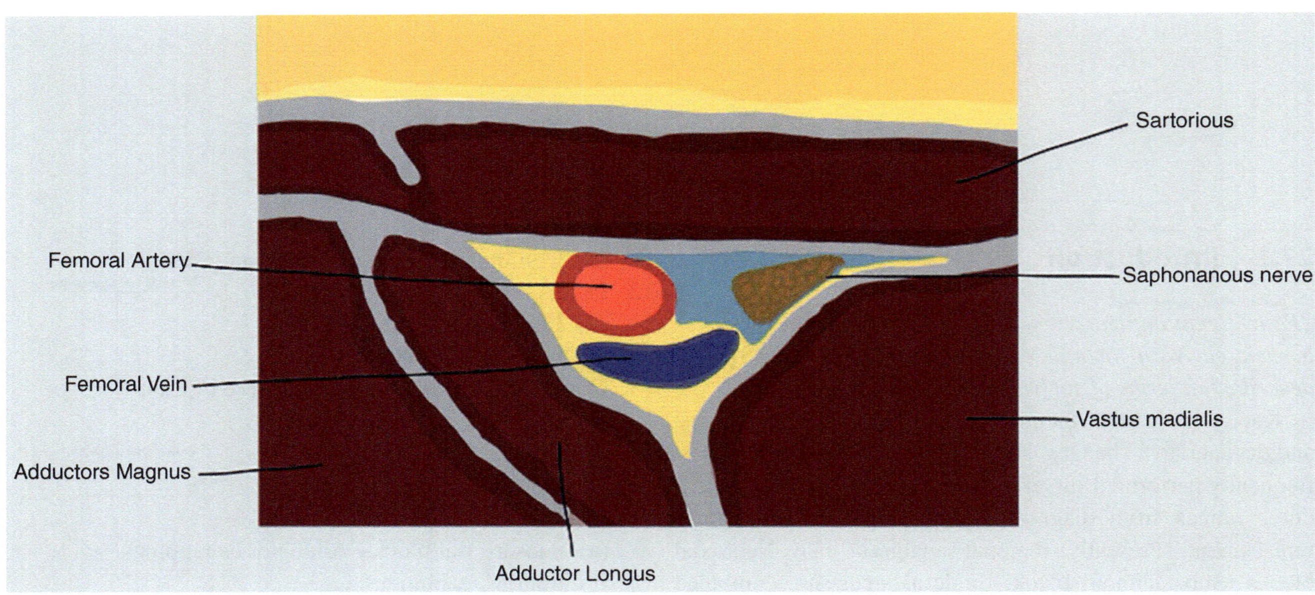


## 27.6 Equipment

- Ultrasound machine with a linear transducer (8–14 MHz), sterile sleeve and gel.
- Standard nerve block tray.
- One 10-mL syringe containing local anaesthetic
- An 80 mm 22–25-gauge needle (Stimuplex, Braun Medical, Melsungen, Germany).
- Sterile gloves.

### 27.6.1 Dose of Local Anaesthetic

1. 1% lignocaine for skin infiltration (1–2 mL)
2. Local anaesthetic for block.
   (a) Ropivacaine Max 3 mg/kg (e.g., 0.5 mL/kg of 0.75%).
   (b) Bupivacaine Max 2 mg/kg (e.g., 0.4 mL/kg of 0.5%).

## 27.7 Technique

1. The patient is positioned supine on operation table with the knee slightly flexed and externally rotated.

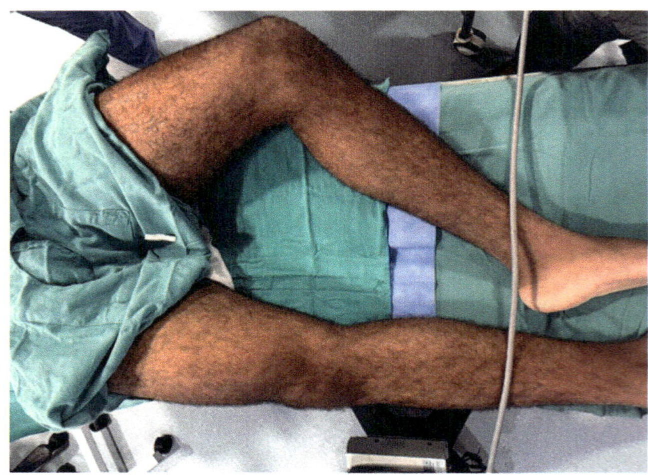

2. The ultrasound machine is positioned opposite to the side of affected leg and the operator on side of the affected leg. This allows the anaesthetist to observe the ultrasound screen comfortably while performing the procedure.
3. The high-frequency linear probe is positioned transversely at the level of mid-thigh in the midline. The probe is then slide medially till the femoral artery is seen with trapezoid shaped sartorius muscle above.
4. The femoral artery is then scanned and followed inferiorly till the point where it posteriorly enters the adductor

hiatus and becomes popliteal artery. The optimal site for the block is just proximal to the adductor hiatus where the nerves is seen anterolateral to the artery but may be difficult to visualized.

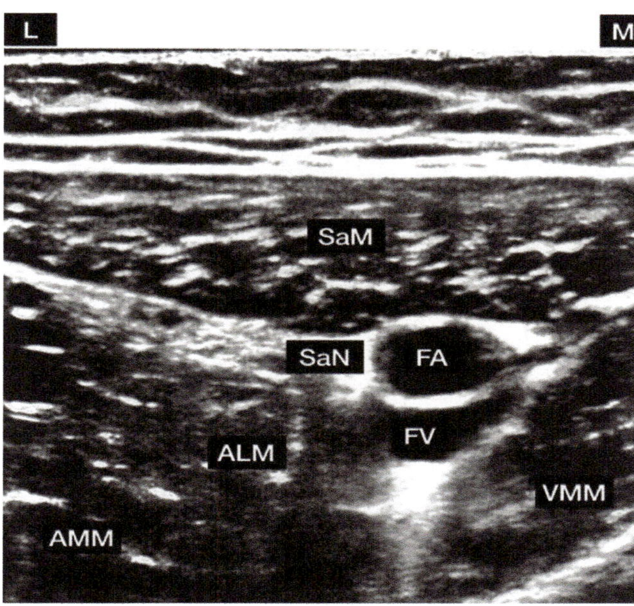


5. The needle is inserted from lateral to medial with an in-plane technique. It can be done at an angle traversing sartorius or horizontally piercing vastus medialis and travelling perpendicular to the ultrasound beam. On entering the Adductor canal, the needle tip should lie immediately lateral or superficial to the femoral artery.

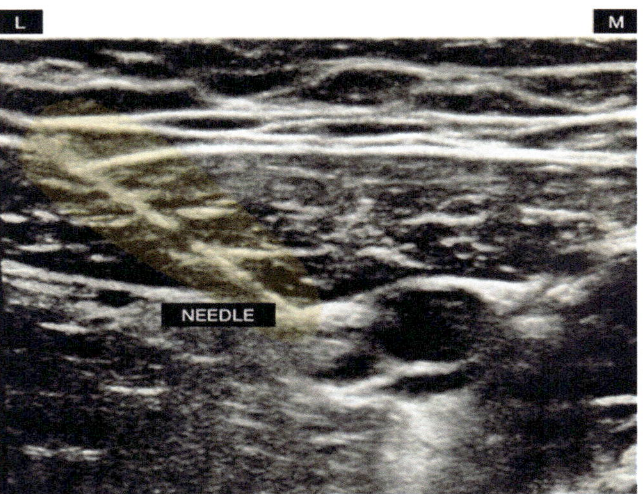


6. After aspirating, test dose of local anaesthetic is injected around the nerve. If the nerve is not visible then the local anaesthetic is given around the artery. After ensuring the correct position of the needle (which is seen as local anaesthetic around the nerve or artery as the condition may be) full dose of the local anaesthetic is given with frequent aspirations to rule out intravascular injection.

## 27.8 Complications

- Motor block of anterior thigh.
- Arterial puncture.
- Bleeding.
- Drug Toxicity,
- Block failure.
- Infection.
- Nerve Injury.

## 27.9 Continuos Adductor Canal Block

1. Using an in-plane ultrasound technique, a 17-gauge Tuohy needle is inserted in the adductor canal with simultaneous injection of 0.9% normal saline (up to 10 mL) for hydro dissection and visualization of nerve and needle tip. The needle is then placed lateral to the superficial femoral artery.
2. Then a 19-gauge open tip epidural catheter is advanced through Tuohy needle into the adductor canal. With 1–2 cm of the catheter placed within the canal, the needle is removed and the catheter is secured with suture. A portable infusion pump (Neofuser) is attached to the catheter.
3. An infusion of 150 ml of 0.2% ropivacaine is administered at 3 mL/h for 24 h.

## 27.10 IPACK

The iPACK stands for infiltration between popliteal artery and capsule of the knee. It is a new regional analgesic technique for postoperatives pain relief to the posterior aspect of the knee after total knee replacement surgery. It provides pain relief by blocking the articular branches of the tibial, common peroneal and obturator nerves in the popliteal region. It is performed under ultrasound guidance and hence has a technical advantage over conventional LIA injection.

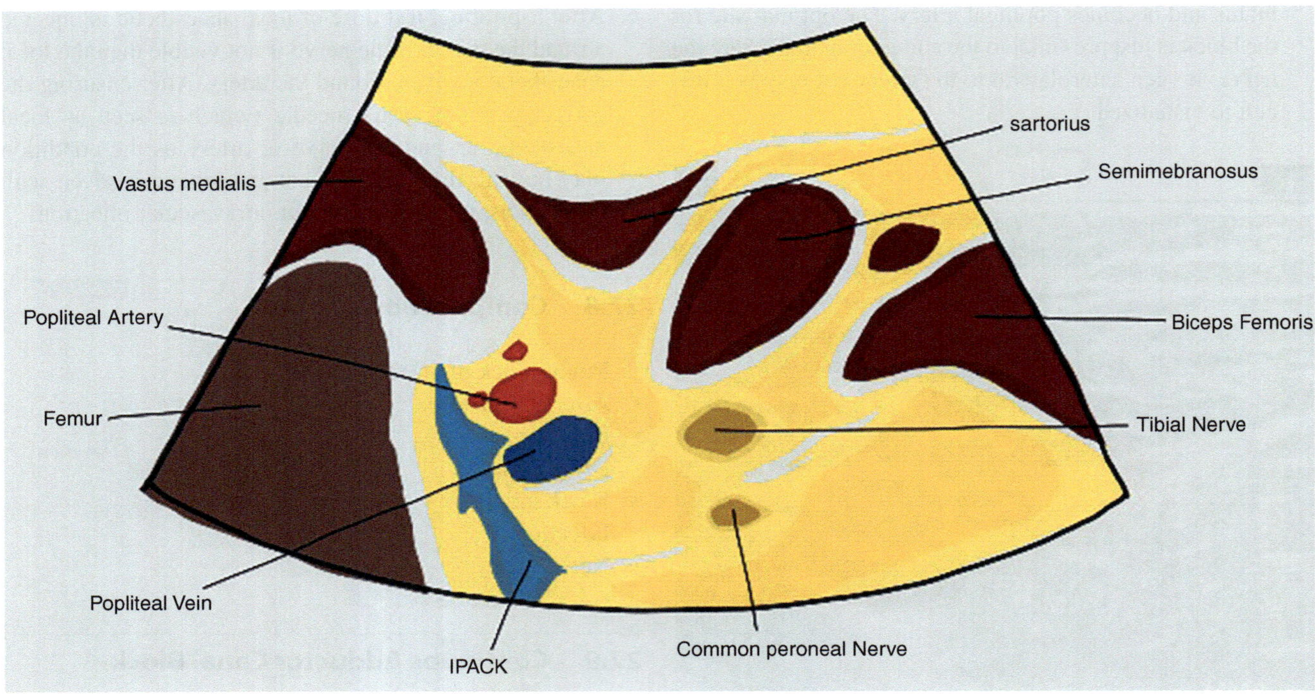


### 27.10.1 Local Anaesthetic Used

1. 1% lignocaine for skin infiltration (1–2 mL)
2. Local anaesthetic for block.
   (a) Ropivacaine Max 3 mg/kg (e.g., 0.5 mL/kg of 0.75%).
   (b) Bupivacaine Max 2 mg/kg (e.g., 0.4 mL/kg of 0.5%).

### 27.10.2 Technique

1. The patient is positioned supine on operation table with the knee slightly flexed and hip abducted.

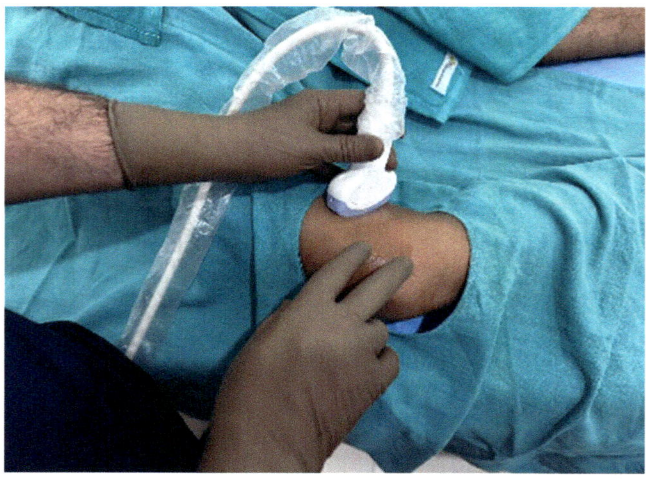

2. The convex probe is positioned transversely (axially) at the level adductor canal to visualize the femoral vessels in cross-section.
3. The transducer is then moved distally observing the femoral artery as it passes through the adductor hiatus into the popliteal fossa to become the popliteal artery.
4. The transducer is then moved posterior and inferiorly to visualize the space between the popliteal artery and the shaft of the femur just superior to the femoral condyles.

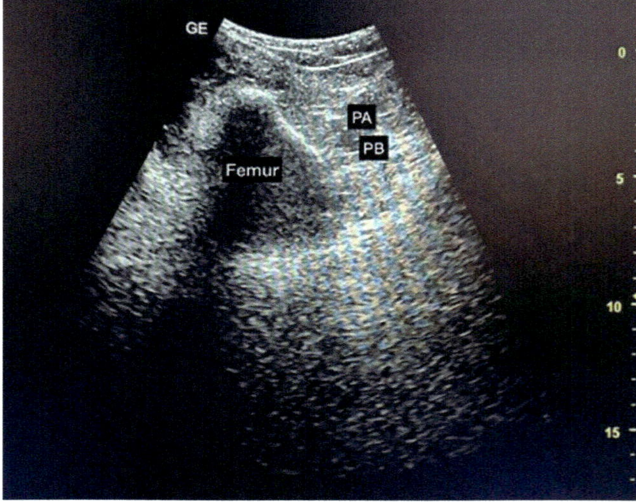


5. Then by using in plane technique, a needle is inserted from medial aspect, the space between the posterior cap-

sule of the knee and the popliteal artery, posterior to the femoral shaft.

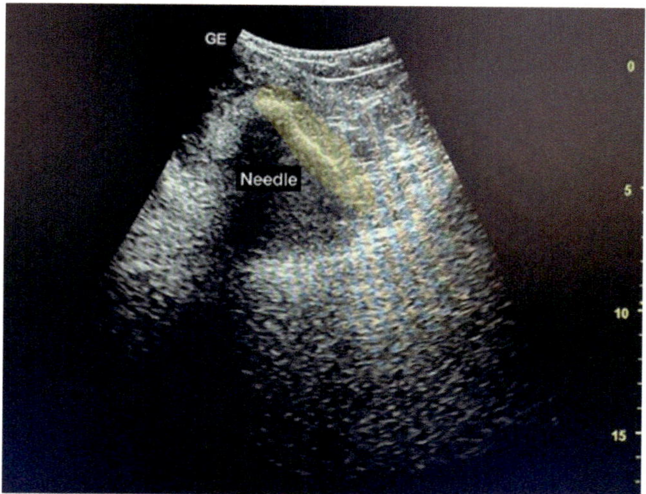


6. A total of 10–15 mL of local anaesthetic is injected incrementally while slowly withdrawing the needle.

As the iPACK block is performed under ultrasound guidance, it reduces the risk of accidental popliteal artery puncture and sciatic nerve block as these are not visualized anterior to the posterior capsule.

## 27.11 Complications

- Block failure.
- Intravascular injection.
- Local anaesthetic toxicity.
- Nerve damage.
- Infection.

## 27.12 LIA (Local Infiltration Analgesia)

Infiltration of the surgical site with local anaesthetic is one of the most widely used method of pain relief used by orthopaedic surgeons. It provides the advantage of blocking pain at the site of its origin.

**Local anaesthetic:** The most commonly used mixture is Ropivacaine-Ketorolac-Adrenaline (RKA) mixture 200 mg ropivacaine 2.0 mg/mL, 30 mg ketorolac and 0.5 mg epinephrine.

### 27.12.1 Technique

The injection is given in three stages intraoperatively by the orthopaedic surgeon.

1. The first injection is done after the bone surfaces have been prepared for implants, but before implants have been inserted. About 30–50 mL is injected through the joint from the front to a depth of 3 mm into the tissues around the posterior joint capsule.
2. The second injection is done after the implants have been inserted, but before both wound closure and tourniquet release. About 35–50 mL is injected into the deep tissues around the medial and lateral collateral ligaments and the wound edges.
3. The third injection of 25–50 mL of the mixture is injected into the subcutaneous tissue.

### 27.12.2 Catheter Placement

1. Immediately before wound closure, a Touhy needle 18-guage is inserted about 10 cm above the incision through the skin, subcutaneous tissue and quadriceps muscles.
2. The tip of the catheter is then inserted through the hub of the needle into the surgical field from the outside to the inside. The catheter is then led along the medial femoral condyle, usually on raw bone, medial to the metal femoral component and adjacent to the medial capsule.
3. Using an artery forceps, the tip is then passed posterior to the medial femoral condyle, so that the tip lies immediately anterior to the posterior capsule.
4. The needle is removed and the catheter is fixed. After wound closure, a further 10–15 mL is injected through the catheter to flood the joint local anaesthetic mixture.

### 27.12.3 Genicular Nerve Blocks

Infiltration of the local anaesthetics around the sensory branches supplying that provide innervation to the knee joint (genicular nerves) before they enter the knee capsule. The genicular nerve block is a motor-sparing technique that anesthetizes the sensory terminal branches innervating the knee joint, resulting in analgesia of the anterior compartment of the knee.

### 27.12.4 Indications

- Chronic knee pain,
- Total knee arthroplasty,
- Procedures associated with moderate to severe postoperative knee pain.

The aim is to deliver local anaesthetic spread next to the genicular arteries (if visible) or at the junction of the epiphysis and diaphysis of the femur and tibia.

### 27.12.5 Innervation of the Knee

1. The superolateral genicular nerves (SLGN) courses around the femur shaft to pass between the vastus lateralis and the lateral epicondyle. It accompanies the superior lateral genicular artery.
2. The superomedial genicular nerves (SMGN) courses around the femur shaft, following the superior medial genicular artery, to pass between the adductor magnus tendon and the medial epicondyle below the vastus medialis.
3. The inferolateral genicular nerves (ILGN) courses around the tibial lateral epicondyle deep to the lateral collateral ligament, following the inferior lateral genicular artery, superior of the fibula head.
4. The Inferomedial genicular nerves (IMGN) courses horizontally below the medial collateral ligament between the tibial medial epicondyle and the insertion of the collateral ligament. It accompanies the inferior medial genicular artery.

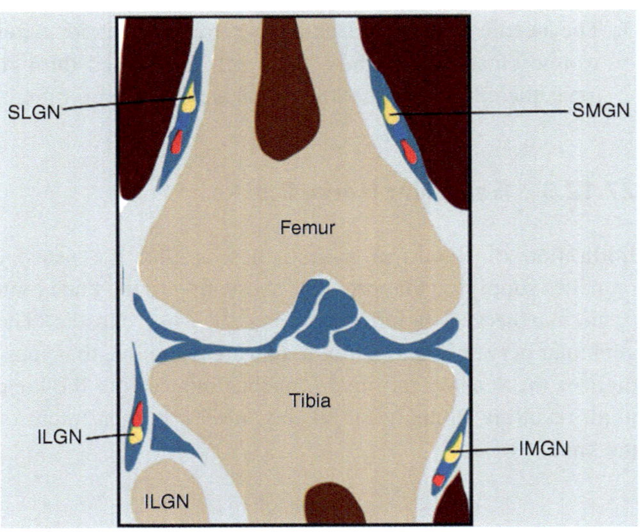


### 27.12.6 Ultrasound View

The ultrasound landmarks are the osteomuscular planes at the level of the metaphysis (the junction between the epiphysis and diaphysis) of the femur and tibia. Additional landmarks are the corresponding arteries, which follow the same path as the nerves and the collateral ligaments.

### 27.12.7 Equipment

- High-frequency, linear transducer.
- 50-mm, 22-gauge, short-bevel needle.

### 27.12.8 Local Anaesthetic

- Bupivacaine(0.25%).
- Ropivacaine (0.25–0.5%) in a volume of 4–5 mL per nerve.

### 27.12.9 Technique

The patient is placed in a supine position with the knee slightly flexed by placing a pillow in the popliteal fossa.

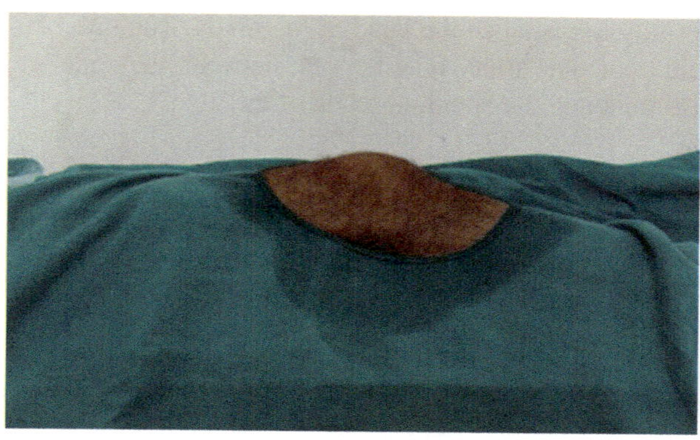

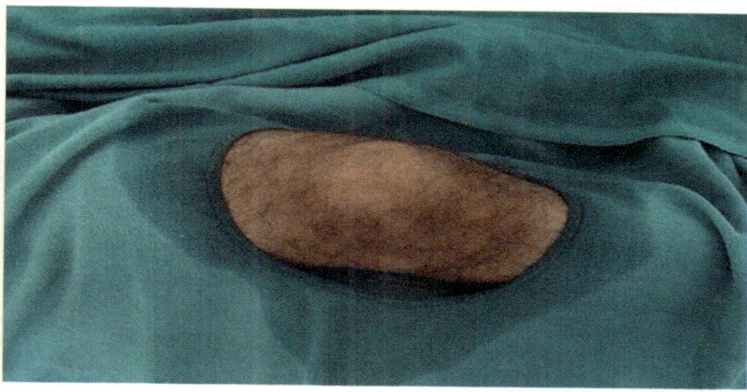

1. **SLGN**: The transducer is placed in a coronal orientation over the lateral epicondyle of the femur and then moved proximally to visualize the metaphysis of the bone. The superolateral genicular artery may be seen between the deep fascia of the vastus lateralis and the femur at this level.

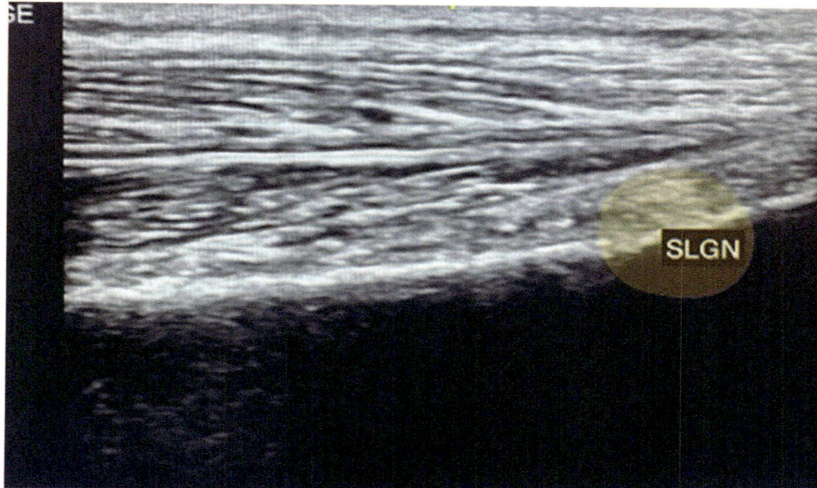


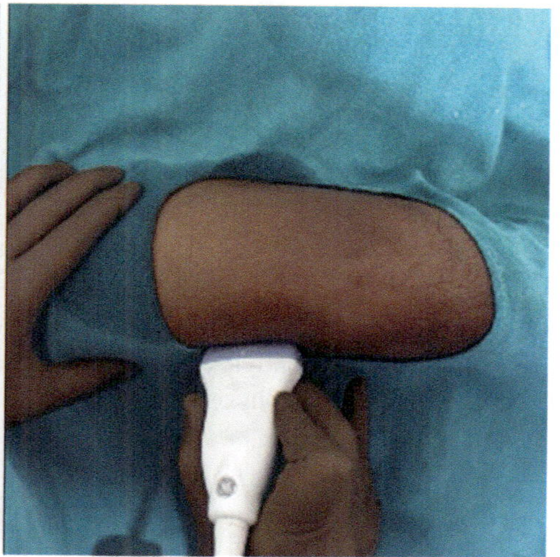

2. **SMGN:** The transducer is placed in a coronal orientation over the medial epicondyle of the femur. The transducer is moved slightly proximally to visualize the metaphysis of the bone just anterior to the adductor tubercle. The SMG artery may be seen at this level between the deep fascia of the vastus medialis and the femur.

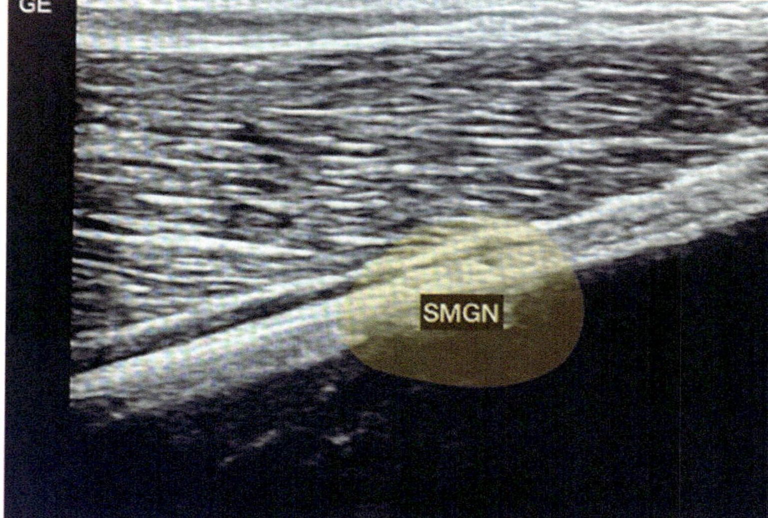


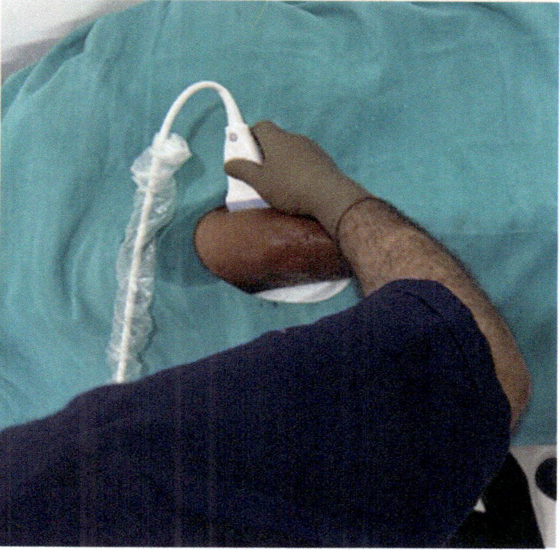

3. **ILGN:** The transducer is placed in a coronal orientation over the lateral side of the distal knee. After identifying the lateral epicondyle of the tibia, the transducer is moved distally to visualize the head of the fibula. The inferolateral genicular artery may be seen between the collateral ligament and the lateral condyle of the tibia.

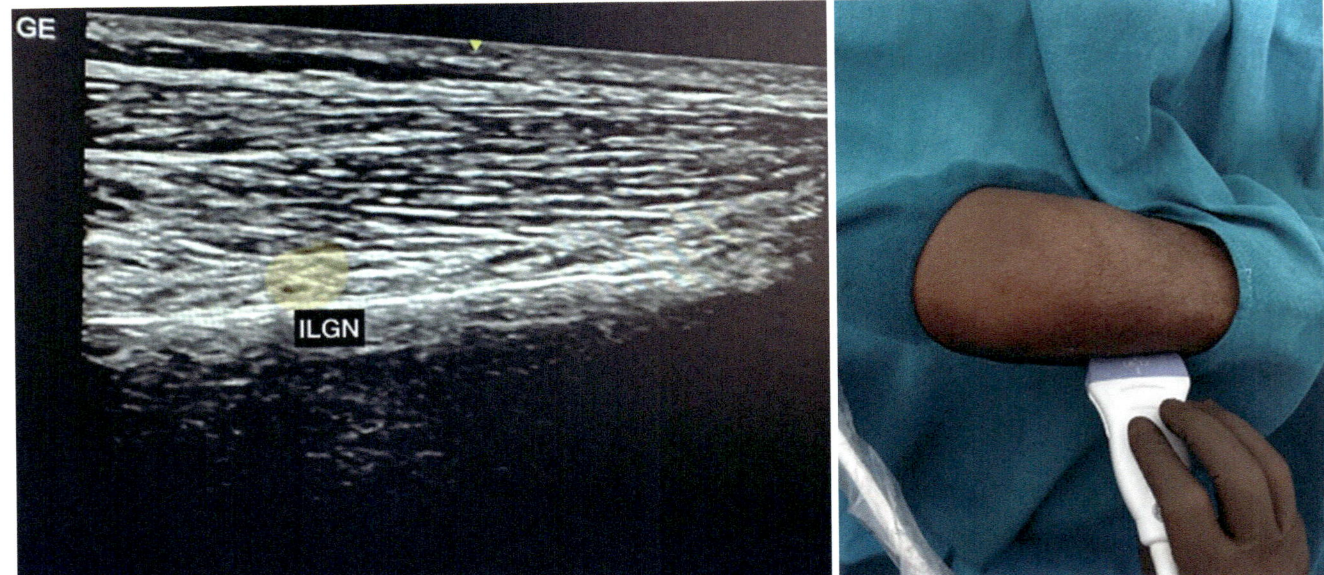


4. **IMGN**: The transducer is placed in a coronal orientation over the medial condyle of the tibia and moved distally to visualize the metaphysis of the bone. At this level, the inferomedial genicular artery is seen beneath the medial collateral ligament.

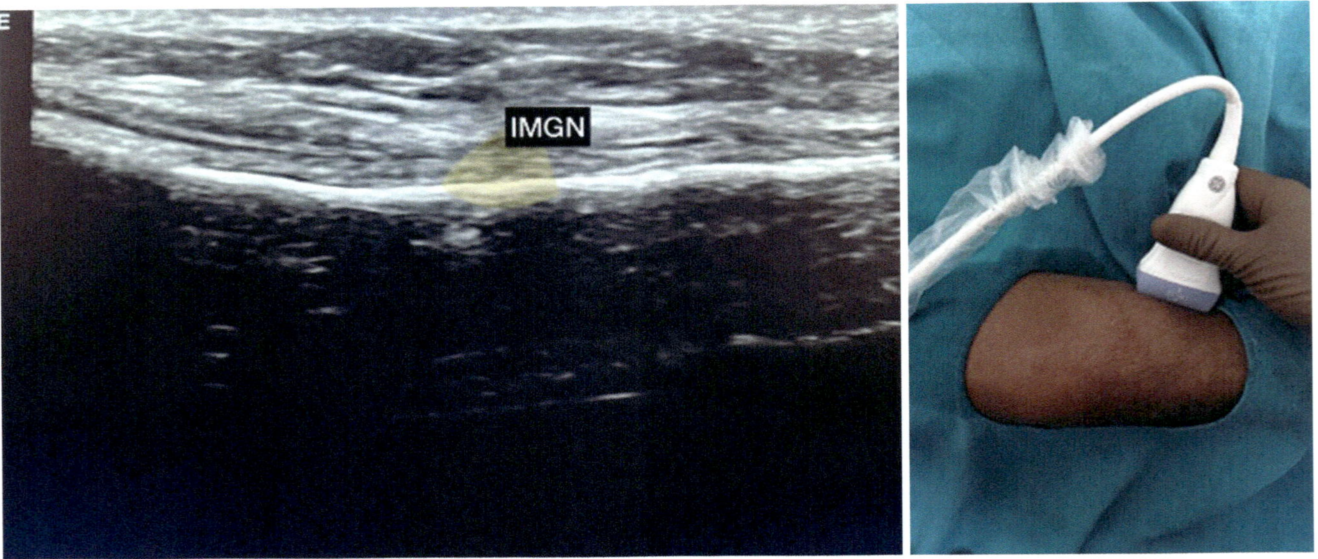

### 27.12.10 Needle Approach and Trajectory

Once the injection site has been identified, the needle tip is advanced next to the vessel (if seen) until bony contact is felt using an in-plane or out-of-plane approach. After confirming the correct position, the LA is injected.

### 27.12.11 Limitations

The genicular nerves vary in number and trajectory and, because of their small size, they are not visualized with the available ultrasound technology.

### 27.12.12 Complications

The proximity of the inferolateral genicular nerve (ILGN) to the common peroneal nerve (CPN) is a risk factor for unintended CPN block resulting in foot drop. Thus, this nerve is spared if denervation is planned to treat chronic pain. Vascular or intraarticular punctures are other potential risks.

# Corrections to: Innovative Techniques of Analgesia for Knee Surgeries

Nitin Bahl, Puja Bahl, and Vikram Arun Mhaskar

**Correction to:**
**Chapter 27 in: V. A. Mhaskar, J. Maheshwari (eds.), *Innovative Approaches in Knee Arthroscopy*, https://doi.org/10.1007/978-981-99-4378-4_27**

The names of the co-authors have been revised to Nitin Bahl and Puja Bahl.

The updated version of this chapter can be found at https://doi.org/10.1007/978-981-99-4378-4_27


V. A. Mhaskar, J. Maheshwari (eds.), *Innovative Approaches in Knee Arthroscopy*,
https://doi.org/10.1007/978-981-99-4378-4_28

GPSR Compliance

*The European Union's (EU) General Product Safety Regulation (GPSR) is a set of rules that requires consumer products to be safe and our obligations to ensure this.*

*If you have any concerns about our products, you can contact us on ProductSafety@springernature.com*

In case Publisher is established outside the EU, the EU authorized representative is:

Springer Nature Customer Service Center GmbH
Europaplatz 3
69115 Heidelberg, Germany

**Batch number: 10371057**

Printed by Printforce, the Netherlands